P9-CFY-286

PROPRIOCEPTIVE NEUROMUSCULAR FACILITATION

Proprioceptive neuromuscular

THIRD EDITION

Dorothy E. Voss, B.Ed., R.P.T.

Associate Professor Emeritus of Rehabilitation Medicine
Northwestern University Medical School
Chicago, Illinois

Marjorie K. Ionta, B.S., R.P.T.

Formerly, Supervisor of Physical Therapy
Massachusetts General Hospital
Special Instructor, Physical Therapy Program
Simmons College
Boston, Massachusetts

Beverly J. Myers, B.S., O.T.R.

Instructor, Department of Occupational Therapy
University of Illinois
Chicago, Illinois

Foreword by Sedgwick Mead, M.D.

HARPER & ROW, PUBLISHERS

PHILADELPHIA

Cambridge   London
New York   Mexico City
Hagerstown   São Paulo
San Francisco   Sydney

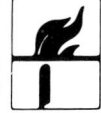

1817

facilitation PATTERNS AND TECHNIQUES

Acquisitions Editor: Lisa A. Biello
Sponsoring Editor: Darlene D. Pedersen
Manuscript Editor: Rosanne Hallowell
Indexer: Catherine Battaglia
Art Director: Maria S. Karkucinski

Designer: Patrick Turner
Production Supervisor: J. Corey Gray
Production Coordinator: Barney Fernandes
Compositor: Progressive Typographers
Printer/Binder: The Murray Printing Company

Third Edition

3 5 6 4

Library of Congress Cataloging in Publication Data

Voss, Dorothy E.
 Proprioceptive neuromuscular facilitation.

 Rev. ed. of: Proprioceptive neuromuscular facilita-
tion/Margaret Knott, Dorothy E. Voss. 2nd ed. 1968.
 Bibliography: p.
 Includes index.
 1. Physical therapy. 2. Muscles. 3. Proprioceptors.
I. Ionta, Marjorie K. II. Myers, Beverly J. III. Knott,
Margaret. Proprioceptive neuromuscular facilitation.
IV. Title. [DNLM: 1. Exercise therapy. WB 541 V969p]
RM700.V66 1984 615.8'2 84-4630
ISBN 0-06-142595-8

 This edition is substantially updated and revised from Proprioceptive Neuromuscular Facilitation, second edition, by Margaret Knott and Dorothy E. Voss, published in 1968.

FOREWORD

Having written the foreword for the first and second editions of this classic work, *Proprioceptive Neuromuscular Facilitation*, I am happy to do so for the current one. My closing comment in the first edition (1956) was, "In time I believe that the basic principles presented here — which any interested person can verify by himself on normal subjects — will be universally accepted as both rational kinesiology and therapeutics." In the second edition (1968) I stated, "Initially skeptical about it [1954], I have come to feel that it exceeds all other methods of therapeutic exercise in speed of improvement, economy of time, and thoroughness of results." For all but 6 years of its existence I have been able to observe the development of proprioceptive neuromuscular facilitation (PNF).

Let me emphasize that while almost all of my experience has been with catastrophic physical impairment in an in-patient setting, I am aware that physical therapists apply the principles and the method in treating orthopaedic patients who constitute the majority in physical therapy in general hospitals.

One of the first questions to be asked about PNF is, what kind of disability is it good for? And, if good for cerebral palsy, as is claimed for a few other competing systems, surely it would not be good for other disease entities, would it? Here is where we patiently reply that the techniques are not doctrinaire, being only an extension of normal physiology and kinesiology. The response of the patient will indeed be modified by the special circumstances of the disease or injury. But though these manifestations may get in the way of and modify recruitment, making it less effective, the mechanism for improved function is still there.

The second question a tough-minded investigator would pose is whether PNF can be subjected to controlled, prospective study. The honest answer is that it cannot be. Neurological conditions are so variable in their pathology and clinical manifestations that setting up reasonable numbers of cohorts would be impossible. There are just too many independent variables. The controls in a single center would not be real controls, for they would soon clamor to join the clearly superior PNF group. A controlled study in two or more centers could be a possibility.

Among orthopaedic conditions, the recurrence of knee injury in athletes deserves study. Has restoration of function following injury or surgery been complete? Athletic trainers are finding PNF useful in prevention of injury as well as in treatment post-injury or post-surgery. The Suggested Readings in this edition include a Sports Physical Therapy section, a new and growing interest.

I have heard therapists in some centers say that they are eclectic, choosing a little PNF here, a little Bobath there. I think this is to misunderstand fundamentally what one is trying to accomplish and the basic neurophysiology involved. PNF *is* empirical.

Our attempts to rationalize it using the neurophysiology currently in our grasp may be drastically modified by future discoveries, but PNF does work and will be just as effective then as now.

Sedgwick Mead, M.D.
Medical Director
Easter Seal Society of Alameda County
Oakland, California;
Formerly Medical Director (1954–1969)
Kaiser Foundation Rehabilitation Center
Vallejo, California;
Chief of Neurology (1969–1977)
Kaiser-Permanente Medical Center
Vallejo, California

PREFACE

Almost 4 decades ago Dr. Herman Kabat began his development of "proprioceptive facilitation" in Washington, DC. The original concepts expressed by Dr. Kabat have been extended far beyond his "treatment for paralysis." To those of us who have applied his ideas more broadly, this approach adds to the understanding of human movement and constitutes a total approach.

I added the word *neuromuscular* to Dr. Kabat's term in 1954, thinking that physical therapists might more easily recognize that the method held meaning for them. The acronym for proprioceptive neuromuscular facilitation, PNF, was readily accepted.

Since the early 1950s physical therapists from around the world have come to the United States to learn PNF. They came principally to the Kaiser Foundation Rehabilitation Center (KFRC), Vallejo, California, beginning in Dr. Kabat's time, and in Margaret Knott's time. The training program at KFRC continues.

Intensive short courses and clinical workshops have been offered here and abroad. Unfortunately, there is no permanent central registry of names and places. Inclusion of PNF in undergraduate educational programs is evidenced by the 1977–1978 Textbook Survey done by the American Physical Therapy Association. The Knott and Voss book, *Proprioceptive*

Neuromuscular Facilitation, second edition, was the leader of ten titles under the heading *Exercise*.

The most objective evidence of the success of PNF is the demand for the Knott and Voss book. The first edition was deemed a success. However, the demand for the second edition has been more than 4 times greater. The increase in demand also reflects to some extent the increase in numbers of physical therapy students.

The first edition emerged in 1956 with a German translation in 1962, and a translation to French in 1968 just ahead of the second edition. Translation of the second edition appeared in German in 1970, in Italian, Spanish (Argentina), and Japanese in 1974, and in Dutch in 1975.

The first edition included the "how to" and the individual patterns. It was written from our understanding of the responses of normal subjects and from experience with the method. We relied upon Dr. Kabat's knowledge of the works of Sherrington. This great man exemplified for all of us the need to understand the components in order to understand the whole without losing sight of the wholeness.

The second edition presented aspects of developing motor behavior. We relied on the works of Hooker, Gesell and his colleagues, and McGraw. This material reflects our belief that learning or relearning the sequence of developmental activities has value for all patients; its use should not be limited to the treatment of the patient having cerebral palsy. The sequence permits treatment by design rather than by haphazard, chance decisions.

In the second edition, all of the procedures suggested for the facilitation of total patterns have a common purpose: to promote motor learning. Again, our understanding of motor learning must be based on work in other fields. We must look to neurophysiology for knowledge of basic mechanisms, to experimental psychology, and to cybernetics and tracking.

This third edition is the sum of the first and the second, and, in addition, contains material new to some, awaited by many. The free active performance of patterns, the scapular patterns in supine and prone, and the thrusting variations and their reversals, the bilateral combinations where the stronger segment reinforces the weaker, should promote the learning of skills.

The learner of PNF needs the balanced antagonism, the resiliency and bounce of the normal subject. The pitfall inherent in trying to learn by working with patients is that, by virtue of previous education and practice, the physical therapist becomes involved with the periphery or focuses on the most severely involved segment or muscle group. PNF enlists the less involved parts to promote a balanced antagonism of reflex activity of muscle groups, and of components of motion. Those who cannot resist the temptation to work with patients before they have acquired understanding and have practiced with normal subjects would do best by beginning with total patterns as presented in mat activities.

Contributions to illustration of this book have been noteworthy. The drawings in the first edition were done by Helen Drew Hipshman, San Francisco; subjects were Margaret Knott and Dorothy E. Voss. The second edition drawings were by James B. Buckley, Chicago, based on photography by Carl Manner, Vallejo. The subjects were Margaret Hennessy, British Columbia; Inge Berlin, Germany; and Lorna Brand, Wales. The supervisor of the photography sessions was Dorothy E. Voss.

In this edition the photography was done by Alan Lucas, Orthopaedic Media Service, Massachusetts General Hospital (MGH); Beverly J. Myers, Co-author; Christine A. McCarthy, R.P.T., Senior Staff Physical Therapist, Department of Rehabilitation Medicine, MGH; and Stanley Bennett, Chief of Photography, Photographic Department, MGH. The subjects were Anastasia Z. Boyd, R.P.T., Physical Therapist for the Head-Injured and Multi-Impaired, Adult Services, Perkins School for the Blind, Watertown, Massachusetts; Amy E. Flynn, R.P.T., Senior Staff Physical Therapist, MGH, and Special Instructor, Department of Physical Therapy, Simmons College, Bos-

ton; Christine A. McCarthy; and Susan B. Perry, R.P.T., Assistant Supervisor and Coordinator of Clinical Education for Physical Therapy, Massachusetts General Hospital (MGH), and Special Instructor, Physical Therapy Program, Simmons College, Boston, Massachusetts. Supervisors of the photography sessions were Marjorie K. Ionta and Dorothy E. Voss.

Those who contributed captions and legends for the illustrations are as follows: Free Active Motion: Paul D. Becker, R.P.T., Physical Therapy Consultant, Visiting Nurse Association, Chicago, Illinois, and Department of Public Health, Chicago, Illinois; Bilateral Combinations for Reinforcement: Theodore Corbitt, R.P.T., Director of Physical Therapy, International Center for the Disabled, New York, and Associate in Physical Therapy, Rehabilitation Medicine, Columbia University, New York, New York; Thomas S. Holland, R.P.T., Director, Orthopaedic Rehabilitation Service, Memorial Hospital of South Bend, South Bend, Indiana; Beverly J. Myers, Co-author; and Susan B. Perry; Scapular Patterns and Thrusting Variations: Marjorie K. Ionta, Co-author; and Vital and Related Functions: Beverly J. Myers, Co-author.

For the first time the use of exercise equipment is presented. The photography of the use of wall pulleys was done at the Orthion Corporation, Costa Mesa, California, by David Tanaka, Student of Telecommunications, San Diego State University, San Diego. The subjects were Patsy Ann Delsman, A.T.C., Athletic Injuy Orthopedic Rehabilitation Center, San Diego; Andrew Einhorn, R.P.T., A.T.C., Southern California Center for Sports Medicine, Long Beach; and Robert P. Engle, R.P.T., A.T.C., Director of Orthopedic and Sports Physical Therapy, Wyomissing, Pennsylvania. The supervisor of the photography was Debra M. Ellison, R.P.T., formerly Staff Therapist, Poudre Valley Hospital, Fort Collins, Colorado. Captions were prepared by Dorothy E. Voss.

Special contributions to this third edition are "PNF: A Brief History" by Dorothy E. Voss (see the Introduction, which follows), and "Coupling PNF and Joint Mobilization," by Thomas S. Holland. References and Suggested Reading were prepared with assistance from Bernice E. Lyford, R.P.T., Formerly Supervisor of Physical Therapy, Youville Hospital, Cambridge, Massachusetts.

A special word of appreciation is owed each of the physicians who confirmed or corrected information and dates in "PNF: A Brief History," and who contributed to the understanding of the use of PNF to the benefit of patients in California and throughout the country, and, because of the therapists who came to learn, around the world. They are Dr. Herman Kabat, M.D., Ph.D., originator of the PNF approach; Dr. Sedgwick Mead, M.D., who succeeded Dr. Kabat as Medical Director, KFRC, Vallejo, and who wrote the foreword for the first, second, and third editions; Dr.

Rene Cailliet, M.D, who worked with Dr. Kabat and Margaret Knott at the Kabat-Kaiser Institute (KKI) in Washington, and who devoted a number of years to the use of PNF at KKI, Santa Monica; and to Dr. Howard Liebgold, M.D., first at KFRC, Vallejo, in 1962, who succeeded Dr. Mead in 1969, and who continues as Chief of KFRC.

We thank our publisher, the J. B. Lippincott Company, Health Professions Publisher of Harper & Row, Publishers, especially Lisa A. Biello, Editor, Medical Books; Darlene D. Pedersen, Associate Editor; Rosanne Hallowell, Manuscript Editor; and Maria Karkucinski, Art Director, for sharing their special knowledge and advice, and for their completion of this long-term task. We thank, too, those who assisted in the reading of galley proof: Bernice E. Lyford, a contributor to the book, and Kathryn J. Shaffer, retired, Director of Physical Therapy, formerly Professor, Department of Physical Therapy, Boston-Bouvé College, Northeastern University, Boston.

And, finally, we are grateful to physical therapists, occupational therapists, physical educators, athletic trainers, kinesiologists, and those from other health-related professions who show growing interest in the PNF approach to therapeutic exercise; and to those who teach, and to their students. As always, we value most highly our broad experience with patients, and our years of teaching. Together they have provided the backdrop for this book.

Dorothy E. Voss, B. ED., R.P.T.
Marjorie K. Ionta, B.S. R.P.T.
Beverly J. Myers, B.S., O.T.R.

INTRODUCTION

PNF: A BRIEF HISTORY

"Proprioceptive facilitation techniques" and "neuromuscular rehabilitation" were terms first used to describe the method now commonly referred to as proprioceptive neuromuscular facilitation (PNF).[7] To report the history of a method, its origins, the course of development, and evidence of maturity must be considered as well as the professional people who contributed in significant ways through the years.

The originator of the PNF method was Dr. Herman Kabat, M.D., Ph.D., a man whose professional background is impressive.[9] In 1932, at 19 years of age, Herman Kabat received the bachelor of science degree from New York University. In 1935, at age 22, he was awarded the doctor of philosophy in neurology by Northwestern University Medical School in Chicago. During the period 1932 to 1936, he was a fellow in neurology and a fellow in anatomy at Northwestern University.

In 1936 Dr. Kabat moved to the University of Minnesota where he served as an instructor in physiology and also studied medicine. He received his medical doctorate in 1942 at age 29. From 1942 to 1943 he was Assistant Professor of Physiology and Neuropsychiatry. With this background, Dr. Kabat became a neurophysiologist and a physician, or, as he once referred to himself, "a clinical neurophysiologist." He was one of a kind in his time.

The 1940s

Coincidentally, while Dr. Kabat was at the University of Minnesota, Sister Elizabeth Kenny arrived from Australia. Sister Kenny, a nurse, came to share her experience in treatment of patients affected by anterior poliomyelitis. She held lectures and demonstrations of the "Kenny method." Orthopaedic surgeons, nurses, and physical therapists came to Minneapolis from many areas of the United States where "polio" had been rampant. Some who came were receptive, others were not. Since 1916, patients with polio had been treated with Lovett's, then Legg and Merrill's "muscle reeducation."[8] This method had its roots in anatomy and its origins in orthopaedics: one motion, one joint, one muscle at a time.

Dr. Kabat, physician and neurophysiologist, was asked to analyze the "Kenny method."* As he observed Sister Kenny at work with patients, he became aware that some facets of her method had a sound base in neurophysiology and some did not. He suggested certain changes to Sister Kenny. She was not receptive to his ideas. His growing interest in the treatment of patients was reinforced by his firm impression that those who had come to learn from Sister Kenny were

---

* Kabat H: Personal communication, 1953

sadly lacking in knowledge of neurophysiology. Dr. Kabat was convinced that neurophysiological principles based on the work of Sherrington should be applied in the treatment of paralysis. He decided to pursue the treatment of patients and so left his post in the physiology department at the university.

From 1943 to 1946 Dr. Kabat held several positions in the Washington, DC area including that of Consultant, Crippled Children's Program, District of Columbia. At this time, he became interested in cerebral palsied patients. In 1946 he became Medical Director of the newly founded Kabat-Kaiser Institute for Neuromuscular Rehabilitation in Washington, DC. Henry Kaiser, the industrialist, became interested in Dr. Kabat's work because his son, Henry J. Kaiser, Jr., suffered from multiple sclerosis. The Kaisers founded a second institute in Vallejo, California, in 1948, and a third in Santa Monica in 1950.

Upon the establishment of the Kabat-Kaiser Institute (KKI) to be opened in July, 1946, Dr. Kabat began his search for physical therapists in 1945. He approached the Office of the Surgeon General, US Army Medical Corps, to discuss with the staff his wish to interview physical therapists, who, upon discharge, might be interested in his method of treating patients with paralysis. Many were, and a staff was employed.

The first physical therapist to be employed by Dr. Kabat and to become his Head Physical Therapist was Margaret (Maggie) Knott. A graduate of Appalachia State Teachers College in North Carolina, she held majors in physical education and biology. After teaching in the public schools for 3 years, and upon the involvement of the United States in World War II, Maggie entered the training program for physical therapists at Walter Reed Army Hospital. She served as a Second Lieutenant for 2½ years until the close of the war. In December 1945 she began working with Dr. Kabat, first in Washington, and then in Vallejo when the center was opened in August 1948.[6,9]

The 1950s

Dr. Kabat developed the PNF method by working with patients until he arrived at combinations that made sense. He combined motions to ascertain the effectiveness of maximal resistance and stretch in facilitating the response of a weak distal muscle by irradiation from a stronger proximal muscle which was related in function. In this way, he identified mass movement patterns that were spiral and diagonal in character. Stretch of synergistic muscles in mass movement patterns is in itself an effective facilitation mechanism.[3] Beginning on March 14, 1950, an intensive effort was made to identify the specific spiral and diagonal patterns. All possible combinations of components of motion were tested with patients, with results recorded on a five-page form bearing the March 14, 1950 date and designated KKI#01. On January 24, 1951, when a two-page form was issued, the patterns were clearly apparent.* The data recorded from each patient had revealed the precise patterns, which were three-dimensional.

During the same period, Kabat developed a battery of techniques based on Sherrington's work in neurophysiology, relying on Sherrington's principles of successive induction, reciprocal innervation and inhibition, and the process of irradiation. On the five-page form, KKI#01, six techniques were listed: maximal resistance, rhythmic stabilization, quick reversal, contract–relax, holding, and stretch. On the January 24, 1951 form, three techniques had been added: slow reversal, slow reversal–hold, and hold–relax–active motion. A total of nine techniques were available and were selected according to the patient's needs.

While Margaret Knott was the first physical therapist employed by Dr. Kabat, a number of those discharged from the Army Medical Corps made up the majority of the KKI staff in Washington. When, in 1948, Dr. Kabat and Margaret Knott moved to head the center in Vallejo, a number of staff members fol-

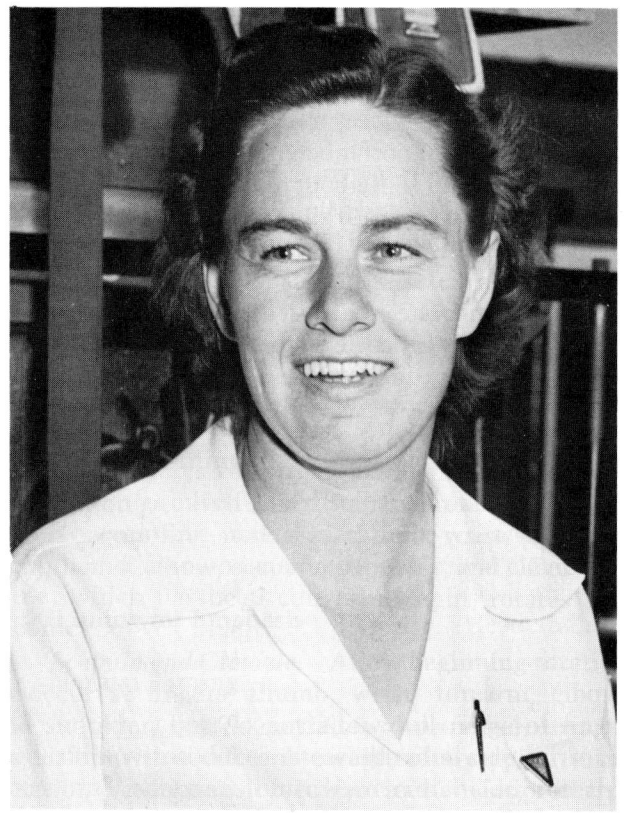

Margaret (Maggie) Knott in the 1940s

* Evaluation forms, KKI#01, March 14, 1950; January 24, 1951.

lowed. Dr. René Cailliet and Dr. Jean Vivino directed the program in Washington with adequate supportive staff. Dr. Kabat and Maggie Knott returned to Washington periodically to introduce new techniques as they were developed, and early in 1951 they presented the spiral and diagonal patterns to the entire staff. Physicians were to examine patients and follow Kabat's method of analysis and program planning. The physicians then relied upon the physical therapists to carry out the programs.

In 1950, while Chief Physical Therapist at George Washington University Hospital (GWUH) in Washington, DC, I became interested in PNF. During a meeting of the District of Columbia Chapter of the American Physical Therapy Association (APTA), held at the Kabat-Kaiser Institute, Dr. Jean Vivino demonstrated the use of PNF with a patient who had multiple sclerosis. Dr. Vivino attempted facilitation of the flexion–adduction–external rotation pattern of the lower extremity. The patient responded and was able to dorsiflex foot and ankle. Someone asked, "Would you do the same with a polio patient?" Dr. Vivino replied simply, "Yes." Dr. Vivino gave me clues enough so that I was able to try to reproduce the technique in order to facilitate response in my polio patient's anterior tibial muscle. The obviously more effective technique applied to a pattern of movement rather than to the individual muscle convinced me to learn the PNF method.

In the fall of 1951, I spent 6 weeks at KKI-Vallejo and learned all that I could. I accompanied Dr. Kabat as he examined patients, analyzed their motor ability, and formulated treatment programs for each. I was greatly impressed by his preciseness, his organization, and his systematic analysis from head to foot. Margaret Knott instructed me in patterns and techniques as she worked with several patients with whom I was to "practice" in order to learn.

When I returned to GWUH in Washington, I applied PNF in treating patients with anterior poliomyelitis, painful shoulders, postoperative knees, and others. To me, PNF was a complete method of therapeutic exercise based in neurophysiology with new concepts of human movement. It was not limited to the treatment of paralysis. As I realized that there was much more to be learned, I decided to accept the offer to become Margaret Knott's assistant, and so joined the KKI staff in April 1952.

The physical therapy staff numbered about thirty qualified therapists trained in the USA and one from Great Britain. The patient population included those with multiple sclerosis and cerebral palsy, ever-increasing numbers of polio patients, and a large group of patients with spinal cord injuries, orthopaedic disabilities, and arthritis. The majority of patients were sponsored by the United Mine Workers of America (UMWA).

In addition to physical therapy, other medically prescribed therapies included occupational therapy, speech therapy, and numerous craft and appliance repair classes and recreational activities.[9] The last two types of activities were available within limits of safety, and if supplemental to the physical therapy program. Evenings and weekends were occupied with classes and recreation, including "out-trips."

A patient's treatment program frequently occupied 5 hours a day. The patient usually required resistive work on a treatment table or on a mat, or both. One half hour, and sometimes one hour, was scheduled and supplemented by self-conducted mat programs, pulley programs, and gait training. Occupational therapy was useful to many patients, and those who needed speech therapy received individual attention.

KKI developed a unique method of financing treatment. The basic charge was for physical therapy according to the time required. All other modalities and therapies were provided without charge. A KKI fund provided additional therapy time for patients who needed financial assistance. Some patients who had substantial resources contributed to this fund.

By 1952 Kabat's method was attracting the interest of physical therapists in the United States to a degree. Perhaps three or four a year would come for 3 months of training. A reasonable tuition was charged. Those trained in foreign countries were seeking training on the job, an "earn, learn, and return" program; the majority came for 6 months, others for a year. They came from Canada; Scandinavia, Great Britain, West Germany, France, Belgium, and other European countries; and Australia, New Zealand, and South America.

Vallejo's KKI offered therapists boundless opportunity to broaden their knowledge and to acquire skill by working with a wide variety of patients. From 1952 to 1954 I assisted Margaret Knott with teaching and supervision of staff therapists. Our first attempt at continuing education was a 2-day workshop presented following the APTA Annual Conference in Philadelphia in 1952. Patterns with techniques superimposed were taught, with therapists working in pairs at and on treatment tables. During that period, in 1953, Dr. Kabat decided that Maggie and I should analyze the patient's problems and develop suitable programs. The staff physicians carried out the more traditional duties of all physicians.

The close of 1953 saw the closing of the program of the UMWA with the opening of their hospitals in the coal-mining regions. This reduced the patient population from about 200 to 50. Consequently, many physical therapists, as did staff physicians and occupational therapists, sought employment elsewhere. The greatest shock was the departure of Dr. Kabat in January 1954. His contributions over the 7 years were many. His one-man research effort resulted in a new, sometimes controversial, but soundly based approach to rehabilitation.

After Dr. Kabat's resignation, the names of the Kabat-Kaiser Institutes were changed to California Rehabilitation Centers at Vallejo and Santa Monica. (The Institute in Washington was closed in the early 1950s.) Several years later the centers were renamed once more to Kaiser Foundation Rehabilitation Center (KFRC).

Fortunately, on July 1, 1954, Dr. Sedgwick Mead, M.D., Associate Professor of Rehabilitation Medicine at Washington University in St. Louis, came to serve as Medical Director. Dr. Mead, a graduate of Harvard College and of Harvard Medical School, was a specialist in neurology and in physical medicine. He was affiliated with the Massachusetts General Hospital, Boston, where I first knew him. I suggested that he be approached for the post of Medical Director of KFRC. He accepted and assumed his duties on July 1, 1954.

In July 1954 Margaret Knott and I presented the first 2-week course in Vallejo following the APTA Annual Conference in Los Angeles. The nineteen therapists attending included one director of a physical therapy school and five who were clinical supervisors. At my request, we taught patterns as active movement before teaching "hands on" techniques. I followed this practice through the years with undergraduate students and in continuing education courses.

Publication of the first edition of the Knott and Voss textbook on PNF was assured by a contract with Paul B. Hoeber, New York, in 1954. I had, since 1952, worked at the analysis of the spiral and diagonal patterns as to topographical alignment of muscles. By 1954 that task was completed and I was well under way in the writing of the textual material. Helen Drew (now Hipshman) had completed the artwork. At this point I received an invitation to travel to Cairo to teach nurses from the University Hospital to treat poliomyelitis patients. I accepted this challenge and therefore decided to leave KFRC in November 1954, since the number of patients had not increased sufficiently to warrant two supervisory positions. I traveled to Chicago to await word on going to Washington for orientation before proceeding to Cairo. During this period I completed the manuscript and submitted it to Paul Hoeber in February 1955. The call to Washington from the International Cooperation Agency came, and on March 10, 1955, I departed for my 5 months in Cairo. My experience there was very interesting, and the teaching of PNF to the class of nurses and working with the mothers of the children who had had polio was extremely gratifying. Communication with those who spoke no English was much easier when I used PNF than when I presented muscle testing to the nurses. All physicians I met understood and spoke English fluently.

Upon my return in September 1955, I accepted a position with the American Physical Therapy Association (APTA), then with headquarters in New York City. My free time for several weeks was occupied with reading galley proof for the Knott and Voss book. The first edition became available in September 1956; it was well received.

During the late 1950s Margaret Knott presented several 2-week courses sponsored by Boston University. Emphasis of content was on individual patterns and techniques.* From 1955 to 1962 as I pursued my APTA duties as a consultant, I visited a number of chapters each year. Frequently I was invited to demonstrate and discuss the merits of PNF as an approach to therapeutic exercise. The need for a second edition of the PNF book became apparent. Broadening of concepts and greater depth of understanding and teaching PNF as a developmental approach became my first priority.

The 1960s

In August 1962 I left the APTA, and in October I returned to Vallejo to refresh my knowledge of PNF and to prepare for writing new material for the second edition. I found that PNF had not changed, but the patient population had. There were very few polio patients. An ever-increasing number of patients with spasticity included stroke victims, the brain-injured, and those with spinal cord lesions due to vehicular and other accidents. There was a substantial number of orthopaedic patients, notably injured fruit-pickers who had fallen from their ladders. A few burn patients, mostly children, needed and benefited from treatment.

Other than a small group of "private" patients, the Kaiser Health Plan and various insurance companies supported the cost of patient care. Therapy programs were for the most part based on the original plan designed by Dr. Kabat. Physical therapy was the foundation of the treatment.

In 1963 72% (13 of 18) of the physical therapy staff comprised qualified therapists from countries around the world. The roster of patients was 79, which seemed a small group for 16 full-time staff therapists. Each patient, however, received individual treatment two to four periods a day in areas of table work, and in mat, gait, and self-care activities.†

There was little opportunity for more than two US-trained therapists to gain entry for 3 months of training. As Margaret Knott said, ". . . those edu-

---

* McDonald R: Personal communication, 1980.
† KFRC: Scheduling of patients, Nov 25, 1963.

cated in America comprised the minority of participants in the training program in Vallejo."[5]

After working for 3 months with a series of patients who were representative of the whole group, I began writing new material and revising the first edition as necessary. The emphasis was on the developmental basis of PNF. Photographs were taken of total patterns of the developmental sequence and several of gait, transfer, and self-care activities. In addition to working on the second edition, each afternoon I treated several patients and supervised or gave guidance to a number of the therapist "trainees."

In August 1962 and 1963 I joined Lois Wellock at Northwestern University in teaching PNF short courses. Elizabeth C. Wood, Director of the Physical Therapy Program, had asked me to join the faculty in 1962. In 1963 I felt that I could complete the work on the second edition and so accepted Miss Wood's offer. We agreed that I should begin on December 15, as I would teach therapeutic exercise during the Winter and Spring Quarters. This I did. Teaching and developing teaching materials were demanding my time, so that the second edition was set aside.

In 1965 Margaret Knott contributed to the second of two symposia on the Child with Central Nervous System Deficit held at Stanford University.[4] Again the focus was on methods for facilitation and inhibition. Funded by grants, the sessions were well attended. I represented Northwestern and was pleased to have an opportunity to talk with Maggie Knott and other presenters of lecture-demonstrations.

In 1965 we at Northwestern began planning a special therapeutic exercise project, NU-STEP, the proper name of which was "An Exploratory and Analytical Survey of Therapeutic Exercise." Supported by grant funds, all but two schools of physical therapy in the United States were represented. Upon our invitation, and at their own expense, all schools in Canada were represented. An outstanding faculty was assembled to present the neurophysiological, developmental, and motor learning aspects of motor behavior. These bases for five methods of facilitation and inhibition of motor activity were analyzed. The *Proceedings* of NU-STEP, edited by Dr. Harry Bouman, M.D., contained more than 1100 pages and has been in demand around the world.[1]

Post NU-STEP, I returned to the second edition on a half-time basis for the fall quarter. I engaged James Buckley to convert the photographs to drawings; Maggie and I selected the sequence. Finally in December 1966, the manuscript and illustrations were sent to the publisher. As with the first, the second edition was begun in Vallejo and completed in Chicago. The second edition made its appearance in June 1968. While the first had been translated to German and French, the second was translated to German, Spanish, Italian, Japanese, and Dutch. With the English-speaking countries included, PNF's contributions through the second edition and NU-STEP have indeed girdled the globe.

In the summer and fall quarters, I taught PNF short courses at Northwestern and elsewhere. Brief periods of teaching undergraduate students were arranged at the University of Wisconsin, the Medical College of Virginia, and the University of Tennessee. The 5-year series at Northwestern, 1969 to 1973, presented a 2-week general course which I followed by three 1-week clinical courses. Participants worked with patients in the afternoons under supervision by the PNF faculty. This series and teaching at other locations in the United States and Canada brought us into the 1970s.

The 1970s

In 1972 Margaret Knott presented the APTA's most prestigious lecture, the eighth Mary McMillan Lecture, at the Annual Conference in Las Vegas. The title, "In the Groove," was Maggie's term used when teaching precision of performance in diagonal direction.[5] She dwelt on international relationships, on the need to free physical therapy education from traditionalism, the merits of PNF, and the profession's need to become involved and to keep abreast with change in society. I was there along with hundreds of others.

The decade of the 1970s was to become one of pain and loss. In 1974 I became disabled by cervicospondylosis and compression fractures of the dorsolumbar spine. In 1975 my need to retire from Northwestern became obvious. In September I moved to Weymouth, Massachusetts. In 1976 and from then onward I gave guidance to those conducting courses and workshops. I had long believed that students and course participants should be taught in a way that they could teach others as well as to treat patients. Also, I made it a practice to enlist graduates and those who had had experience in Vallejo to assist in teaching. Rarely did anyone decline. Using the developmental approach, beginning with total patterns rather than with complex individual patterns, made learning and teaching easier. More could be taught, and learned, in less time. Thus, "faculties" were easily recruited.

Maggie and I talked on the telephone on such matters as the second edition and the possibility of a third, or to learn one another's opinion of the ability of a certain physical therapist; our meeting in Las Vegas was the last time I saw the person called "Maggie" from Vallejo eastward or westward and around the world. On December 18, 1978, she died at her home in Vallejo. Her health had failed over a period of years. She taught, but, more than a teacher, she was a patient's advocate. She was honored by her professional organization, the APTA, by the Chartered Society of

Physiotherapy (England), and by the Canadian Physiotherapy Association.

The 1980s

At this writing in 1982, the decade is new. The needs of the profession, for the development of teachers, for emphasis on newer concepts and methods in the curricula, and for clinical research, continue. For me, the new decade permitted me to use the mobility I had worked hard to gain.

In August 1980 I traveled to Dubuque, Iowa, to be present for the 2-week course I helped to plan. All went well, and in August 1981 a similar course was held in Ann Arbor, Michigan. Also, in 1981 I was invited to present the 17th Mary McMillan Lecture in Anaheim, California, in June 1982.

My topic, "Everything Is There Before You Discover It," intrigued me when Bill Stipe, Assistant Professor of Art, Northwestern University, used it in one of his creative works. To me the topic was fitting because I had enjoyed my career, especially when I "discovered" new combinations that made sense.[10] As with previous recipients of the McMillan Lecture Award, I devoted months to the searching and writing. In the end, the presenting of the lecture to an enthusiastic audience was a thoroughly rewarding experience.

I dwelt on education, and on the fact that in 1965 the mean number of hours given to teaching PNF was six, whereas in 1980 the median number of hours was 20 to 29. Continuing education is not an alternative to basic education, but is the only cure for obsolescence. I emphasized the need for clinical research and for clinical books on PNF. I reminded the listeners that Mary McMillan was a hands-on-the-patient physical therapist and, in effect, said that patients need what she offered, and that physical therapy education must meet patients' needs.

The occasion to travel to California gave me an opportunity to visit the new KFRC facility within the Kaiser Hospital in Vallejo. I was greeted by a friendly staff, all but four of whom were new to me. They, of course, would not have been new to Maggie. The desire to maintain Margaret Knott's standards was apparent, and the facility was aglow with its newness.

Dr. Howard Liebgold, M.D., a graduate of the University of California Medical School, joined the KFRC staff in 1962. He was an associate physician at that time I first met him. Now he is Chief at KFRC, a post he assumed in 1969 as successor to Dr. Mead.

Closing Comments

This brief recounting of my experience with PNF and with those who developed it in the beginning is inadequate. A search, or even the reading of reference lists, in the physical and occupational therapy literature, in journals of physical medicine, sports medicine, physical education, in kinesiology, and no doubt in other areas, reflects the impact of Dr. Kabat's work. His clinical application of neurophysiology and his identification of the spiral and diagonal patterns extended the knowledge of human movement far beyond his "treatment of paralysis."

To mention only the names of those who have contributed through clinical work and teaching efforts, clinical and academic, would not do them justice. Although a number of therapists have spoken for themselves through publication, patients, students, and colleagues will speak for many in unpublished tributes.

THE METHOD

In the development of PNF techniques, greatest emphasis was placed on the application of maximal resistance throughout the range of motion, using many combinations of motions that were related to primitive patterns and the employment of postural and righting reflexes. These motions allowed for two component actions of muscles as well as permitting action to occur at two or more joints. For example, the peroneals were allowed to contract in plantar flexion and eversion instead of straight eversion, and the anterior tibial was stimulated in combination with hip and knee flexion. Positioning of a part was considered valuable in that it helped to obtain a stronger contraction in the desired muscle groups. Motion was performed first in the strongest part of the range, progressing toward the weaker parts of the range of motion. Stretch was applied to groups of muscles, usually synergists, for greater proprioceptive stimulation. The process of overflow, referred to as reinforcement, was used throughout in whatever combination of motions achieved the desired response. The technique of repeated contractions was used to gain range as well as to improve endurance. Stimulation of many types of reflexes was incorporated in treatment programs.

These methods were used for several years. In 1949, a valuable contribution was made when it was learned that having a patient contract isometrically the agonist, then the antagonist, resulted in increased response of the agonist. Upon evaluation, it was realized that Sherrington's law of successive induction had a definite place in techniques of facilitation. This technique was named "rhythmic stabilization." Soon, following the use of rhythmic stabilization, it was found that applying the same procedure of alternating resistance to isotonic contractions of antagonist and agonist also had a facilitating effect. This technique was named "slow reversal."

Early in 1951, the combinations of motion being used were analyzed carefully. It was found that the most effective combinations were those that permitted maximum elongation of related muscle groups so that the stretch reflex could be elicited throughout a "pattern." These patterns were spiral and diagonal in character, and, upon study, their similarity to normal, functional patterns of motions was noted. Since 1951, application of specific techniques has been made in mat, gait, and self-care activities as a means of accelerating the learning process as well as improving strength and balance.

DEFINITIONS

Techniques of PNF are used to place specific demands in order to secure a desired response. Facilitation, by definition, means, "(1) the promotion or hastening of any natural process; the reverse of inhibition; (2) specifically, the effect produced in nerve tissue by the passage of an impulse; the resistance of the nerve is diminished so that a second application of the stimulus evokes the reaction more easily."[2] Proprioceptive means "receiving stimulation within the tissues of the body." Neuromuscular (neuromyal) means "pertaining to the nerves and muscles."[3] Therefore, techniques of proprioceptive neuromuscular facilitation may be defined as methods of promoting or hastening the response of the neuromuscular mechanism through stimulation of the proprioceptors.

PRINCIPLES

By definition and demonstration, PNF related to normal responses of the neuromuscular mechanism. Knowledge of the normal neuromuscular mechanism, including motor development, anatomy, neurophysiology, and kinesiology, is basic to the learning of the method. Knowledge of the abilities and limitations of the normal subject from birth to maturity is basic to intelligent application in the treatment of patients who present motor dysfunction.

The normal neuromuscular mechanism is capable of a wide range of motor activities within the limits of the anatomical structure, the developmental level, and inherent and previously learned neuromuscular responses. The innumerable combinations of motion available to the mature, normal subject in meeting the demands of life have been acquired through a well-established developmental pattern and many learning situations requiring physical effort and skill. The normal subject is endowed with reserves of power which may be tapped in stress situations, as evidenced in acts of self-preservation or heroism. The normal subject is also endowed with potentials which may be developed in accordance with environmental influences and voluntary decisions. Extreme evidences of this are the child and octogenarian prodigies.

The normal neuromuscular mechanism becomes integrated and efficient without awareness of individual muscle action, reflex activity, and a multitude of other neurophysiological reactions. Variations occur in relation to coordination, strength, rate of movement, and endurance, but these variations do not prevent adequate response to the ordinary demands of life.

The deficient neuromuscular mechanism is inadequate to meet the demands of life, in proportion to the degree of the deficiency. Response may be limited as a result of faulty development, trauma, or disease of the nervous or the musculoskeletal systems. Deficiencies present themselves in terms of limitation of movement as evidenced by weakness, incoordination, adaptive shortening or immobility of joints, muscle spasm, or spasticity.

It is the deficient neuromuscular mechanism that becomes the concern of the medical profession and the physical therapist. Specific demands placed by the physical therapist have a facilitating effect upon the patient's neuromuscular mechanism. The facilitating effect is the means used by the physical therapist to reverse the limitations of the patient.

PLAN OF VOLUME

Part 1 presents patterns of motion, which include patterns as free active motion; facilitation and reinforcement of unilateral (individual) patterns and bilateral combinations; and total patterns. These four series reflect diagonal patterns and the rotation patterns of head and neck, and trunk. No series is all-inclusive. However, a series may be expanded by selecting patterns for combinations from another series and adapting them as necessary.

Free active performance is intended as a device for learners: teachers, students, patients, athletes, nurses, physicians who are interested in assessment of movement, and, of course, physical therapists and occupational therapists. The brief commands may be used for self-instruction or for teaching or directing others. The individual learner may use a mirror in order to correct his performance.

The unilateral (individual) patterns in this edition, as in the first and second editions, provide detail of motion components and major muscle components. The manual contacts, normal timing, timing for emphasis of specific pivots of action, and the commands are given for each pattern. The illustrations are designed to show the physical therapist's approach to the patient, the manual contacts, the motion characteristics of the patterns through full range, and the motion characteristics of the physical therapist.

The unilateral patterns, presented as the first series in facilitation and reinforcement, precede bilateral combinations and total patterns. This order is not in keeping with the developmental approach; the order is reversed. Because the spiral and diagonal patterns of irradiation are the unique feature of the method, they must be learned as free active motion and will then be understood. They are combined for reinforcement and are identified in total patterns.

New material integrated with unilateral patterns portrays manual contacts for emphasis of scapular patterns, thrusting variations, mass closing and opening of the hand, and foot and ankle patterns.

The bilateral combinations are shown in lengthened, middle, and shortened ranges. The therapist selects combinations that produce increased strength of response through irradiation and resistance, and the point in the range in need of emphasis. Bilateral combinations are numerous. When points in the range are considered, combinations and possibilities are innumerable. Ipsilateral and contralateral combinations can be gleaned from Reference Tables 4 and 5.

The final series on the use of total patterns of movement and posture may be performed as free active motion. Related aspects of normal motor behavior are discussed, and an adapted sequence of developmental activities is given. Many of the activities are illustrated with text that is intended to be helpful to the therapist's learning. Greatest emphasis has been given to mat activities because their use prepares for more advanced activities. Again, the therapist must apply the methods according to the needs of the individual patient.

Part 2 is devoted to the various techniques used to promote the desired response, and to hasten motor learning. An attempt is made to describe the "how to" of the various techniques. It is not possible, within the limitations of a manual, to present in complete detail the application and modifications of the techniques according to specific clinical diagnoses. General knowledge can be applied to a specific situation by an intelligent physical therapist. The summary of techniques presents a partial guide to the selection of techniques, their indications and contraindications. A brief discussion of the use of cold, electrical stimulation, and mechanical vibration as adjunctive agents is included.

Part 3 includes application of the method for improvement of vital and related functions. The location of this material in the book does not indicate its relative importance. These functions are of primary importance in the treatment of many patients.

Part 4 is new; this is the first time that coupling PNF with joint mobilization has appeared in this book.

Part 5 presents suggestions for evaluation of the patient's performance and for planning a treatment program.

Part 6 gives suggestions for teaching, and presents the 2×2 rule for varying practice.

Following Part 6 are references and suggested readings supportive of the understanding and application of the method.

The Reference Tables present suggested combinations of patterns for reinforcement, optimal patterns for individual muscles, and a listing of muscles according to peripheral innervation and in relation to individual patterns.

The use of acronyms has been introduced in several areas of content. Acronyms such as PNF should be useful as time and space savers.

Dorothy E. Voss, B.ED., R.P.T.

CONTENTS

LIST OF ILLUSTRATIONS AND TABLES

List of Illustrations

Total Patterns

Mat Activities

Rolling: supine toward prone:

Rolling: prone toward supine:

Activities for lower trunk (inferior region):

Prone progression: crawling:

Prone progression: on elbows and knees:

Prone progression: on hands and knees:

Prone progression: on hands and feet:

Sitting:

Kneeling progression:

Bipedal progression:

List of Tables

List of Reference Tables

PROPRIOCEPTIVE NEUROMUSCULAR FACILITATION

PATTERNS OF MOTION

1

Introduction

The patterns of motion for proprioceptive neuromuscular facilitation (PNF) are mass movement patterns. Mass movement is a characteristic of normal motor activity and is in keeping with Beevor's axiom that the brain knows nothing of individual muscle action but knows only of movement. In normal, functional motor activity various combinations of motion, or mass movements, require shortening and lengthening reactions of many muscles in varying degrees. Mass movement that is to be a means of placing a specific demand must be a specific combination of motions that is optimum for the specific sequence of muscles primarily responsible for the movement, and it must allow these muscles to contribute their components of action consistently. When performed against resistance, patterns of facilitation promote selective irradiation, a process demonstrated by Sherrington.[44]

The mass movement patterns of facilitation are spiral and diagonal in character and closely resemble the movements used in sports and in work activities. The spiral and diagonal character is in keeping with the spiral and rotatory characteristics of the skeletal system of bones and joints and the ligamentous structures. This type of motion is also in harmony with the topographical alignment of the muscles from origin to insertion and with the structural characteristics of the individual muscles.

There are two diagonals of motion for each of the major parts of the body: the head and neck, the upper trunk, the lower trunk, and the extremities. Each diagonal is made up of two patterns that are antagonistic to each other. Each pattern has a major component of

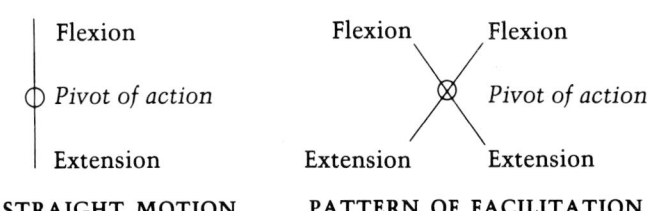

STRAIGHT MOTION   PATTERN OF FACILITATION

flexion or one of extension, there being two flexion and two extension patterns for each of the major parts. These major components are always combined with two other components.

MOTION COMPONENTS

Each spiral and diagonal pattern is a three-component motion with respect to all of the joints or pivots of action participating in the movement. The three components include flexion or extension, motion toward and across the midline or across and away from the midline, and rotation.

In describing patterns of facilitation, flexion is always referred to as flexion and extension is always referred to as extension. Motion toward and across the midline has its counterpart of adduction with reference to extremity pivots. Motion across and away from the midline has its counterpart of abduction. External rotation has its counterparts, supination and inversion. Internal rotation has its counterparts of pronation and eversion.

Head and Neck and Trunk

The patterns of the head and neck and the upper trunk are described as flexion or extension with rotation to the left or to the right. The head and neck patterns are the key to the upper trunk patterns, and the components of a specific head and neck pattern are continued in the homologous pattern of the upper trunk. The head, neck, and trunk rotate toward the left or right, and flexion or extension are combined with motion of the head across the midline of the trunk. For example, the pattern of upper trunk flexion to the right has a starting position in which the head, neck, and upper trunk are rotated to the left and hyperextended laterally as though the subject were looking up and above the left shoulder. The pattern proceeds with the head rotating toward the right, the neck flexing and rotating toward the right so that the chin crosses the midline of the body as the upper trunk begins to flex with rotation toward the right. The left shoulder approaches the right hip as the motion is completed. The entire motion is one of looking up and above the left shoulder, then turning and pulling the head toward the right hip. The directly antagonistic pattern, upper trunk extension with rotation to the left, proceeds from the completed or shortened range of the described motion of upper trunk flexion with rotation to the right. Upper extremity patterns are combined in bilateral asymmetry as reinforcement for diagonal patterns of the upper trunk.

The rotation patterns of the head and neck and the upper trunk are spiral in character. The major component is one of rotation from extreme left to extreme right or vice versa, thereby passing through a flexion phase and into an extension phase. Just as in the diagonal patterns, head and neck rotation is the key to upper trunk rotation. The motion is one of looking down and behind one shoulder, then turning to look down and behind the opposite shoulder. The head and neck rotate as far as possible, and the trunk rotates from lateral hyperextension on one side to lateral hyperextension on the other side.

The lower trunk patterns are described as flexion or extension with rotation to the left or to the right. The bilateral asymmetrical lower extremity patterns are the key to the lower trunk patterns and contribute their respective components of motion. The distal parts of the extremities move across the midline of the trunk. Motions of the pelvis include elevation of the pelvic brim as the counterpart of flexion, depression of the pelvic brim as the counterpart of extension, and rotation toward the left or right.

Tables 1-1 and 1-2 list the patterns for the head and neck, the trunk, and the upper and lower extremities, along with their acronyms (see Table 1-3, p. 8).

Upper and Lower Extremities

Proximal Pivots

The patterns of the extremities are named for the three components of motion occurring at the proximal joints or pivots of action: the shoulder and the hip. Each extremity pattern includes a component of flexion or extension, adduction or abduction, and external

Table 1-1. Head and Neck and Trunk Patterns and Their Acronyms

Head and Neck and Upper Trunk			Lower Trunk		
Pattern	Acronym	Upper Extremities*	Pattern	Acronym	Lower Extremities*
Flexion with rotation to right	D fl, R	D1 ex, R; D2 ex, L	Flexion with rotation to left	D fl, L	D2 fl, L; D1 fl, R
Extension with rotation to left	D ex, L	D2 fl, L; D1 fl, R	Extension with rotation to right	D ex, R	D1 ex, R; D2 ex, L
Flexion with rotation to left	D fl, L	D1 ex, L; D2 ex, R	Flexion with rotation to right	D fl, R	D2 fl, R; D1 fl, L
Extension with rotation to right	D ex, R	D2 fl, R; D1 fl, L	Extension with rotation to left	D ex, L	D1 ex, L; D2 ex, R
Rotation to left	Ro, L	D1 ex, L; D1 fl, R	Rotation to left	Ro, L	D1 ex, L; D1 fl, R
Rotation to right	Ro, R	D1 ex, R; D1 fl, L	Rotation to right	Ro, R	D1 ex, R; D1 fl, L

Bilateral asymmetrical (BA) combinations for reinforcement of diagonal patterns of upper trunk require contact between upper extremities. Forearm and wrist of leading arm are grasped by hand of following arm.

Rotation patterns of upper trunk are reinforced by bilateral reciprocal D1 patterns. Rotation patterns of lower trunk are reinforced by BA patterns of lower extremities (supine position).

Reinforcement of lower trunk by BA combinations of lower extremities requires contact between the extremities.

* See Table 1-2, and Bilateral Combinations for Reinforcement.

(After Voss DE: Proprioceptive neuromuscular facilitation. Am J Phys Med 46:846–848, 1967)

Table 1-2. Upper and Lower Extremities Patterns and Their Acronyms

Patterns	Acronym	Patterns	Acronym
Upper Extremity		**Lower Extremity**	
Flexion – adduction – external rotation	D1 fl	Flexion – adduction – external rotation	D1 fl
Extension – abduction – internal rotation	D1 ex	Extension – abduction – internal rotation	D1 ex
Flexion – abduction – external rotation	D2 fl	Flexion – abduction – internal rotation	D2 fl
Extension – adduction – internal rotation	D2 ex	Extension – adduction – external rotation	D2 ex

There are two pairs of antagonistic, diagonal patterns in upper and in lower extremities. One pair of diagonal patterns has been designated "the first diagonal"; the second pair is "the second diagonal." The acronyms are derived from the first (D1) and second (D2) diagonals combined with the names of the major components, flexion (fl) and extension (ex). The names of the patterns and their respective acronyms are listed: See Evaluation Forms as an example of use.

(After Voss DE: Proprioceptive neuromuscular facilitation. Am J Phys Med 46:846 – 848, 1967)

or internal rotation. There are certain variations between the upper and lower extremity patterns because of the complexity of the upper extremity. In the upper extremity, shoulder flexion and extension are combined with adduction and abduction. External rotation is consistent with flexion, and internal rotation is consistent with extension. In the lower extremity, hip flexion and extension are combined with adduction and abduction and with external and internal rotation. However, adduction is consistent with external rotation, and abduction is consistent with internal rotation.

Intermediate Pivots

The intermediate joints, the elbow and knee, may remain straight or they may flex or extend. The rotation and gliding motions of these joints are consistently in line with the rotation and adduction or abduction occurring at the shoulder or hip. This is true regardless of whether the intermediate action is that of flexion or extension.

Distal Pivots

Distal components of motion are consistent with proximal components regardless of intermediate joint action. In the upper extremity, supination of the forearm and motion of the wrist toward the radial side are consistent with flexion and external rotation of the shoulder. Pronation and motion of the wrist toward the ulnar side are consistent with extension and internal rotation. Wrist flexion is consistent with shoulder adduction, and wrist extension is consistent with shoulder abduction.

In the lower extremity, plantar flexion of the ankle and foot is consistent with hip extension, and dorsiflexion is consistent with hip flexion. Inversion of the foot and motion toward the tibial side is consistent with hip adduction and external rotation. Eversion of the foot with motion toward the fibular side is consistent with abduction and internal rotation.

Digital Pivots

Digital motions are always consistent with the proximal joint motions and with those of the wrist and hand or the ankle and foot, regardless of intermediate joint action. In the upper extremity, flexion with adduction of the fingers occurs with flexion of the wrist and shoulder adduction. Extension with abduction of the fingers occurs with wrist extension and shoulder abduction. The fingers rotate or glide toward the radial side consistently with radial motions of the wrist, supination, shoulder flexion, and external rotation. They rotate or glide toward the ulnar side with ulnar motions of the wrist, pronation, shoulder extension, and internal rotation.

Thumb flexion with adduction and external rotation of the first metacarpal occurs in the flexion – adduction – external rotation pattern. Thumb extension with adduction and external rotation of the first metacarpal occurs in the flexion – abduction – external rotation pattern. Thumb palmar abduction with abduction and internal rotation of the first metacarpal is combined with thumb extension in the extension – abduction – internal rotation pattern. Thumb opposition with abduction and internal rotation of the first metacarpal occurs in the extension – adduction – internal rotation pattern. Therefore, adduction of the thumb is consistent with external rotation and flexion of the shoulder; abduction of the thumb is consistent with internal rotation and extension of the shoulder; flexion of the thumb is consistent with adduction of the shoulder; and extension of the thumb is consistent with abduction of the shoulder.

In the lower extremity, extension with abduction of the toes is combined with dorsiflexion of the foot and ankle and is consistent with flexion of the hip. Flexion with adduction of the toes is combined with plantar flexion and is consistent with hip extension. The toes rotate or glide toward the tibial side with inversion of the foot, and hip adduction and external rotation. The toes rotate or glide toward the fibular side with eversion, and hip abduction and internal rotation.

MAJOR MUSCLE COMPONENTS

The major muscle components of a given pattern are related by their topographical alignment upon the skeletal system and are primarily responsible for the movement. As an example, the flexion–adduction–external rotation pattern of the lower extremity consists primarily of muscles that are anteriorly and medially located. Specifically, the hip muscles are the iliopsoas group, the gracilis, the adductores longus and brevis, the obturatorius externus, the pectineus, and the sartorius. When this pattern is performed with the knee straight or with knee extension, the medial portion of the rectus femoris contributes its component of hip flexion. When knee extension is performed, the vastus medialis and the medial portion of the rectus femoris are primarily responsible. When the knee flexes, the medially located hamstrings, the semitendinosus, and the semimembranosus are primarily responsible. Distally, the anteriorly and medially located muscles are responsible for dorsiflexion with inversion of the ankle and foot, and extension with abduction of the toes toward the tibial side. The muscles include the anterior tibial, the extensor hallucis longus, the extensor digitorum longus, the abductor hallucis, the extensor digitorum brevis, the interossei dorsales, and the lumbricales.

When the lower extremity is positioned with the hip in extension, abduction, and internal rotation, the knee straight, extended, or flexed, the ankle and foot plantar flexed in eversion, and the toes flexed and adducted toward the fibular side, the topographical relationship of these muscles may be visualized. These are the major muscle components. Their action and cooperation is essential to performance of the described pattern.

The muscles secondarily responsible for a pattern are those most closely related by location and function. These muscles provide overlapping between patterns having one or two common components of action. The portions of muscles whose fibers are aligned with the muscles of a related pattern will contribute to that pattern, although it may not be the optimal pattern for that particular muscle. For example, the extension–adduction–external rotation pattern is optimal for the gluteus maximus, but it may contribute to the extension component of the extension–abduction–internal rotation pattern. The glutei medius and minimus are primarily responsible for this pattern, but those fibers of the gluteus maximus that are aligned with those of the glutei medius and minimus will cooperate.

This type of overlapping is characteristic of the major muscle components of the proximal parts: the trunk, shoulder, and hip. It contributes to the stability of these parts and is a sign of the versatility of muscles, that is, of their ability to contribute several components of action and their ability to contribute to several combinations of motion.

The versatility of muscles in patterns of facilitation is seen to progress from proximal to distal. Whereas proximally a portion of a muscle may contribute to a related pattern, the muscles of the intermediate joints contribute specifically to two patterns related by two common components with reference to the proximal pivot. For example, the vastus medialis contributes to those patterns having components of adduction and external rotation, thereby combining with hip flexion and hip extension. Overlapping of the proximal type occurs but to a lesser degree.

Distal muscles are more versatile in that they contribute specifically to two patterns, which are related by only one component with reference to the proximal joint. For example, the toe extensors contribute to both hip flexion patterns. The lumbricales are the most versatile of all muscles since they contribute to all patterns. This distal versatility contributes to dexterity and speed of movement, as compared with proximal versatility, which makes for stability.

NOTE: The analysis of major muscle components is based upon study of the alignment characteristics of the individual muscles as they are portrayed in the anatomy textbooks, observation and palpation of muscle action in normal and pathological subjects, and an elementary study determining the position of maximal stretch. The analysis of the position of maximal stretch was performed by placing a suitably sized piece of sheet elastic on the human skeleton at the points of origin and insertion of the individual muscles. The part was then moved from the anatomical position through all possible components of motion: flexion versus extension, adduction versus abduction, and external rotation versus internal rotation, or their counterparts of supination and pronation. In the head and neck and the trunk, flexion versus extension and rotation with lateral motion toward the same or opposite sides were considered.

LINE OF MOVEMENT

The spiral and diagonal patterns of facilitation provide for an optimal contraction of the major muscle components. A pattern of motion that is optimal for a specific "chain" of muscles allows these muscles to contract from their completely lengthened state to their completely shortened state, when the pattern is performed through the full range of motion. The optimal patterns for the individual muscles are shown in Reference Tables 8 to 11 at the back of this book.

In the starting position of a given pattern (termed the lengthened range, the range of initiation, or the stretch range), the major muscle components are in their completely lengthened state; the fibers of related muscles may be subjected to maximal stretch for facilitation. When the major muscle components contract, the subject, or patient, moves the part from the lengthened range through the available range of motion to the shortened range. In the shortened range of the pattern, the major muscle components have reached their completely shortened state within the limits of the anatomical structure. The halfway point or midpoint between the lengthened and shortened ranges is referred to as the middle range.

Positioning of a part in the lengthened range of a pattern requires consideration of all the components of motion from proximal to distal. The major components of flexion or extension are considered first. If a pattern has a component of flexion, the part is moved toward extension. Motion relative to the midline is next considered; if the pattern has a component of adduction, the part is moved toward abduction. Rotation is always considered last; if the pattern has a component of external rotation, the part is placed in internal rotation. In subjects who present a less-than-normal range of passive motion, rotation should be considered first and last. Finally, positioning of the part is done smoothly, with all three components considered and combined for diagonal placement.

As a pattern of motion is initiated, rotation enters the motion first as the spiral characteristic of the pattern, and the other two components combine to give the pattern a diagonal direction. A figurative cross may be drawn through the proximal joint or pivot to show the diagonal direction of the pattern. A cross having a perpendicular pole bisected at 90° by a horizontal pole should be rotated 45° either clockwise or counterclockwise to give the direction of the diagonals.

The diagonal line of movement is referred to as the "groove" of the pattern. It is the optimal line of movement produced by the optimal or maximal contraction of the major muscle components from their lengthened state to the shortened state. The normal subject readily demonstrates greater strength when he performs in the groove of the pattern than when the line of movement is to either side of the diagonal.

COOPERATIVE FUNCTION OF MUSCLES

Since three components of motion are considered with reference to all joints or pivots participating in a pattern, the major muscle components cooperatively contribute to the three components as far as their topographical location and structure will permit. The function of an individual muscle is a three-component action. The motion component that places the most stretch on a muscle determines its primary action component. The other motion components determine the secondary and tertiary action components. Thus, a muscle may be primarily a flexor, secondarily an adductor, and thirdly an external rotator.

Such a muscle is the psoas major, a major muscle component of the flexion – adduction – external rotation pattern of the lower extremity. Extension achieves the greatest amount of stretch, abduction the second greatest amount, and, finally, internal rotation completes the stretch. The psoas major has a primary action component of flexion, a secondary action component of adduction, and a tertiary action component of external rotation. When the pattern is performed from the lengthened range to the shortened range, the psoas major has contributed three components of action at the hip joint in cooperation with all major muscle components of the pattern.

A single muscle is not solely responsible for a single motion component. The individual muscle is augmented by other related muscles and, in turn, augments the action components of related muscles. The interrelationship of action components with reference to a specific pivot is finely shaded and graded and contributes to smoothness of motion. Following the example above, the psoas major is related topographically and functionally with the psoas minor and iliacus. This relationship is so close that they are commonly referred to as the iliopsoas group. These three muscles have common components of action in slightly varying degrees. The remaining muscle components of the pattern, the gracilis, the adductores longus and brevis, the pectineus, the rectus femoris, the sartorius, and the obturator externus, all contribute flexion components even though minimal. These same muscles contribute adduction components in varying degrees and external rotation components in varying degrees. The obturator externus and the sartorius are the primary intrinsic and extrinsic external rotators. The adductores longus and brevis, the pectineus, and the gracilis are the muscles having primary components of adduction. The gracilis contributes minimal external rotation. Deficiency of any muscle lessens the power with which the pattern is performed and disrupts the smoothness of the movement. A single motion component may be relatively weak while the other two are relatively strong depending on the primary action of the deficient major muscle components.

In the mature, normal subject, optimal contraction of the major muscle components occurs in sequence when the pattern is performed through the available range of motion. The normal timing is from distal to proximal. In the flexion – adduction – external rotation pattern of the lower extremity, the motion is that of pulling the foot up and across the midline of the body as far as possible. This is true whether the knee remains straight, flexes, or extends. The range of motion occurring at the hip must necessarily vary in accordance with the knee motion used, but the direction and goal of the pattern are the same. Smoothness of motion is dependent upon the foot moving first. If the foot moves last, the motion appears to be an afterthought. The contraction of muscles in sequence is related to coordination and is acquired in the developmental process.

Agonists and Antagonists

Optimal, sequential contractions of a "chain" of muscles implies true synergy of these muscles as they move the part through the available range of the pattern of motion. The pattern of muscles contracting toward their shortened state is termed the agonistic pattern. The pattern of muscles approaching their lengthened state in cooperation with those of the agonistic pattern is termed the antagonistic pattern.

The antagonistic pattern is composed of a "chain" of major muscle components having components of action that are exactly the opposite of those of the agonistic pattern. Their location is diagonally opposite those of the agonistic pattern. If a pattern is composed primarily of muscles that are anteriorly and medially located, the muscles of the antagonistic pattern are located posteriorly and laterally. When flexion – adduction – external rotation of the lower extremity is considered the agonistic pattern, extension – abduction – internal rotation is the antagonistic pattern. Its major muscle components with reference to the hip pivot are the glutei medius and minimus. These muscles have action components of extension, abduction, and internal rotation, and they are the direct antagonists of the iliopsoas group.

The lengthening reaction of the antagonistic pattern occurs from distal to proximal as demanded by the range of motion occurring in the agonistic pattern. As the shortened state of the agonistic pattern is reached, as the range of motion is completed, tension occurs in the antagonistic pattern as a range-limiting factor. This is most evident when the two-joint muscles are required to lengthen rather than to shorten. When the action of two-joint muscles is not considered, soft-tissue contact or ligamentous structures may become the range-limiting factor. The muscles of closely related patterns must also contribute lengthening reactions in line with the overlapping of muscle components. For example, in order for complete range of dorsiflexion and inversion of the foot and ankle to be achieved, the peroneus longus and peroneus brevis, among others, must lengthen. The first is primarily responsible to the extension – abduction – internal rotation pattern, while the latter is primarily responsible to the flexion – abduction – internal rotation pattern.

Summary of Muscle Function

In patterns of facilitation, the individual muscle contracts from its completely lengthened state to its completely shortened state in cooperation with the major muscle components of the pattern wherein it is located.

The individual muscle contributes three components of action as far as its topographical location and structure will allow.

The individual muscle lengthens completely in cooperation with its antagonists, which are located diagonally opposite and have opposite components of action.

The individual muscle contributes to a related pattern as far as common components of motion and topographical location will allow. This contribution may be a shortening or lengthening reaction depending upon whether the related pattern is considered an agonist or an antagonist.

The individual muscle is not solely responsible for a single motion component of a pattern but is augmented by related muscles and, in turn, augments the action components of related muscles.

Deficiency of an individual muscle expresses itself to the greatest degree in relation to its primary action component, and to a lesser degree in relation to its secondary and tertiary components of action.

TYPES OF MUSCLE CONTRACTION

In techniques of PNF, two types of muscle contraction are employed. An attempt by the subject to perform a pattern through any part of the range of motion is referred to as active motion, with isotonic contraction of the muscles responsible for the motion. When a technique involves an attempt by the subject to hold a part still without permitting motion to occur, the muscular contraction is referred to as a "hold," or isometric contraction.

Kabat defined the terms of muscle contraction as used in PNF as follows[29]:

> Isotonic: active voluntary shortening of a muscle
> Isometric: static hold against equal resistance
> Eccentric: active voluntary lengthening of a muscle

The various terms used to describe muscle contraction have origins in several languages and in several scientific fields. Arrangement of synonymous terms may add clarity.

> Isotonic — dynamic — movement
> Shortening — concentric — positive work
> Lengthening — eccentric — negative work
> Isometric — static — stable position

The terms derived principally from the Greek language are *isotonic, isometric,* and *dynamic.* Those principally from Latin are *static, concentric, eccentric, positive,* and *negative.*[37]

The terms *isotonic* and *isometric* are frequently used in the fields of medicine, physiology, and neurophysiology.[6] *Static* and *dynamic, concentric* and *eccentric*, and *positive* and *negative* are terms used in the physiology of exercise and in physical education.[1] At times, terms are used interchangeably.[39]

PNF techniques employ either isotonic or isometric contraction, and in most instances both types are used. Normal persons are capable of performing both. Isotonic contractions are clearly related to movement; isometric contractions clearly contribute to posture. In developing motor behavior, the ability to move precedes the ability to maintain posture. Thus, isotonic contractions may be considered more primitive than isometric ("hold") contractions. In mature neuromuscular activity there must be a neat intermixture of both; movement is necessary to posture, and posture is necessary to movement.

Examples of Types and Terms

Rising to stand and lowering to sit in a chair are total patterns that use the concentric and eccentric phases of isotonic contraction. Rising to stand is an extensor-dominant activity. To achieve appropriate stretch of extensor muscle groups, the person should draw his feet under the chair as he flexes his knees, head and neck, trunk, and hips, thereby stretching and activating extensor groups. Hands placed on chair arms permit stretch of shoulder and elbow extensors as the person assumes maximum flexion. The command, "Look up and stand up!" should produce results through mass extension. The shortening or concentric phase of isotonic contraction is used to produce positive work.

Lowering to sit, a reversal of direction, is flexor dominant, and uses the eccentric phase of isotonic contraction of extensor muscle groups. The controlled lengthening of extensors permits flexion of the total pattern. While standing close to the chair the person flexes head and neck as he reaches for the chair arms. Elbows and shoulders flex slowly as trunk, hips, and knees flex until the chair seat is reached. The lengthening or eccentric phase of isotonic contraction is used to produce negative work.

If, while lowering to sit, the person is called to the telephone, must he continue lowering before rising to stand? Or may he shift from lowering (eccentric) to rising (concentric) by "holding" at the point of reversal of direction? Static (isometric) and dynamic (isotonic) contractions are mutually facilitory.[20]

INDICATIONS FOR PATTERNS

Patterns of facilitation are used as free active motion, guided active motion, or resisted motion depending upon the indications for exercise. The patterns serve, too, as passive motion for determination of limitation of range of motion. The goal of treatment is the coordi-

nated performance of patterns of facilitation through a full, or complete, range of motion with a balance of power between antagonistic patterns of both diagonals of motion.

Patterns may be performed, and usually should be, in any position that allows the desired range of motion to occur with the greatest ease and strength. As the normal subject changes his position, the relationship with gravitational pull is altered accordingly. The influence and interaction of reflex mechanisms that underlie movement and posture are factors to be considered.

Thus, positioning for performance is a means of increasing or lessening demands. Visual cues, too, influence performance, and in some instances positioning to permit vision to lead or follow movement may be of primary importance, and may lessen the demand in performance. The changing and grading of demands introduces varied motor experiences that may help to build the patient's abilities.

When movement cannot be voluntarily initiated in a position which demands that gravitational pull be overcome, the patient should be positioned so that gravity assists initiation of movement. By positioning the patient in this way, other factors will automatically contribute to the ease of performance, and procedures will become more effective as follows:

> Tonus will be enhanced through the tonic labyrinthine reflex
> Manual contacts with the patient's body will provide appropriate sensory input through pressure over the agonistic muscle groups rather than the antagonistic muscle groups
> Stretch can be used more adequately to increase response
> Resistance can be used to recruit more motor units and to strengthen the response

Such positioning will exclude, for the most part, the need for "assistive exercise." During assistive exercise, the therapist helps the patient to overcome gravitational pull. The therapist has difficulty in sensing or monitoring the patient's effort, and the four factors as listed will be negative influences rather than contributing to ease of performance.

An example of positioning for facilitation is as follows:

> *Movement to be performed:* hip flexion with knee flexion
> *Position for gravity to assist:* Prone (segment over edge of table or patient in creeping position)
> *Tonic labyrinthine reflex:* Prone posture increases flexor tonus
> *Manual contacts:* Over anterior surface of thigh and foot

Stretch: Lifting part into complete extension (hyperextension) provides stretch to hip flexors and lower trunk flexors

Resistance: Weak hip flexors can be resisted; this also may be reinforced by stronger trunk and knee flexors and ankle dorsiflexors

See Table 1-7, Support by Postural and Righting Reflexes.

REMINDERS FOR LEARNING PATTERNS

Learn the components of motion by performing patterns as free active motion in accordance with normal timing.

Did rotation enter the motion first so that the motion was truly diagonal?

Did the distal parts complete their full range of motion before the middle range was reached?

Proceed from one pattern to its directly antagonistic pattern, a reversal of direction.

Begin with the head and neck and the upper trunk and proceed to the upper extremities, the lower trunk, and the lower extremities.

Practice patterns in as many positions as possible: supine, sidelying (lateral), prone, hands–knees (creeping), sitting, kneeling, and standing.

Practice combining patterns as outlined in Reference Tables 1 to 7, and in patterns as free active motion.

Instruct and criticize other normal subjects in performance of patterns in free active motion, in accordance with normal timing.

Learn the major muscle components of each pattern with regard to each pivot of action or joint.

Learn to use the full name as well as the acronym for each pattern (see Table 1-3).

Table 1-3. Acronyms

Reinforcements

BA	Bilateral asymmetrical
BS	Bilateral symmetrical
BR	Bilateral reciprocal
S, O	Same, opposite side
S, CD	Same, crossed diagonals
EH	Eyes follow hand(s)
HE	Hand(s) follow eyes

Range (R) for Initiation (I), Emphasis (E)

Le-RI, Le-RE	Lengthened
Mid-RI, Mid-RE	Middle
Sh-RI, Sh-RE	Shortened

Points in Range (R)

Le-R	Lengthened
Mid-R	Middle
Sh-R	Shortened

Total Patterns of Posture

Su	Supine
Pr	Prone
Sl	Sidelying
Si	Sitting
HK	Hands–knees
Kn	Kneeling
Sta	Standing

Directions

L	Left
R	Right
F	Forward
B	Backward
C	Circle
S	Sideward
DF	Diagonally forward
DB	Diagonally backward

Techniques

Ap	Approximation
CR	Contract–relax
HR	Hold–relax
HRA	Hold–relax–active motion
MC	Manual contact
MR	Maximal resistance
QR	Quick reversal
RC	Repeated contractions
RI	Rhythmic initiation
RRo	Rhythmic rotation
RS	Rhythmic stabilization
SR	Slow reversal
SRH	Slow reversal–hold
SRHR	Slow reversal–hold–relax
Str	Stretch
Str-R	Repetitive stretch
TE	Timing for emphasis
Tr	Traction

Diagonal Patterns

Upper Extremity

D1 fl	Flexion–adduction–external rotation
D1 ex	Extension–abduction–internal rotation
D2 fl	Flexion–abduction–external rotation
D2 ex	Extension–adduction–internal rotation

Lower Extremity

D1 fl	Flexion–adduction–external rotation
D1 ex	Extension–abduction–internal rotation
D2 fl	Flexion–abduction–internal rotation
D2 ex	Extension–adduction–external rotation

The initial phase of learning PNF is the active performance of spiral and diagonal patterns. Repetition with self-correction before a mirror or correction by expert teachers is necessary to motor learning. Varying practice, that is, performing a pattern or a combination two or three times and then changing to another combination, promotes learning.[49] The pattern or combination previously performed should be performed again with improved form and skill. Speaking commands aloud and directing them to one's self hastens learning.[37] "I will open my hands, look up, and lift my arms up and away. And I will close my hands, look down, and pull my arms down and across" (D2 fl, D2 ex).

Active performance by students, patients, and others is a useful means to assess motor abilities and coordination, and to identify limitations of range of motion when many combinations are compared. The therapist, a teacher, a trainer of athletes, all leaders, must become skilled performers, keen observers, and analyzers. They must serve as models to learners. The learner tracks the leader. In visually tracking the leader, the learner may limit the movement of his head and neck. The leader may offset this limitation by halting his own performance and commanding learners to look in the desired direction. Vision leads movement.

Diagonal patterns may be performed in any position that permits the desired range to occur. Varying the position of the body, using as many developmental total patterns as possible, will alter demands. The demands are varied through the influence of gravity and by postural and righting reflexes. Changing and grading demands introduces a new combination of motor experiences which may build the patient's abilities.

While standing, all head and neck, upper trunk, and unilateral and combinations of upper extremity patterns may be performed. All unilateral patterns of the lower extremity may be done as weight is borne by the opposite limb. For security, a group of persons may join hands. For the individual, contact with a railing, table, or chair back may help. Hands and feet lead the extremity movements.

In the sitting position, all upper extremity patterns and combinations as well as head and neck and upper trunk patterns may be performed. Lower extremity combinations of knee, foot, and ankle patterns can be carried out. Mass flexion and extension of hips and knees cannot be done.

In the supine posture, on a mat, the range of patterns may be limited by contact with the surface. Nevertheless, the components of the patterns may be learned and performed insofar as the surroundings permit. Another limiting factor is that vision cannot be used to complete advantage as the leader of the movement. Proprioception and kinesthetic sense must be relied upon for placement of parts that cannot be seen. In the treatment of patients, elevation of the head may be necessary if the patient is to learn with minimal frustration.

In the hands – knees position (prone posture), intermediate joints of the extremity patterns, elbow and knee, may flex and extend as in mass flexion and extension (hip flexes, knee flexes; hip extends, knee extends). In this prone posture, the lengthened ranges of patterns are assisted by gravity. This adds to the ease of rhythmic movement.

The PNF patterns have certain consistencies that promote learning. The patterns of head and neck and upper trunk are movements to one side or the other, to L or to R. They are asymmetrical, as are the related patterns of the upper extremities during chopping and lifting, BA ex and BA fl. The abduction patterns, D1 ex, and D2 fl, lead with the open hand. The adduction patterns, D1 fl and D2 ex, follow with the hand closed on, or gripping, the leading forearm. All diagonal patterns have asymmetry; movement is toward L or R. When the eyes engage the hand, a diagonal pattern of head and neck is elicited. Again, vision leads movement.

The diagonal thrusts of the upper extremity are inconsistent with other patterns. Thrusting movements represent primitive reaching and grasping, also pushing away from and pulling toward the body. The hand and forearm motions are exactly reversed when compared with diagonal patterns, where forearm supination occurs with external rotation of the shoulder; pronation occurs with internal rotation. In thrusting, counterrotation requires pronation with external rotation and supination with internal rotation. Thrusting is fast and powerful, an all-or-none movement. Reversals of thrusting have exactly opposite components of motion.

In reality, there are innumerable combinations with varying ranges or points in the range.

Illustrations (Figs. 1-1 to 1-32)

For ease in self-instruction and in teaching, two postural patterns were selected, standing and sitting. Head and neck, upper trunk, and upper extremity patterns including unilateral patterns of the lower extremity were performed while standing. Sitting was used for pattern combinations of feet, ankles, and knees. A wide range of lower extremity patterns is portrayed in the section entitled Bilateral Combinations for Reinforcement, as are those of the upper extremity.

All patterns are presented with the subject facing forward in a symmetrical posture. A diagonal position was used in addition for selected upper extremity patterns. These two positions provide opportunity for study and observation of the more complex upper extremity.

Each pattern or combination of patterns is portrayed from the lengthened range (Le-R) to the shortened range (Sh-R). Then, with a few exceptions, the direction is reversed showing the antagonistic pattern from lengthened to shortened range.

In a series of five photographs, A to E, the first, A, and the last, E, are the same, that is, the lengthened range of A begins with the shortened range of E.

The second of the series, B, and the fourth, D, show the timing and the movement of the distal pivots, hands or feet. These phases should be repeated and corrected during practice because they influence the precise path or direction to the shortened range, A to C.

In the series of three, A to C, the first, A, and the third, C, are the same. B is the shortened range of A to B. The antagonistic pattern with reversal of direction is shown in B to C.

COMMANDS

Concise commands are given for each phase in a series. Commands in greater detail are included under Unilateral Patterns and under Bilateral Combinations for Reinforcement. See also Commands and Communication (under Basic Procedures in Chap. 2, Techniques for Facilitation).

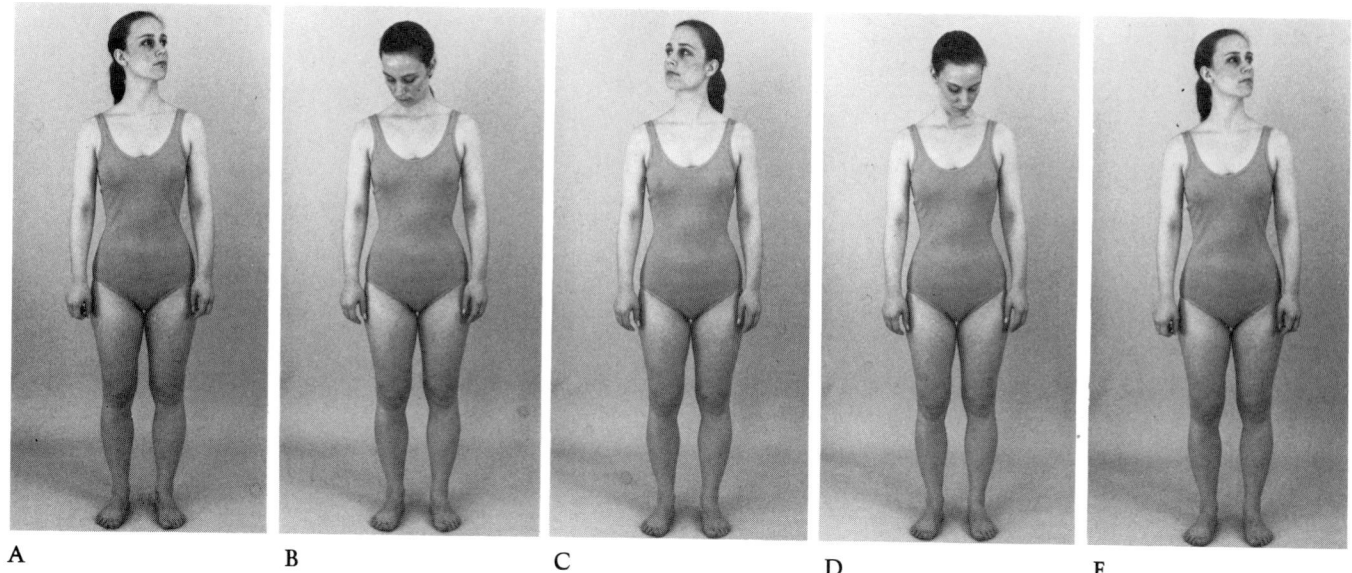

A B C D E

FIG. 1-1. Head and neck, diagonal patterns: D ex, L; D fl, R; D ex, R; D fl, L; D ex, L.

Commands (left to right)

A. "Ready! Look up and away to your left!"
B. "Look down and across to your right hip."
C. "Now change, look up and away to your right."
D. "And look down and across to your left hip."
E. "Now change, look up and away to your left! And repeat! And again!" (Speak the commands as your perform.)

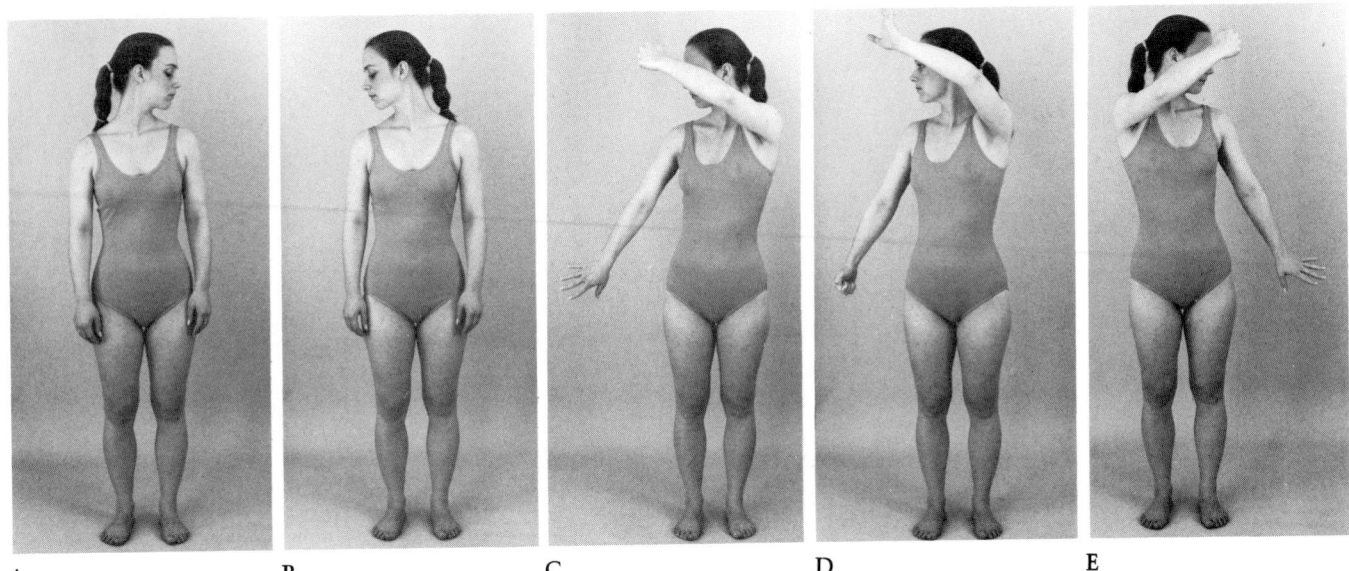

A   B   C   D   E

FIG. 1-2. Head and neck, rotation (Ro) patterns: Ro, L; Ro, R; Ro, L.

Upper extremities, bilateral reciprocal (BR): D1 fl, R; D1 ex, L
Head: Ro, L; D1 ex, L; D1 fl, R; Ro, R; D1 ex, R; D1 fl, L

Commands (left to right)

A. "Ready!"
B. "Turn your head to your right and look down behind your right shoulder."
C. "Now open your right hand down and away as you close your left up and across your eyes."
D. "And close the right! Open the left!"
E. "Now turn your head and upper body to your left, and push your left hand down and away as you pull the right up and across your eyes! And repeat with head to right! And again!" (Speak the commands as you perform.)

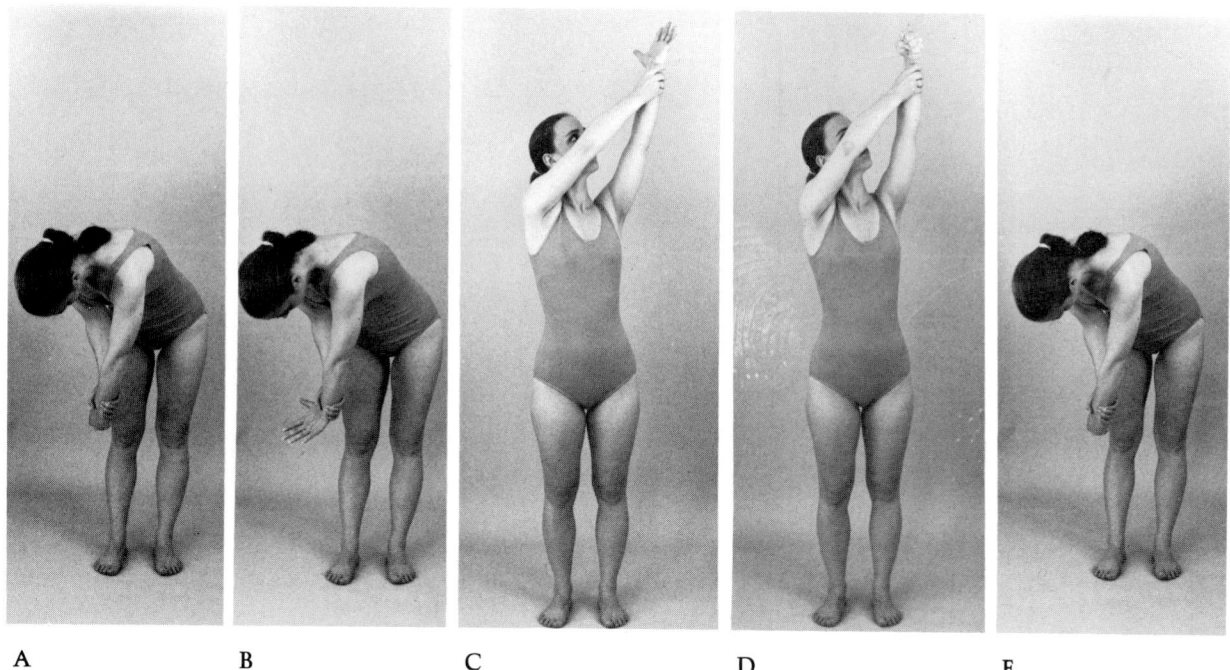

A   B   C   D   E

FIG. 1-3. Upper trunk, diagonal patterns: extension with lifting (BA) to left.

Head and neck, and upper trunk: D fl, R; D ex, L; D fl, R
Upper extremities: D1, R; D2, L, (BA fl, L); reverse (BA ex, R)

Commands (left to right)

A. "Ready! Your right hand grasps your left wrist."
B. "Open your left hand; thumb toward your face!"
C. "And lift your head and hands up toward the left. Look at your hands!"
D. "Now close your left hand!"
E. "Look down and across as you pull your left hand down toward your right knee! And repeat with lifting to left! And reversal to right." (Speak commands as you perform.)

NOTE: Transpose direction for upper trunk extension with lifting to right with reversal to left.

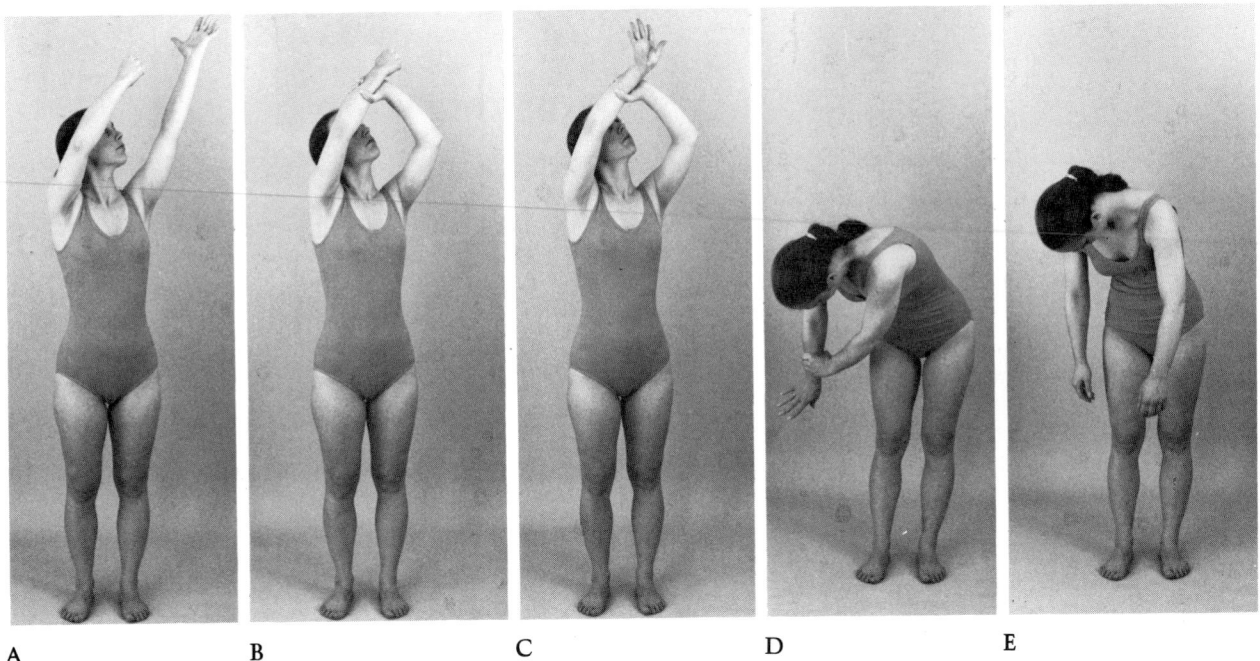

FIG. 1-4. Upper trunk, diagonal patterns: Flexion with chopping (BA) to right.

Head, neck, and trunk: D ex, L; D fl, R
Upper extremities: D1, R; D2, L (BA fl, L); reverse (BA ex, R)

Commands (left to right)

A. "Ready! Close your right hand across your face and open your left hand up and out, thumb back!"
B. "Now your left grasps the right wrist."
C. "Open your right hand, thumb down and out."
D. "Look down and across as you push your right hand down and out."
E. "Look down and across to your right hip as you let your arms hang free." (Speak the commands as you perform.)

NOTE: Transpose direction for upper trunk flexion with chopping to left with reversal to right.

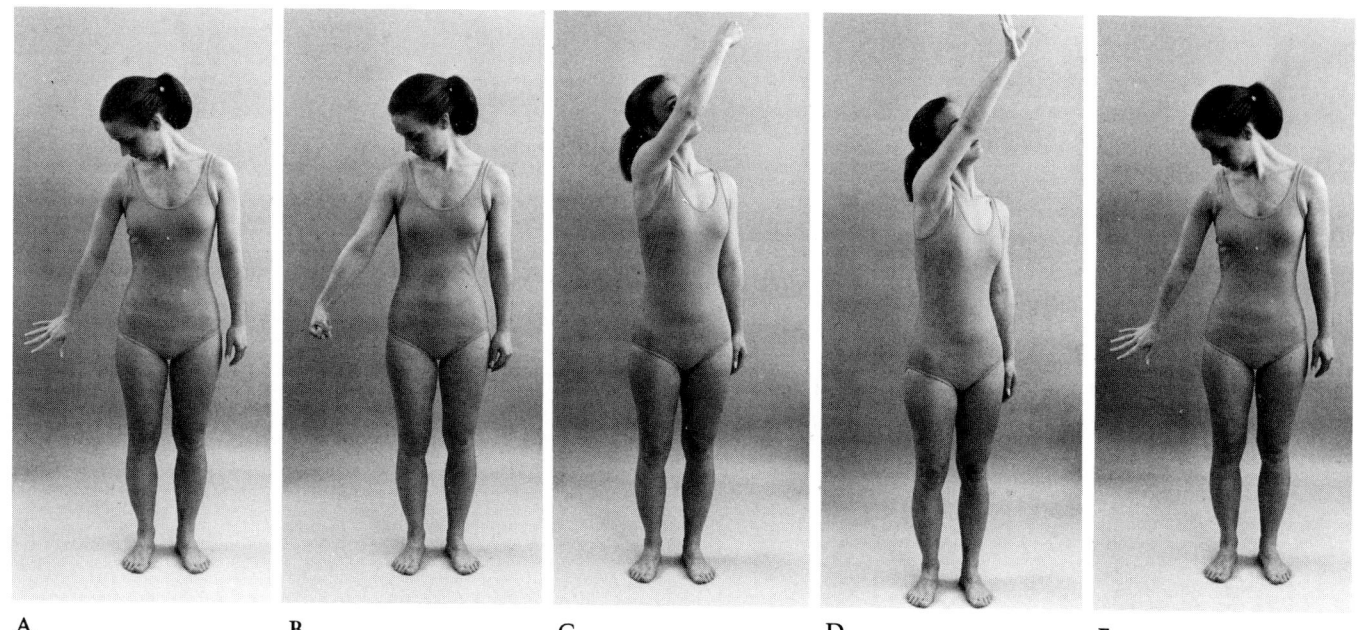

A   B   C   D   E

FIG. 1-5.

D1 fl and D1 ex, elbow straight
Head and neck: D fl, R; D ex, L

Commands (left to right)

A. "Ready! Look at your hand!"
B. "Close and turn your right hand toward your face."
C. "Pull up and across!"
D. "Now open your hand."
E. "And push down and away! And repeat! And again!" (Speak the commands as you perform.)

Upper Extremities, Unilateral Patterns

FACE FORWARD

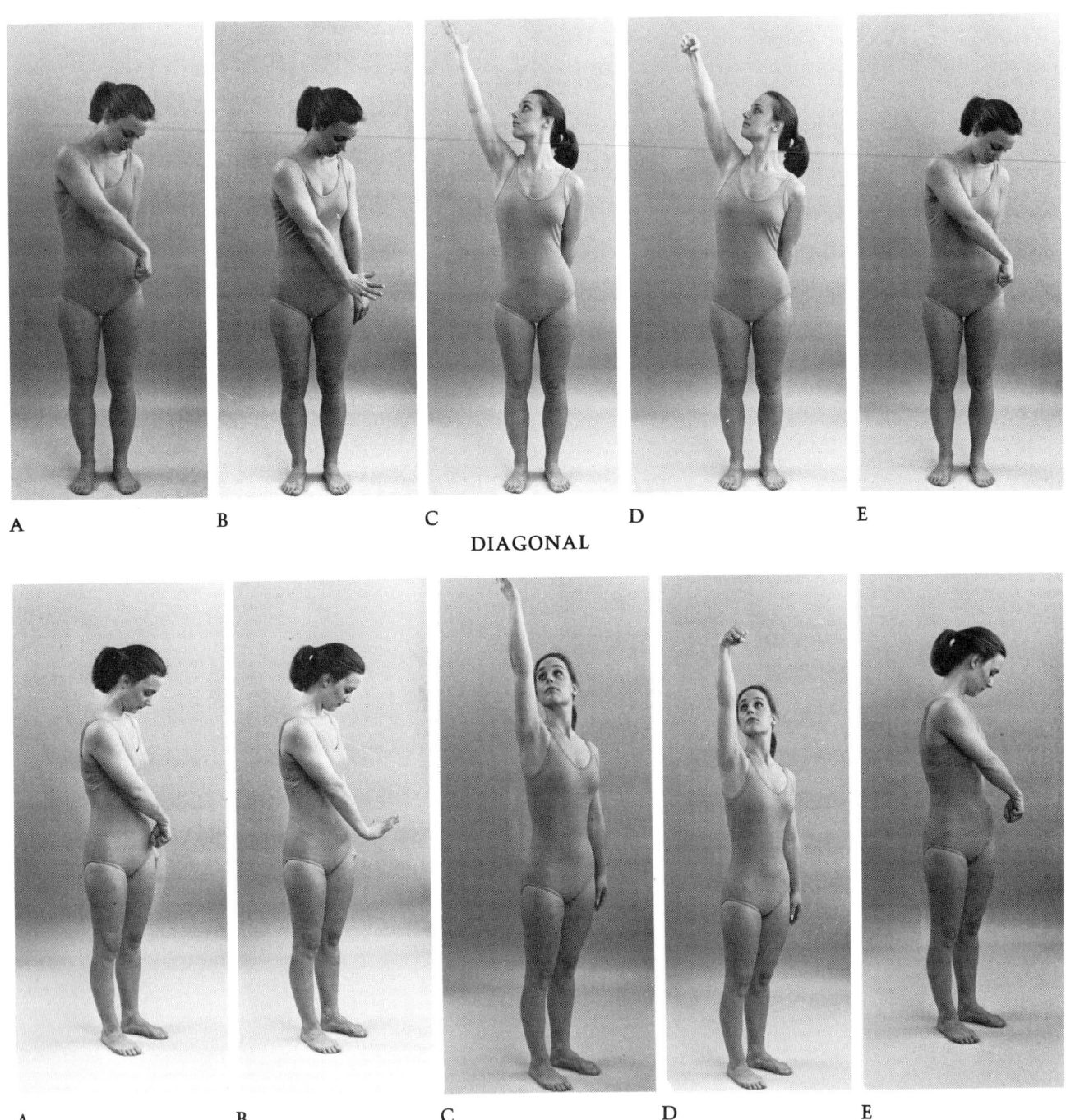

A B C D E

DIAGONAL

A B C D E

FIG. 1-6.

D2 fl and D2 ex, elbows straight
Head and neck: D ex, R; D fl, L

Commands (left to right)

A. "Ready! Look at your hand!"
B. "Open and turn your right hand, thumb toward your face!"
C. "Lift up and out!"

D. "Now close your hand!"
E. "And pull down and across! And repeat! And again!" (Speak the commands as you perform.)

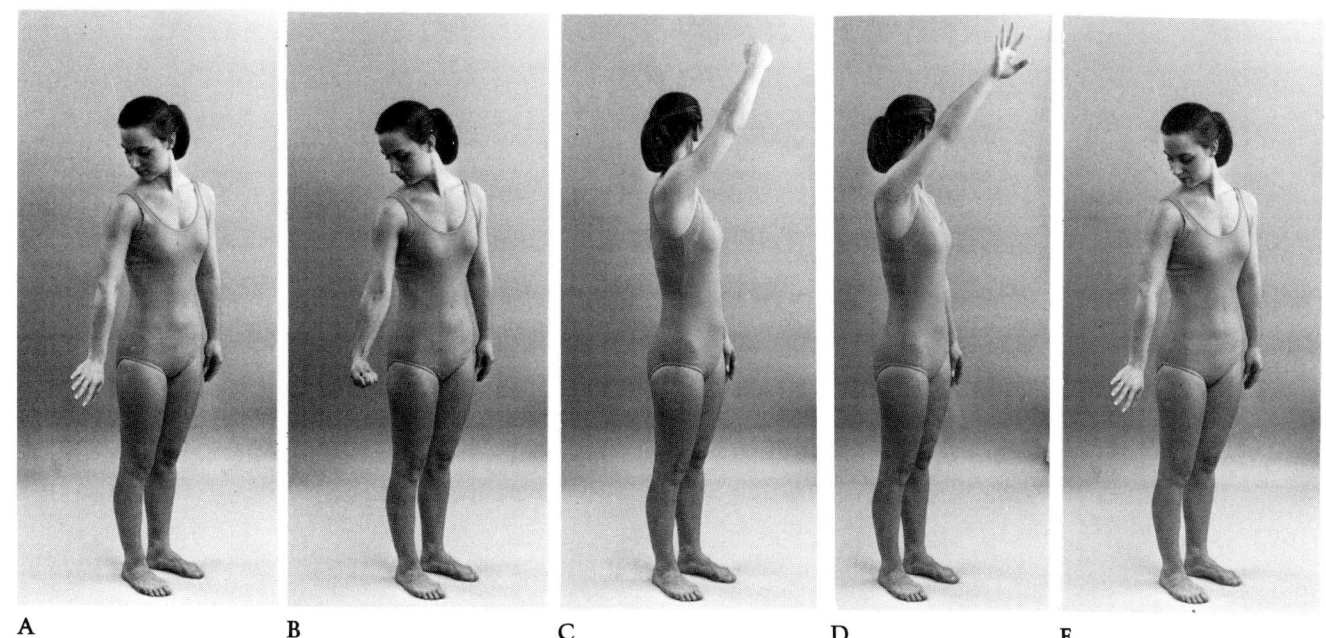

A B C D E

FIG. 1-7.

D1 fl and D1 ex, elbows straight
Head and neck: Ro, R; Ro, L; Ro, R

Commands (left to right)

A. "Ready! Look behind your right shoulder!"
B. "Close and turn your right hand toward your face."
C. "Turn your head and look behind your left shoulder as you pull your hand up and across."
D. "Now open your hand."
E. "And turn your head and look behind your right shoulder as you push down and away! And repeat! And again! (Speak the commands as you perform.)

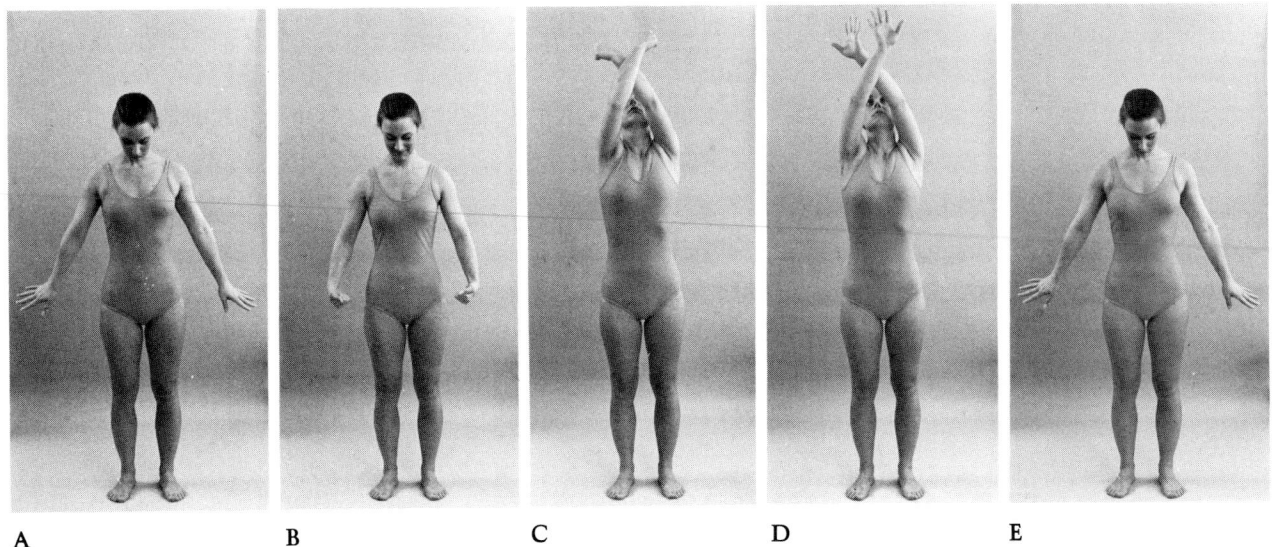

A   B   C   D   E

FIG. 1-8.   D1 fl and D1 ex, elbows straight.

Commands (left to right)

A. "Ready!"
B. "Close your hands and turn them toward your face!"
C. "Pull up and across the face!"
D. "Now open your hands and turn away from your face!"
E. "And push down and away! And repeat! And again!" (Speak the commands as you perform.)

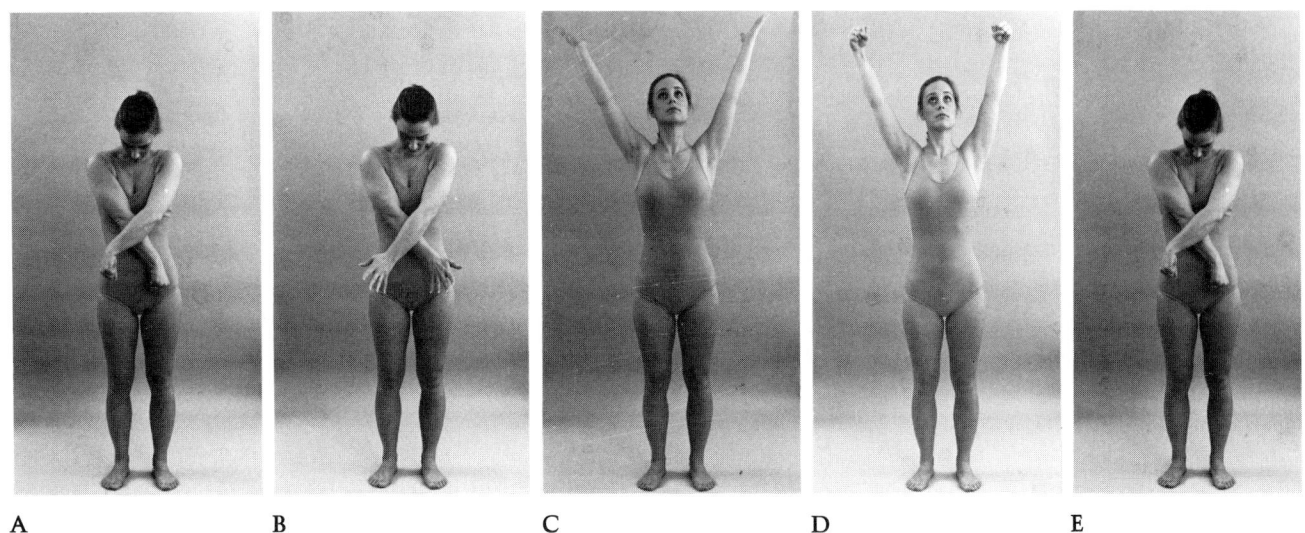

A   B   C   D   E

FIG. 1-9.   D2 fl and D2 ex, elbows straight.

Commands (left to right)

A. "Ready!"
B. "Open your hands, and turn the thumbs up and out!"
C. "Now raise your arms, and reach up and away!"
D. "Close your hands, and bend your wrists toward the little finger side!"
E. "And pull down and across to the opposite hip! And repeat! And again!" (Speak the commands as you perform.)

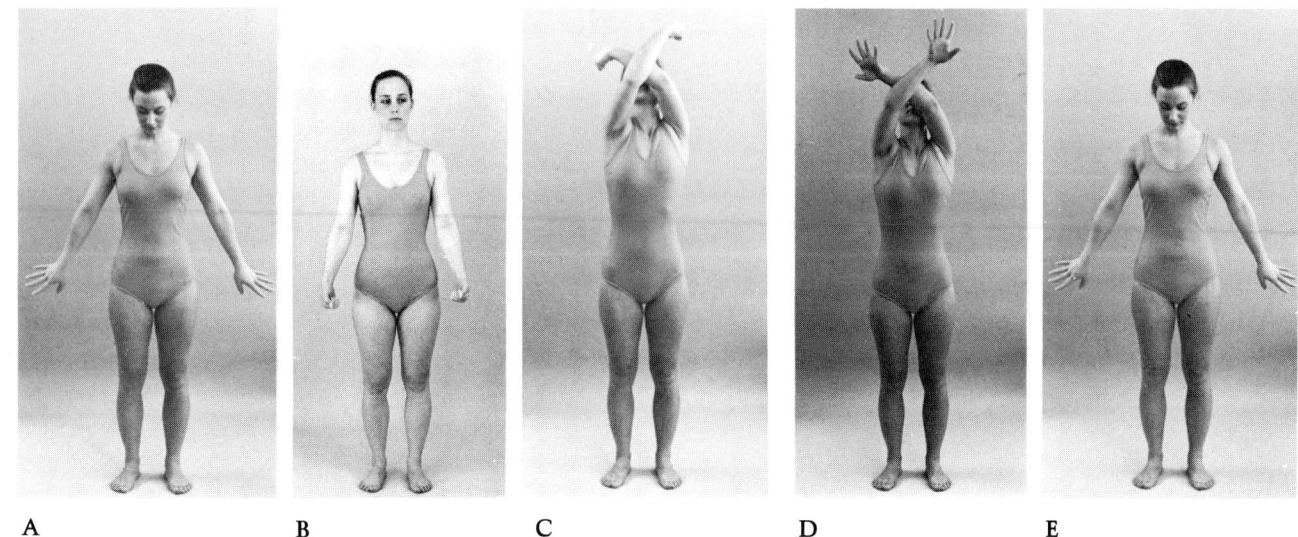

A   B   C   D   E

FIG. 1-10. D1 fl, elbow fl; D1 ex, elbow ex.

Commands (left to right)

A. "Ready!"

B. "Close your hands, and turn toward your face!"

C. "Now pull your arms up and across as you bend your elbows across your face!"

D. "Open your hands! Thumbs turn down and away!"

E. "Now reach down and out as you straighten your elbows! And repeat! And again!" (Speak the commands as you perform.)

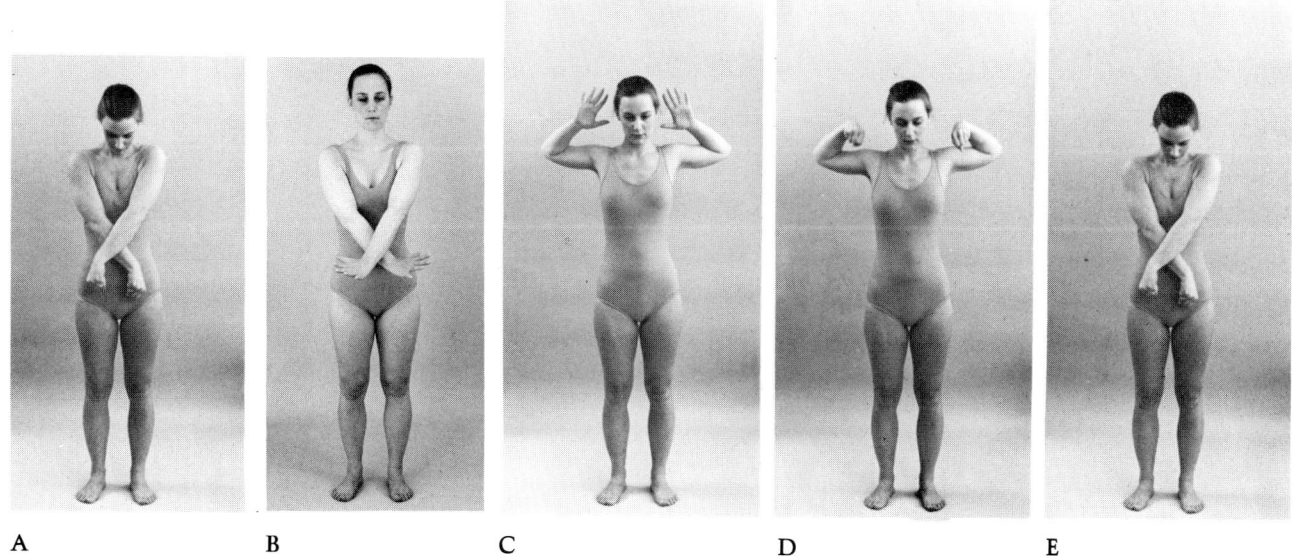

FIG. 1-11. D2 fl, elbow fl; D2 ex, elbow ex.

Commands (left to right)

A. "Ready!"

B. "Open your hands! Thumbs turn up and away!"

C. "Now bend your elbows as you raise your arms up and away! Point the elbows up and out!"

D. "Close your hands, and bend your wrists toward the little finger side!"

E. "Now reach down and across to the opposite hip as you straighten your elbows! And repeat! And again!" (Speak the commands as you perform.)

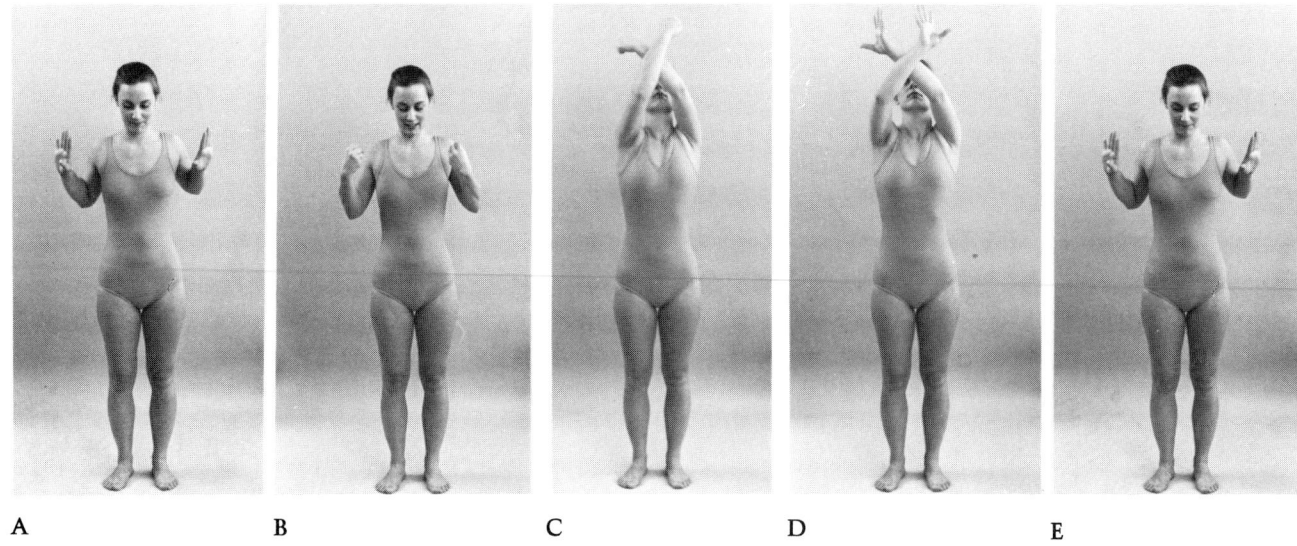

FIG. 1-12. D1 fl, elbows ex; D1 ex, elbows fl.

Commands (left to right)

A. "Ready!"
B. "Close your hands and turn them toward your face!"
C. "Now reach up and across! Straighten your elbows across your face!"
D. "Open your hands and turn the thumbs down and away!"
E. "Now bend your elbows and pull down and out to the side! And repeat! And again!" (Speak the commands as you perform.)

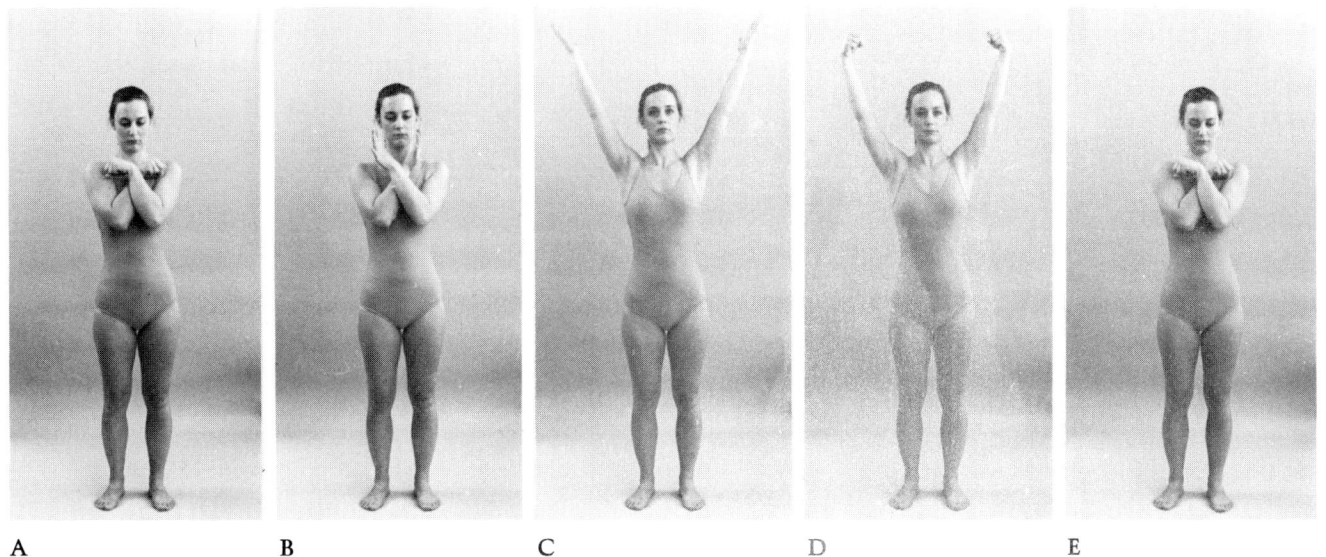

A   B   C   D   E

FIG. 1-13. D2 fl, elbows ex; D2 ex, elbows fl.

Commands (left to right)

A. "Ready!"
B. "Open your hands! Thumbs toward your ears!"
C. "Now raise your arms, straighten your elbows, as hands reach up and away. Reach as far as you can!"
D. "Close your hands, and bend your wrists toward the little finger side."
E. "And pull your elbows toward your middle so that each points to the opposite hip. And repeat! And again!" (Speak the commands as you perform.)

FACE FORWARD

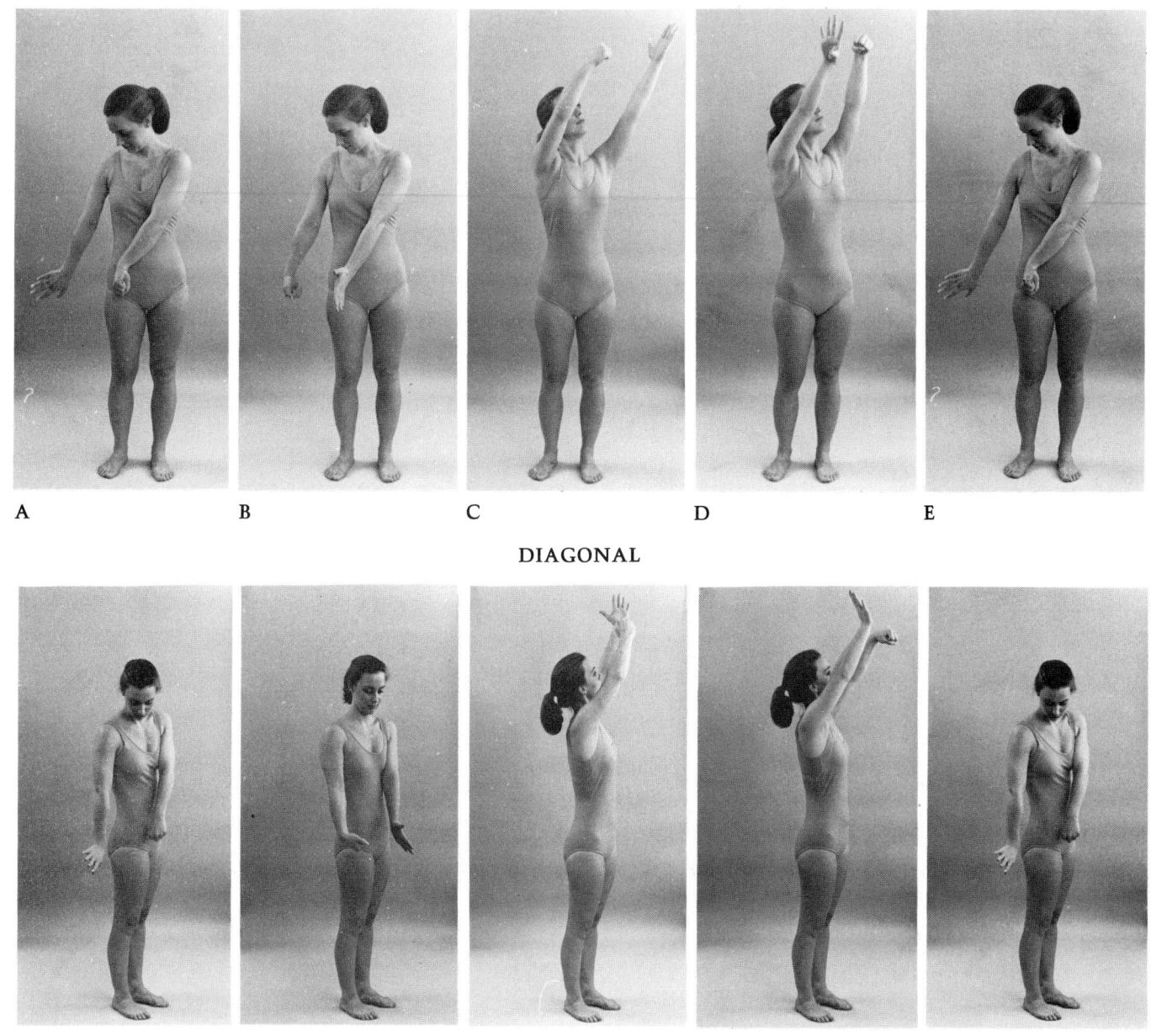

DIAGONAL

FIG. 1-14.   D1, R; D2, L; elbows straight.

Commands (left to right)

A. "Ready! Look at your hands all of the way!"
B. "Open the left hand and close the right!"
C. "Now lift your arms up and across to the left!"
D. "Close the left hand and open the right!"
E. "Now reach down and across to the right! And re-peat! And again!" (Speak the commands as you perform.)

Upper Extremities, Bilateral Reciprocal (BR, CD) Patterns

FACE FORWARD

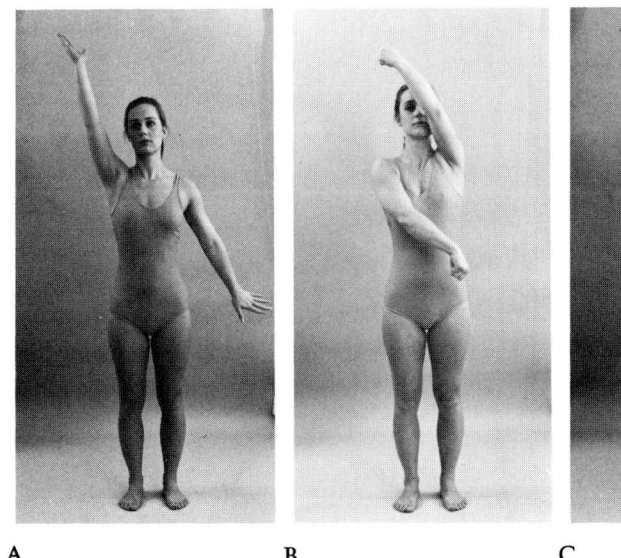

A   B   C

DIAGONAL

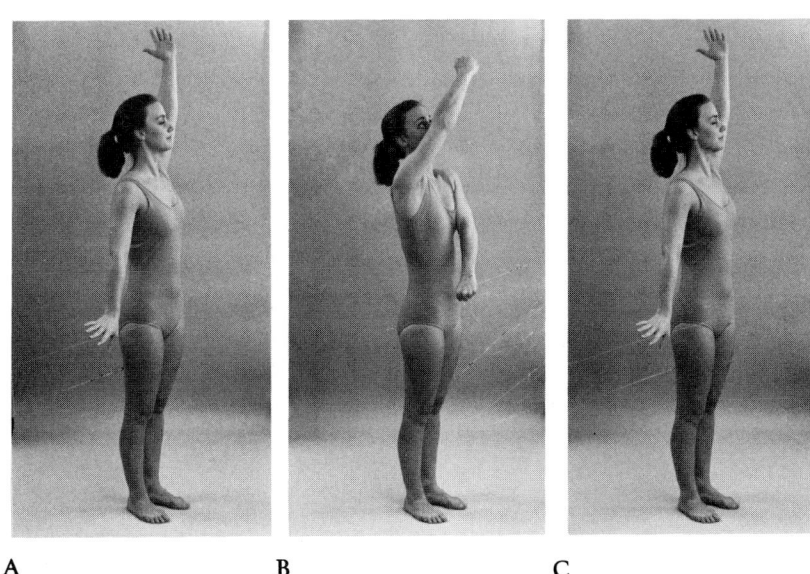

A   B   C

FIG. 1-15.

D1, L; D2, R; elbows straight (face forward positions)
D1, R; D2, L; elbows straight (diagonal positions)

Commands (left to right)

A. "Ready!"
B. "Close your hands and pull across!"
C. "Now reverse! Open your hands and spread apart!
And repeat! And again!" (Speak the commands as
you perform.)

FACE FORWARD

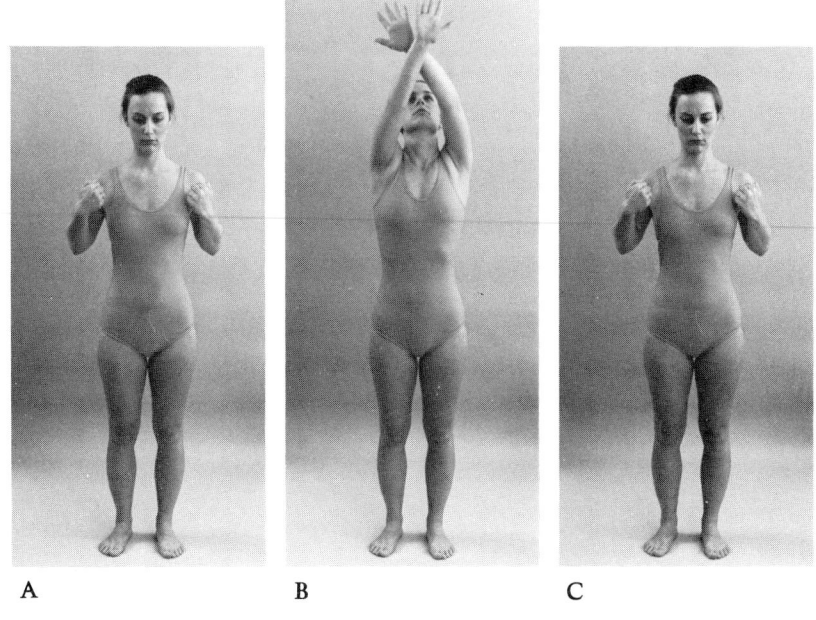

A   B   C

DIAGONAL

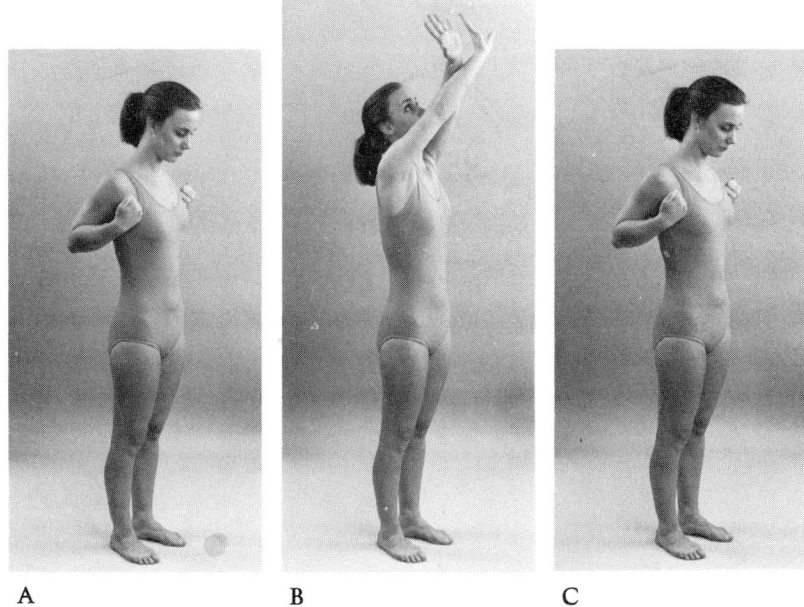

A   B   C

FIG. 1-16. D1 fl, ulnar extensor thrust.

Commands (left to right)

A. "Ready!"
B. "Open your hands! Push up and across! And hold!"
C. "Now reverse! Close your hands toward the thumb side and pull to your side. Bend your elbows! And repeat! And thrust again!" (Speak the commands as you perform.)

Upper Extremities, Bilateral Symmetrical (BS) Thrusting Patterns

FACE FORWARD

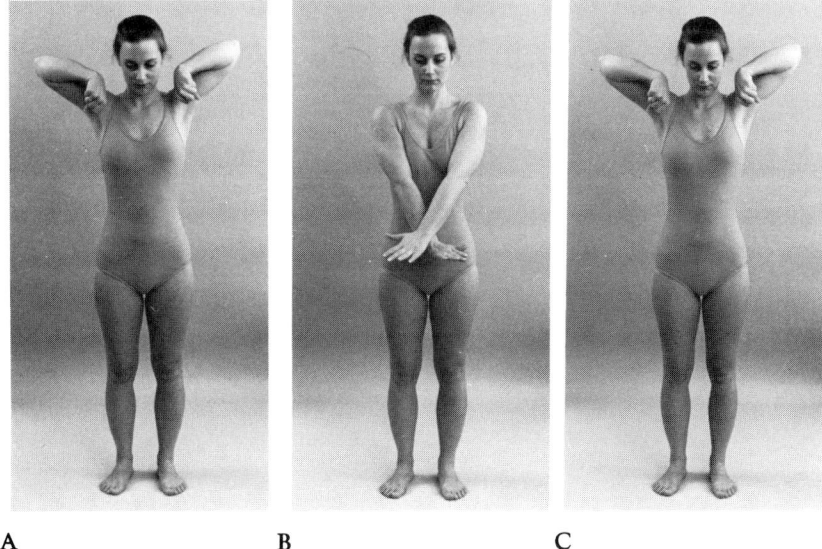

A   B   C

DIAGONAL

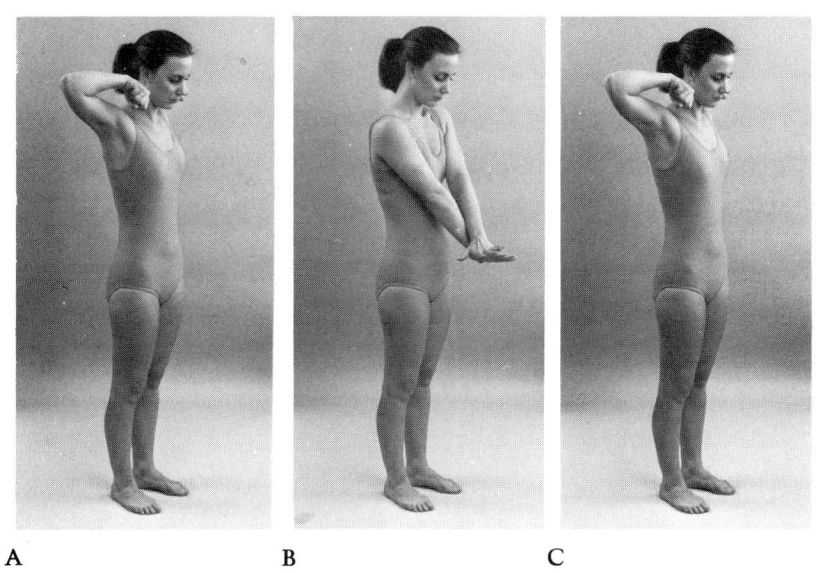

A   B   C

FIG. 1-17. D2 ex, radial extensor thrust.

Commands (left to right)

A. "Ready!"
B. "Open your hands! Push down and across! And hold!"
C. "Now reverse! Close your hands to the little finger side! Bend your elbows! And repeat! And thrust again!" (Speak the commands as you perform.)

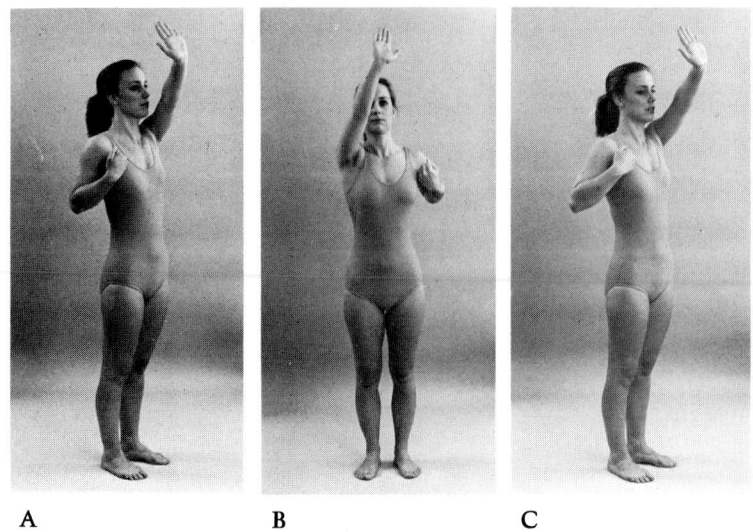

A   B   C

FIG. 1-18. D1 fl, ulnar extensor thrust; D1 ex, reversal thrust

Commands (left to right)

A. "Ready!"
B. "Shove up with the right! And pull down with the left!"
C. "Change! Push the left and pull the right! And repeat! And again!" (Speak the commands as you perform.)

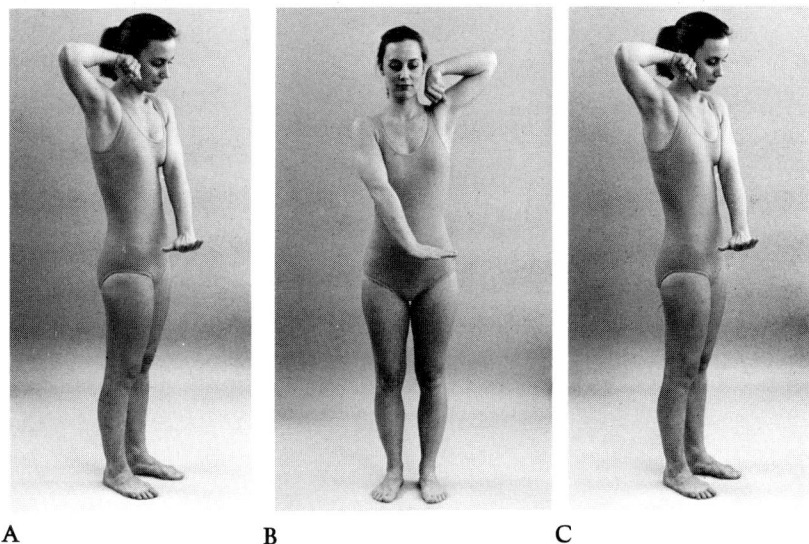

A   B   C

FIG. 1-19. D2, radial extensor thrust.

Commands (left to right)

A. "Ready!"

B. "Open your right hand and thrust as you close your left, and reverse!"

C. "Now! Close your left hand to the little finger side, and open your right to the thumb side! Pull with the left as you push with the right! And repeat! And again!" (Speak the commands as you perform.)

FACE FORWARD

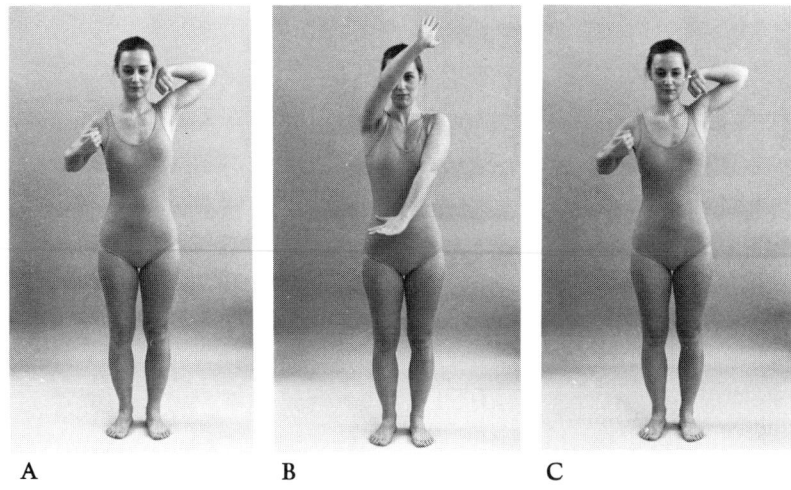

A   B   C

DIAGONAL

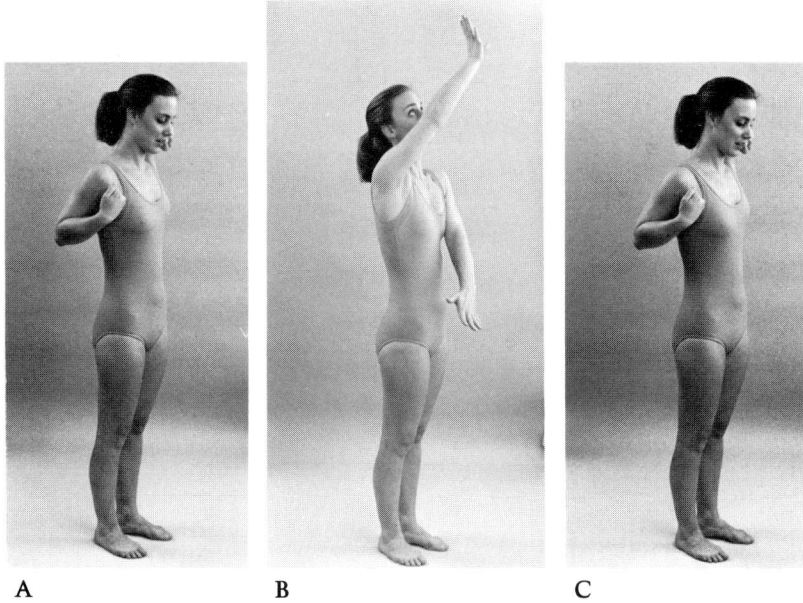

A   B   C

FIG. 1-20. D1, R; D2, L.

Commands (left to right)

A. "Ready!"
B. "Open your hands! Push up and across with the right! And down and across with the left! And hold!" (*Note:* As subject looks at right hand, wrist extension becomes complete on the right, but not on the left.)
C. "Now reverse! Close your right toward the thumb side, and close your left toward the little finger side. Bend your elbows! Right, down and out! Left, up and out! And repeat! And thrust again!" (Speak the commands as you perform.)

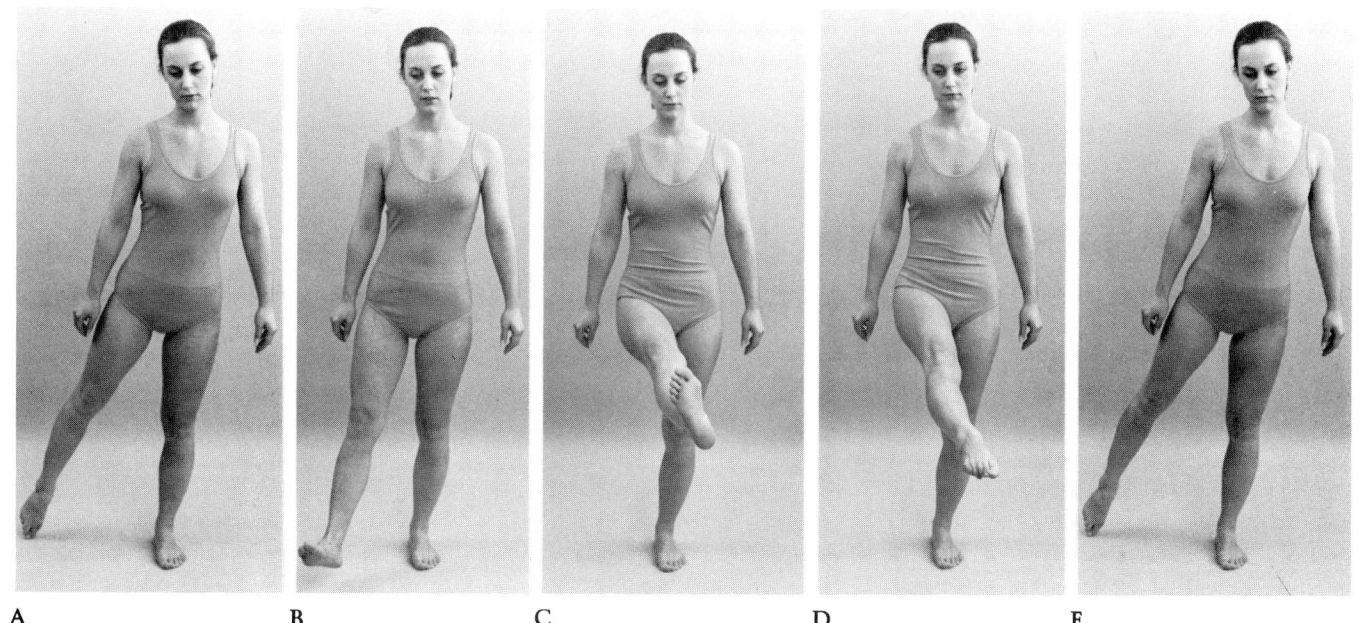

A   B   C   D   E

FIG. 1-21.   D1 fl and D1 ex, knee straight.

Commands (left to right)

A. "Ready!"
B. "Pull your toes up and in! Turn your heel!"
C. "Now pull up and across!"
D. "Point your toes down and away! Turn your heel!"
E. "And push your foot down and away! And repeat!
   And again!" (Speak the commands as you perform.)

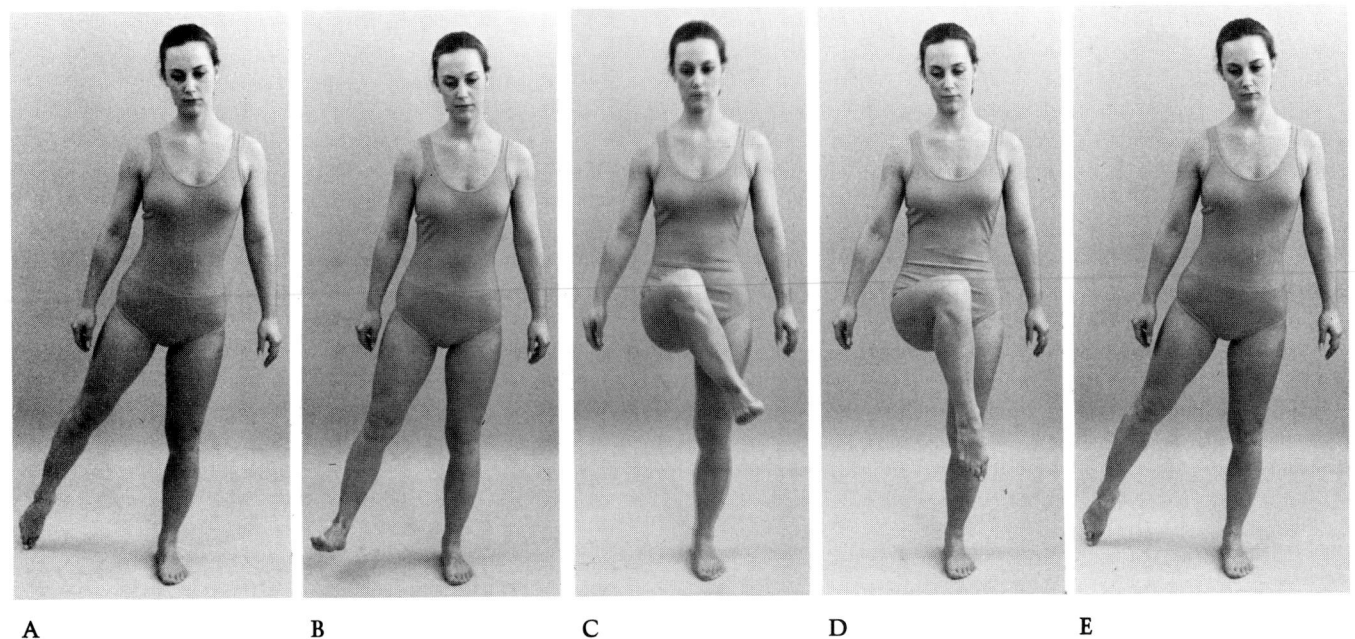

A   B   C   D   E

FIG. 1-22. D1 fl, knee fl; D1 ex, knee ex.

Commands (left to right)

A. "Ready! Point your toes down and out!"
B. "Pull your toes and foot up and in!"
C. "Now pull up and across, as you bend your knee!"
D. "Point your toes down and out! And push down and out at the hip and knee!"
E. "All the way! Knee straight! And repeat! And again." (Speak the commands as you perform.)

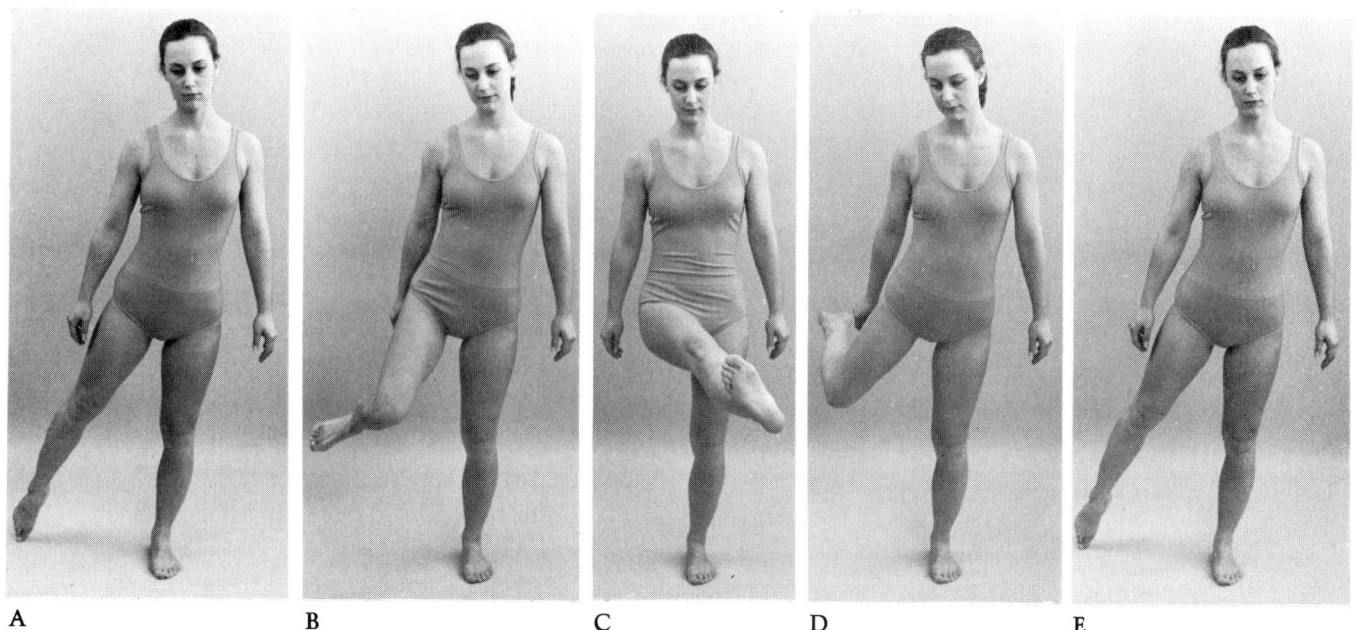

A   B   C   D   E

FIG. 1-23.   D1 fl, knee ex; D1 ex, knee fl.

Commands (left to right)

A. "Ready!"
B. "Bend your knee as you pull your foot up!"
C. "Straighten your knee as you kick up and across!"
D. "Point your toes down and away and bend your knee!"
E. "Now lower your foot and straighten your knee. And repeat! And again!" (Speak the commands as you perform.)

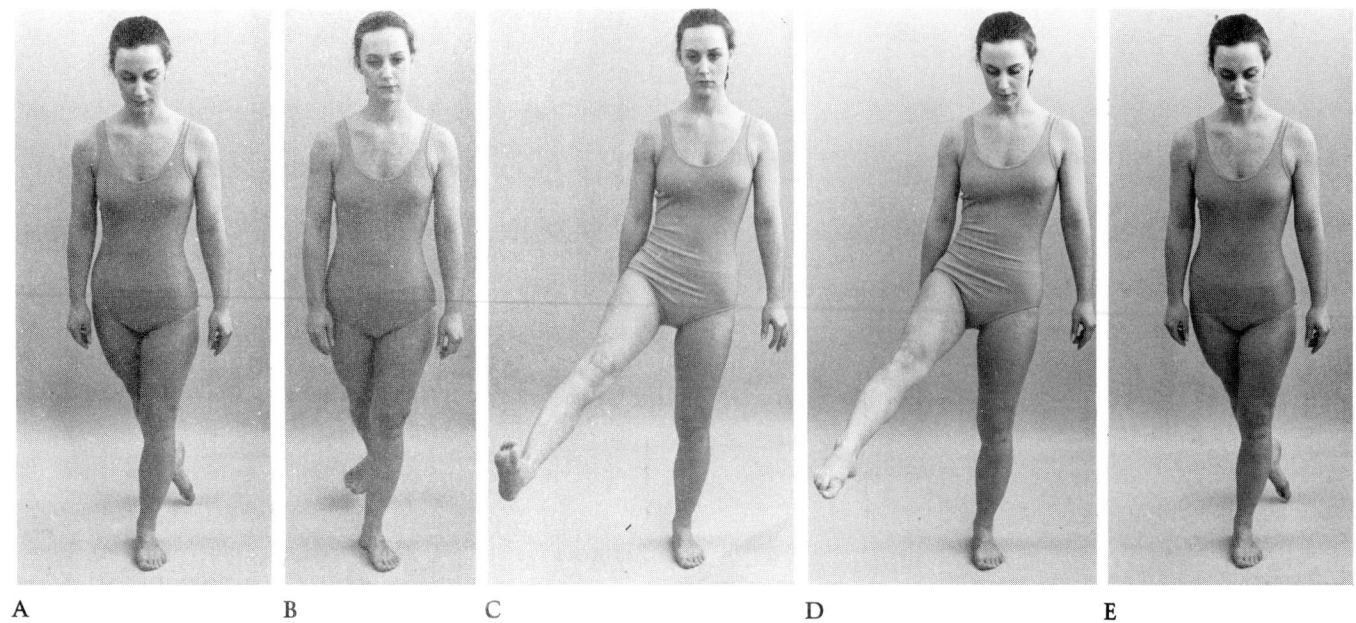

A   B   C   D   E

FIG. 1-24.   D2 fl and D2 ex, knee straight.

Commands (left to right)

A. "Ready!"
B. "Pull your toes up and out! Turn your heel!"
C. "Now kick up and out!"
D. "Point your toes down and in! Turn your heel!"
E. "And reach your foot back and across! And repeat!
   And again!" (Speak the commands as you perform.)

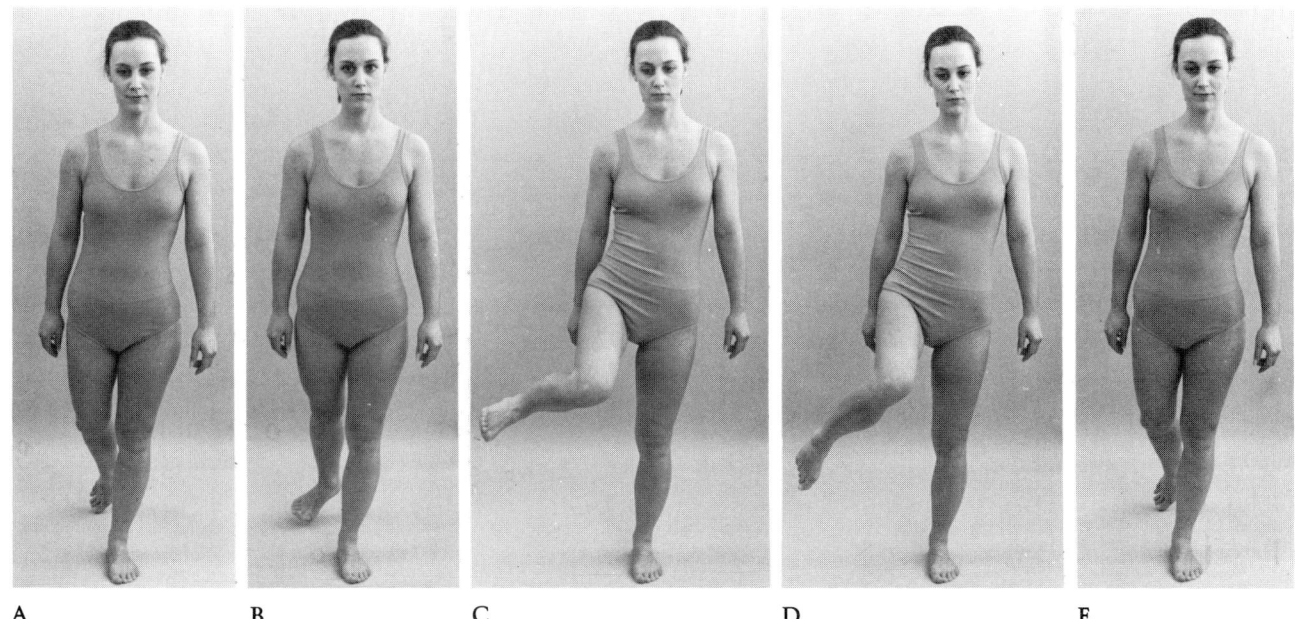

A   B   C   D   E

FIG. 1-25.   D2 fl, knee fl; D2 ex, knee ex.

Commands (left to right)

A. "Ready!"
B. "Pull your toes and foot up and out!"
C. "Now pull up and out, as you bend your knee!"
D. "Point your toes down and in!"
E. "And reach your foot back and across as you straighten your knee! And repeat! And again!" (Speak the commands as you perform.)

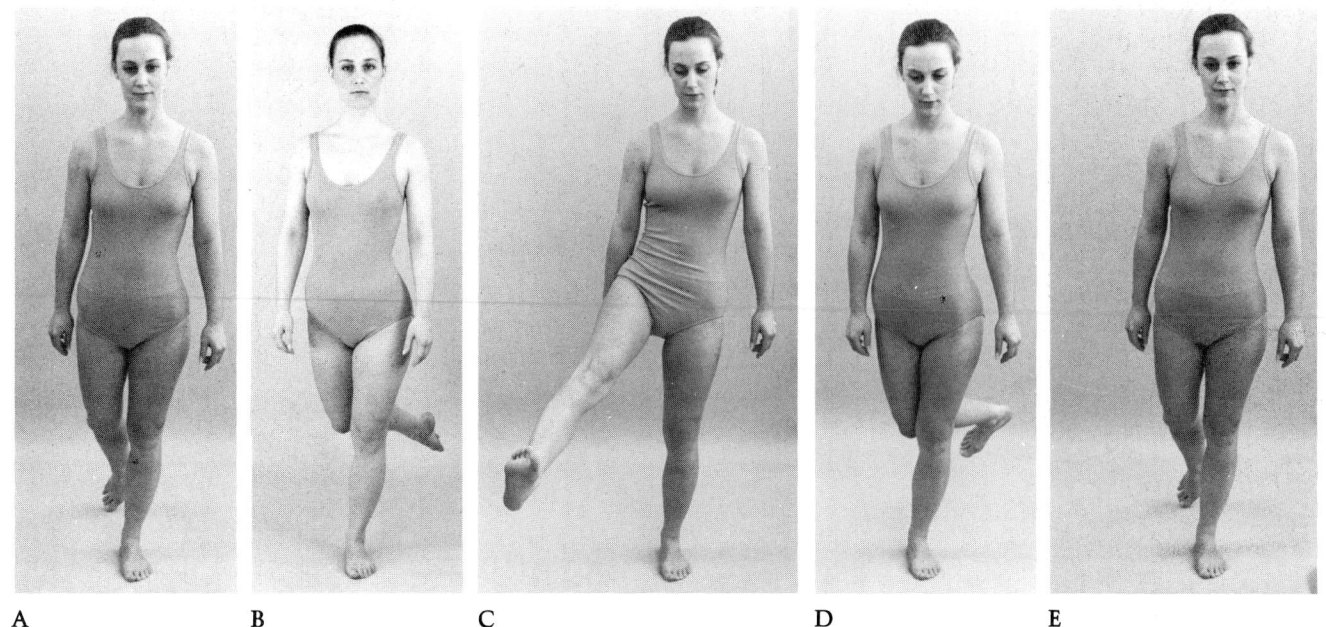

A B C D E

FIG. 1-26. D2 ex, knee fl; D2 fl, knee ex.

Commands (left to right)

A. "Ready!"
B. "Point your toes down and in, and bend your knee!"
C. "Now pull your foot up and out, and kick forward! Knee straight!"
D. "Point your toes down and in as you reach back at the hip." (In *D*, plantar flexion is delayed.)
E. "And reach your foot back and across as you straighten your knee! And repeat! And again." (Speak the commands as you perform.)

Lower Extremities, Bilateral Symmetrical (BS) Patterns

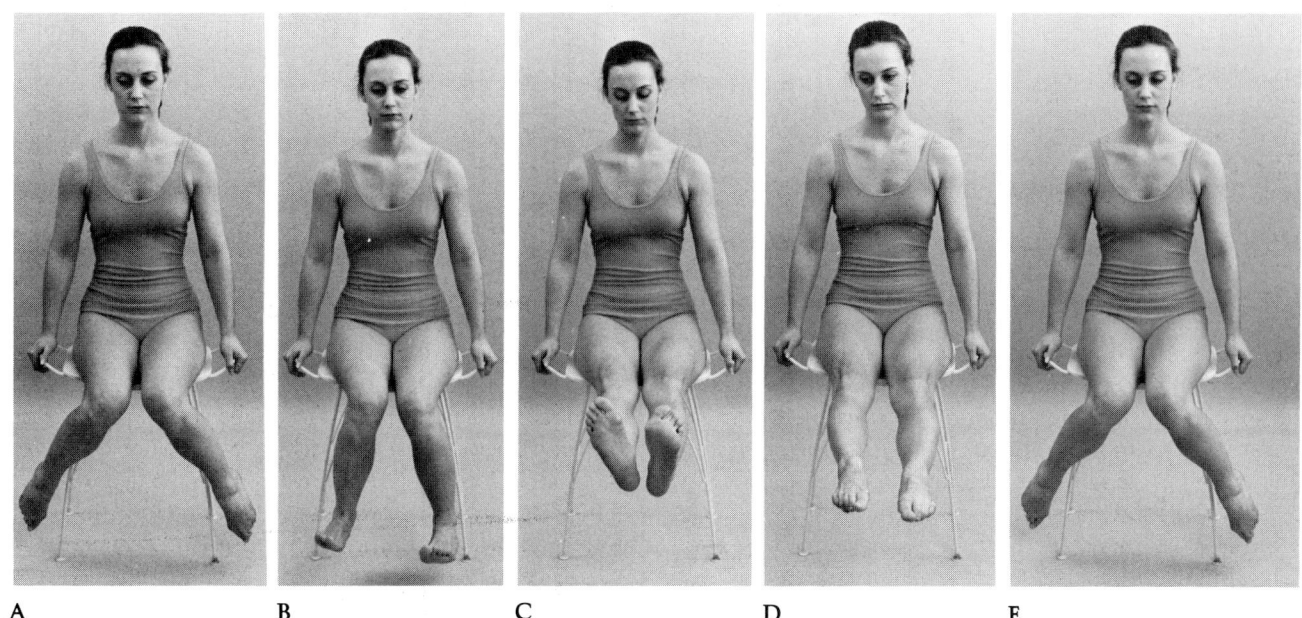

A   B   C   D   E

FIG. 1-27.   D1 fl, knee ex; D1 ex, knee fl.

Commands (left to right)

A. "Ready!"
B. "Pull your toes up and in! Turn your heels!"
C. "Now kick up and together! Knees straight!"
D. "Turn your heels! Point your toes down and away!"
E. "And push your feet down and away! Bend your knees. And repeat! And again!" (Speak the commands as you perform.)

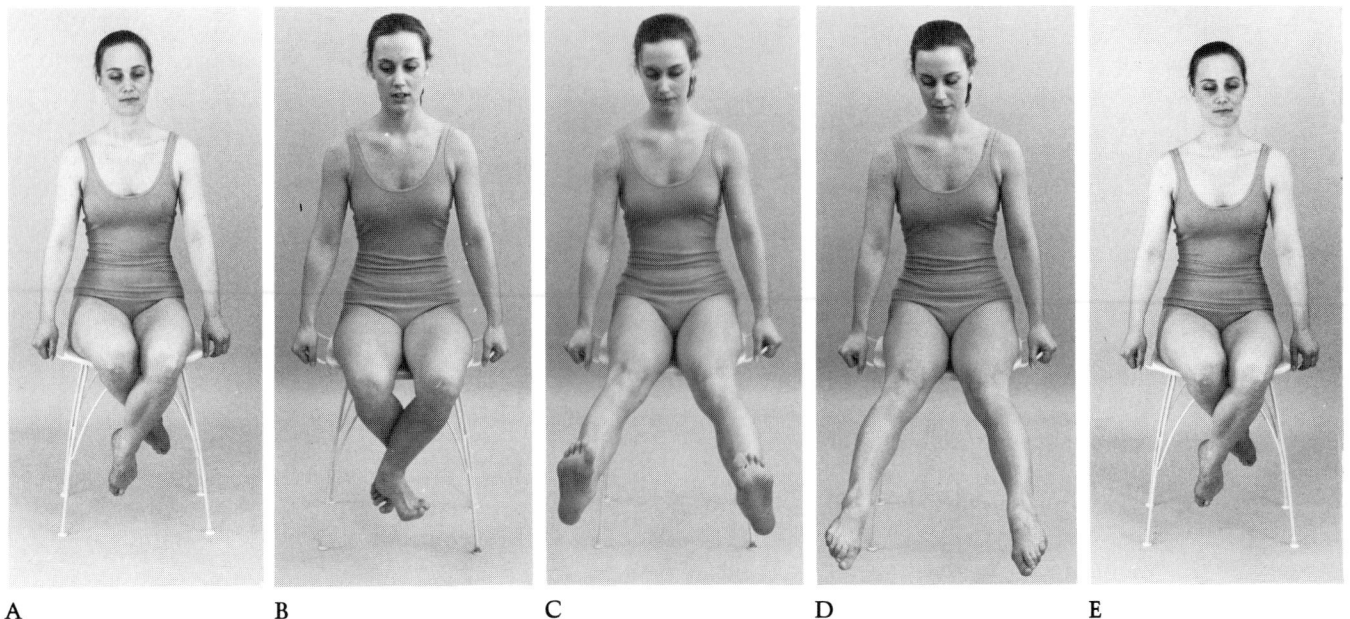

A   B   C   D   E

FIG. 1-28. D2 fl, knee ex; D2 ex, knee fl.

Commands (left to right)

A. "Ready!"
B. "Pull your toes up and out! Turn your heels!"
C. "Now kick up and out!"
D. "Point your toes down and in! Turn your heels!"
E. "And push your feet down and across! Bend your knees! And repeat! And again!" (Speak the commands as you perform.)

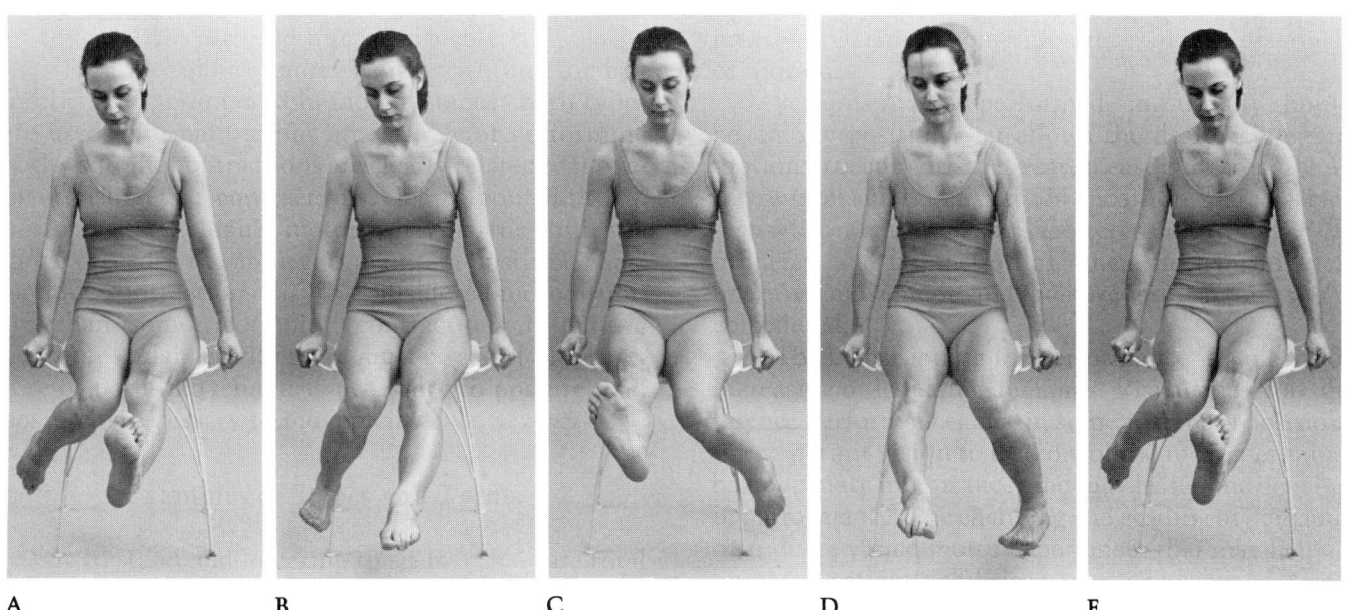

A   B   C   D   E

FIG. 1-29. D1 fl with knee ex; D1 ex with knee fl.

Commands (left to right)

A. "Ready!"
B. "Push your left foot down and away, and pull your right foot up and in!"
C. "Bend your left knee and push down and away! And kick up and in with your right!"
D. "And reverse! Down and out with the right foot! And up and in with the left!"
E. "Bend your right knee! Straighten your left! And repeat! And again!" (Speak the commands as you perform.)

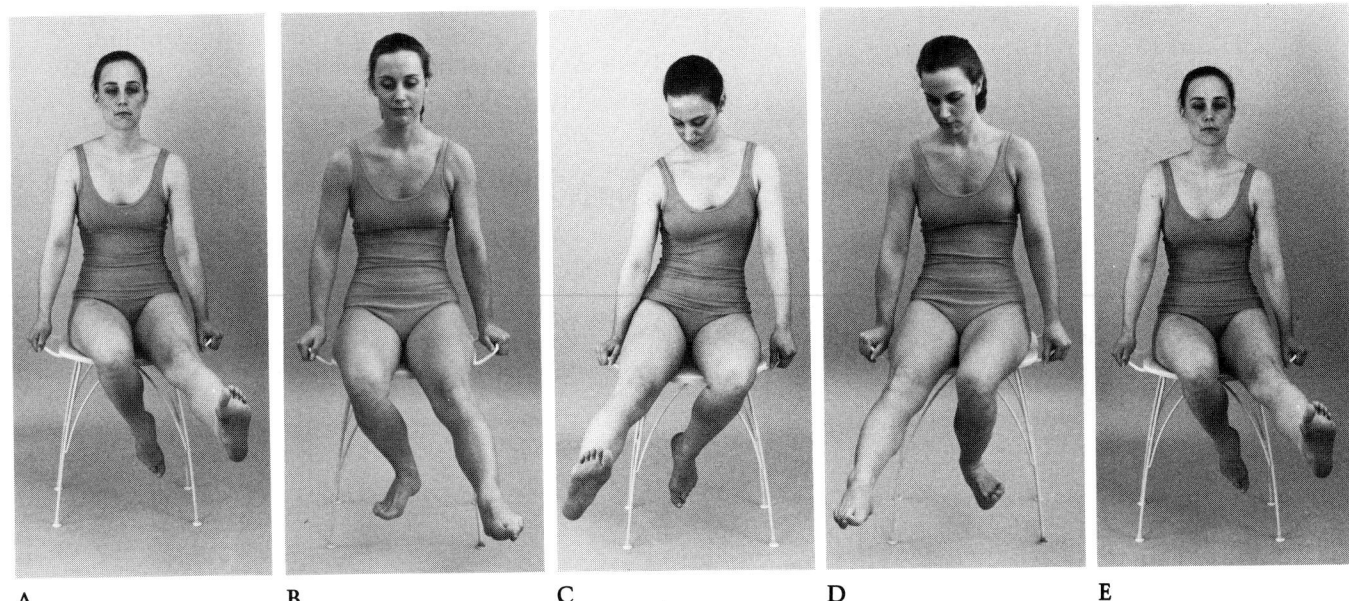

A   B   C   D   E

FIG. 1-30.   D2 fl with knee ex; D2 ex with knee fl.

Commands (left to right)

A. "Ready!"
B. "Push your left foot down and across, and pull your right foot up and out!"
C. "Bend your left knee and push down and across! And kick up and out with your right!"
D. "And reverse! Push your right foot down and across, and pull your left foot up and out!"
E. "Bend your right knee and push down and across! Kick up and out with your left! And repeat! And again!" (Speak the commands as you perform.)

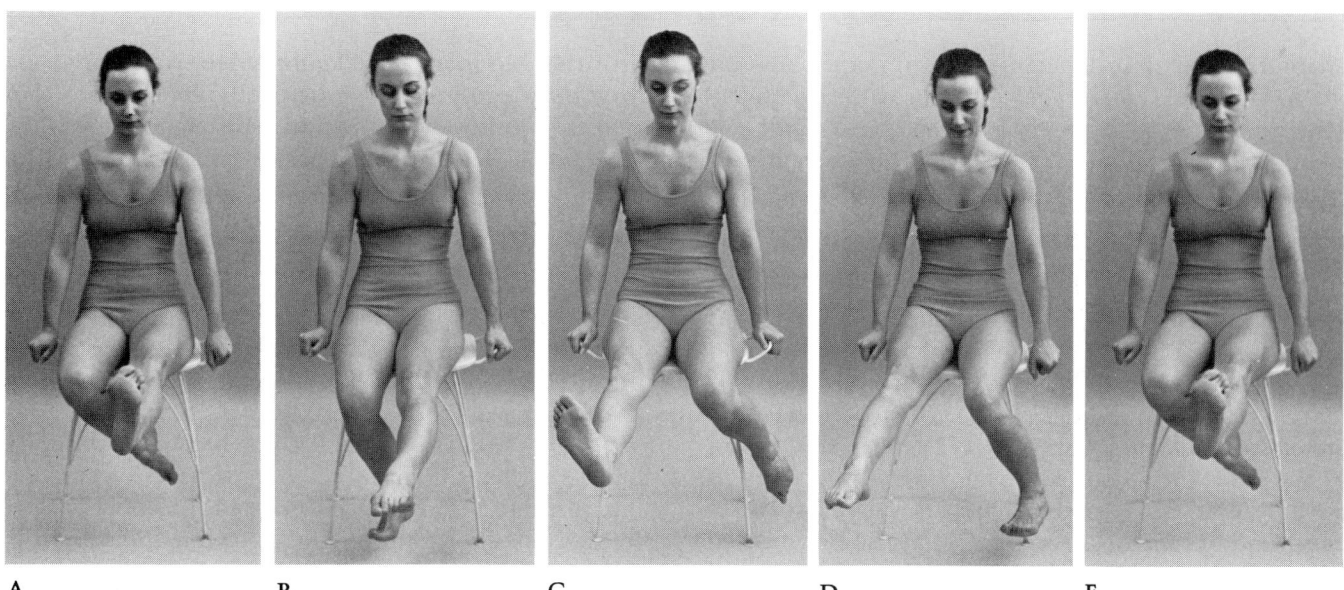

A B C D E

FIG. 1-31.   D1, L; D2, R; knees fl and ex.

Commands (left to right)

A. "Ready!"
B. "Push your left foot down and away, and pull your right foot up and out!"
C. "Bend your left knee and push down and away! And kick up and out with your right!"
D. "And reverse! Down and in with the right foot, up and in with the left!"
E. "And bend your right knee, and straighten the left! And repeat! And again!" (Speak the commands as you perform.)

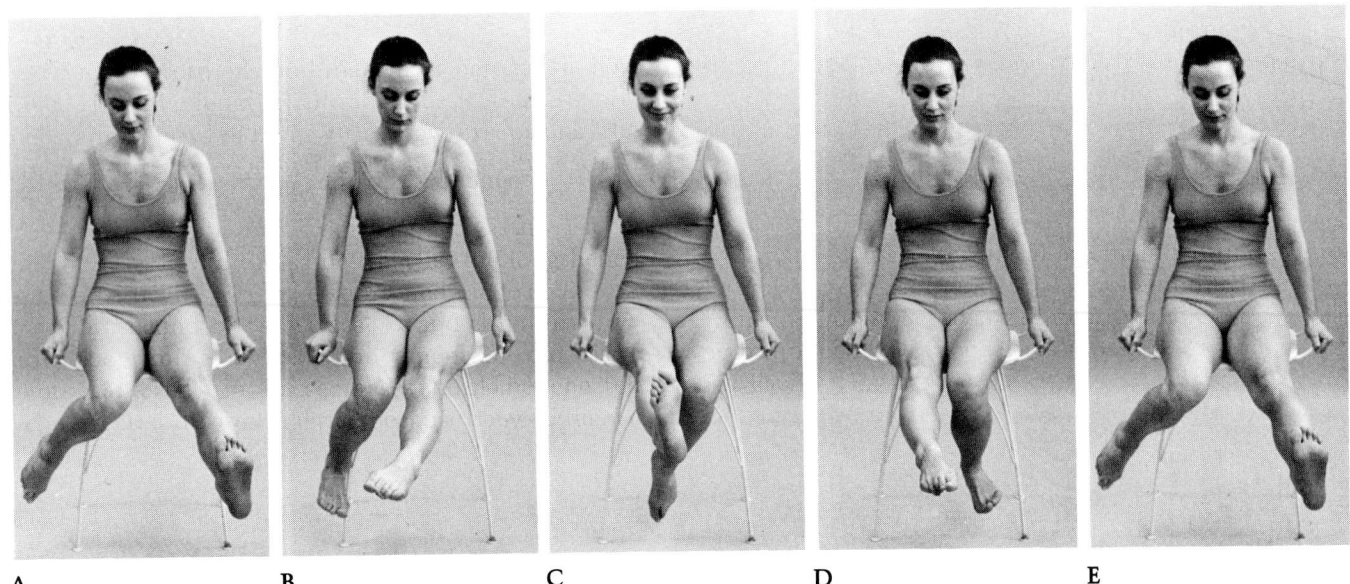

A   B   C   D   E

FIG. 1-32.   D2, L; D1 R; knees fl and ex.

Commands (left to right)

A. "Ready! Left foot up and out, right foot down and out."
B. "Left foot down and in, right foot up and in!"
C. "Bend your left knee, foot down and in, as you kick your right foot up and in!"
D. "And reverse! Up and out with the left foot, and down and out with the right!"
E. "Straighten your left knee! Bend the right! And repeat! And again!" (Speak the commands as you perform.)

UNILATERAL PATTERNS

Illustrations (Figs. 1-33 to 1-81)

Each drawing portrays the full range of motion of a specific pattern. The initial position of the physical therapist, showing the lengthened range of the pattern, is in black. The middle range of the pattern is depicted by the dark gray figure and the shortened range of the pattern is shown by the light gray figure. The three positions show the motion characteristics of the pattern and the motion characteristics of the physical therapist. The physical therapist moves his body in order to allow the desired range of motion to occur.

The manual contacts portrayed in each illustration are optimum for the specific pattern. Certain variations are included, for example, the use of both hands distally, shifting to one hand proximally and one hand distally. The proximal hand may be shifted as needed during the patient's performance. Adaptations of manual contacts must be made when combinations of patterns are used during reinforcement. See Bilateral Combinations for Reinforcement.

The normal timing of the pattern is portrayed. The distal pivots of action have completed their range of motion by the time the middle range of the pattern is reached. Timing for emphasis, as a technique, will alter the range of motion of the proximal pivot when distal pivots are emphasized. The combination of motions and direction of the pattern remain unchanged. This variation in range is shown in Figures 1-76 and 1-81.

The spiral characteristic of the pattern is shown by the dotted lines placed medially or laterally on the extremities. The dotted lines on the trunk are intended to show the diagonal directions of the pattern with motion of the distal parts crossing the midline of the body.

The subject is portrayed in the supine position. Patterns may be performed in any position that permits the desired range of motion to occur.

Normal reinforcements by related patterns are not included in the unilateral pattern illustrations that follow; see Bilateral Combinations for Reinforcement, and Reference Tables 1 through 7.

All information concerning a specific pattern is given for left or right extremities, or the trunk and neck motions to the left or right. For the specific pattern of the opposite side, left and right must be interchanged.

Components of Motion

Description is from distal to proximal in accordance with normal timing.

Description, for the purpose of simplification, is limited to parts and major joints, rather than naming each individual joint that participates in the pattern of motion. Minor components of joint motion, such as gliding motions of metacarpal and carpal joints, contribute to the rotation and medial or lateral components of motion.

Normal Timing

Action occurs from distal to proximal. Normal timing may be used with maximal resistance or may be performed as free active motion without contact with the subject by the physical therapist. See discussion of techniques of facilitation.

Timing for Emphasis

Description is from proximal to distal in accordance with the normal process of development. Timing for emphasis alters range of motion of the proximal pivots when distal pivots are emphasized. This is illustrated in Figures 1-76 and 1-81. See the discussion of techniques of facilitation (Chap. 2, Basic Procedures). See also Emphasis on Scapular Motions (Figs. 1-56 to 1-59), Elbow Extensor Thrust and Reversal (Figs. 1-60 to 1-63), Mass Closing and Opening of the Hand (Figs. 1-76 to 1-80), and Foot and Ankle Patterns (Figs. 1-64, 1-67, 1-70, 1-73, and 1-81).

Commands

Preparatory commands must be varied in accordance with the age level and abilities of the subject to cooperate. They may become superfluous after the subject has learned the desired patterns.

Action commands may be repeated as necessary in order to stimulate the patient to further effort. Sequence of commands used in applying other techniques must be learned in conjunction with those techniques.

Although commands are described in terms of words and voice, other sensory cues are equally important, and in many instances are more effective. Luring the child or urging the patient to look in the direction of the movement may be more meaningful than a dozen words of explanation or instruction. Quickly touching a part of the body will provide another clue to the patient. For example, a brisk tap on the upper left region of the chest will guide a patient as he performs neck flexion with rotation to the left. One externally applied stimulus may not be enough to facilitate response; two or three types of stimulus may produce far more response.

Pattern Analysis

The motion components and major muscle components are presented from proximal to distal in keeping with anatomical description.

The origins, insertions, and innervation of muscles are not included since this information is readily available to all. Optimal patterns according to peripheral innervation are presented in Reference Tables 12 and 13 in the back of the book.

The distal components of motion and major muscle components are listed only once for each pattern. They are presented with the patterns that require no motion of the intermediate joint or pivot.

Range-limiting factors are expressed in terms of the major muscle components of the antagonistic pattern. When the two-joint action of major muscles is not considered, soft tissue contact may become the range-limiting factor. Limitation by ligaments and joint structures is minimal unless hypermobility is present. Those ligaments that underlie the tendinous attachments of the major muscle components of the antagonistic pattern are potential range-limiting factors.

Flexion with Rotation to the Right (D fl, R)

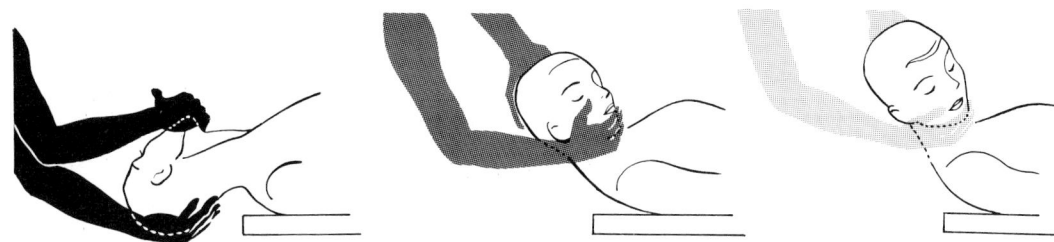

FIG. 1-33

Antagonistic Pattern

Extension with rotation to left (Fig. 1-34).

Components of Motion

Head rotates toward right (axis on atlas), mandible depresses toward right, atlanto-occipital joint flexes toward right, and cervical spine flexes with rotation toward right so that chin approximates right clavicle.

Normal Timing

Action occurs from distal to proximal, that is, head rotates toward right (atlas on axis), mandible depresses as atlanto-occipital joint flexes toward right, and cervical spine, which has been convex to right, flexes with rotation to right, and becomes convex to left.

Timing for Emphasis

Head Rotation Toward Right. Allow beginning flexion to occur at atlanto-occipital joint with depression of mandible, and allow beginning flexion of cervical spine to occur, but do not allow full range of cervical flexion with rotation toward right to occur, until head begins to rotate toward right.

NOTE: Resist stronger components of neck flexion.

Depression of Mandible and Flexion of Atlanto-Occipital Joint. Allow beginning rotation of head and beginning flexion with rotation of cervical spine toward right to occur, but do not allow full range of head rotation and cervical flexion with rotation to occur, until mandible depresses with flexion occurring at atlanto-occipital joint.

NOTE: Resist stronger components of neck flexion, but guide weaker components through their optimal range of motion in accordance with normal timing.

Cervical Flexion with Rotation Toward Right. Allow beginning head rotation and depression of mandible with flexion of atlanto-occipital joint to occur, but do not allow full range of head rotation and mandibular depression with atlanto-occipital flexion to occur, until cervical spine begins to flex with rotation toward right.

NOTE: Resist stronger components of neck flexion, but guide weaker components through their optimal range of motion in accordance with normal timing.

Manual Contacts

Right Hand. Pressure of medial palmar surface of hand and fingers under inferior surface of mandible on right between symphysis and right angle (Fig. 1-33).

Left Hand. Palmar surface of hand and fingers on left posterior–lateral aspect of skull to control rotation (Fig. 1-33).

Commands

Preparatory. "You are going to turn your head to the right, and pull it down and over toward the right, so that your chin touches your chest."

Action. "Turn your head! Pull your chin down! Pull your head down!"

Pattern Analysis

Head Rotation. Major muscle components: Right sternocleidomastoid, left rectus capitis lateralis, right rectus capitis anterior, right longus capitis (rotation component).

Depression of Mandible. Major muscle components: Right suprahyoid and infrahyoid, platysma.

Atlanto-Occipital Joint Flexion. Major muscle components: Right longus capitis (flexion component), right sternocleidomastoid.

Cervical Flexion with Rotation. Major muscle components: Right sternocleidomastoid, longus capitis (flexion component), longus colli, scaleni (posterior, medius, anterior).

NOTE: The sternocleidomastoids are the most versatile of all neck muscles, and both muscles enter in when flexion is performed to right or left. When flexion is performed to right, right sternocleidomastoid contracts first, and as head approaches midline of body, left sternocleidomastoid contracts. Pattern of flexion to right must be first initiated by intrinsic muscles of pattern; if only sternocleidomastoids and supra- and infrahyoid muscles contract, motion is superficial, and shortened range of pattern will lack stability. Those supra- and infrahyoid muscles on left, the fibers of which are stretched by demanding neck flexion to right, will contribute to motion. Most closely related extremity pattern is extension–adduction–internal rotation of left upper extremity.

Range-Limiting Factors

Tension or contracture of any of muscles of extension with rotation to left pattern (Fig. 1-34).

Head and Neck

Extension with Rotation to the Left (D ex, L)

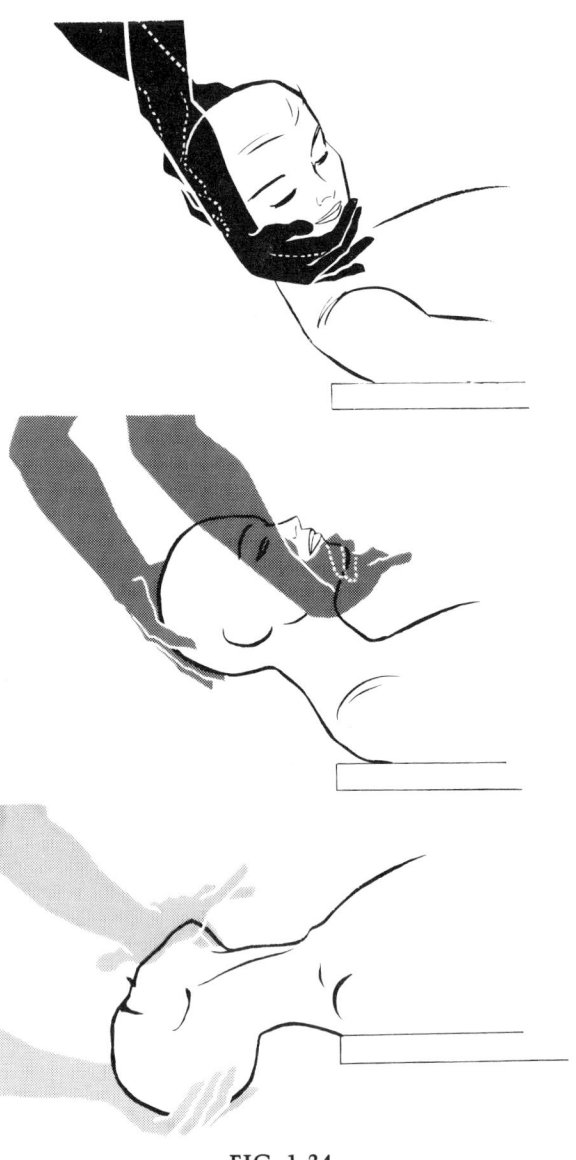

FIG. 1-34

Antagonistic Pattern

Flexion with rotation to right (Fig. 1-33).

Components of Motion

Head rotates toward left, atlanto-occipital joint extends toward left, mandible elevates toward left, and cervical spine extends with rotation toward left, so that chin moves up and away from right clavicle.

Normal Timing

Action occurs from distal to proximal, that is, head rotates toward left, mandible elevates as atlanto-occipital joint extends, and cervical spine, which has been convex to left, extends with rotation to left, and becomes convex to right.

Timing for emphasis

Head Rotation Toward Left. Allow beginning extension to occur at atlanto-occipital joint with elevation of mandible, but do not allow full range of cervical extension with rotation toward left to occur, until head begins to rotate toward left.

NOTE: Resist stronger components of neck extension.

Elevation of Mandible and Extension of Atlanto-Occipital Joint. Allow beginning rotation of head and beginning extension with rotation of cervical spine to occur toward left, but do not allow full range of head rotation and cervical extension with rotation to occur, until mandible elevates with extension occurring at atlanto-occipital joint.

NOTE: Resist stronger components of neck extension, but guide weaker components through their optimal range of motion in accordance with normal timing.

Cervical Extension with Rotation Toward Left. Allow beginning head rotation and elevation of mandible with extension of atlanto-occipital joint to occur, but do not allow full range of head rotation and mandibular elevation with atlanto-occipital extension to occur, until cervical spine begins to extend with rotation toward left.

NOTE: Resist stronger distal components of pattern but guide weaker components through their optimal range of motion in accordance with normal timing.

Manual Contacts

Right Hand. Pressure of lateral palmar surface of hand and fingers on superior surface of mandible on left between symphysis and left angle (Fig. 1-34).

Left Hand. Pressure of palmar surface of hand and fingers on left posterior–lateral surface of the occiput and cervical region (Fig. 1-34).

Commands

Preparatory. "You are going to turn your head to the left, and lift your chin up and away from your chest."

Action. "Turn your head. Lift your chin up! Push your head back!"

Pattern Analysis

Head Rotation. Major muscle components: Left obliquus capitis superior, obliquus capitis inferior (rotation component), splenius capitis, longissimus capitis, semispinalis capitis, trapezius (upper portion).

Elevation of Mandible and Atlanto-Occipital Joint Extension. Major muscle components: Left obliquus capitis inferior (extension component), rectus capitis posterior major, rectus capitis posterior minor, semispinalis capitis, longissimus capitis, splenius capitis.

Cervical Extension with Rotation. Major muscle components: Left semispinalis capitis, longissimus capitis, longissimus cervicis, iliocostalis cervicis, splenius capitis, splenius cervicis, interspinales, intertransversarii, trapezius (upper portion). Right semispinalis cervicis, multifidus.

NOTE: Since rotation of vertebral column becomes more evident when motion of entire column is considered, rotation characteristic of components of muscle action becomes apparent when pattern is performed through full range. Major cervical muscles contribute component of rotation as well as component of flexion or extension. Also, because of overlapping of origins and insertions, there is overlapping of components in contributing muscle groups. More laterally located extensor muscles have stronger component of rotation, but intrinsic rotation is responsibility of specific rotator muscles such as obliquus capitis inferior and multifidus. Overlapping of action between muscles of left and muscles of right is apparent in flexion and extension patterns and is also characteristic of upper trunk patterns. The most closely related extremity pattern is flexion–abduction–external rotation of left upper extremity.

Range-Limiting Factors

Tension or contracture of any of muscles of flexion with rotation to right pattern (Fig. 1-33).

Head and Neck

Rotation to the Right (Ro, R)

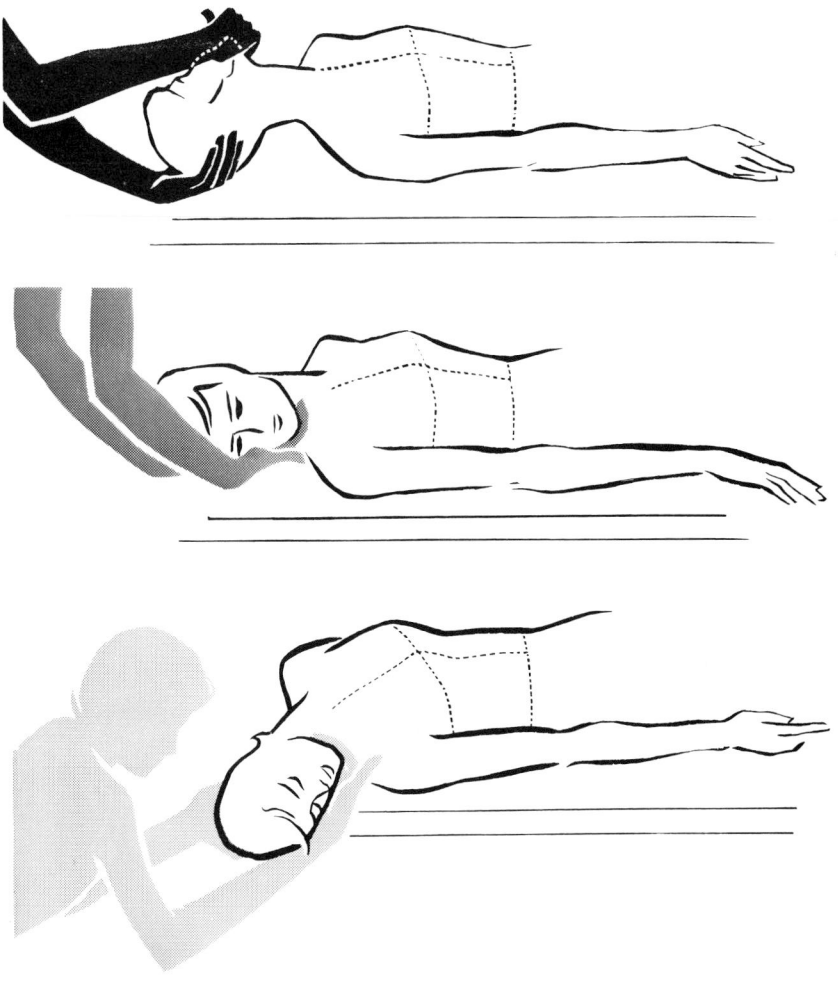

FIG. 1-35

Antagonistic Pattern

Rotation to left (motion components, major muscle components, and manual contacts are exactly opposite).

Components of Motion

Head rotates toward right, mandible depresses and rotates from left to right, atlanto-occipital joint flexes toward right, and cervical spine rotates through flexion and into extension toward right. Cervical spine, which has been convex to right, rotates and becomes convex to left.

Normal Timing

Action occurs from distal to proximal, that is, head rotates toward right as atlanto-occipital joint flexes, and right mandible depresses and approaches right shoulder as cervical spine rotates and becomes convex to left.

Timing for Emphasis

Head Rotation Toward Right. Allow beginning flexion of atlanto-occipital joint and mandibular depression with rotation of cervical spine, but do not allow full range of mandibular depression and cervical rotation to occur, until head begins to rotate.

NOTE: Resist stronger components of neck rotation.

Depression of Mandible and Flexion of Atlanto-Occipital Joint. Allow beginning head rotation and cervical spine rotation through flexion to occur, but do not allow full range of head rotation and cervical spine rotation to occur, until mandible begins to depress with flexion of atlanto-occipital joint.

NOTE: Resist stronger components of neck rotation, but guide weaker components through their optimal range of motion in accordance with normal timing.

Cervical Spine Rotation (Through Flexion into Extension). Allow beginning head rotation and mandibular depression with atlanto-occipital flexion to occur toward the right, but do not allow full range of head rotation and mandibular depression with atlanto-occipital flexion to occur, until cervical spine begins to rotate through flexion and toward extension to right.

NOTE: Resist stronger components of head and neck rotation, but guide weaker components through their optimal range of motion in accordance with normal timing.

Manual Contacts

Right Hand. Pressure of medial palmar surface of hand and fingers under inferior border of mandible on right; tips of fingers near symphysis, to control flexion and rotation components (Fig. 1-35).

Left Hand. Pressure of lateral palmar surface of hand and fingers on right posterior – lateral surface of skull, between mastoid process and occiput, and extending downward to lateral cervical extensors (Fig. 1-35).

Commands

Preparatory. "You are going to turn your head, so that your chin is touching your right shoulder, as if you were going to look down and behind your shoulder."

Action. "Turn it! Get your chin on your shoulder! Push your head back!"

Pattern Analysis

Head Rotation. Major muscle components: Right rectus capitis anterior, left rectus capitis lateralis, right sternocleidomastoid.

Depression of Mandible and Flexion of Atlanto-Occipital Joint. Major muscle components: More lateral right supra- and infrahyoid muscles and right sternocleidomastoid.

Cervical Spine Rotation (Through Flexion into Extension). Major muscle components: Right scaleni medius and posterior, longissimus capitis, longissimus cervicis, iliocostalis cervicis, splenius capitis, splenius cervicis, and semispinalis capitis.

NOTE: Both sternocleidomastoids act in rotation of neck to left or to right. When neck is rotated from left to right, right sternocleidomastoid acts first, and as head passes midline of body, left sternocleidomastoid contracts and maintains head in shortened range of rotation to right. Rotation cannot be separated from major components of flexion or extension of vertebral column. In rotation pattern, first components are related to flexion with rotation in initiation of pattern, shortened range of pattern requires components of extension with rotation. More lateral muscles contribute most strongly to rotation. Rotation pattern is optimum for rotation components of contributing muscles, but is not optimum for flexion or extension components. Most closely related extremity patterns are extension – abduction – internal rotation of right upper extremity and flexion – adduction – external rotation of left upper extremity.

Range-Limiting Factors

Tension or contracture of any muscles of rotation to left pattern and of flexion to left pattern and neck extension to left pattern.

Flexion with Rotation to the Right (D fl, R)

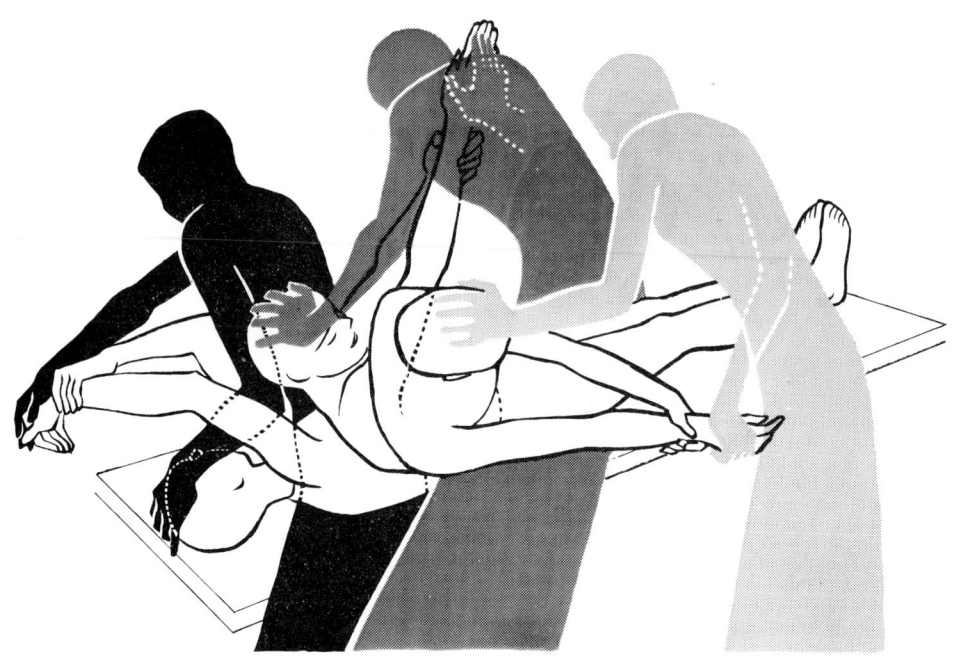

FIG. 1-36

Antagonistic Pattern

Upper trunk extension with rotation to the left (Fig. 1-37).

Components of Motion

Head rotates toward right, atlanto-occipital joint flexes with mandible depressing toward right, cervical and dorsal regions of spine, which have been convex to right, flex with rotation and become convex to left. Forehead approaches right hip.

Normal Timing

Action occurs from distal to proximal, that is, head rotation, then atlanto-occipital flexion with mandibular depression, then cervical spine flexion with rotation, and dorsal spine flexion with rotation.

Timing for Emphasis

Dorsal Spine Flexion with Rotation. Allow beginning contraction of components of neck flexion with rotation to right pattern, in accordance with normal timing, but do not allow full range of these components to occur, until abdominals contract and dorsal spine begins to flex and rotate toward right.

NOTE: Resist stronger components of neck flexion, but guide weaker components through their optimal range of motion in accordance with normal timing.

Manual Contacts

Left Hand. Pressure of palmar surface of hand and fingers on right anterior–lateral aspect of patient's forehead (Fig. 1-36).

Right Hand. Palmar surface of hand and fingers cupped over dorsal–ulnar aspect of fingers and wrist of patient's right hand (Fig. 1-36).

Commands

Preparatory. "You are going to turn your head, and pull yourself up and over toward your right hip."

Action. "Pull up and over! Turn it! Pull your chin down! Pull your head down! Pull your arms toward your right hip!"

Pattern Analysis

Motion components and major muscle components of neck flexion with rotation to the right (Fig. 1-33).

Dorsal Spine Flexion with Rotation. Major muscle components: Left external oblique, right internal oblique, rectus abdominis (right portion), left transversus thoracis, right internal intercostals, right subcostals (quadratus lumborum).

NOTE: Most closely related extremity patterns are extension–adduction–internal rotation of left upper extremity, extension–abduction–internal rotation of right upper extremity, flexion–adduction–external rotation of right lower extremity, and flexion–abduction–internal rotation of left lower extremity. Lower trunk pattern that is most closely related is lower trunk flexion with rotation to left. When this pattern is combined with upper trunk flexion with rotation to right, crossing of rotation components occurs at dorsolumbar junction of vertebral column. When upper trunk flexion with rotation to right is combined with lower trunk flexion with rotation to right, all the oblique abdominal muscles contract.

Range Limiting Factors

Tension or contracture of any muscles of upper trunk extension with rotation to left pattern (Fig. 1-37).

ILLUSTRATION NOTE: Figure 1-36 portrays reinforcement of upper trunk flexion with rotation to right by combined upper extremity patterns that are most closely related: those of extension–adduction–internal rotation of left upper extremity and extension–abduction–internal rotation of right upper extremity. Extension–adduction–internal rotation pattern contributes to flexion component of upper trunk while extension–abduction–internal rotation pattern contributes to rotation of upper trunk. These combined patterns are referred to as "chopping."

If pattern is to be performed without resistance to "chopping," manual contacts for head and neck flexion with rotation to right pattern may be used.

Upper Trunk (Superior Region)

Extension with Rotation to the Left (D ex, L)

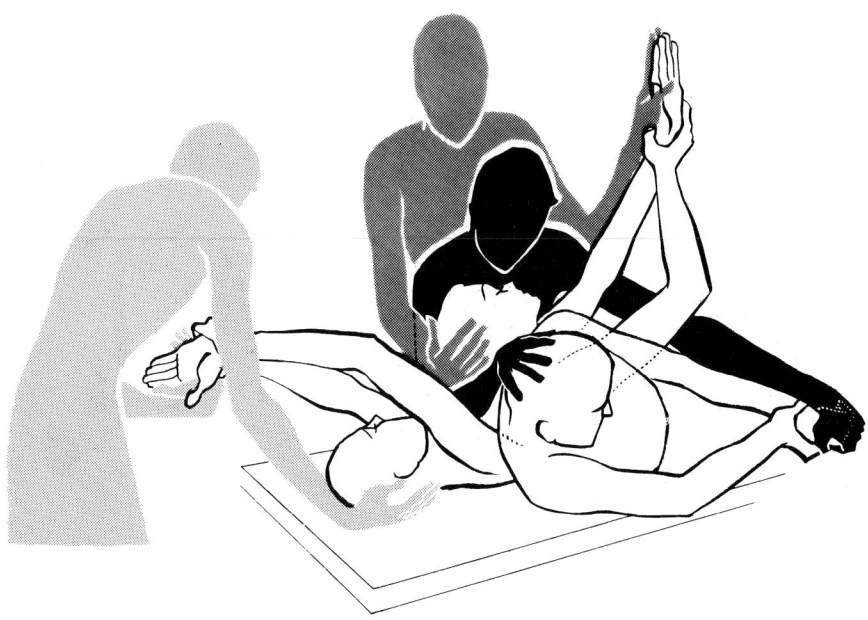

FIG. 1-37

Antagonistic Pattern

Upper trunk flexion with rotation to the right (Fig. 1-36).

Components of Motion

Head rotates toward left, atlanto-occipital joint extends toward left with mandible elevating toward left, cervical and dorsal regions of spine, which have been convex to left, extend with rotation and become convex to right. Forehead moves away from right hip.

Normal Timing

Action occurs from distal to proximal, that is, head rotation, then atlanto-occipital extension with mandibular elevation, then cervical spine extension with rotation, and dorsal spine extension with rotation.

Timing for Emphasis

Dorsal Spine Extension with Rotation. Allow beginning contraction of all components of neck extension with rotation to left, in accordance with normal timing, but do not allow full range of their components to occur, until dorsal extensors on left contract and dorsal spine begins to extend and rotate toward left.

NOTE: Resist components of neck extension, but guide weaker components through their optimal range of motion in accordance with normal timing.

Manual Contacts

Left Hand. Palmar surface of hand and fingers cupped over dorsal–radial aspect of fingers and wrist of patient's left hand (Fig. 1-37).

Right Hand. Pressure of palmar surface of hand and fingers on left posterior–lateral aspect of patient's head (Fig. 1-37).

Commands

Preparatory. "You are going to turn your head, and push it up and away from your right hip, so that you are looking up and over your left shoulder."

Action. "Push up and over! Turn your head! Lift your arms up! Push your head away and up! Straighten your back!"

Pattern Analysis

Motion components and major muscle components of neck extension with rotation to left (Fig. 1-34).

Dorsal Spine Extension with Rotation. Major muscle components: Left spinalis dorsi, longissimus dorsi, iliocostalis dorsi, iliocostalis lumborum, quadratus lumborum, interspinales, intertransversarii, serratus posterior superior, external intercostals. Right semispinalis dorsi, levatores costarum, multifidus, rotatores, serratus posterior inferior. Transversus abdominis.

NOTE: Most closely related patterns are flexion–abduction–external rotation of left upper extremity, flexion–adduction–external rotation of right upper extremity, extension–abduction–internal rotation of left lower extremity, and extension–adduction–external rotation of right lower extremity. When lower trunk extension with rotation to left is combined with upper trunk extension to left, entire spine extends with rotation toward left with right convexity occurring in shortened range of combined patterns. When lower trunk extension with rotation to right is combined with upper trunk extension with rotation to left, dorsal spine becomes convex to right and lumbar spine becomes convex to left with crossing of rotation occurring at dorsolumbar junction.

ILLUSTRATION NOTE: Illustration portrays reinforcement of upper trunk extension with rotation to left by combined upper extremity patterns that are most closely related: those of flexion–abduction–external rotation of left upper extremity and flexion–adduction–external rotation of right upper extremity. Flexion–abduction–external rotation pattern contributes to component of extension of upper trunk, while flexion–adduction–external rotation pattern contributes to rotation of upper trunk. These combined upper extremity patterns are referred to as "lifting."

If pattern is to be performed without resistance to "lifting," manual contacts for head and neck extension with rotation to left pattern may be used.

Range-Limiting Factors

Tension or contracture of any muscles of upper trunk flexion with rotation to right pattern (Fig. 1-36).

Upper Trunk (Superior Region)

Rotation to the Right (Ro, R)

Antagonistic Pattern

Upper trunk rotation to the left. (Motion components, major muscle components, and manual contacts are exactly opposite.)

Components of Motion

Head rotates toward right, atlanto-occipital joint flexes with depression and rotation of the mandible from left to right, cervical and dorsal spine rotates through flexion and into extension toward right. Cervical and dorsal regions of spine, which have been convex to right, rotate and become convex to left.

Normal Timing

Action occurs from distal to proximal, that is, head rotation, atlanto-occipital flexion with mandibular depression and rotation, then cervical and dorsal spine rotation through flexion into extension.

Timing for Emphasis

Upper Trunk Rotation to Right. Allow beginning contraction of all components of head and neck rotation to right, in accordance with normal timing, but do not allow full range to occur, until contraction proceeds in abdominals and laterally into extensors.

NOTE: Resist stronger components of rotation, but guide weaker components through their optimal range of motion in accordance with normal timing.

Manual Contacts

Left and right hands as in head and neck rotation to the right (Fig. 1-35).

Commands

Preparatory. "You are going to turn your head to the right, and twist your body to look down and behind your right shoulder."
Action. "Turn! Pull your chin to your shoulder! Pull your chin down! Push your head back!"

Pattern Analysis

Motion components and major muscle components of head and neck rotation to right.
Upper Trunk Rotation to Right. Major muscle components: Rotation components of trunk flexors: left external oblique, right internal oblique, transversus abdominus. Rotation component of trunk extensors: right iliocostalis dorsi, iliocostalis lumborum, quadratus lumborum.

NOTE: Upper extremity patterns most closely related to upper trunk rotation to right are extension–abduction–internal rotation of right upper extremity and flexion–adduction–external rotation of left upper extremity. These are the patterns that contribute to rotation of upper trunk flexion to right pattern and upper trunk extension to right pattern. Since upper trunk rotation to right is primarily a pattern of rotation but has components of flexion and extension, these upper extremity patterns combine most effectively to reinforce rotation of upper trunk. Pattern may be performed with manual contacts applied to head and one upper extremity, or to both upper extremities with free active motion of head and neck. This pattern is optimum for quadratus lumborum on right. Extension–abduction–internal rotation of right lower extremity is most closely related.

Range-Limiting Factors

Tension or contracture of any muscles of rotation to left pattern.

Lower Trunk (Inferior Region)

Flexion with Rotation to the Left (D fl, L)

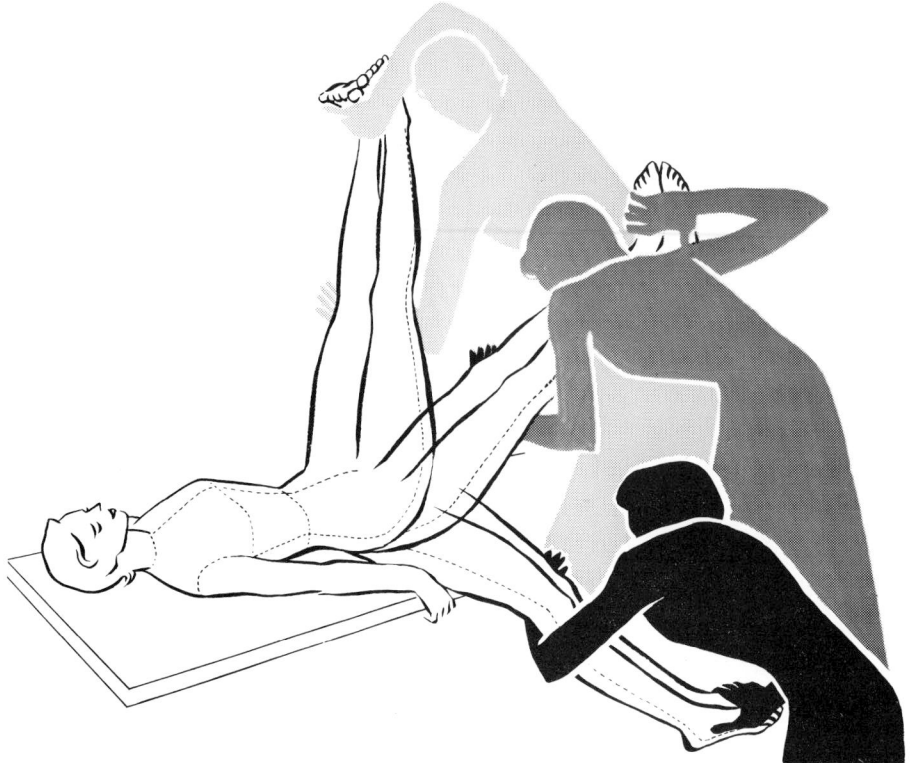

FIG. 1-38. With knees straight.

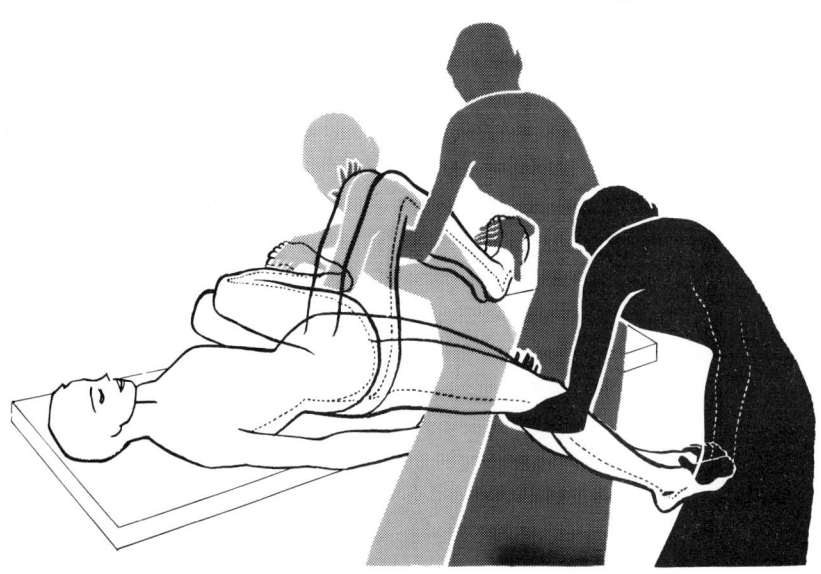

FIG. 1-39. With knees flexing.

Antagonistic Pattern

Lower trunk extension with rotation to right (Figs. 1-41 to 1-43).

Components of Motion

Lower extremities, in close approximation, flex and rotate to left, requiring flexion–abduction–internal rotation of left lower extremity and flexion–adduction–external rotation of right lower extremity including all of their respective components of motion. Intermediate joints, knees, may remain straight, flex, or extend. Pelvis rotates, brim moving upward and to left. Lumbar spine, which has been convex to left, flexes with rotation and becomes convex to right.

Normal Timing

Action occurs from distal to proximal, that is, action proceeds from distal to proximal in relation to

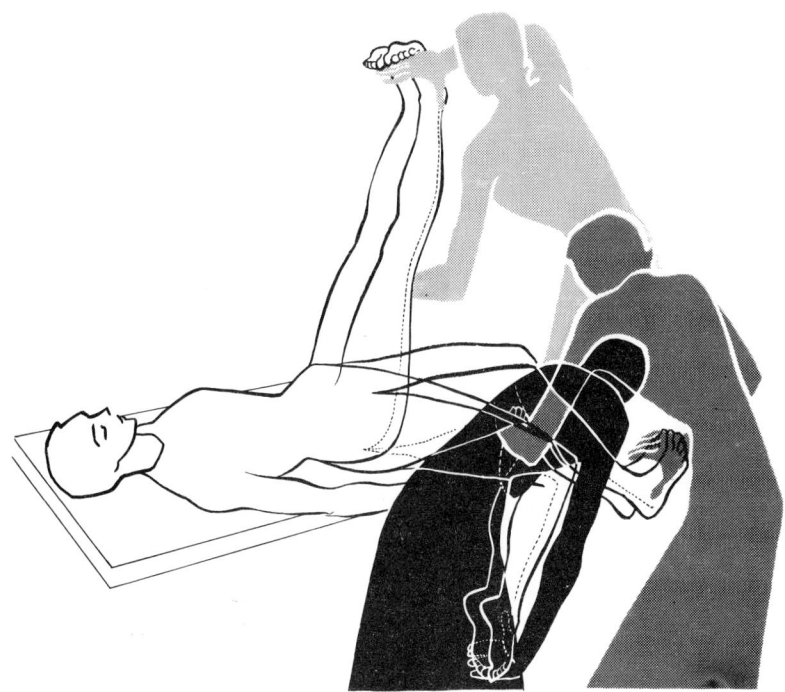

FIG. 1-40. With knees extending.

lower extremities, toes, feet, ankles, knees (if intermediate joint motion is desired), then hips, pelvic rotation, and lumbar flexion with rotation to left.

Timing for Emphasis

Allow beginning rotation to occur at toes, ankles, knees, and hips, but do not allow full range of lower extremity components to occur, until pelvis begins to rotate toward left and lumbar spine begins to flex with rotation toward left.

NOTE: When intermediate joint action is used, that is, knee flexion or extension, pelvic rotation and lumbar flexion is delayed because of time required for action of intermediate joints.

Manual Contacts

Right Hand. Pressure of palmar surface of hand and fingers on dorsal aspect of both feet, especially left foot. Internal malleoli should be in close approximation (Fig. 1-40). If patient has no active motion below ankles, right hand may be used to grip both heels, to control rotation at hips.

Left Hand. Pressure of palmar surface of hand, fingers, and forearm on anterior surface of both thighs proximal to knee joint. Patient's knees should be in close approximation. If patient has difficulty in initiating range of hip motions, left hand may be placed on posterior aspect of thighs proximal to popliteal spaces (Fig. 1-40).

Commands

Preparatory. "You are going to turn your heels away from me, and pull your feet up and across your body. Keep your knees straight." ("Bend your knees," or "Straighten your knees.")

Action. "Pull! Pull your feet up! Keep your knees straight!" ("Bend your knees!" or "Straighten your knees!") "Pull them up and away from me!"

Pattern Analysis

Lower Extremities. Motion components and major muscle components: Same as flexion – abduction – internal rotation of left (Figs. 1-70 to 1-72), and flexion – adduction – external rotation of right (Figs. 1-64 to 1-66).

Pelvic Rotation and Lumbar Spine Flexion with Rotation to Left. Major muscle components: Left external oblique, rectus abdominis (left portion), quadratus lumborum. Right internal oblique.

NOTE: Most closely related upper extremity patterns are extension – adduction – internal rotation of left and flexion – adduction – external rotation of right. Extension – adduction – internal rotation of left contributes to flexion component; flexion – adduction – external rotation of right contributes to rotation component. Upper trunk flexion with rotation to right requires action of same oblique abdominal muscles, and upper trunk flexion with rotation to left requires action of all abdominal muscles. Neck flexion with rotation to right and to left are related in the same manner as upper trunk flexion patterns.

Range-Limiting Factors

Tension or contracture of any muscles of lower trunk extension with rotation to right pattern (Figs. 1-41 to 1-43).

Extension with Rotation to the Right (D ex, R)

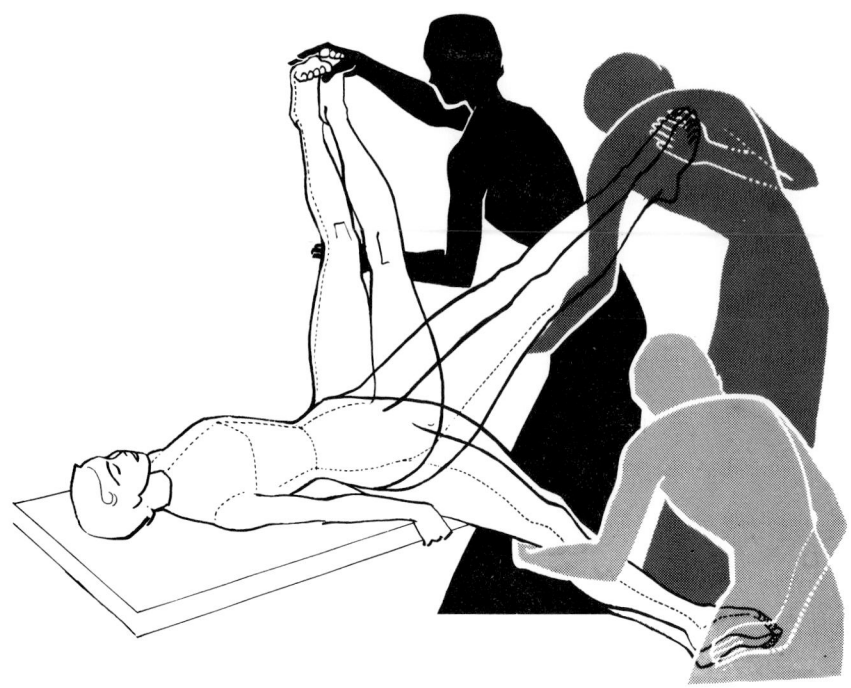

FIG. 1-41. With knees straight.

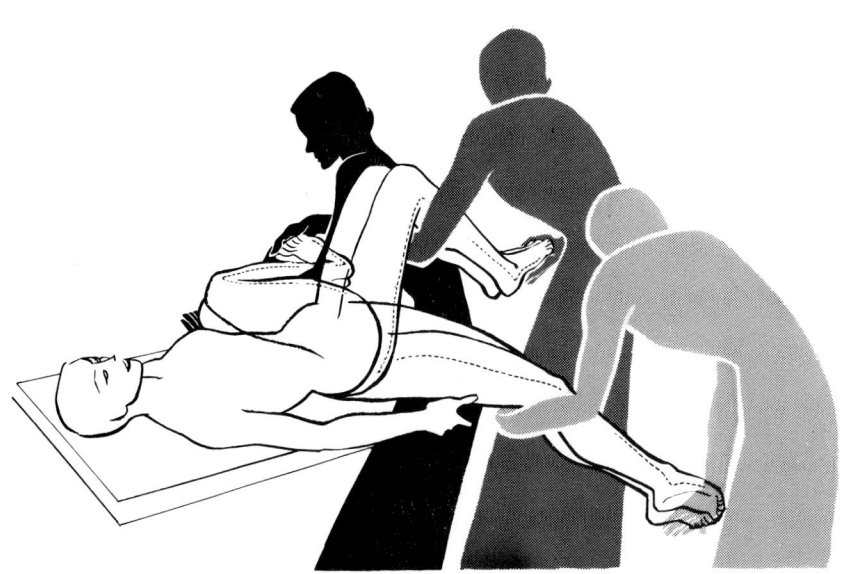

FIG. 1-42. With knees extending.

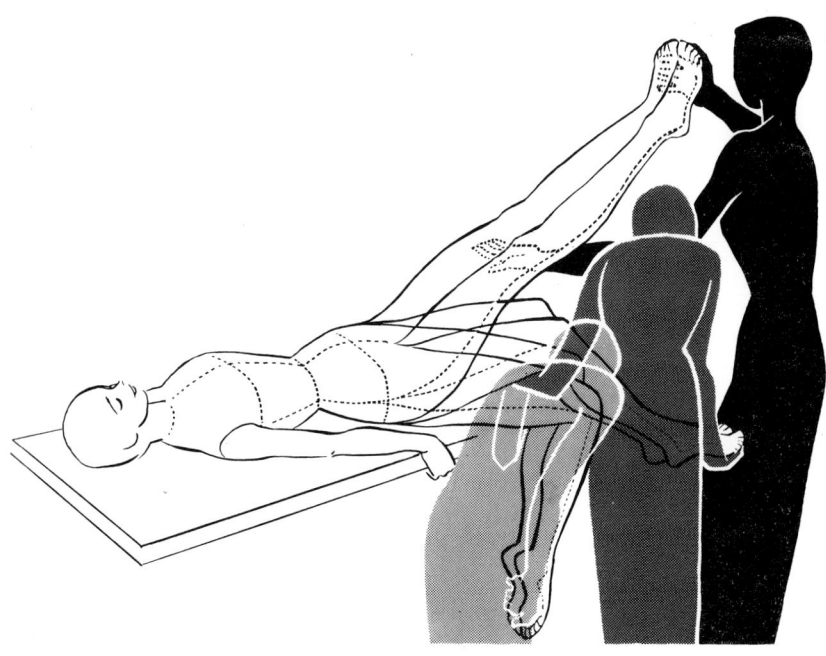

FIG. 1-43. With knees flexing.

Antagonistic Pattern

Lower trunk flexion with rotation to the left (Figs. 1-38 to 1-40).

Components of Motion

Lower extremities, in close approximation, extend and rotate to right, requiring extension–abduction–internal rotation of right lower extremity and extension–adduction–external rotation of left lower extremity, including all of their respective components of motion. Intermediate joints may remain straight, flex, or extend. Pelvis rotates, brim moving downward and to right. Lumbar spine, which has been convex to right, extends with rotation and becomes convex to left.

Normal Timing

Action occurs from distal to proximal, that is, action proceeds from distal to proximal in relation to lower extremities, toes, feet, ankles, knees (if intermediate joint motion is desired), then hips, pelvic rotation, and lumbar extension with rotation to right.

Timing for Emphasis

Allow beginning rotation to occur at toes, ankles, knees, and hips, but do not allow full range of lower extremity components to occur, until pelvis rotates toward right and lumbar spine begins to extend with rotation toward right.

NOTE: When intermediate joint action is used, that is, knee flexion or knee extension, pelvic rotation and lumbar spine extension is delayed because of time required for action of intermediate joints. Resist stronger distal components, but guide weaker distal components through their optimal range of motion in accordance with normal timing.

Manual Contacts

Right Hand. Pressure of palmar surface of hand and fingers on plantar surface of both feet, especially right foot. Internal malleoli should be in close approximation (Fig. 1-43). If patient has no active motion below ankle, right hand may be used to grip both heels, to control rotation at hips.

Left Hand. Pressure of palmar surface of hand, fingers, and forearm on posterior surface of both thighs proximal to popliteal space. Patient's knees should be in close approximation (Fig. 1-43).

Commands

Preparatory. "You are going to turn your heels toward me, and push your feet down and over toward me. Keep your knees straight." ("Bend your knees," or "Straighten your knees.")

Action. "Push! Turn your heels! Push your feet down! "Push toward me! Keep your knees straight!" ("Bend your knees!" or "Straighten your knees!")

Pattern Analysis

Lower Extremities. Motion components and major muscle components: Same as extension–abduction–internal rotation pattern of the right (Figs. 1-67 to 1-69) and extension–adduction–external rotation of left (Figs. 1-73 to 1-75).

Pelvic Rotation and Lumbar Spine Extension with Rotation to Right. Major muscle components: Right sacrospinalis, iliocostalis lumborum, quadratus lumborum, interspinales, intertransversarii, longissimus dorsi, spinalis dorsi; left multifidus, rotatores. Right dorsal extensors and rotators will enter motion if pattern is initiated from range sufficient to demand their response.

NOTE: Upper trunk extension with rotation to right is most closely related upper trunk pattern; neck extension with rotation to right is most closely related neck pattern. Most closely related upper extremity patterns are flexion–abduction–external rotation of left upper extremity, which reinforces extension component, and extension–abduction–internal rotation of right upper extremity, which reinforces rotation component.

Range-Limiting Factor

Tension or contracture of any muscles of lower trunk flexion with rotation to left pattern (Figs. 1-38 to 1-40).

Flexion–Adduction–External Rotation (D1 fl), with Elbow Straight

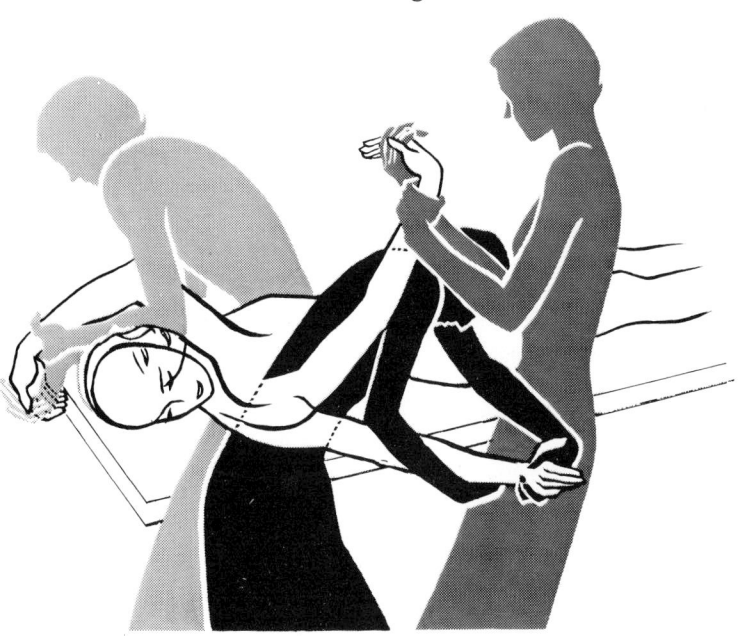

FIG. 1-44

Antagonistic Pattern

Extension–abduction–internal rotation (with elbow straight) pattern (Fig. 1-47).

Components of Motion

Fingers flex and adduct toward radial side (lateral fingers more than medial); thumb externally rotates, flexes, and adducts toward radial side; wrist supinates and flexes toward radial side; forearm supinates; elbow remains straight; shoulder flexes, adducts, and externally rotates with scapula rotating, abducting (inferior angle), and elevating anteriorly (acromion); and clavicle approximates sternum with rotation and elevation anteriorly.

Normal Timing

Action is from distal to proximal, that is, action occurs first at fingers, thumb, wrist, and forearm, then at shoulder, scapula, and clavicle.

Timing for Emphasis

Scapula and Clavicle. Allow beginning rotation to occur at fingers, wrist, forearm, and shoulder, but do not allow full range of finger flexion with adduction toward radial side, wrist flexion toward radial side, forearm supination, and shoulder flexion–adduction–external rotation to occur, until scapula begins to rotate, abduct, and elevate anteriorly.

NOTE: If normal timing is prevented by excessive resistance to weak distal components, action cannot occur proximally. Resist stronger distal components, but guide weaker distal components through their optimal range of motion in accordance with normal timing.

Shoulder. Allow beginning rotation to occur at fingers, wrist, forearm, and shoulder, but do not allow full range of finger flexion with adduction toward radial side, wrist flexion toward radial side, and forearm supination to occur, until shoulder begins to flex and adduct in external rotation.

NOTE: Resist stronger proximal and distal components, but guide weaker distal components through their optimal range of motion in accordance with normal timing.

Forearm. Allow beginning rotation to occur at fingers, thumb, wrist, forearm, and shoulder, but do not allow full range of finger flexion with adduction toward radial side, wrist flexion toward radial side, and shoulder flexion–adduction–external rotation to occur, until forearm begins to supinate.

NOTE: Resist stronger proximal and distal components, but guide weaker distal components through their optimal range of motion in accordance with normal timing.

Wrist. Allow beginning rotation to occur at fingers, thumb, wrist, forearm, and shoulder, but do

D1 fl, LeR for Closing   REVERSAL: D1 ex, Sh-R for Opening

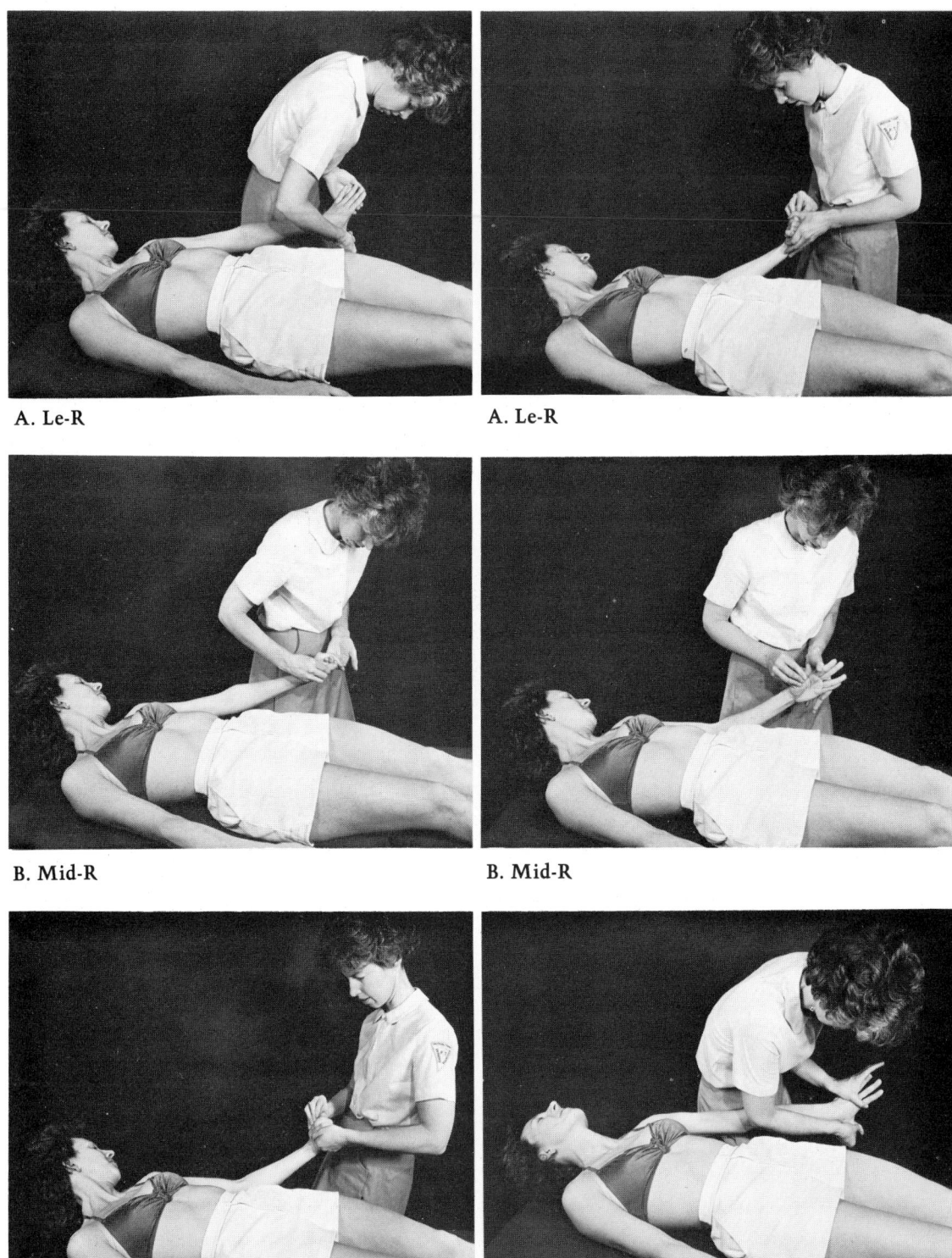

A. Le-R   A. Le-R

B. Mid-R   B. Mid-R

C. Sh-R   C. Sh-R

FIG. 1-44, *continued*

not allow full range of finger flexion toward radial side, forearm supination, and shoulder flexion–adduction–external rotation to occur, until wrist begins to flex toward radial side.

NOTE: Resist stronger proximal and distal components, but guide weaker distal components through their optimal range of motion in accordance with normal timing.

Fingers. Allow beginning rotation to occur at fingers, thumb, wrist, forearm, and shoulder, but do not allow full range of wrist flexion toward radial side, forearm supination, and shoulder flexion–adduction–external rotation to occur, until fingers begin to flex and adduct toward radial side.

NOTE: Resist stronger proximal components. Emphasis may be placed on metacarpal–phalangeal joints, or interphalangeal joints, or emphasis may be placed upon a specific joint of an individual digit.

Thumb. Allow beginning rotation to occur at fingers, wrist, forearm, and shoulder, but do not allow full range of other components to occur, until thumb begins to flex and adduct. Components of fingers and wrist must be allowed to move through range after motion is initiated at thumb. In shortened range of pattern, thumb is flexed, adducted and externally rotated toward second metacarpal.

NOTE: Resist stronger finger, wrist, and proximal components.

Manual Contacts

Left Hand. Placed in palm of patient's right hand, so that patient may grasp with fingers and thumb, and so that wrist may flex toward radial side (Fig. 1-44).

Right Hand. *For emphasis of distal joints:* Grip with pressure of palmar surface over distal anterior aspect of forearm, to control supination and proximal components of motion (Fig. 1-44).

For emphasis of shoulder: Pressure of palmar surface on anterior–medial surface of patient's arm, to control external rotation and proximal components of motion.

For emphasis of scapula: Pressure of palmar surface of hand over anterior aspect of patient's shoulder proximal to acromion process.

For mass closing of hand and for emphasis of thumb motion: Grasp right thumb of patient with thumb and index finger of left hand, with contact of thumb and finger medially and laterally at interphalangeal joint of thumb. Place right fingers and hand on palmar surface of fingers of patient's right hand. Flexion of all fingers and thumb flexion–adduction may be resisted. Physical therapist's right hand prevents range of motion occurring proximally until fingers flex and adduct.

Commands

Preparatory. "You are to squeeze my hand, turn it, and pull my hand up and across your face, keeping your elbow straight."
Action. "Pull! Squeeze my hand! Turn it! Pull up across your face! Keep your elbow straight!"

Pattern Analysis

Scapula. *Motion components:* Rotation, abduction (inferior angle), elevation anteriorly (acromion). *Major muscle components:* Serratus anterior.
Shoulder. *Motion components:* Flexion, adduction, external rotation. *Major muscle components:* Pectoralis major (clavicular portion), deltoid (anterior portion), coracobrachialis, biceps brachii (shoulder flexion component).
Forearm. *Motion components:* Supination. *Major muscle components:* Supinator.
Wrist. *Motion components:* Flexion toward radial side. *Major muscle components:* Flexor carpi radialis, palmaris longus.
Fingers. *Motion components:* Flexion, adduction toward radial side. *Major muscle components:* Flexor digitorum superficialis, flexor digitorum profundus, flexor digiti quinti brevis, opponens digiti quinti, palmar interossei, lumbricales.
Thumb. *Motion components:* Flexion, adduction with rotation toward second metacarpal. *Major muscle components:* Flexor pollicis longus, flexor pollicis brevis, adductores pollicis.

Range-Limiting Factor

Tension or contracture of any muscles of the extension–abduction–internal rotation (with elbow straight) pattern (Fig. 1-47).

Flexion – Adduction – External Rotation (D1 fl), with
Elbow Flexion

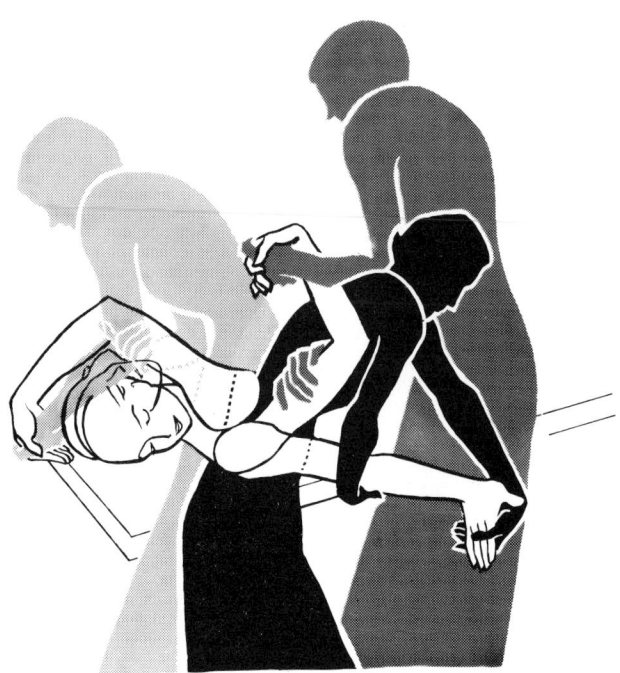

FIG. 1-45

Antagonistic Pattern

Extension – abduction – internal rotation (with elbow extension) pattern (Fig. 1-48).

Components of Motion

Fingers flex and adduct toward radial side (lateral fingers more than medial); thumb externally rotates, flexes, and adducts toward radial side; wrist supinates and flexes toward radial side; forearm supinates; elbow flexes; shoulder flexes, adducts, and externally rotates with scapula rotating, abducting (inferior angle), and elevating anteriorly (acromion); and clavicle approximates sternum with rotation and elevation anteriorly.

Normal Timing

Action is from distal to proximal, that is, action occurs first at fingers, thumb, wrist, forearm, and elbow, then at shoulder, scapula, and clavicle.

Timing for Emphasis

Scapula and Clavicle. Allow beginning rotation to occur at fingers, thumb, wrist, forearm, elbow, and shoulder, but do not allow full range of finger flexion with adduction toward radial side, wrist flexion toward radial side, forearm supination, elbow flexion, and shoulder flexion – adduction to occur, until scapula begins to rotate, abduct, and elevate anteriorly.

NOTE: If normal timing is prevented by excessive resistance to weak distal components, action cannot occur proximally. Resist stronger distal components, but guide weaker distal components through their optimal range of motion in accordance with normal timing.

Shoulder. Allow beginning rotation to occur at fingers, thumb, wrist, forearm, elbow, and shoulder, but do not allow full range of finger flexion with adduction toward radial side, wrist flexion toward radial side, forearm supination, elbow flexion, and scapular rotation to occur, until shoulder begins to flex and adduct in external rotation.

NOTE: Resist stronger proximal and distal components, but guide weaker distal components through their optimal range of motion in accordance with normal timing.

Elbow. Allow beginning rotation to occur at fingers, thumb, wrist, forearm, elbow, and shoulder, but do not allow full range of finger flexion with adduction toward radial side, wrist flexion toward radial side, forearm supination, shoulder flexion – adduction, and scapular rotation to occur, until elbow begins to flex.

NOTE: Resist stronger distal and proximal components, but guide weaker distal components through their optimal range of motion in accordance with normal timing.

Forearm. Allow beginning rotation to occur at fingers, thumb, wrist, forearm, elbow, and shoulder, but do not allow full range of finger flexion with adduction toward radial side, wrist flexion toward radial side, elbow flexion, and shoulder flexion – adduction with scapular rotation to occur, until forearm begins to supinate.

NOTE: Resist stronger proximal and distal components, but guide weaker components through their optimal range of motion in accordance with normal timing.

Wrist. Allow beginning rotation to occur at fingers, thumb, wrist, forearm, elbow, and shoulder, but do not allow full range of finger flexion with adduction toward radial side, forearm supination, elbow flexion, and shoulder flexion – adduction with scapular rotation to occur, until wrist begins to flex toward radial side.

NOTE: Resist stronger distal and proximal components, but guide weaker distal components through their optimal range of motion in accordance with normal timing.

Fingers. Allow beginning rotation to occur at fingers, thumb, wrist, forearm, elbow, and shoulder, but do not allow full range of wrist flexion toward radial side, forearm supination, elbow flexion, and shoulder flexion – adduction to occur, until fingers begin to flex and adduct toward radial side.

NOTE: Resist stronger proximal components. Emphasis may be placed upon metacarpal – phalangeal joints or interphalangeal joints, or emphasis may be placed upon a specific joint of an individual digit.

Thumb. Allow beginning rotation to occur at fingers, thumb, wrist, forearm, elbow, and shoulder, but do not allow full range of finger flexion with adduction toward radial side, wrist flexion toward radial side, forearm supination, elbow flexion, and shoulder flexion – adduction to occur, until thumb begins to flex and adduct. Components of fingers and wrist must be allowed to move through range after motion is initiated at thumb. In shortened range of pattern, thumb is flexed, adducted, and externally rotated toward second metacarpal.

NOTE: Resist stronger finger, wrist, and proximal components.

Manual Contacts

Left Hand. Placed in palm of patient's right hand, so that patient may grasp with fingers and thumb, and so that wrist may flex toward radial side (Fig. 1-45).

Right Hand. *For emphasis of distal joints:* Grip with pressure of palmar surface over distal anterior aspect of forearm, to control supination and proximal components of motion.

For emphasis of elbow: Pressure of palmar surface of hand on anterior – medial surface of arm, to control external rotation and proximal components of motion (Fig. 1-45).

For emphasis of shoulder: Same as for elbow emphasis.

For emphasis of scapula: Pressure of palmar surface of hand over anterior aspect of shoulder proximal to acromion process.

For mass closing of hand and for emphasis of thumb motion: Grasp right thumb of patient with thumb and index finger of left hand. Place right fingers and hand on palmar surface of fingers of patient's right hand. Flexion of all fingers and thumb flexion – adduction may be resisted. Physical therapist's right hand prevents range of motion occurring proximally until fingers flex and adduct.

Commands

Preparatory. "You are to squeeze my hand, turn it, and bend your elbow, and pull my hand up and across your face."

Action. "Pull! Squeeze my hand! Turn it! Bend your elbow! Pull up across your face!"

Pattern Analysis

Scapula. *Motion components:* Rotation, abduction (inferior angle), elevation anteriorly (acromion). *Major muscle components:* Serratus anterior.

Shoulder. *Motion components:* Flexion, adduction, external rotation. *Major muscle components:* Pectoralis major (clavicular portion), deltoid (anterior portion), coracobrachialis, biceps brachii (shoulder flexion component).

Elbow. *Motion components:* Flexion with forearm supination. *Major muscle components:* Biceps brachii (long and short heads), brachialis.

Forearm. *Motion components:* Supination. *Major muscle components:* Supinator.

Wrist, Fingers, and Thumb. See flexion – adduction – external rotation (with elbow straight) pattern.

Range-Limiting Factors

Tension or contracture of any muscles of extension – abduction – internal rotation (with elbow extension) pattern (Fig. 1-48).

Flexion–Adduction–External Rotation (D1 fl), with
Elbow Extension

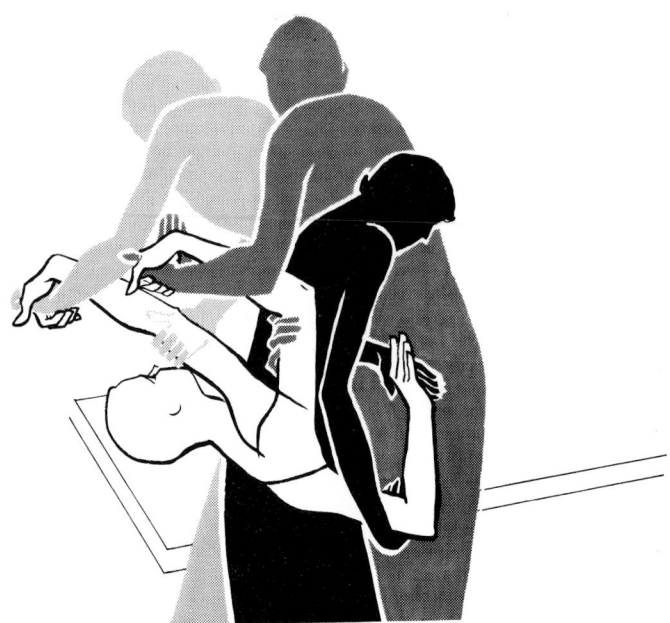

FIG. 1-46

Antagonistic Pattern

Extension–abduction–internal rotation (with elbow flexion) pattern (Fig. 1-49).

Components of Motion

Fingers flex and adduct toward radial side (lateral fingers more than medial); thumb externally rotates, flexes, and adducts toward radial side; wrist supinates and flexes toward radial side; forearm supinates; elbow extends; shoulder flexes, adducts, and externally rotates with scapula rotating, abducting (inferior angle), and elevating anteriorly (acromion); and clavicle approximates sternum with rotation and elevation anteriorly.

Normal Timing

Action is from distal to proximal, that is, action occurs first at fingers, thumb, wrist, forearm, and elbow, then at shoulder, scapula, and clavicle.

Timing for Emphasis

Scapula and Clavicle. Allow beginning rotation to occur at fingers, thumb, wrist, forearm, elbow, and shoulder, but do not allow full range of finger flexion with adduction toward radial side, wrist flexion toward radial side, forearm supination, elbow extension, and shoulder flexion–adduction to occur, until scapula begins to rotate, abduct, and elevate anteriorly.

NOTE: If normal timing is prevented by excessive resistance to weak distal components, action cannot occur proximally. Resist stronger distal components, but guide weaker distal components through their optimal range of motion in accordance with normal timing.

Shoulder. Allow beginning rotation to occur at fingers, thumb, wrist, forearm, elbow, and shoulder, but do not allow full range of finger flexion with adduction toward radial side, wrist flexion toward radial side, forearm supination, elbow extension, and scapular rotation to occur, until shoulder begins to flex and adduct in external rotation.

NOTE: Resist stronger distal components, but guide weaker distal components through their optimal range of motion in accordance with normal timing.

Elbow. Allow beginning rotation to occur at fingers, thumb, wrist, forearm, elbow, and shoulder, but do not allow full range of finger flexion with adduction toward radial side, wrist flexion toward radial side, forearm supination, and shoulder flexion–adduction to occur, until elbow begins to extend.

NOTE: Resist stronger proximal and distal components, but guide weaker distal components through their optimal range of motion in accordance with normal timing.

Forearm. Allow beginning rotation to occur at fingers, thumb, wrist, forearm, elbow, and shoulder, but do not allow full range of finger flexion with adduction toward radial side, wrist flexion toward radial side, elbow extension, and shoulder flexion – adduction to occur, until forearm begins to supinate.

NOTE: Resist stronger proximal and distal components, but guide weaker distal components through their optimal range of motion in accordance with normal timing.

Wrist. Allow beginning rotation to occur at fingers, thumb, wrist, forearm, elbow, and shoulder, but do not allow full range of finger flexion with adduction toward radial side, forearm supination, elbow extension, and shoulder flexion – adduction to occur, until wrist begins to flex toward radial side.

NOTE: Resist stronger proximal and distal components, but guide weaker distal components through their optimal range of motion in accordance with normal timing.

Fingers. Allow beginning rotation to occur at fingers, thumb, wrist, forearm, elbow, and shoulder, but do not allow full range of wrist flexion toward radial side, forearm supination, elbow extension, and shoulder flexion – adduction to occur, until fingers begin to flex and adduct toward the radial side.

NOTE: Resist stronger proximal components. Emphasis may be placed on metacarpal – phalangeal joints, or emphasis may be placed on a specific joint of an individual digit.

Thumb. Allow beginning rotation to occur at fingers, thumb, wrist, forearm, elbow, and shoulder, but do not allow full range of finger flexion with adduction toward radial side, wrist flexion toward radial side, forearm supination, elbow extension, and shoulder flexion – adduction to occur, until thumb begins to flex and adduct. Components of fingers and wrist must be allowed to move through range after motion is initiated at thumb. In shortened range of pattern, the thumb is flexed, adducted, and externally rotated toward the second metacarpal.

NOTE: Resist stronger finger, wrist, and proximal components.

Manual Contacts

Left Hand. Placed in palm of patient's right hand so that patient may grasp with fingers and thumb and so that wrist may flex toward radial side (Fig. 1-46).

Right Hand. *For emphasis of distal joints:* Grip with pressure of palmar surface of hand over distal anterior aspect of forearm, to control supination and proximal components of motion.

For emphasis of elbow: Pressure of palmar surface on anterior – medial surface of arm, to control external rotation and proximal components of motion (Fig. 1-46).

For emphasis of shoulder: Same as for elbow emphasis.

For emphasis of scapula: Pressure of palmar surface of hand over the anterior aspect of shoulder proximal to acromion process.

For mass closing of hand and for emphasis of thumb motion: Grasp right thumb of patient with thumb and index finger of left hand; place right fingers and hand on palmar surface of fingers of patient's right hand. Flexion of all fingers and thumb flexion – adduction may be resisted. Physical therapist's right hand prevents range of motion occurring proximally until fingers flex and adduct.

Commands

Preparatory. "You are to squeeze my hand, turn it, and straighten your elbow as you pull my hand up and across your face."

Action. "Pull! Squeeze my hand! Turn it! Straighten your elbow! Pull it up across your face!"

Pattern Analysis

Scapula. *Motion components:* Rotation, abduction (inferior angle), elevation anteriorly (acromion). *Major muscle components:* Serratus anterior.

Shoulder. *Motion components:* Flexion, adduction, external rotation. *Major muscle components:* Pectoralis major (clavicular portion), deltoid (anterior portion), coracobrachialis.

Elbow. *Motion components:* Extension with forearm supination. *Major muscle components:* Triceps (lateral portion), anconeus.

Forearm. *Motion components:* Supination. *Major muscle components:* Supinator.

Wrist, Fingers, and Thumb. See flexion – adduction – external rotation (with elbow straight) pattern.

Range-Limiting Factors

Tension or contracture of any muscles of extension – abduction – internal rotation (with elbow flexion) pattern (Fig. 1-49).

Extension–Abduction–Internal Rotation (D1 ex), with Elbow Straight

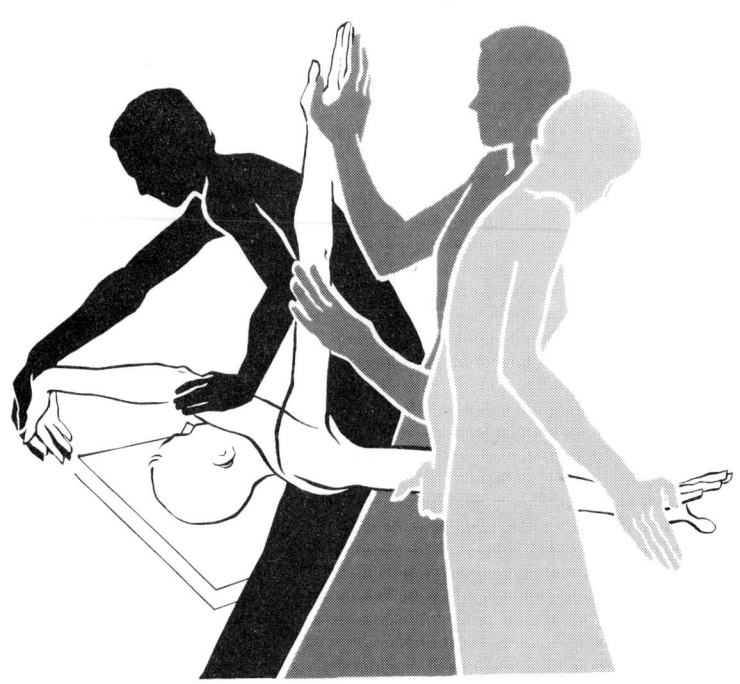

FIG. 1-47

Antagonistic Pattern

Flexion–adduction–external rotation (with elbow straight) pattern (Fig. 1-44).

Components of Motion

Fingers extend and abduct toward ulnar side (medial fingers more than lateral); thumb extends, abducts, and internally rotates toward ulnar side (palmar abduction); wrist pronates and extends toward ulnar side; forearm pronates; elbow remains straight; shoulder extends, abducts, and internally rotates with scapula rotating, adducting (inferior angle) and depressing posteriorly (acromion); and clavicle rotates and depresses anteriorly away from sternum.

Normal Timing

Action is from distal to proximal, that is, action occurs first at fingers, thumb, wrist, and forearm, then at scapula, and clavicle.

Timing for Emphasis

Scapula and Clavicle. Allow beginning rotation to occur at fingers, thumb, wrist, forearm, and shoulder, but do not allow full range of finger exten-sion with abduction toward ulnar side, wrist pronation and extension toward ulnar side, forearm pronation, and shoulder extension–abduction to occur, until scapula begins to rotate, adduct, and depress posteriorly.

NOTE: If normal timing is prevented by excessive resistance to weak components, action cannot occur proximally. Resist stronger distal components, but guide weaker distal components through their optimal range of motion in accordance with normal timing.

Shoulder. Allow beginning rotation to occur at fingers, thumb, wrist, forearm, shoulder, and scapula, but do not allow full range of finger extension with abduction toward ulnar side, wrist pronation and extension toward ulnar side, forearm pronation, and scapular rotation to occur, until shoulder begins to extend and abduct in internal rotation.

NOTE: Resist stronger proximal and distal components, but guide weaker distal components through their optimal range of motion in accordance with normal timing.

Forearm. Allow beginning rotation to occur at fingers, thumb, wrist, forearm, and shoulder, but do

D1 ex, Le-R for Opening

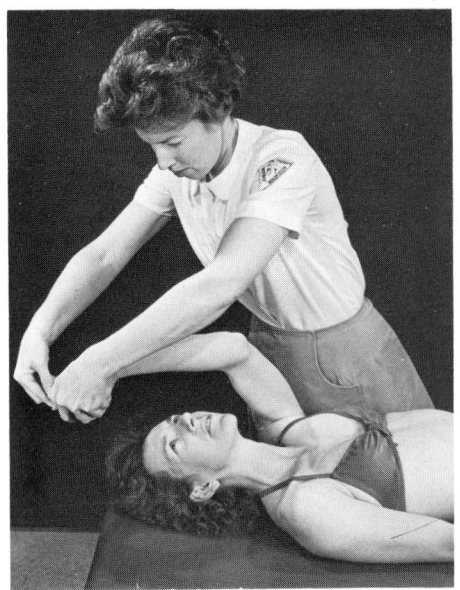
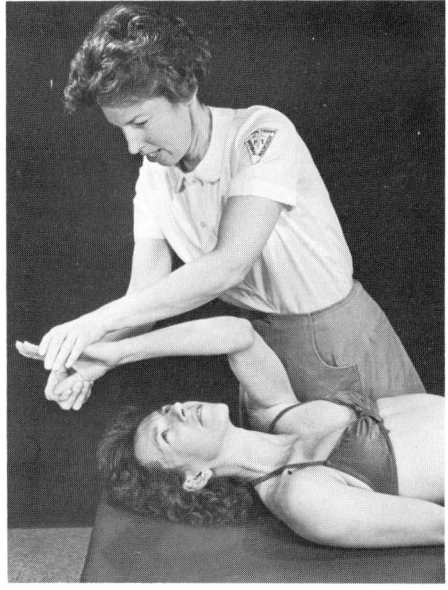
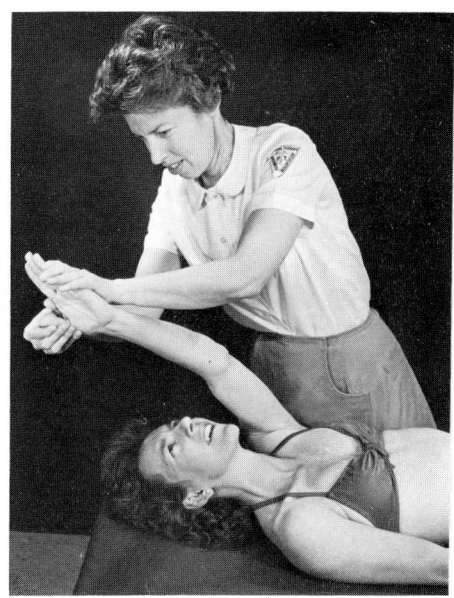

A. Le-R

B. Mid-R

C. Sh-R

REVERSAL: D1 fl, Sh-R for Closing

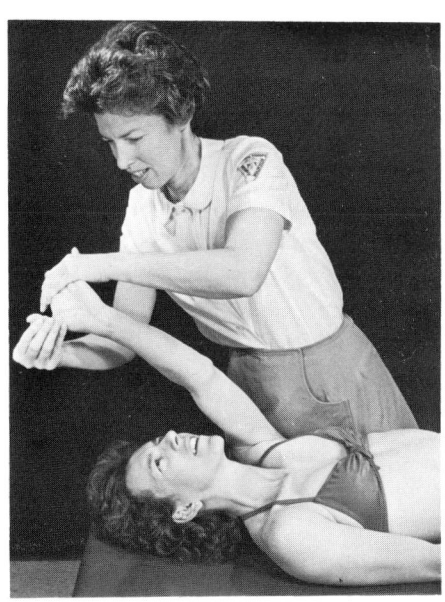
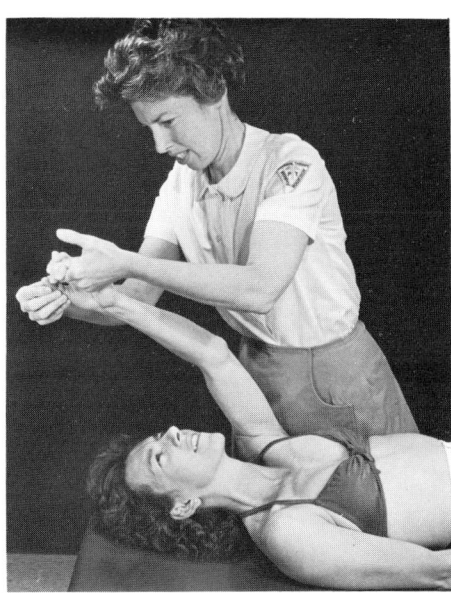
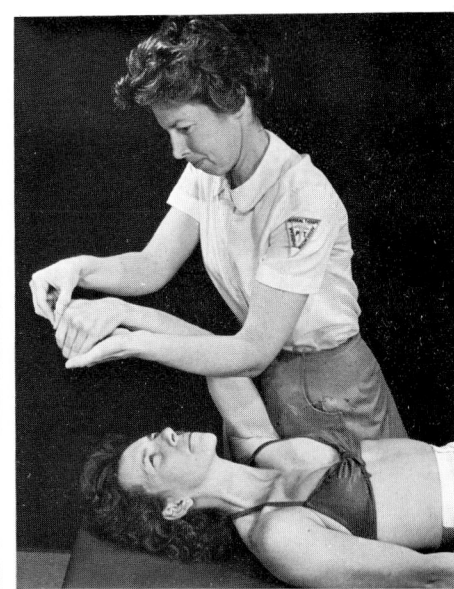

A. Le-R

B. Mid-R

C. Sh-R

FIG. 1-47, *continued*

not allow full range of finger extension with abduction toward ulnar side, wrist extension toward ulnar side, and shoulder extension–abduction to occur, until forearm begins to pronate.

NOTE: Resist stronger proximal and distal components, but guide weaker distal components through their optimal range of motion in accordance with normal timing.

Wrist. Allow beginning rotation to occur at fingers, thumb, wrist, forearm, and shoulder, but do not allow full range of finger extension with abduction toward ulnar side, forearm pronation, and shoulder extension–abduction to occur, until wrist begins to pronate and extend toward ulnar side.

NOTE: Resist stronger proximal and distal components, but guide weaker distal components through their optimal range of motion in accordance with normal timing.

Fingers. Allow beginning rotation to occur at fingers, thumb, wrist, forearm, and shoulder, but do not allow full range of wrist pronation with extension toward ulnar side, forearm pronation, and shoulder extension–abduction to occur, until fingers begin to extend and abduct toward ulnar side.

NOTE: Resist stronger proximal components. Emphasis may be placed upon metacarpal–phalangeal joints, or interphalangeal joints, or emphasis may be placed upon a specific joint of an individual digit.

Thumb. Allow beginning rotation to occur at fingers, thumb, wrist, forearm, and shoulder, but do not allow full range of finger extension with abduction toward ulnar side, wrist pronation with extension toward ulnar side, forearm pronation, and shoulder extension–abduction to occur, until thumb begins to extend and abduct toward ulnar side. Components of fingers and wrist must be allowed to move through range after motion is initiated at thumb. In shortened range of pattern, thumb is extended, abducted, and internally rotated away from second metacarpal.

NOTE: Resist stronger finger, wrist, and proximal components.

Manual Contacts

Right Hand. Palmar surface of hand and fingers cupped over dorsal–ulnar aspect of fingers and wrist of patient's right hand (Fig. 1-47).

Left Hand. For emphasis of distal joints: Grip with pressure of palmar surface over dorsal–ulnar aspect of forearm, to control pronation and proximal components of motion.

For emphasis of shoulder: Pressure of palmar surface on posterior–lateral surface of arm, to control internal rotation and proximal components of motion (Fig. 1-47).

For emphasis of scapula: Pressure of palmar surface of hand over the scapula between spine and inferior angle, to control rotation and adduction.

For mass opening of hand and for emphasis of thumb motion: Grasp the patient's right thumb with thumb and index finger of left hand; contact of physical therapist's thumb and finger should be medially and laterally at interphalangeal joint of patient's thumb, to control rotation of patient's thumb as well as extension and abduction components. Physical therapist's right hand should be cupped over dorsal and ulnar aspect of patient's right hand, to resist wrist extension toward ulnar side and finger extension and abduction toward ulnar side. Right hand of physical therapist also controls and resists proximal components.

Commands

Preparatory. "You are to open your hand, turn it, and push it down and away from your face.

Action. "Push! Open your hand! Turn it! Push it down toward me! Keep your elbow straight!"

Pattern Analysis

Scapula. Motion components: Rotation, adduction (inferior angle), depression posteriorly (acromion). *Major muscle components:* Levator scapulae, rhomboidei minor and major.

Shoulder. Motion components: Extension, abduction, internal rotation. *Major muscle components:* Teres major, latissimus dorsi, deltoid (posterior portion), long head of triceps brachii (shoulder extension component).

Forearm. *Motion components:* Pronation. *Major muscle components:* Pronator quadratus.

Wrist. *Motion components:* Extension toward ulnar side. *Major muscle components:* Extensor carpi ulnaris.

Fingers. *Motion components:* Extension, abduction toward ulnar side. *Major muscle components:* Extensor digitorum communis, extensor digiti quinti proprius, abductor digiti quinti, dorsal interossei, lumbricales.

Thumb. *Motion components:* Extension with abduction and rotation toward ulnar side (palmar abduction). *Major muscle components:* Abductor pollicis brevis, extensor pollicis longus.

Range-Limiting Factors

Tension or contracture of any muscles of flexion – adduction – external rotation (with elbow straight) pattern (Fig. 1-44).

Extension–Abduction–Internal Rotation (D1 ex),
with Elbow Extension

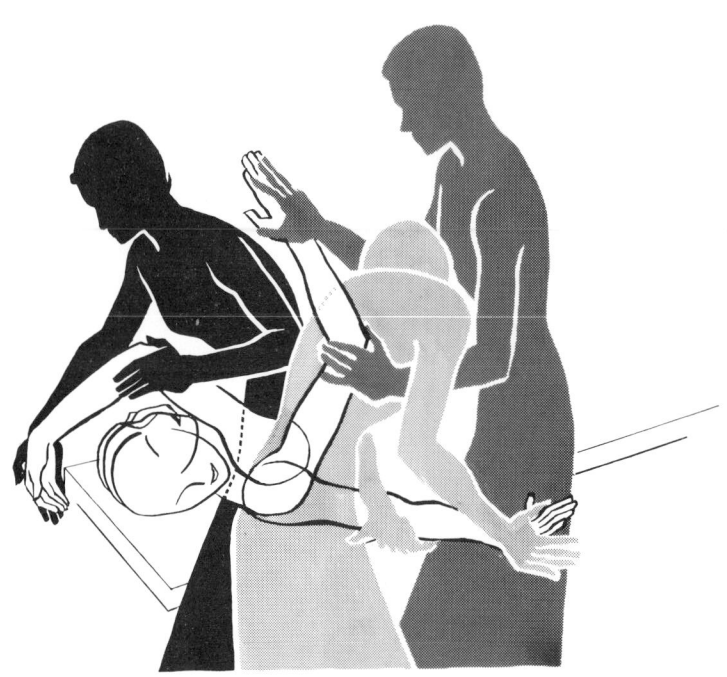

FIG. 1-48

Antagonistic Pattern

Flexion–adduction–external rotation (with elbow flexion) pattern (Fig. 1-45).

Components of Motion

The fingers extend and abduct toward ulnar side (medial fingers more than lateral); thumb extends, abducts, and internally rotates toward ulnar side (palmar abduction); wrist pronates and extends toward ulnar side; forearm pronates; elbow extends; shoulder extends, abducts, and internally rotates with scapula rotating, adducting (inferior angle) and depressing posteriorly (acromion); and clavicle rotates and depresses anteriorly away from sternum.

Normal Timing

Action is from distal to proximal, that is, action occurs first at fingers, thumb, wrist, and forearm, then at elbow, scapula, shoulder, and clavicle.

Timing for Emphasis

Scapula and Clavicle. Allow beginning rotation to occur at fingers, thumb, wrist, forearm, elbow, and shoulder, but do not allow full range of finger extension with abduction toward ulnar side, wrist pronation with extension toward ulnar side, forearm pronation, elbow extension, and shoulder extension–abduction to occur, until scapula begins to rotate, adduct, and depress posteriorly.

NOTE: If normal timing is prevented by excessive resistance to weak distal components, action cannot occur proximally. Resist stronger distal components, but guide weaker distal components through their optimal range of motion in accordance with normal timing.

Shoulder. Allow beginning rotation to occur at fingers, thumb, wrist, forearm, elbow, and shoulder, and scapula, but do not allow full range of finger extension with abduction toward ulnar side, wrist pronation with extension toward ulnar side, forearm pronation, elbow extension, and scapular rotation to occur, until shoulder begins to extend and abduct in internal rotation.

NOTE: Resist stronger proximal and distal components, but guide weaker distal components through their optimal range of motion in accordance with normal timing.

Elbow. Allow beginning rotation to occur at fingers, thumb, wrist, forearm, elbow, and shoulder, but do not allow full range of finger extension with abduction toward ulnar side, wrist pronation with extension toward ulnar side, forearm pronation, and shoulder extension–abduction to occur, until elbow begins to extend.

NOTE: Resist stronger proximal and distal components, but guide weaker distal components through their optimal range of motion in accordance with normal timing.

Forearm. Allow beginning rotation to occur at fingers, thumb, wrist, forearm, elbow, and shoulder, but do not allow full range of finger extension with abduction toward ulnar side, wrist pronation with extension toward ulnar side, elbow extension, and shoulder extension–abduction to occur, until forearm begins to pronate.

NOTE: Resist stronger proximal and distal components, but guide weaker distal components through their optimal range of motion in accordance with normal time.

Wrist. Allow beginning rotation to occur at fingers, thumb, wrist, forearm, elbow, and shoulder, but do not allow full range of finger extension with abduction toward ulnar side, forearm pronation, elbow extension, and shoulder extension–abduction to occur, until wrist begins to pronate and extend toward ulnar side.

NOTE: Resist stronger proximal and distal components, but guide weaker distal components through their optimal range of motion in accordance with normal timing.

Fingers. Allow beginning rotation to occur at fingers, thumb, wrist, forearm, elbow, and shoulder, but do not allow full range of wrist pronation with extension toward ulnar side, forearm pronation, elbow extension, and shoulder extension–abduction to occur, until fingers begin to extend and abduct toward ulnar side.

NOTE: Resist stronger proximal components. Emphasis may be placed on metacarpal–phalangeal joints, or interphalangeal joints, or emphasis may be placed on a specific joint of an individual digit.

Thumb. Allow beginning rotation to occur at fingers, thumb, wrist, forearm, elbow, and shoulder, but do not allow full range of finger extension with abduction toward ulnar side, wrist pronation with extension toward ulnar side, forearm pronation, elbow extension, and shoulder extension–abduction to occur, until thumb begins to extend and abduct toward ulnar side. Components of fingers and wrist must be allowed to move through range after motion is initiated at thumb. In shortened range of pattern, thumb is extended, abducted, and internally rotated away from second metacarpal.

NOTE: Resist stronger finger, wrist, and proximal components.

Manual Contacts

Right Hand. Palmar surface of hand and fingers cupped over dorsal–ulnar aspect of fingers and wrist of patient's right hand (Fig. 1-48).

Left Hand. For emphasis of distal joints: Grip with pressure of palmar surface over dorsal–ulnar aspect of forearm, to control pronation and proximal components of motion.

For emphasis of shoulder and elbow: Apply pressure of palmar surface to posterior–lateral surface of arm, to control internal rotation and proximal components of motion (Fig. 1-48).

For emphasis of scapula: Apply pressure of palmar surface of hand over scapula between spine and inferior angle, to control rotation and adduction.

For mass opening of hand and for emphasis of thumb motion: Grasp patient's right thumb with thumb and index finger of left hand; contact of physical therapist's thumb and finger should be medially and laterally at interphalangeal joint of patient's thumb, to control rotation of patient's thumb as well as extension and abduction components. Physical therapist's right hand should be cupped over dorsal and ulnar aspect of patient's right hand, to resist wrist extension toward ulnar side and finger extension and abduction toward ulnar side. Right hand of physical therapist also controls and resists proximal components of extension–abduction–internal rotation pattern.

Commands

Preparatory. "You are going to open your hand, turn it, push it down and away from your face, and extend your elbow."

Action. "Push! Open your hand! Turn it! Straighten your elbow! Push it down and out toward me!"

Pattern Analysis

Scapula. Motion components: Rotation, adduction (inferior angle), depession posteriorly (acromion). *Major muscle components:* Levator scapulae, rhomboidei minor and major.

Shoulder. Motion components: Extension, abduction, internal rotation. *Major muscle components:* Teres major, latissimus dorsi, deltoid (posterior portion), long head of triceps brachii (shoulder extension component.)

Elbow. Motion component: Extension. *Major muscle components:* Triceps brachii, anconeus and subanconeus.

Forearm. Motion components: Pronation. *Major muscle components:* Pronator quadratus.

Wrist, Fingers, and Thumb. See extension–abduction–internal rotation (with elbow straight) pattern.

Range-Limiting Factors

Tension or contracture of any muscles of flexion–adduction–external rotation (with elbow flexion) pattern (Fig. 1-45).

Extension–Abduction–Internal Rotation (D1 ex),
with Elbow Flexion

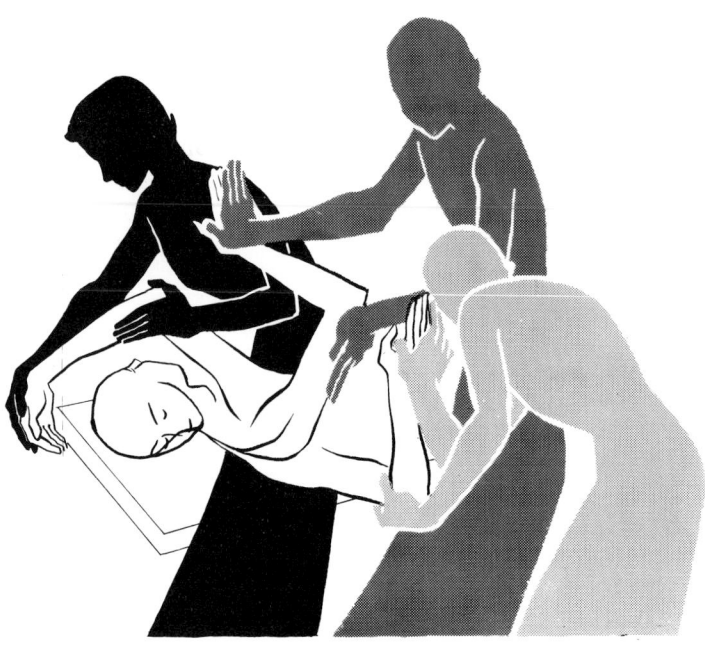

FIG. 1-49

Antagonistic Pattern

Flexion–adduction–external rotation (with elbow extension) pattern (Fig. 1-46).

Components of Motion

Fingers extend and adduct toward ulnar side (medial fingers more than lateral); thumb extends, abducts, and internally rotates toward ulnar side (palmar abduction); wrist pronates and extends toward ulnar side; forearm pronates; elbow flexes; shoulder extends, abducts, and internally rotates with scapula rotating, adducting (inferior angle), and depressing posteriorly (acromion); and clavicle rotates and depresses anteriorly away from sternum.

Normal Timing

Action is from distal to proximal, that is, action occurs first at fingers, thumb, wrist, and forearm, then at elbow, scapula, shoulder, and clavicle.

Timing for Emphasis

Scapula and Clavicle. Allow beginning rotation to occur at fingers, thumb, wrist, forearm, elbow, and shoulder, but do not allow full range of finger extension with abduction toward ulnar side, wrist pronation and extension toward ulnar side, forearm pronation, elbow flexion, and shoulder extension–abduction to occur, until scapula begins to rotate, adduct, and depress posteriorly.

NOTE: If normal timing is prevented by excessive resistance to weak distal components, action cannot occur proximally. Resist stronger distal components, but guide weaker distal components through their optimal range of motion in accordance with normal timing.

Shoulder. Allow beginning rotation to occur at fingers, thumb, wrist, forearm, elbow, shoulder, and scapula, but do not allow full range of finger extension with abduction toward ulnar side, wrist pronation with extension toward ulnar side, forearm pronation, elbow flexion, and scapular rotation to occur, until shoulder begins to extend and abduct in internal rotation.

NOTE: Resist stronger proximal and distal components, but guide weaker distal components through their optimal range of motion in accordance with normal timing.

Elbow. Allow beginning rotation to occur at fingers, thumb, wrist, forearm, elbow, and shoulder, but do not allow full range of finger extension with abduction toward ulnar side, wrist pronation with extension toward ulnar side, forearm pronation, and shoulder extension–abduction to occur, until elbow begins to flex.

NOTE: Resist stronger proximal and distal components, but guide weaker distal components through their optimal range of motion in accordance with normal timing.

Forearm. Allow beginning rotation to occur at fingers, thumb, wrist, forearm, elbow, and shoulder, but do not allow full range of finger extension with abduction toward ulnar side, wrist extension toward ulnar side, elbow flexion, and shoulder extension–abduction to occur, until forearm begins to pronate.

NOTE: Resist stronger proximal components, but guide weaker distal components through their optimal range of motion in accordance with normal timing.

Wrist. Allow beginning rotation to occur at fingers, thumb, wrist, forearm, elbow, and shoulder, but do not allow full range of finger extension with abduction toward ulnar side, forearm pronation, elbow flexion, and shoulder extension–abduction to occur, until wrist begins to pronate and extend toward ulnar side.

NOTE: Resist stronger proximal and distal components, but guide weaker distal components through their optimal range of motion in accordance with normal timing.

Fingers. Allow beginning rotation to occur at fingers, thumb, wrist, forearm, elbow, and shoulder, but do not allow full range of wrist pronation with extension toward ulnar side, forearm pronation, elbow flexion, and shoulder extension–abduction to occur, until fingers begin to extend and abduct toward ulnar side.

NOTE: Resist stronger proximal components. Emphasis may be placed on metacarpal–phalangeal joints, or interphalangeal joints, or emphasis may be placed on a specific joint of an individual digit.

Thumb. Allow beginning rotation to occur at fingers, thumb, wrist, forearm, elbow, and shoulder, but do not allow full range of finger extension with abduction toward ulnar side, wrist pronation with extension toward ulnar side, forearm pronation, elbow flexion, and shoulder extension–abduction to occur, until thumb begins to extend and abduct toward ulnar side. Components of fingers and wrist must be allowed to move through range after motion is initiated at thumb. In shortened range of pattern, thumb is extended, abducted, and internally rotated away from second metacarpal.

NOTE: Resist stronger finger, wrist, and proximal components.

Manual Contacts

Right Hand. Cup palmar surface of hand and fingers over dorsal–ulnar aspect of fingers and wrist of patient's right hand (Fig. 1-49).

Left Hand. *For emphasis of distal joints:* Grip with pressure of palmar surface over dorsal–ulnar aspect of forearm, to control pronation and proximal components of motion.

For emphasis of shoulder and elbow: Apply pressure of palmar surface on posterior–lateral surface of arm, to control internal rotation and proximal components of motion (Fig. 1-49).

For emphasis of scapula: Apply pressure of palmar surface of hand over scapula between spine and inferior angle, to control rotation and adduction.

For mass opening of hand and for emphasis of thumb motion: Grasp patient's right thumb with thumb and index finger of the left hand; contact of physical therapist's thumb and finger should be medially and laterally at interphalangeal joint of patient's thumb, to control rotation of patient's thumb as well as extension and abduction components. Physical therapist's right hand should be cupped over dorsal and ulnar aspect of patient's right hand, to resist wrist extension toward ulnar side and finger extension and abduction toward ulnar side. Right hand of physical therapist also controls and resists proximal components of extension–abduction–internal rotation pattern.

Commands

Preparatory. "You are going to open your hand, turn it, push it down and away from your face, and bend your elbow."

Action. "Push! Open your hand! Turn it! Bend your elbow! Push it toward me!"

Pattern Analysis*

Scapula. Motion components: Rotation, adduction (inferior angle), depression posteriorly (acromion). *Major muscle components:* Levator scapulae, rhomboidei minor and major.

Shoulder. Motion components: Extension, abduction, internal rotation. *Major muscle components:* Teres major, latissimus dorsi, deltoid (posterior portion).

Elbow. Motion component: Flexion. *Major muscle components:* Brachialis, biceps brachii (lateral portion).

Forearm. Motion component: Pronation. *Major muscle component:* Pronator quadratus.

Wrist, Fingers, and Thumb. See extension–abduction–internal rotation (with elbow straight) pattern.

Range-Limiting Factors

Tension or contracture of any muscles of flexion–adduction–external rotation (with elbow extension) pattern (Fig. 1-46).

---

* If extension–abduction–internal rotation is continued posteriorly, the motion components combine with those of the extension–adduction–internal rotation pattern. The fingers and wrist flex toward the ulnar side, the elbow may remain straight or flex, and the shoulder extends, adducts and internally rotates with the scapula rotating, adducting (inferior angle), and depressing anteriorly (acromion process). This movement is important to the complete reeducation of the latissimus dorsi with consideration given to the adduction component of this muscle.

*Flexion–Abduction–External Rotation (D2 fl), with
Elbow Straight*

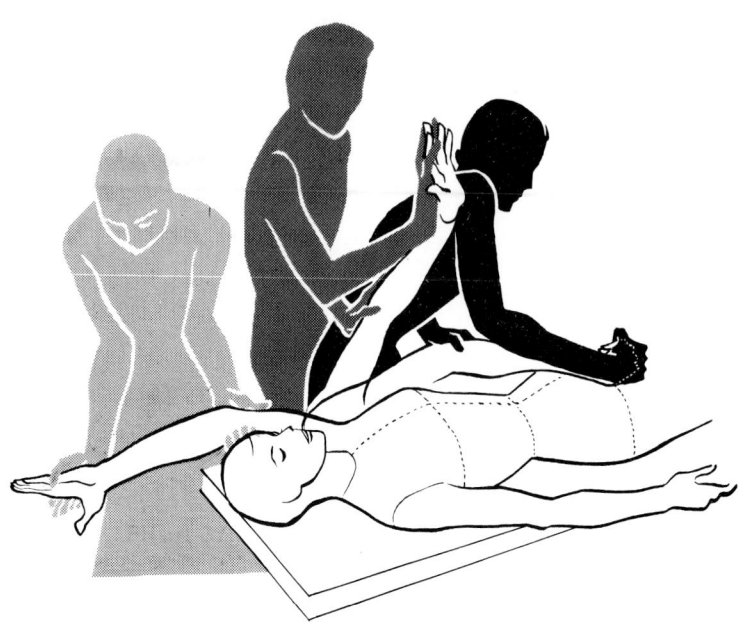

FIG. 1-50

Antagonistic Pattern

Extension–adduction–internal rotation (with elbow straight) pattern (Fig. 1-53).

Components of Motion

Fingers extend and abduct toward radial side (lateral fingers more than medial); thumb extends, adducts, and externally rotates toward radial side; wrist supinates and extends toward radial side; forearm supinates; elbow remains straight; shoulder flexes, abducts, and externally rotates with scapula rotating, adducting (medial angle), and elevating posteriorly (acromion); and clavicle rotates and elevates anteriorly away from sternum.

Normal Timing

Action is from distal to proximal, that is, action occurs first at fingers, thumb, wrist, and forearm, then at scapula, shoulder, and clavicle.

Timing for Emphasis

Scapula and Clavicle. Allow beginning rotation to occur at fingers, thumb, wrist, forearm, and shoulder, but do not allow full range of finger extension with abduction toward radial side, wrist supination with extension toward radial side, forearm supination, and shoulder flexion–abduction to occur, until scapula begins to rotate, adduct, and elevate posteriorly.

NOTE: If normal timing is prevented by excessive resistance to weak components, action cannot occur proximally. Resist stronger distal components, but guide weaker distal components through their optimal range of motion in accordance with normal timing.

Shoulder. Allow beginning rotation to occur at fingers, thumb, wrist, forearm, shoulder, and scapula, but do not allow full range of finger extension with abduction toward radial side, wrist supination with extension toward radial side, forearm supination, and scapular rotation to occur, until shoulder begins to flex and abduct in external rotation.

NOTE: Resist stronger proximal and distal components, but guide weaker distal components through their optimal range of motion in accordance with normal timing.

Forearm. Allow beginning rotation to occur at fingers, thumb, wrist, forearm, and shoulder, but do not allow full range of finger extension with abduction toward radial side, wrist supination with extension toward radial side, and shoulder flexion–abduction to occur, until forearm begins to supinate.

NOTE: Resist stronger proximal and distal components, but guide weaker distal components through their optimal range of motion in accordance with normal timing.

Wrist. Allow beginning rotation to occur at fingers, thumb, wrist, forearm and shoulder, but do

D2 fl, Le-R for Opening   REVERSAL: D2 ex, Le-R for Closing

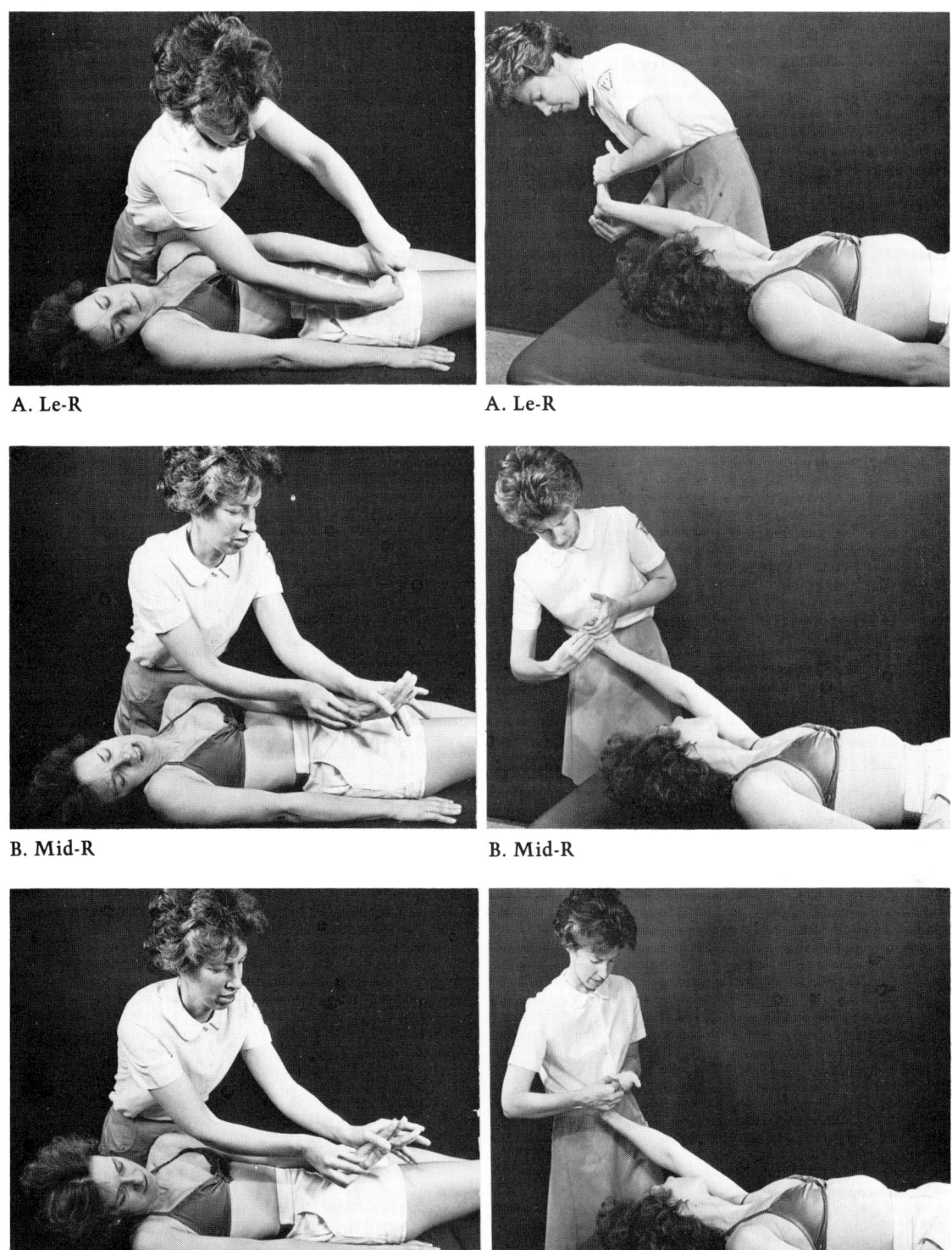

A. Le-R   A. Le-R

B. Mid-R   B. Mid-R

C. Sh-R   C. Sh-R

FIG. 1-50, *continued*

not allow full range of finger extension with abduction toward radial side, forearm supination, and shoulder flexion – abduction to occur, until wrist begins to supinate and extend toward radial side.

NOTE: Resist stronger proximal and distal components, but guide weaker distal components through their optimal range of motion in accordance with normal timing.

Fingers. Allow beginning rotation to occur at fingers, thumb, wrist, forearm, and shoulder, but do not allow full range of wrist supination with extension toward radial side, forearm supination, and shoulder flexion – abduction to occur, until fingers begin to extend and abduct toward radial side.

NOTE: Resist stronger proximal components. Emphasis may be placed on metacarpal – phalangeal joints or upon interphalangeal joints, or emphasis may be placed on a specific joint of an individual digit.

Thumb. Allow beginning rotation to occur at fingers, thumb, wrist, forearm, and shoulder, but do not allow full range of finger extension with abduction, wrist supination with extension toward radial side, forearm supination, and shoulder flexion – abduction to occur, until thumb begins to extend and adduct toward radial side. Components of fingers and wrist must be allowed to move through range after motion is initiated at thumb. In shortened range of

pattern, thumb is extended, adducted, and externally rotated toward second metacarpal.

NOTE: Resist stronger finger, wrist, and proximal components.

Manual Contacts

Right Hand. Palmar surface of hand and fingers cupped over dorsal – radial aspect of fingers and wrist of patient's left hand (Fig. 1-50).

Left Hand. For emphasis of distal joints: Grip with pressure of palmar surface over dorsal – radial aspect of forearm, to control supination and proximal components of motion.

For emphasis of shoulder: Apply pressure of palmar surface on anterior – lateral surface of patient's arm, to control rotation and proximal components of motion (Fig. 1-50).

For emphasis of scapula: Apply pressure of palmar surface of hand over scapula at medial angle, to control rotation and adduction.

For mass opening of hand and for emphasis of thumb motion: Grasp patient's left thumb with thumb and index finger of right hand; contact of physical therapist's thumb and finger should be medially and laterally at interphalangeal joint of patient's thumb, to control rotation of patient's thumb as well as extension and adduction components. Physical therapist's left hand should be cupped over dorsal and radial aspect of patient's left hand, to resist wrist extension toward radial side and finger extension with abduction toward radial side. Right hand of physical therapist also controls and resists proximal components of flexion – abduction – external rotation pattern.

Commands

Preparatory. "You are going to open your hand, turn it, and lift it up and out toward me, keeping your elbow straight."

Action. "Lift! Open your hand! Turn it! Keep your elbow straight! Lift it up toward me!"

Pattern Analysis

Scapula. *Motion components:* Rotation, adduction (medial angle), elevation posteriorly (acromion). *Major muscle components:* Trapezius (upper, middle, and lower portions).

Shoulder. *Motion components:* Flexion, abduction, external rotation. *Major muscle components:* Teres minor, supraspinatus, infraspinatus, deltoid (middle portion).

Forearm. *Motion component:* Supination. *Major muscle component:* Brachioradialis.

Wrist. *Motion component:* Extension toward radial side. *Major muscle components:* Extensor carpi radialis longus, extensor carpi radialis brevis.

Fingers. *Motion components:* Extension, abduction toward radial side. *Major muscle components:* Extensor digitorum communis, extensor indicis proprius, dorsal interossei, lumbricales.

Thumb. *Motion components:* Extension with adduction and rotation toward radial side. *Major muscle components:* Extensor pollicis longus, abductor pollicis longus, extensor pollicis brevis, first dorsal interosseus.

Range-Limiting Factors

Tension or contracture of any muscles of extension – adduction – internal rotation (with elbow straight) pattern (Fig. 1-53).

Flexion – Abduction – External Rotation (D2 fl), with
Elbow Flexion

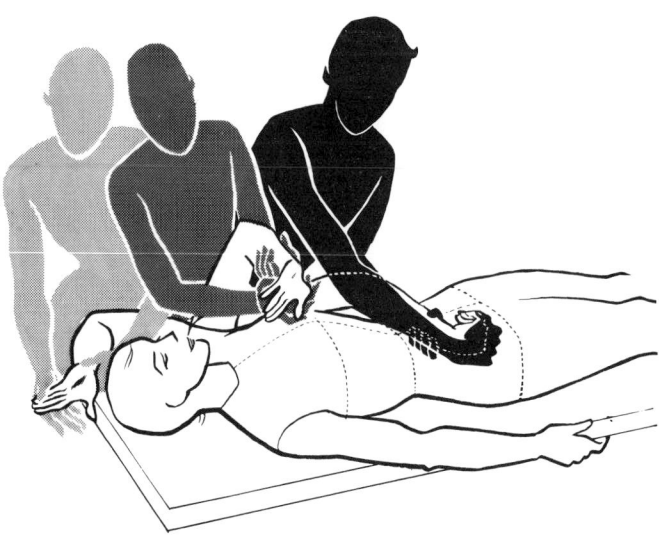

FIG. 1-51

Antagonistic Pattern

Extension – adduction – internal rotation (with elbow extension) pattern (Fig. 1-54).

Components of Motion

Fingers extend and abduct toward radial side (lateral fingers more than medial); thumb extends, adducts, and externally rotates toward radial side; wrist supinates and extends toward radial side; forearm supinates; elbow flexes; shoulder flexes, abducts, and externally rotates with scapula rotating, adducting (medial angle), and elevating posteriorly (acromion); and clavicle rotates and elevates anteriorly away from sternum.

Normal Timing

Action is from distal to proximal, that is, action occurs first at fingers, thumb, wrist, and forearm, then at elbow, scapula, shoulder, and clavicle.

Timing for Emphasis

Scapula and Clavicle. Allow beginning rotation to occur at fingers, thumb, wrist, forearm, elbow, and shoulder, but do not allow full range of finger extension with abduction toward radial side, wrist supination with extension toward the radial side, forearm supination, elbow flexion, and shoulder flexion – abduction to occur, until scapula begins to rotate, adduct, and elevate posteriorly.

NOTE: If normal timing of pattern is prevented by excessive resistance to weak components, action cannot occur proximally. Resist stronger distal components, but guide weaker distal components through their optimal range of motion in accordance with normal timing.

Shoulder. Allow beginning rotation to occur at fingers, thumb, wrist, forearm, elbow, shoulder, and scapula, but do not allow full range of finger extension with abduction toward radial side, wrist supination with extension toward radial side, forearm supination, elbow flexion, and scapular rotation to occur, until shoulder begins to flex and abduct in external rotation.

NOTE: Resist stronger proximal and distal components, but guide weaker distal components through their optimal range of motion in accordance with normal timing.

Elbow. Allow beginning rotation to occur at fingers, thumb, wrist, forearm, elbow, and shoulder, but do not allow full range of finger extension with abduction toward radial side, wrist supination with extension toward radial side, forearm supination, and shoulder flexion – abduction to occur, until elbow begins to flex.

NOTE: Resist stronger proximal and distal components, but guide weaker distal components through their optimal range of motion in accordance with normal timing.

Forearm. Allow beginning rotation to occur at fingers, thumb, wrist, forearm, elbow, and shoulder, but do not allow full range of finger extension with abduction toward radial side, wrist supination with extension toward radial side, elbow flexion, and shoulder flexion–abduction to occur, until forearm begins to supinate.

NOTE: Resist stronger proximal and distal components, but guide weaker distal components through their optimal range of motion in accordance with normal timing.

Wrist. Allow beginning rotation to occur at fingers, thumb, wrist, forearm, elbow, and shoulder, but do not allow full range of finger extension with abduction toward radial side, forearm supination, elbow flexion, and shoulder flexion–abduction to occur, until wrist begins to supinate and extend toward radial side.

NOTE: Resist stronger proximal and distal components, but guide weaker components through their optimal range of motion in accordance with normal timing.

Fingers. Allow beginning rotation to occur at fingers, thumb, wrist, forearm, elbow, and shoulder, but do not allow full range of wrist supination with extension toward radial side, forearm supination, elbow flexion, and shoulder flexion–abduction to occur, until fingers begin to extend and abduct toward radial side.

NOTE: Resist stronger proximal components. Emphasis may be placed upon metacarpal–phalangeal joints, or interphalangeal joints, or emphasis may be placed upon a specific joint of an individual digit.

Thumb. Allow beginning rotation to occur at fingers, thumb, wrist, forearm, elbow, and shoulder, but do not allow full range of finger extension with abduction toward radial side, wrist supination with extension toward radial side, forearm supination, elbow flexion, and shoulder flexion–abduction to occur, until thumb begins to extend and adduct toward radial side. Components of fingers and wrist must be allowed to move through range after motion is initiated at thumb. In shortened range of pattern, thumb is extended, adducted, and externally rotated toward second metacarpal.

NOTE: Resist stronger finger, wrist, and proximal components.

Manual Contacts

Right Hand. Palmar surface of hand and fingers cupped over dorsal–radial aspect of fingers and wrist of patient's left hand (Fig. 1-51).

Left Hand. *For emphasis of distal joints:* Grip with pressure of palmar surface over dorsal–radial aspect of forearm, to control supination and proximal components of motion (Fig. 1-51).

For emphasis of shoulder and elbow: Apply pressure of palmar surface on anterior–lateral surface of patient's arm, to control rotation and proximal components of motion.

For emphasis of scapula: Apply pressure of palmar surface of hand over scapula at medial angle, to control rotation and adduction.

For mass opening of hand and for emphasis of thumb motion: Grasp patient's left thumb with thumb and index finger of right hand; contact of physical therapist's thumb and finger should be medially and laterally at interphalangeal joint of patient's thumb, to control rotation of patient's thumb as well as extension and adduction components. Physical therapist's left hand should be cupped over dorsal and radial aspect of patient's left hand, to resist extension toward radial side and finger extension with abduction toward radial side. Right hand of physical therapist also controls and resists proximal components of flexion–abduction–external rotation pattern.

Commands

Preparatory. "You are going to open your hand, turn it, and lift it up and out toward me, bending your elbow."

Action. "Pull! Open your hand! Turn it! Bend your elbow! Pull it up here toward me!"

Pattern Analysis

Scapula. *Motion components:* Rotation, adduction (medial angle), elevation posteriorly (acromion). *Major muscle components:* Trapezius (upper, middle, and lower portions).

Shoulder. *Motion components:* Flexion, abduction, external rotation. *Major muscle components:* Teres minor, supraspinatus, infraspinatus, deltoid (middle portion), biceps brachii (long head: shoulder flexion component).

Elbow. *Motion component:* Flexion. *Major muscle components:* Biceps brachii (long head, lateral portion), brachioradialis.

Forearm. *Motion component:* Supination. *Major muscle component:* Brachioradialis.

Wrist, Fingers, and Thumb. See flexion–abduction–external rotation (with elbow straight) pattern.

Range-Limiting Factors

Tension or contracture of any muscles of extention–adduction–internal rotation (with elbow extension) pattern (Fig. 1-54).

*Flexion–Abduction–External Rotation (D2 fl), with
Elbow Extension*

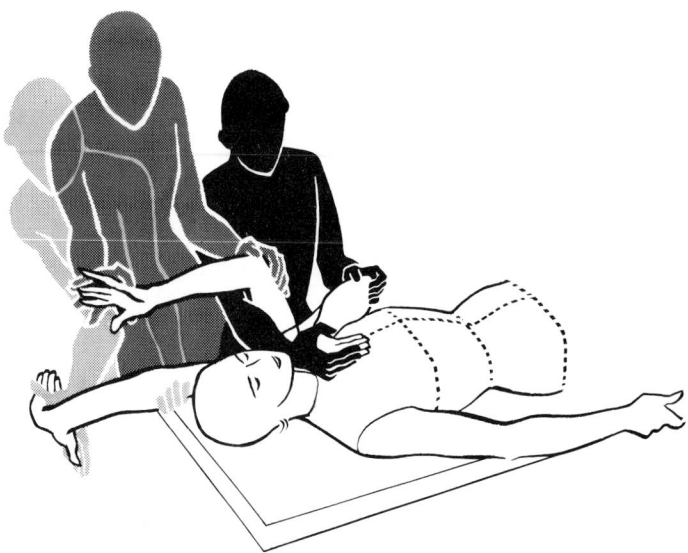

FIG. 1-52

Antagonistic Pattern

Extension–adduction–internal rotation (with elbow flexion) pattern (Fig. 1-55).

Components of Motion

Fingers extend with abduction toward radial side (lateral fingers more than medial); thumb extends, adducts, and externally rotates toward radial side; wrist supinates and extends toward radial side; forearm supinates; elbow extends; shoulder flexes, abducts, and externally rotates with scapula rotating, adducting (medial angle), and elevating posteriorly (acromion); and clavicle rotates and elevates anteriorly away from sternum.

Normal Timing

Action occurs from distal to proximal, that is, action occurs first at fingers, thumb, wrist, and forearm, then at elbow, scapula, shoulder, and clavicle.

Timing for Emphasis

Scapula and Clavicle. Allow beginning rotation to occur at fingers, thumb, wrist, forearm, elbow, and shoulder, but do not allow full range of finger extension with abduction toward radial side, wrist supination with extension toward radial side, forearm supination, elbow extension, and shoulder flexion–abduction to occur, until scapula begins to rotate, ad-

duct, and elevate posteriorly.

NOTE: If normal timing is prevented by excessive resistance to weak components, action cannot occur proximally. Resist stronger distal components, but guide weaker distal components through their optimal range of motion in accordance with normal timing.

Shoulder. Allow beginning rotation to occur at fingers, thumb, wrist, forearm, elbow, shoulder, and scapula, but do not allow full range of finger extension with abduction toward radial side, wrist supination with extension toward radial side, forearm supination, elbow extension, and scapular rotation to occur, until shoulder begins to flex and abduct in external rotation.

NOTE: Resist stronger proximal and distal components, but guide weaker distal components through their optimal range of motion in accordance with normal timing.

Elbow. Allow beginning rotation to occur at fingers, thumb, wrist, forearm, elbow, and shoulder, but do not allow full range of finger extension with abduction toward radial side, wrist supination with extension toward radial side, forearm supination, and shoulder flexion–abduction to occur, until elbow begins to flex.

NOTE: Resist stronger proximal and distal components, but

guide weaker distal components through their optimal range of motion in accordance with normal timing.

Forearm. Allow beginning rotation to occur at fingers, thumb, wrist, forearm, elbow, and shoulder, but do not allow full range of finger extension with abduction toward radial side, wrist supination with extension toward radial side, elbow extension, and shoulder flexion–abduction to occur, until forearm begins to supinate.

NOTE: Resist stronger proximal and distal components, but guide weaker distal components through their optimal range of motion in accordance with normal timing.

Wrist. Allow beginning rotation to occur at fingers, thumb, wrist, forearm, elbow, and shoulder, but do not allow full range of finger extension with abduction toward radial side, forearm supination, elbow extension, and shoulder flexion–abduction to occur, until wrist begins to supinate and extend toward radial side.

NOTE: Resist stronger proximal and distal components, but guide weaker distal components through their optimal range of motion in accordance with normal timing.

Fingers. Allow beginning rotation to occur at fingers, thumb, wrist, forearm, elbow, and shoulder, but do not allow full range of wrist supination with extension toward radial side, forearm supination, elbow extension, and shoulder flexion–abduction to occur, until the fingers begin to extend and abduct toward radial side.

NOTE: Resist stronger proximal components. Emphasis may be placed upon metacarpal–phalangeal joints, or interphalangeal joints, or emphasis may be placed upon a specific joint of an individual digit.

Thumb. Allow beginning rotation to occur at fingers, thumb, wrist, forearm, elbow, and shoulder, but do not allow full range of finger extension with abduction toward radial side, wrist supination with extension toward radial side, forearm supination, elbow extension, and shoulder flexion–abduction to occur, until thumb begins to extend and adduct toward radial side. Components of fingers and wrist must be allowed to move through range after motion is initiated at thumb. In shortened range of pattern thumb is extended, adducted, and externally rotated toward second metacarpal.

NOTE: Resist stronger finger, wrist, and proximal components.

Manual Contacts

Right Hand. Cup palmar surface of hand and fingers over dorsal–radial aspect of fingers and wrist of patient's left hand (Fig. 1-52).

Left Hand. For emphasis of distal joints: Grip with pressure of palmar surface over dorsal–radial aspect of forearm, to control supination and proximal components of motion.

For emphasis of shoulder and elbow: Apply pressure of palmar surface on anterior–lateral surface of patient's arm, to control rotation and proximal components of motion (Fig. 1-52).

For emphasis of scapula: Apply pressure of palmar surface of hand over scapula at medial angle, to control rotation and adduction.

For mass opening of hand and for emphasis of thumb motion: Grasp patient's left thumb with thumb and index finger of right hand; contact of physical therapist's thumb and finger should be medially and laterally at interphalangeal joint of patient's thumb, to control rotation of patient's thumb as well as extension and adduction components. Physical therapist's left hand should be cupped over dorsal and radial aspect of patient's left hand, to resist wrist extension toward radial side and finger extension with abduction toward radial side. Right hand of physical therapist also controls and resists proximal components of flexion–abduction–external rotation pattern.

Commands

Preparatory. "You are going to open your hand, turn it, and push it up and out toward me, straightening your elbow."

Action. "Push! Open your hand! Turn it! Push it up and out toward me! Straighten your elbow!"

Pattern analysis

Scapula. Motion components: Rotation, adduction (medial angle), elevation posteriorly (acromion). *Major muscle components:* Trapezius (upper, middle and lower portions).

Shoulder. Motion components: Flexion, abduction, external rotation. *Major muscle components:* Teres minor, supraspinatus, infraspinatus, deltoid (middle portion).

Elbow. Motion component: Extension. *Major muscle components:* Triceps brachii (lateral portion), anconeus.

Forearm. Motion component: Supination. *Major muscle component:* Brachioradialis.

Wrist, Fingers, and Thumb. See flexion–abduction–external rotation (with elbow straight) pattern.

Range-Limiting Factors

Tension or contracture of any muscles of extension–adduction–internal rotation (with elbow flexion) pattern (Fig. 1-55).

Extension–Adduction–Internal Rotation (D2 ex),
with Elbow Straight

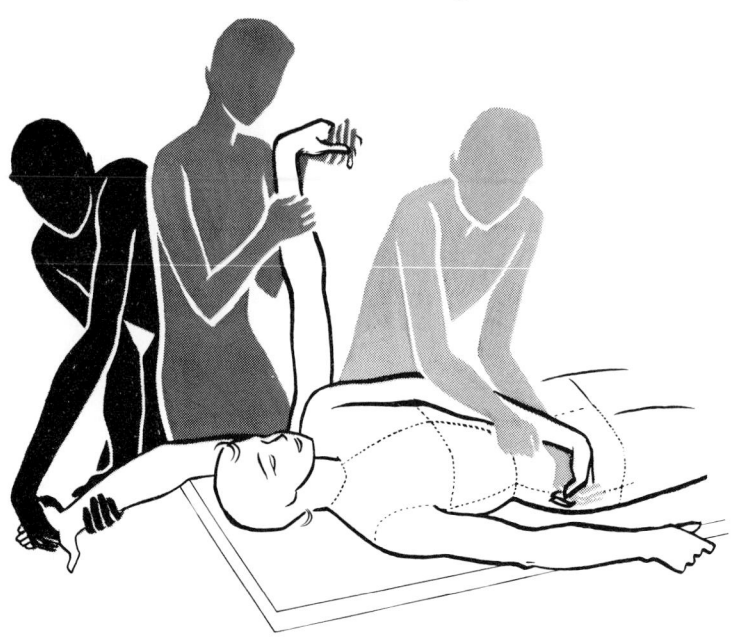

FIG. 1-53

Antagonistic Pattern

Flexion – abduction – external rotation (with elbow straight) pattern (Fig. 1-50).

Components of Motion

Fingers flex and adduct (medial fingers more than lateral) toward ulnar side; thumb flexes, abducts, and internally rotates toward ulnar side (opposition); wrist pronates and flexes toward ulnar side; forearm pronates; elbow remains straight; shoulder extends, adducts, and internally rotates with scapula rotating, abducting (medial angle) and depressing anteriorly (acromion); and clavicle rotates and depresses anteriorly in approximation with sternum.

Normal Timing

Action is from distal to proximal, that is, action occurs first at fingers, thumb, wrist, and forearm, then at shoulder, scapula, and clavicle.

Timing for Emphasis

Scapula and Clavicle. Allow beginning rotation to occur at fingers, thumb, wrist, forearm, and shoulder, but do not allow full range of finger flexion with adduction toward ulnar side, wrist pronation and flexion toward ulnar side, forearm pronation, and shoulder extension – adduction to occur, until scapula begins to rotate, abduct, and depress anteriorly.

NOTE: If normal timing is prevented by excessive resistance to weak components, action cannot occur proximally. Resist stronger distal components, but guide weaker components through their optimal range of motion in accordance with normal timing.

Shoulder. Allow beginning rotation to occur at fingers, thumb, wrist, forearm, and shoulder, but do not allow full range of finger flexion with adduction toward ulnar side, wrist pronation with flexion toward ulnar side, and forearm pronation to occur, until shoulder begins to extend and adduct in internal rotation.

NOTE: Resist stronger distal components, but guide weaker components through their optimal range of motion in accordance with normal timing.

Forearm. Allow beginning rotation to occur at fingers, thumb, wrist, forearm, and shoulder, but do not allow full range of finger flexion with adduction toward ulnar side, wrist pronation with flexion toward ulnar side, and shoulder extension – adduction to occur, until forearm begins to pronate.

NOTE: Resist stronger proximal and distal components, but guide weaker distal components through their optimal range of motion in accordance with normal timing.

Wrist. Allow beginning rotation to occur at fingers, thumb, wrist, forearm, and shoulder, but do

D2 ex, Le-R for Closing   REVERSAL: D2 fl, Sh-R for Opening

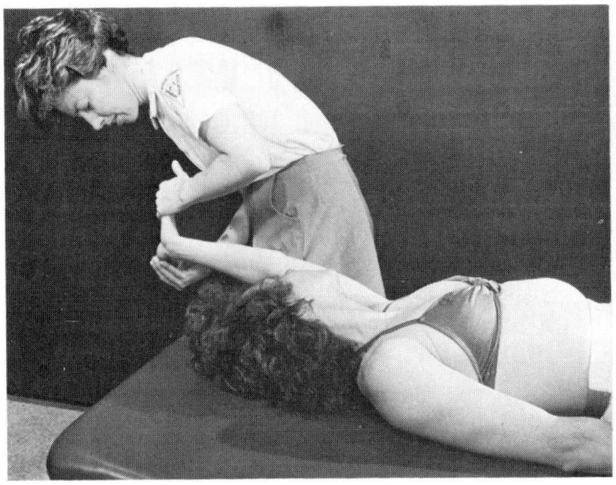

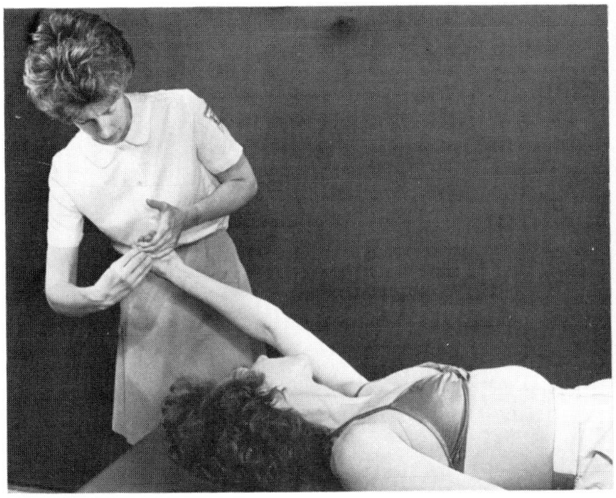

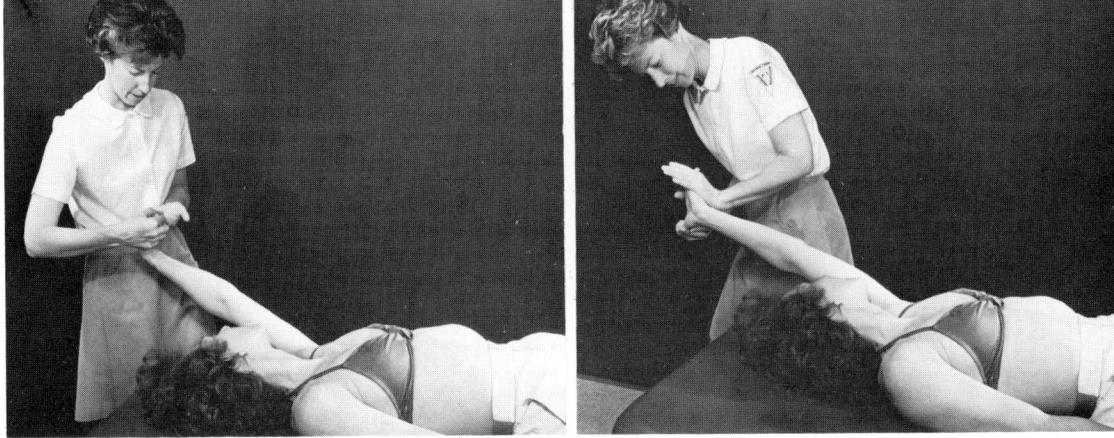

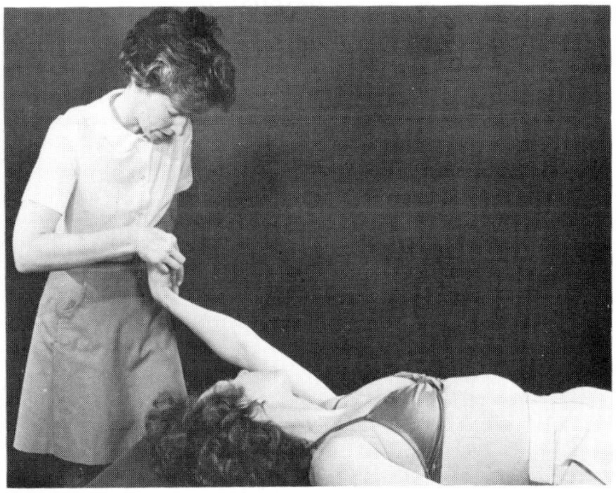

A. Le-R   A. Le-R

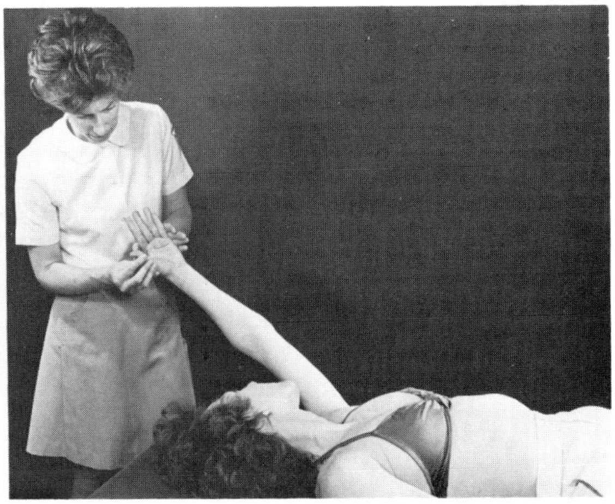

B. Mid-R   B. Mid-R

C. Sh-R   C. Sh-R

FIG. 1-53, *continued*

not allow full range of finger flexion with adduction toward ulnar side, forearm pronation, and shoulder extension–adduction to occur, until wrist begins to pronate and flex toward ulnar side.

NOTE: Resist stronger proximal and distal components, but guide weaker distal components through their optimal range of motion in accordance with normal timing.

Fingers. Allow beginning rotation to occur at fingers, thumb, wrist, forearm, and shoulder, but do not allow full range of wrist pronation with flexion toward ulnar side, forearm pronation, and shoulder extension–adduction to occur, until fingers begin to flex and adduct toward ulnar side.

NOTE: Resist stronger proximal components. Emphasis may be placed upon metacarpal–phalangeal joints, or interphalangeal joints, or emphasis may be placed upon a specific joint of an individual digit.

Thumb. Allow beginning rotation to occur at fingers, thumb, wrist, forearm, and shoulder, but do not allow full range of finger flexion with adduction toward ulnar side, wrist pronation with flexion toward ulnar side, forearm pronation, and shoulder extension–adduction to occur, until thumb begins to flex and abduct toward ulnar side. Components of fingers and wrist must be allowed to move through range after motion is initiated at thumb. In shortened range of pattern, thumb is flexed, abducted, and internally rotated away from second metacarpal and toward fifth metacarpal.

NOTE: Resist stronger components of fingers and wrist, and all proximal components.

Manual Contacts

Left Hand. Place in palm of patient's left hand so that patient may grasp with fingers and thumb, and so that wrist may flex toward ulnar side (Fig. 1-53).

Right Hand. For emphasis of distal joints: Grip with pressure of palmar surface over anterior–ulnar aspect of patient's forearm, to control pronation and proximal components of motion (Fig. 1-53).

For emphasis of shoulder: Apply pressure of palmar surface on posterior–medial surface of patient's arm, to control internal rotation and proximal components of motion.

For emphasis of scapula: Apply pressure of palmar surface of hand over anterior–medial axillary space and acromion process.

For mass closing of hand and for emphasis of thumb motion: Grasp patient's left thumb with thumb and index finger of right hand; contact of physical therapist's thumb and index finger should be medially and laterally at interphalangeal joint of patient's thumb, to control rotation of patient's thumb as well as the flexion and abduction components. Physical therapist's left hand should be placed with palmar surface of hand and fingers on palmar surface of hand and fingers of patient's left hand. Physical therapist's left hand prevents range of motion occurring proximally until fingers flex and adduct toward ulnar side. Flexion of all fingers and thumb flexion–adduction may be resisted.

Commands

Preparatory. "You are going to squeeze my hand, turn it, and pull it down toward your right hip, keeping your elbow straight."

Action. "Pull! Squeeze my hand! Turn it! Keep your elbow straight! Pull it down toward your right hip!"

Pattern Analysis

Scapula. *Motion components:* Rotation, abduction (medial angle), depression anteriorly (acromion). *Major muscle components:* Pectoralis minor, subclavius (acting upon clavicle).

Shoulder. *Motion components:* Extension, adduction, internal rotation. *Major muscle components:* Subscapularis, pectoralis major (sternal portion).

Forearm. *Motion component:* Pronation. *Major muscle component:* Pronator teres.

Wrist. *Motion components:* Pronation, flexion toward ulnar side. *Major muscle components:* Flexor carpi ulnaris, palmaris longus.

Fingers. *Motion components:* Flexion, adduction toward ulnar side. *Major muscle components:* Flexor digitorum superficialis, flexor digitorum profundus, palmar interossei, lumbricales.

Thumb. *Motion components:* Flexion, abduction, rotation away from second metacarpal. *Major muscle components:* Flexor pollicis longus, flexor pollicis brevis, opponens pollicis, palmaris brevis.

Range-Limiting Factors

Tension or contracture of any muscles of the flexion–abduction–external rotation (with elbow straight) pattern (Fig. 1-50).

Extension–Adduction–Internal Rotation (D2 ex), with Elbow Extension

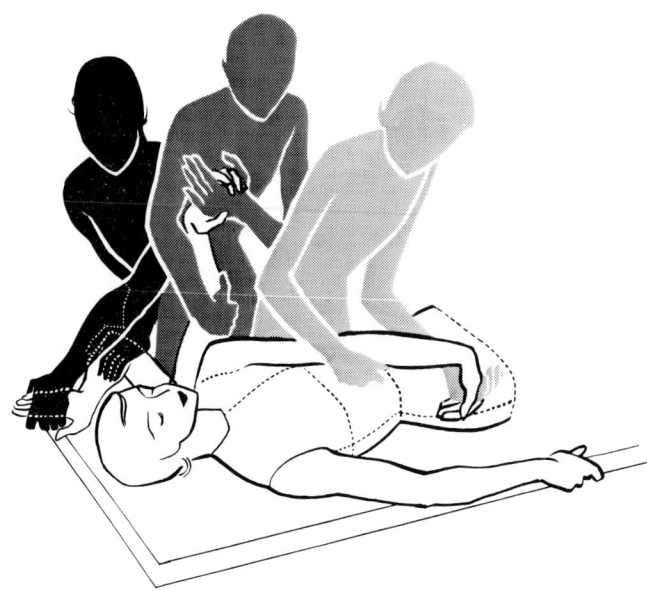

FIG. 1-54

Antagonistic Pattern

Flexion–abduction–external rotation (with elbow flexion) pattern (Fig. 1-51).

Components of Motion

Fingers flex and adduct (medial fingers more than lateral) toward ulnar side; thumb flexes, abducts, and internally rotates toward ulnar side (opposition); wrist pronates and flexes toward ulnar side; forearm pronates; elbow extends; shoulder extends, adducts, and internally rotates with scapula rotating, abducting (medial angle), and depressing anteriorly (acromion); and clavicle rotates and depresses anteriorly in approximation with sternum.

Normal Timing

Action is from distal to proximal, that is, action occurs first at fingers, thumb, wrist, and forearm, then at elbow, shoulder, scapula, and clavicle.

Timing for Emphasis

Scapula and Clavicle. Allow beginning rotation to occur at fingers, thumb, wrist, forearm, elbow, and shoulder, but do not allow full range of finger flexion with adduction toward ulnar side, wrist pronation with flexion toward ulnar side, forearm pronation, elbow extension, and shoulder extension–adduction to occur, until scapula begins to rotate, abduct, and depress anteriorly.

NOTE: If the normal timing is prevented by excessive resistance to weak components, action cannot occur proximally.

Resist stronger distal components, but guide weaker distal components through their optimal range of motion in accordance with normal timing.

Shoulder. Allow beginning rotation to occur at fingers, thumb, wrist, forearm, elbow, and shoulder, but do not allow full range of finger flexion with adduction toward ulnar side, wrist pronation with flexion toward ulnar side, forearm pronation, and elbow extension to occur, until shoulder begins to extend and adduct in internal rotation.

NOTE: Resist stronger distal components, but guide weaker components through their optimal range.

Elbow. Allow beginning rotation to occur at fingers, thumb, wrist, forearm, elbow, and shoulder, but do not allow full range of finger flexion with adduction toward ulnar side, wrist pronation with flexion toward ulnar side, forearm pronation, and shoulder extension–adduction to occur, until elbow begins to extend.

NOTE: Resist stronger proximal and distal components, but guide weaker distal components through their optimal range of motion in accordance with normal timing.

Forearm. Allow beginning rotation to occur at fingers, thumb, wrist, forearm, elbow, and shoulder, but do not allow full range of finger flexion with adduction toward ulnar side, wrist pronation with flexion toward ulnar side, elbow extension, and shoulder extension–adduction to occur, until forearm begins to pronate.

NOTE: Resist stronger proximal and distal components, but guide weaker distal components through their optimal range of motion in accordance with normal timing.

Wrist. Allow beginning rotation to occur at fingers, thumb, wrist, forearm, elbow, and shoulder, but do not allow full range of finger flexion with adduction toward ulnar side, forearm pronation, elbow extension, and shoulder extension–adduction to occur, until wrist begins to pronate and flex toward ulnar side.

NOTE: Resist stronger proximal and distal components, but guide weaker distal components through their optimal range of motion in accordance with normal timing.

Fingers. Allow beginning rotation to occur at fingers, thumb, wrist, forearm, elbow, and shoulder, but do not allow full range of wrist pronation with flexion toward ulnar side, forearm pronation, elbow extension, and shoulder extension–adduction to occur, until fingers begin to flex and adduct toward ulnar side.

NOTE: Resist all stronger proximal components. Emphasis may be placed upon metacarpal–phalangeal joints, or interphalangeal joints, or emphasis may be placed upon a specific joint of an individual digit.

Thumb. Allow beginning rotation to occur at fingers, thumb, wrist, forearm, elbow, and shoulder, but do not allow full range of finger flexion with adduction toward ulnar side, wrist pronation with flexion toward ulnar side, forearm pronation, elbow extension, and shoulder extension–adduction to occur, until thumb begins to flex and abduct toward ulnar side. Components of finger and wrist must be allowed to move through range after motion is initiated at thumb. In shortened range of pattern, thumb is flexed, abducted, and internally rotated away from second metacarpal and toward fifth metacarpal.

NOTE: Resist all stronger finger, wrist, and proximal components.

Manual Contacts

Left Hand. Place in palm of patient's left hand, so that patient may grasp with fingers and thumb, and so that wrist may flex toward ulnar side (Fig. 1-54).

Right Hand. *For emphasis of distal joints:* Grip with pressure of palmar surface over anterior–ulnar aspect of patient's forearm, to control pronation and proximal components of motion (Fig. 1-54).

For emphasis of shoulder and elbow: Apply pressure of palmar surface on posterior–medial surface of patient's arm, to control internal rotation and proximal components of motion.

For emphasis of scapula: Apply pressure of palmar surface of hand over anterior–medial axillary space and acromion process.

For mass closing of hand and for emphasis of thumb motion: Grasp patient's left thumb with thumb and index finger of right hand; contact of physical therapist's thumb and index finger should be medially and laterally at interphalangeal joint of patient's thumb, to control rotation of patient's thumb as well as flexion and abduction components. Physical therapist's left hand should be placed with palmar surface of hand and fingers on palmar surface of hand and fingers of patient's left hand. Physical therapist's left hand prevents range of motion occurring proximally until fingers flex and adduct toward ulnar side. Flexion of all fingers and thumb flexion–abduction may be resisted.

Commands

Preparatory. "You are to squeeze my hand, turn it, and push it down and toward your right hip, straightening your elbow."

Action. "Push! Squeeze my hand! Turn it! Straighten your elbow! Push it toward your right hip!"

Pattern Analysis

Scapula. *Motion components:* Rotation, abduction (medial angle), depression anteriorly (acromion). *Major muscle components:* Pectoralis minor, subclavius (acting upon clavicle).

Shoulder. *Motion components:* Extension, adduction, internal rotation. *Major muscle components:* Subscapularis, pectoralis major (sternal portion), triceps brachii (long head, shoulder extension component).

Elbow. *Motion component:* Extension. *Major muscle components:* Triceps brachii, anconeus, subanconeus.

Forearm. *Motion component:* Pronation. *Major muscle component:* Pronator teres.

Wrist, Fingers, and Thumb. See extension–adduction–internal rotation (with elbow straight) pattern.

Range-Limiting Factors

Tension or contracture of any muscles of the flexion–abduction–external rotation (with elbow flexion) pattern (Fig. 1-51).

Extension–Adduction–Internal Rotation (D2 ex),
with Elbow Flexion

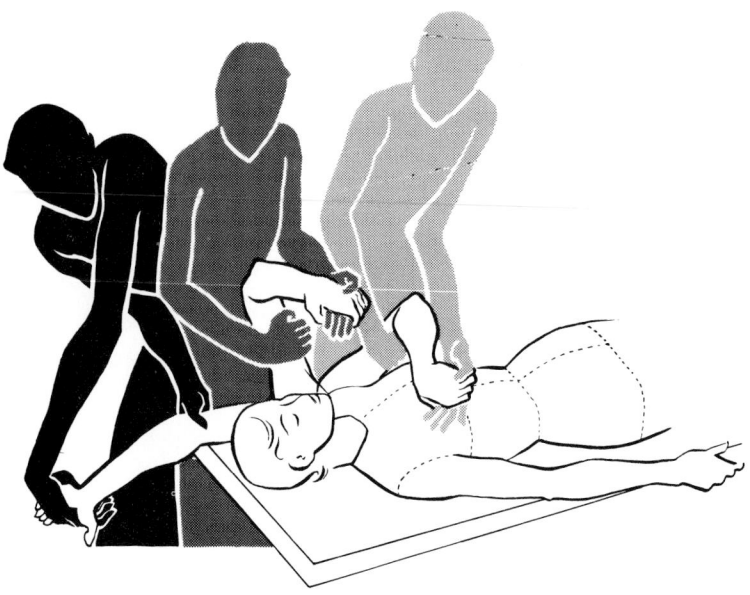

FIG. 1-55

Antagonistic Pattern

Flexion–abduction–external rotation (with elbow extension) pattern (Fig. 1-52).

Components of Motion

Fingers flex and adduct (medial fingers more than lateral) toward ulnar side; thumb flexes, abducts, and internally rotates toward ulnar side (opposition); wrist pronates and flexes toward ulnar side; forearm pronates; elbow flexes; shoulder extends, adducts, and internally rotates with scapula rotating, abducting (medial angle), and depressing anteriorly (acromion); and clavicle rotates and depresses anteriorly in approximation with sternum.

Normal Timing

Action is from distal to proximal, that is, action occurs first at fingers, thumb, wrist, and forearm, then at elbow, shoulder, scapula, and clavicle.

Timing for Emphasis

Scapula and Clavicle. Allow beginning rotation to occur at fingers, thumb, wrist, forearm, elbow, and shoulder, but do not allow full range of finger flexion with adduction toward ulnar side, wrist pronation with flexion toward ulnar side, forearm pronation, elbow flexion, and shoulder extension–adduction to occur, until scapula begins to rotate, abduct, and depress anteriorly.

NOTE: If normal timing is prevented by excessive resistance to weak components, action cannot occur proximally. Resist stronger distal components, but guide weaker distal components through their optimal range of motion in accordance with normal timing.

Shoulder. Allow beginning rotation to occur at fingers, thumb, wrist, forearm, elbow, and shoulder, but do not allow full range of finger flexion with adduction toward ulnar side, wrist pronation with flexion toward ulnar side, forearm pronation, and elbow flexion to occur, until shoulder begins to extend and adduct in internal rotation.

NOTE: Resist stronger distal components, but guide weaker distal components through their optimal range of motion in accordance with normal timing.

Elbow. Allow beginning rotation to occur at fingers, thumb, wrist, forearm, elbow, and shoulder, but do not allow full range of finger flexion with adduction toward ulnar side, wrist pronation with flexion toward ulnar side, forearm pronation, and shoulder extension–adduction to occur, until elbow begins to flex.

NOTE: Resist stronger proximal and distal components, but guide weaker distal components through their optimal range of motion in accordance with normal timing.

Forearm. Allow beginning rotation to occur at fingers, thumb, wrist, forearm, elbow, and shoulder, but do not allow full range of finger flexion with ad-duction toward ulnar side, wrist pronation with flex-ion toward ulnar side, elbow flexion, and shoulder ex-tension – adduction to occur, until forearm begins to pronate.

NOTE: Resist stronger proximal and distal components, but guide weaker distal components through their optimal range of motion in accordance with normal timing.

Wrist. Allow beginning rotation to occur at fingers, thumb, wrist, forearm, elbow, and shoulder, but do not allow full range of finger flexion with ad-duction toward ulnar side, forearm pronation, elbow flexion, and shoulder extension – adduction to occur, until wrist begins to pronate and flex toward ulnar side.

NOTE: Resist stronger proximal and distal components, but guide weaker distal components through their optimal range of motion in accordance with normal timing.

Fingers. Allow beginning rotation to occur at fingers, thumb, wrist, forearm, elbow, and shoulder, but do not allow full range of wrist pronation with flexion toward ulnar side, forearm pronation, elbow flexion, and shoulder extension – adduction to occur, until fingers begin to flex and adduct toward ulnar side.

NOTE: Resist stronger proximal and distal components, but guide weaker distal components through their optimal range of motion in accordance with normal timing. Emphasis may be placed upon metacarpal – phalangeal joints, or interpha-langeal joints, or emphasis may be placed upon a specific joint of an individual digit.

Thumb. Allow beginning rotation to occur at fingers, thumb, wrist, forearm, elbow, and shoulder, but do not allow full range of finger flexion with ad-duction toward ulnar side, wrist pronation with flex-ion toward ulnar side, forearm pronation, elbow flex-ion, and shoulder extension – adduction to occur, until thumb begins to flex and abduct toward ulnar side. Components of fingers and wrist must be allowed to move through range after motion is initiated at thumb. In shortened range of pattern, thumb is flexed, abducted, and internally rotated away from second metacarpal and toward fifth metacarpal.

NOTE: Resist stronger components of fingers, wrist, and proximal components.

Manual Contacts

Left Hand. Place in palm of patient's left hand so that patient may grasp with fingers and thumb and so that wrist may flex toward ulnar side (Fig. 1-55).

Right Hand. *For emphasis of distal joints:* Grip with pressure of palmar surface over anterior – ulnar aspect of patient's forearm, to control pronation and proximal components of motion.

For emphasis of shoulder and elbow: Apply pres-sure of palmar surface on posterior – medial surface of patient's arm, to control internal rotation and proxi-mal components of motion (Fig. 1-55).

For emphasis of scapula: Pressure of palmar sur-face of hand over anterior – medial axillary space and acromion process.

For mass closing of hand and for emphasis of thumb motion: Grasp patient's left thumb with thumb and index finger of right hand; contact of physical ther-apist's thumb and index finger should be medially and laterally at interphalangeal joint of patient's thumb, to control rotation of patient's thumb as well as flexion and abduction components. Physical therapist's left hand should be placed with palmar surface of hand and fingers on palmar surface of hand and fingers of pa-tient's left hand. Physical therapist's left hand pre-vents range of motion occurring proximally until fingers flex and adduct to ulnar side. Flexion of fingers and thumb flexion – abduction may be resisted.

Commands

Preparatory. "You are to squeeze my hand, turn it, and pull it down and toward your chest, bending your elbow."

Action. "Pull! Squeeze my hand! Turn it! Bend your elbow! Pull it down to your chest!"

Pattern Analysis

Scapula. *Motion components:* Rotation, abduc-tion (medial angle), depression anteriorly (acromion). *Major muscle components:* Pectoralis minor, subcla-vius (acting upon clavicle).

Shoulder. *Motion components:* Extension, ad-duction, internal rotation. *Major muscle components:* Subscapularis, pectoralis major (sternal portion).

Elbow. *Motion component:* Flexion. *Major muscle components:* Biceps brachii (short head), brachialis.

Forearm. *Motion component:* Pronation. *Major muscle component:* Pronator teres.

Wrist, Fingers, and Thumb. See extension – adduction – internal rotation (with elbow straight) pattern.

Range-Limiting Factors

Tension or contracture of any muscles of the flexion – abduction – external rotation (with elbow ex-tension) pattern (Fig. 1-52).

Upper Extremity Scapular Patterns

Emphasis on Scapula with Elbow Straight Pattern

FLEXION – ADDUCTION – EXTERNAL ROTATION
(D1 fl)

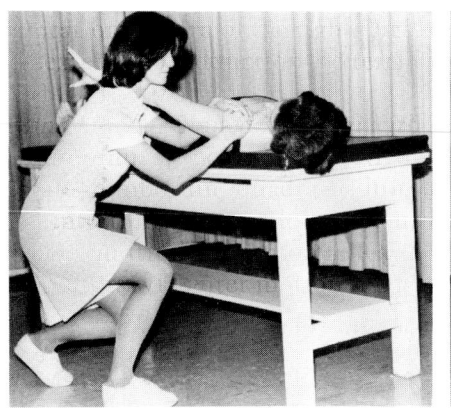 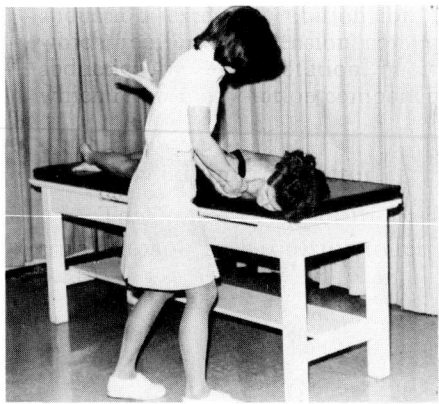

A   A

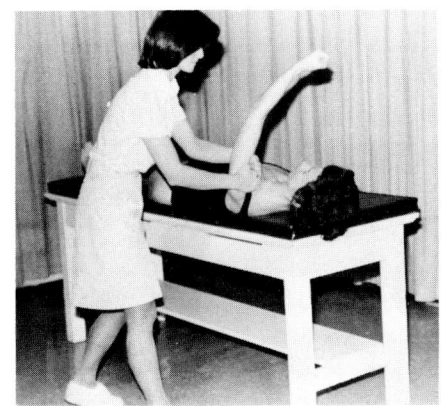 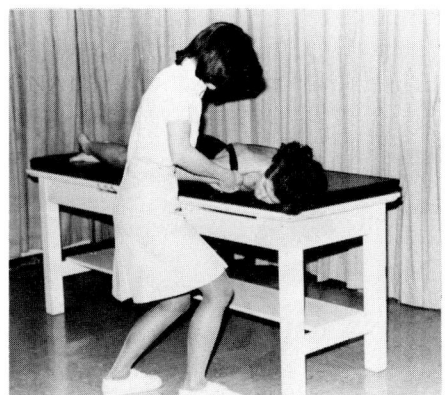

B   B

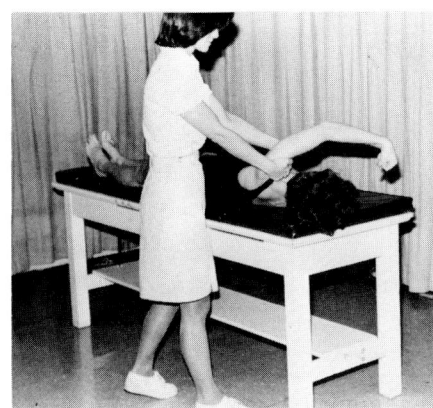 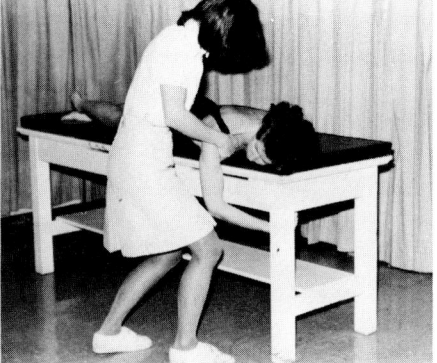

C   C

SUPINE: Left Scapula   PRONE: Right Scapula

FIG. 1-56

Antagonistic Pattern

Extension – abduction – internal rotation (D1 ex).

Components of Motion

Free. In supine position with head rotated toward left, eyes engage hand (A). Head rotates toward right, eyes follow hand (B), causing rotation of head and neck to right (C). Hand is open to ulnar side (A). Hand closes to radial side as wrist flexes toward radial side (B). Shoulder flexes in external rotation, and adducts (C). As therapist permits shoulder to flex, head rotates toward right.

In prone position head is rotated toward right in the lengthened range; hand is open and wrist extended toward ulnar side (A). Hand closes to radial side (B). Elbow flexes as shoulder flexes in external rotation and adducts (C). In supine, the head turns to the right as the left extremity flexes with support by the asymmetric tonic neck reflex. (Manual contacts and commands must be adapted to the prone position and use of the right extremity.) Alternative postures: sitting, side-lying.

Resisted. Scapula rotates with inferior angle abducting and acromion elevating anteriorly. Therapist resists scapula (A and B), and repeats resistance by flexing, then extending hips and knees as subject "holds" at shoulder (C).

SUPINE POSITION

A. Lengthened Range

Commands. *Preparatory.* "You are to look at your left hand and keep your eyes on it." *Action.* "Close your hand, turn it!"

Suggested Techniques. Stretch and resistance.

B. Approaching Middle Range

Commands. "Pull up and across! Hold! Now, pull! Now, pull! Hold!"

Suggested Techniques. Resistance, rhythmic stabilization, and repeated contractions for emphasis.

C. Approaching Shortened Range

Commands. "Pull all the way! Keep your elbow straight! Hold! Now, pull! Now, pull! Hold! Open your hand and push down and out to me. Push! Push again! Hold! Now, pull up and across! Hold! Let go!"

Suggested Techniques. Resistance, repeated contractions for emphasis; slow reversal – hold.

Related Patterns

Unilateral Upper Extremity. *Fig. 1-44:* D1 fl emphasis on shoulder. *Fig. 1-47:* D1 ex with elbow straight, antagonistic pattern.

Total (Mat Activities). *Fig. 1-154:* Rolling: supine toward prone. Head and neck rotation to right. D1 fl of upper extremity. (Shift manual contacts to scapula.) *Fig. 1-170:* Balance on hands and knees. (Shift manual contacts to scapula.) Therapist shifts position to resist D1 fl on left through range.

Upper Extremity Scapular Patterns

Emphasis on Scapula with Elbow Straight Pattern

EXTENSION – ABDUCTION – INTERNAL ROTATION
(D1 ex)

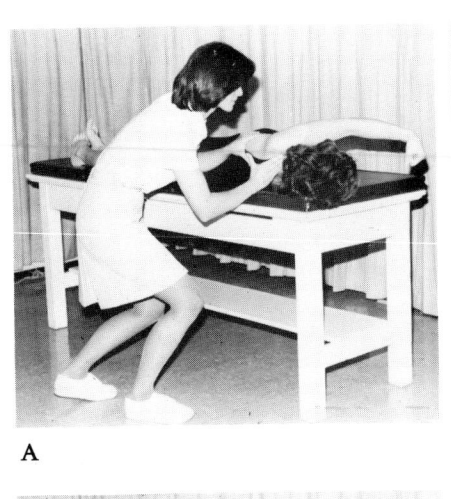

A

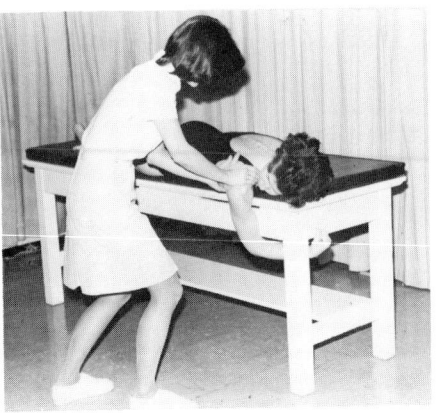

A

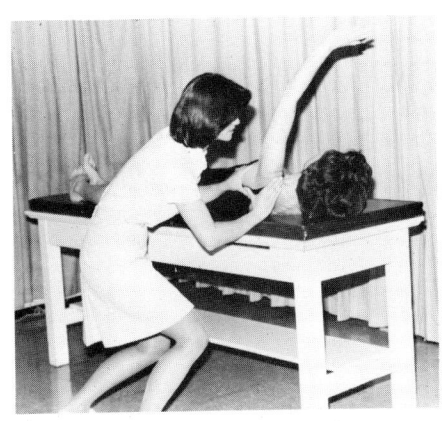

B

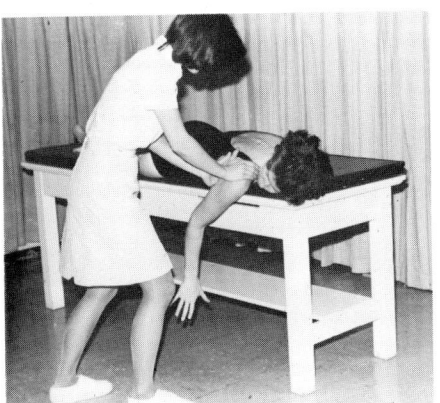

B

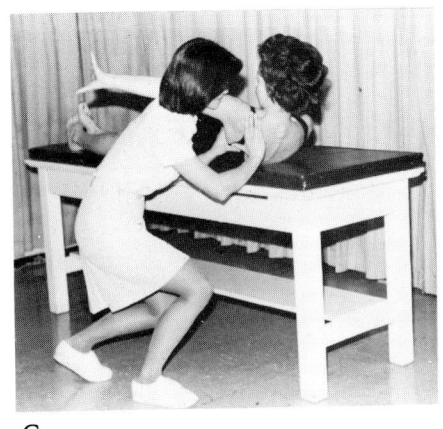

C

SUPINE: Left Scapula

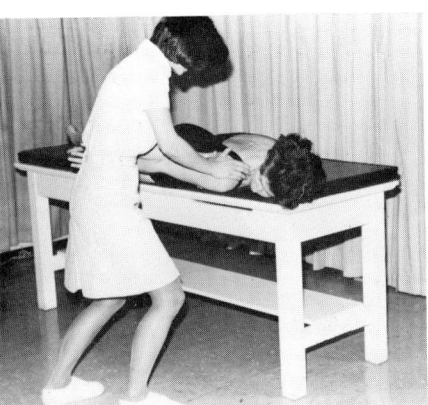

C

PRONE: Right Scapula

FIG. 1-57

Antagonistic Pattern

Flexion – adduction – external rotation (D1 fl).

Components of Motion

Free. In supine position with head rotated toward right, eyes engage left hand (*A*). Head rotates toward left, eyes follow left hand (*B*), causing flexion of head and neck (*C*). Hand is closed to radial side (*A*). Hand opens toward ulnar side as wrist extends toward ulnar side (*B*). Left shoulder extends in internal rotation, and abducts (*C*). As therapist permits shoulder to extend, head rotates toward left.

In prone position with head rotated toward right in the lengthened range, hand is closed and wrist flexed toward radial side (*A*). Hand opens toward ulnar side and elbow extends (*B*), as shoulder extends in internal rotation and abducts (*C*). In supine and in prone, the head turns toward the extending extremity with support by the asymmetric tonic neck reflex. (Manual contacts and commands must be adapted to prone position and use of right extremity.) Alternative postures: sitting, sidelying.

Resisted. Scapula rotates with inferior angle adducting, and acromion depressing posteriorly. Therapist resists scapula (*A* and *B*), and repeats resistance by flexing, then extending hips and knees as subject "holds" at shoulder (*C*).

SUPINE POSITION

A. Lengthened Range

Commands. *Preparatory:* "You are to look at your closed left hand and keep your eyes on it as you open it toward the little finger side. Now, turn your open hand toward me, thumb toward the floor, and put your arm on my shoulder." *Action:* "Open your hand, turn it!"

Suggested Techniques. Stretch and resistance.

B. Approaching Middle Range

Commands. "Push down and out to me!"

Suggested Techniques. Resistance, rhythmic stabilization.

C. Approaching Shortened Range

Commands. "Keep your arm on my shoulder, and push! Hold! Now, push! Again! And relax."

Suggested Techniques. Repeated contractions for emphasis, rhythmic stabilization, slow reversal, slow reversal – hold.

Related Patterns

Unilateral Upper Extremity. *Fig. 1-47:* D1 ex emphasis on shoulder. *Fig. 1-44:* D1 fl with elbow straight, antagonistic pattern.

Upper Trunk Rotation to Left. *Fig. 1-35:* Head and neck, rotation to right. Transpose components for rotation to left.

Total (Mat Activities). *Fig. 1-160:* Rolling: prone toward supine. Head and neck rotation toward left. D1 ex of left upper extremity. (Shift manual contacts to scapula.) *Fig. 1-161:* As for Fig. 1-160.

Upper Extremity Scapular Patterns

Emphasis on Scapula with Elbow Straight Pattern

FLEXION – ABDUCTION – EXTERNAL ROTATION
(D2 fl)

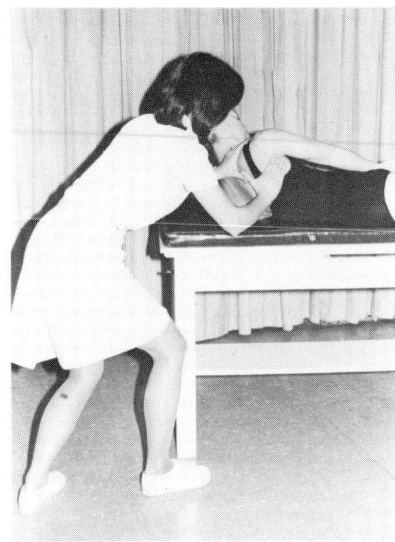 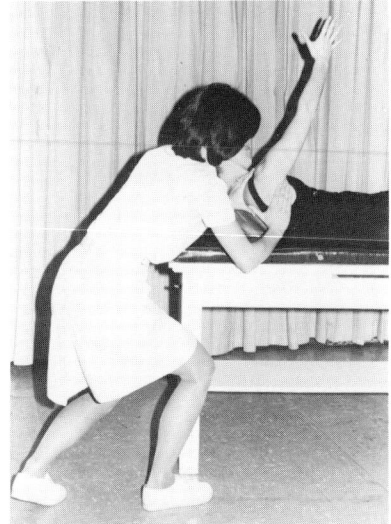 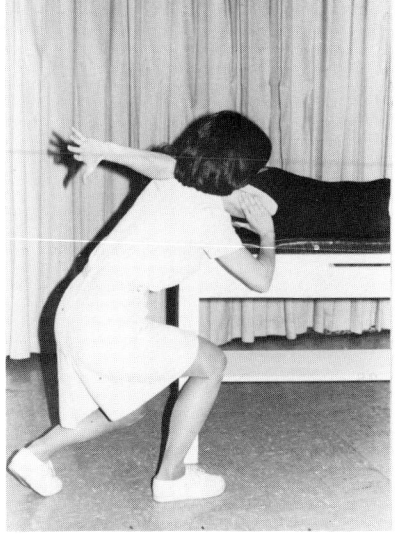

A   B   C

SUPINE: Right Scapula

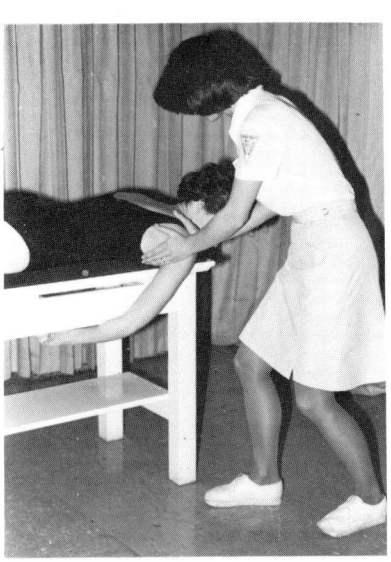 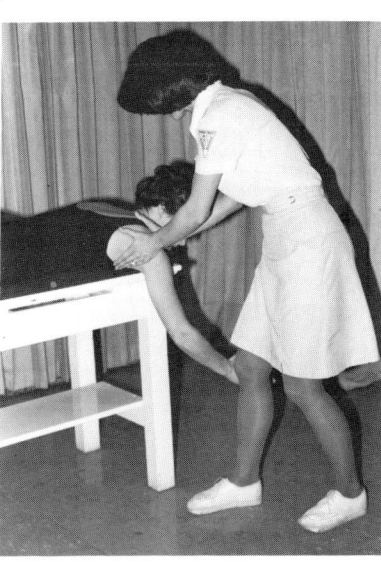 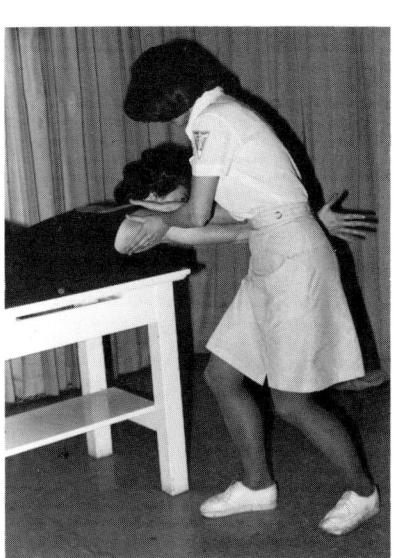

A   B   C

PRONE: Right Scapula

FIG. 1-58

Antagonistic Pattern

Extension – adduction – internal rotation (D2 ex).

Components of Motion

Free. In supine position with head flexed and rotated toward left, eyes engage hand (A). Head extends toward right, eyes follow hand (B), causing extension of head and neck (C). Hand is closed to ulnar side (A). Hand opens toward radial side as wrist extends toward radial side (B). Shoulder flexes in external rotation and abducts (C). As therapist permits shoulder to flex, and as eyes follow hand, head will extend with rotation toward right.

In prone position, head is rotated toward right in the lengthened range (A). Hand opens and wrist extends toward radial side (B). Elbow extends as shoulder flexes in external rotation and abducts (C). In supine and prone positions, head turns toward flexing extremity as eyes follow hand. (Manual contacts and commands must be adapted to prone position and use of right extremity.) Alternative postures: sitting and sidelying.

Resisted. Scapula rotates with medial angle adducting, and acromion elevating posteriorly. Therapist resists scapula (A and B), and repeats resistance by flexing, then extending hips and knees as subject "holds" at shoulder (C).

SUPINE POSITION

A. Lengthened Range

Commands. *Preparatory:* "You are to look down at your closed right hand and keep your eyes on it as you open it toward the thumb side. Then turn your open hand toward me, thumb leading, and lift up toward my shoulder." *Action:* "Open your hand, turn it! Lift up and out toward me."

Suggested Techniques. Stretch and resistance.

B. Approaching Middle Range

Commands. "Lift up and out to me! Hold! hold! hold! Now, lift up! Lift again! and lift! Hold!"

Suggested Techniques. Resistance, rhythmic stabilization, repeated contractions for emphasis.

C. Approaching Shortened Range

Commands. "Keep lifting up and out! Hold! And lift! And lift! And lift! Hold! Close your hand and pull down and across to your left hip. Hold! Now, open your hand and lift up and out. Hold! Let go!"

Suggested Techniques. Resistance, repeated contractions for emphasis, slow reversal, slow reversal – hold, rhythmic stabilization.

Related Patterns

Unilateral Upper Extremity. *Fig. 1-50:* D2 fl emphasis on shoulder. *Fig. 1-53:* D2 ex with elbow straight, antagonistic pattern.

Upper Trunk Rotation to Right. *Fig. 1-37:* Head and neck extension to right. Shift manual contacts to scapula. Upper extremities asymmetrical flexion to right.

Total (Mat Activities). *Fig. 1-178:* Upper trunk extension with rotation to right. Upper extremities asymmetrical flexion to right (lifting). *Fig. 1-159:* Rolling: prone toward supine. Head and neck: extension with rotation, bilateral asymmetrical upper extremities. (Shift manual contacts to scapula.)

Emphasis on Scapula with Elbow Straight Pattern

EXTENSION – ADDUCTION – INTERNAL ROTATION
(D2 ex)

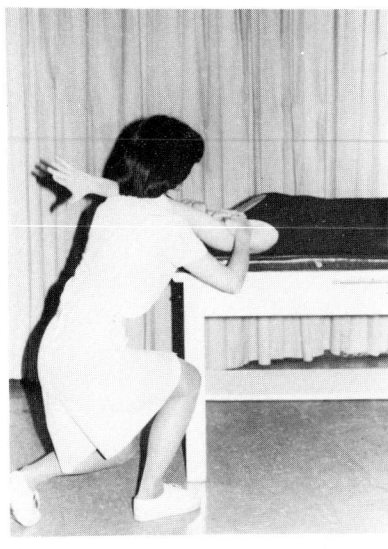 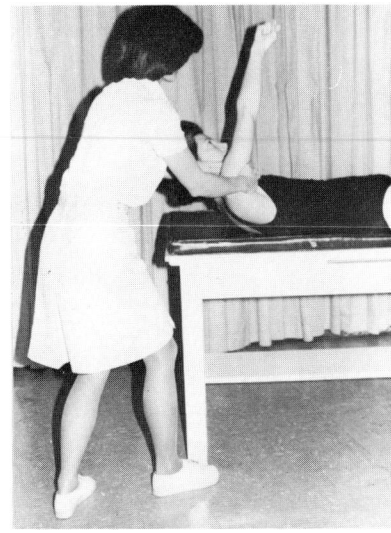 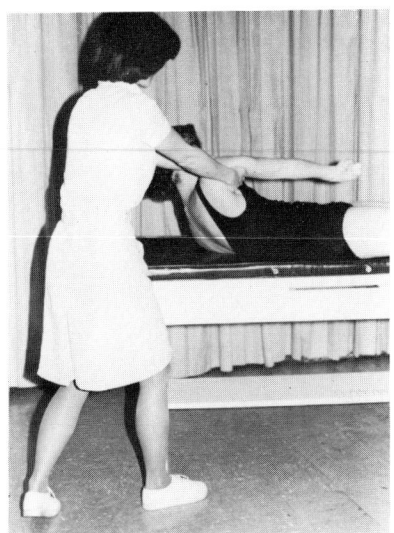

A   B   C

SUPINE: Right Scapula

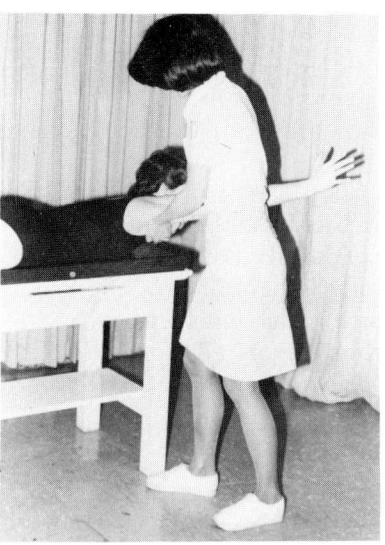 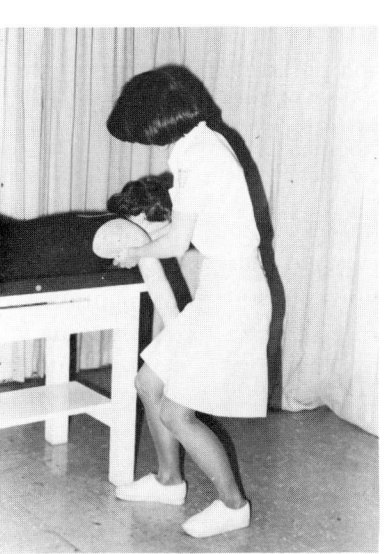 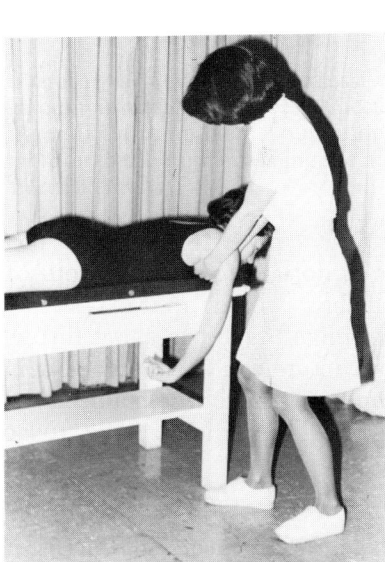

A   B   C

PRONE: Right Scapula

FIG. 1-59

Antagonistic Pattern

Flexion – abduction – external rotation (D2 fl).

Components of Motion

Free. In the supine position with head rotated toward right, eyes engage right hand (A). Head rotates toward left, eyes follow hand (B), causing flexion of head and neck (C). Hand closes to ulnar side as wrist flexes toward ulnar side (B). shoulder extends in internal rotation and adducts (C). As therapist permits shoulder to extend, head will rotate toward left.

In prone position, head is extended toward right in lengthened range (A). Hand closes and wrist flexes toward ulnar side, right forearm and hand hidden from view (B). Shoulder extends in internal rotation and adducts toward left hip (C). In supine and prone positions, the head turns towards the extending extremity. (Manual contacts, commands and position of therapist must be adapted to prone position and use of right extremity.) Alternative postures: sitting and sidelying.

Resisted. Scapula rotates with medial angle abducting and acromion depressing anteriorly. Therapist resists scapula (*A* and *B*), and repeats resistance by flexing, then extending hips and knees as subject holds at shoulder (*C*).

SUPINE POSITION

A. Lengthened Range

Commands. Preparatory: "You are to look at your open right hand. Keep your eyes on it as you close it toward your little finger side. Then pull your closed hand toward your opposite hip." *Action:* "Close your hand! Turn it away from your face! Turn it!"

Suggested Techniques. Stretch and resistance.

B. Approaching Middle Range

Commands. "Pull down and across to your opposite hip! Pull! And pull!

Suggested Technique. Resistance.

C. Approaching Shortened Range

Commands. "Hold! Pull! Pull again! Hold! Hold! Hold! Pull again! All the way! Let go!"

Suggested Techniques. Resistance, approximation, rhythmic stabilization, repeated contractions.

Related Patterns

Unilateral Upper Extremity. Fig. 1-50: D2 ex emphasis on shoulder. *Fig. 1-53:* D2 fl with elbow straight, antagonistic pattern.

Total (Mat Activities). Fig. 1-151: Rolling: Supine toward prone. Head and neck flexion with rotation to the right. D2 ex of upper extremity. (Shift manual contacts to scapula; therapist takes a position in the diagonal at the left shoulder.)

Wheelchair and Transfer Activities. Fig. 1-196: Use of hand brake, D2 extension with elbow extension of left upper extremity (shift manual contacts to scapula; therapist takes a position in the diagonal behind the left shoulder).

Upper Extremity Thrusting Variations

Thrusting patterns of the upper extremity are primitive in that they are closely related to locomotion in the prone posture when the elbows are fully extended and weight is supported on the hands. These movements are a part of "push-ups." They also promote reaching for an object with extending elbow and with the hand opening in preparation for grasp. As with all patterns, thrusting may be performed in any position or posture that permits the desired range of motion to be performed. Thrusting patterns may be initiated by use of the stretch reflex; the response is a rapid and forceful movement. In the shortened range, approximation may be applied by manual contact at the base of the palm. The command to "thrust" is always given sharply and is timed with stretch reflex; or, when approximation is used in the shortened range, the command is "hold."

Thrusting is a variation of the upper extremity patterns. Whereas in the specific patterns of facilitation, opening of the hand is consistent with abduction of the shoulder, in thrusting, opening of the hand is consistent with adduction of the shoulder. In the specific patterns, all rotation occurs in the same direction; in thrusting, the rotation of shoulder and forearm are opposite. The more distal joints move in harmony with the rotation of the forearm. The wrist and elbow always extend. The scapula moves in the direction of the thrust and is, therefore, protracted. The serratus anterior muscle is primarily responsible for the movement of the scapula. The pectoral muscles contribute strongly to the shoulder movement. Thrusting movements may be reversed. During reversal, all components of motion are exactly opposite.

ULNAR EXTENSOR THRUST (D1 fl)

The proximal and intermediate components of motion are those of the flexion–adduction–external rotation with elbow extension pattern. The distal components are those of the extension–abduction–internal rotation pattern. In the lengthened range, or starting position, the hand is closed and the wrist is flexed toward the radial side; the forearm is supinated; the elbow is completely flexed; and the shoulder is extended in abduction. As the subject thrusts, the hand opens and the wrist extends toward the ulnar side, the forearm pro-

nates, the elbow extends, and the shoulder flexes and adducts so that the open hand reaches upward and across the nose and eyes.

RADIAL EXTENSOR THRUST (D2 ex)

The proximal and intermediate components are those of the extension–adduction–internal rotation with elbow extension pattern. The distal components are those of the flexion–abduction–external rotation pattern. In the lengthened range, or starting position, the hand is closed toward the ulnar side; the forearm is pronated; the elbow is completely flexed; and the shoulder is flexed in abduction. As the subject thrusts, the hand opens and the wrist extends toward the radial side, the forearm supinates, the elbow extends, and the shoulder extends and adducts so that the open hand reaches downward and across the body toward the opposite hip.

Thrusting may be performed in any position that permits the desired range of motion. Resisting the thrust may enhance the patient's ability to advance the upper extremities during prone locomotion. One extremity may be exercised as the patient leans on the opposite elbow, or both extremities may participate with alternating reciprocal movements. As the patient reverses the movements, resistance will help him to advance his trunk on the mat.

A powerful thrust, as in boxing and in putting a shot, is an all-or-none movement. Reversal of the thrust, too, is a strong, smooth motion, as in scaling a mountain wall or pulling a branch from a tree.

The illustrations include three points in the range. The middle range may seem superfluous and interruptive; however, when weakness of elbow extensors and flexors exists, emphasis at mid-range may be necessary to completion of the range.

The position of the therapist in Figures 1-60 and 1-61 is optimal. The subject moves toward the therapist as in pushing a person or an object away from one's body, or pushing a loaded cart down the hall, or an object onto the upper shelf. Reversals may include snatching a child from a hot or burning object, or pulling unwanted plants from the garden (see text accompanying figures).

In Figures 1-62 and 1-63 the position of the therapist is less than optimal. In certain surroundings, as in working with the patient at bedside, the therapist may need to use these positions. (Commands are given.)

Upper Extremity Thrusting Variations

*Emphasis on Ulnar Extensor Thrust for
Elbow Extension*

FLEXION – ADDUCTION – EXTERNAL ROTATION
(D1 fl), LEFT

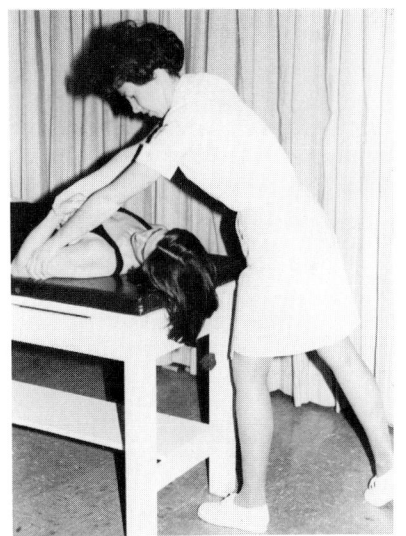 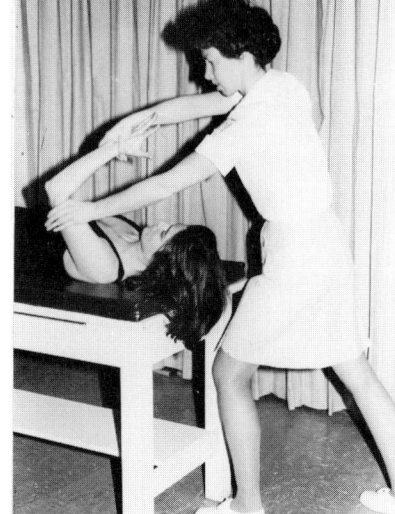 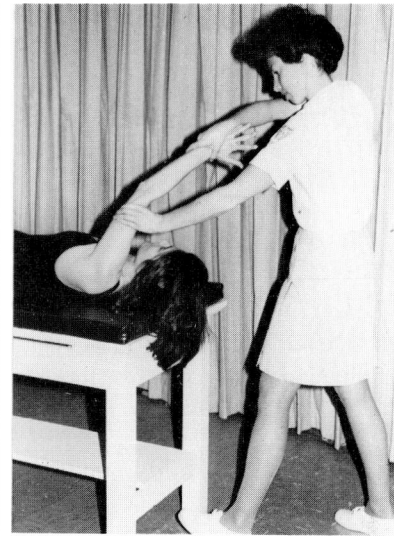

A
THRUST
B
C

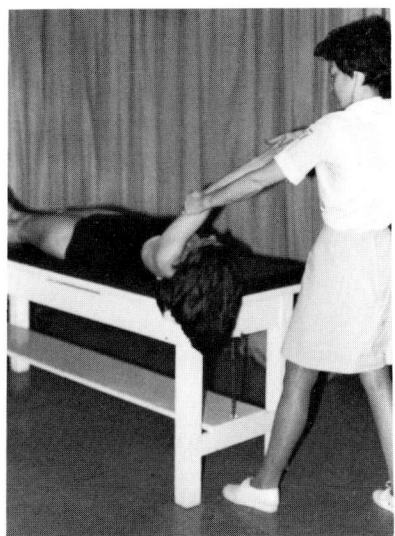 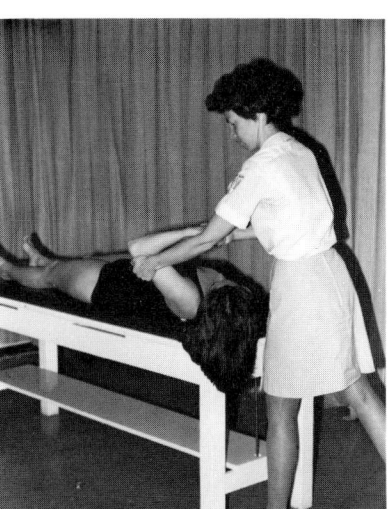 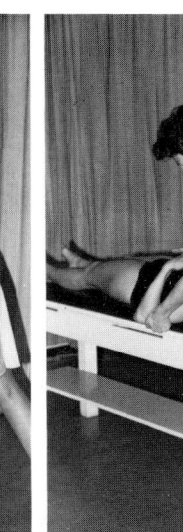

A
REVERSAL
B
C

FIG. 1-60

Components of Motion

Free. With eyes regarding therapist, who stands near right shoulder, head and neck rotate slightly to left. Right hand grips table edge. Alternative position of therapist, standing at subject's left hip, is less than optimal (see Fig. 1-62).

Resisted. Hand opens toward ulnar side as wrist extends toward ulnar side and forearm pronates; elbow extends as shoulder flexes in external rotation and adducts.

A. Lengthened Range

Commands. *Preparatory:* "You are to open your hand, and shove it toward me." *Action:* "Now, shove it toward me!"

Suggested Techniques. Abrupt stretch and resistance.

B. Middle Range

Commands. "Straighten your elbow! Shove it!"
Suggested Technique. Sustained resistance.

C. Shortened Range

Commands. "Shove it! All the way! Hold it!" ("Let go!" or "Reverse!")
Suggested Techniques. Resistance; approximation at command to hold; reversal; or hold–relax active motion.

REVERSAL OF THRUST: EXTENSION – ABDUCTION – INTERNAL ROTATION (D1 ex), LEFT

With eyes regarding therapist, who stands at right shoulder, head and neck rotate slightly to right. Right hand grips table edge.

Resisted. Hand closes to radial side as wrist flexes toward radial side and forearm supinates; elbow flexes as shoulder extends in internal rotation and abducts.

A. Lengthened Range

Commands. *Preparatory:* "You are to close your hand, and pull your elbow down and away from me." *Action:* "Ready! Close your hand!"
Suggested Techniques. Stretch and resistance.

B. Middle Range

Commands. "Bend your elbow! Pull down and away and hold! Hold! Now, pull! Now, pull!"
Suggested Techniques. Resistance, repeated contractions for emphasis.

C. Shortened Range

Commands. "Pull! Keep pulling all the way! Hold it!" ("Let go!" or "Reverse!")
Suggested Techniques. Resistance; reversal or hold–relax active motion.

Related Patterns

Unilateral. *Fig. 1-46:* D1 fl, elbow extension. Hand closes to radial side. In D1 fl thrust, hand is closed toward radial side (*A*) and opens toward ulnar side, with forearm pronation (*B*). *Figs. 1-172 to 1-173:* D1 thrust and reversal may be performed in the prone-on-elbows position.

Upper Extremity Thrusting Variations

Emphasis on Radial Extensor Thrust for Elbow Extension

EXTENSION – ADDUCTION – INTERNAL ROTATION
(D2 ex), LEFT

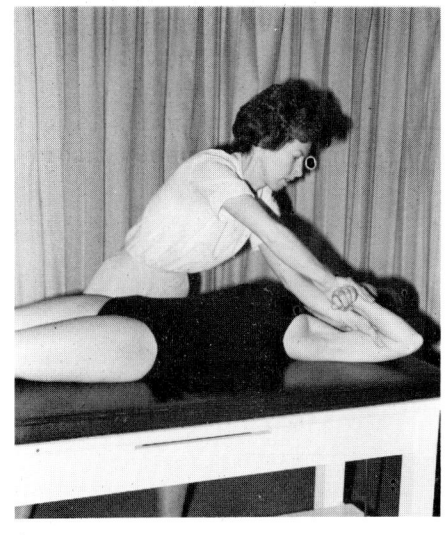 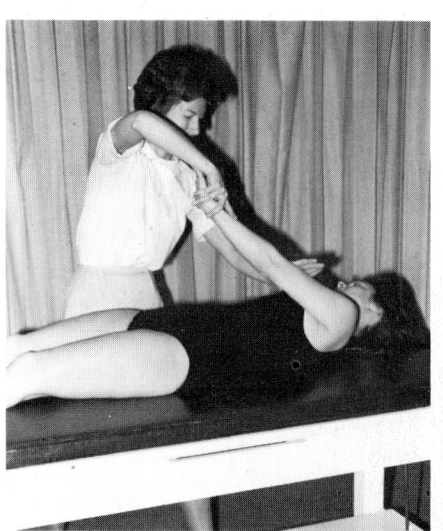 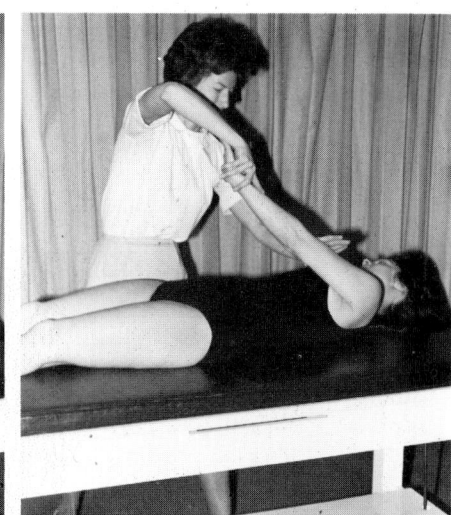

A
THRUST

B

C

FIG. 1-61

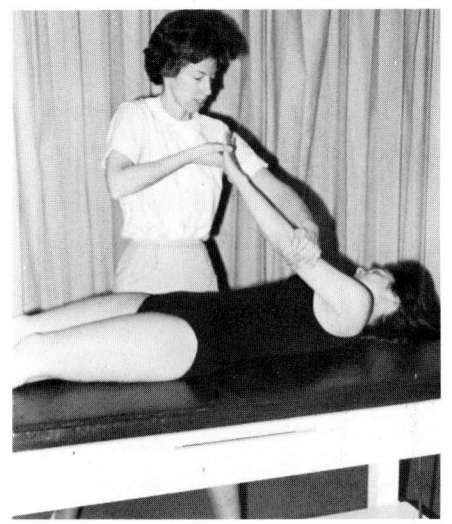 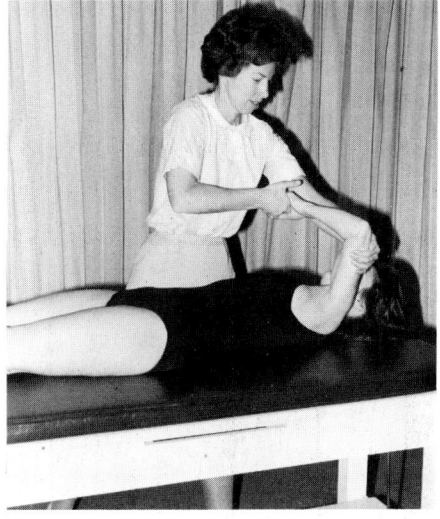 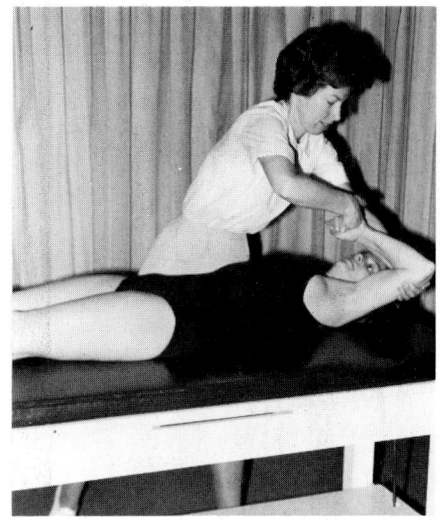

A   B   C

REVERSAL

Components of Motion

Free. With eyes regarding therapist, who stands near subject's right hip, head and neck rotate slightly toward right. Right hand grips table edge. Alternative position of therapist, standing at subject's left shoulder, is less than optimal (see Fig. 1-63).

Resisted. Hand opens toward radial side as wrist extends toward radial side and as forearm supinates; elbow extends as shoulder extends in internal rotation and adducts.

A. Lengthened Range

Commands. Preparatory: "You are to open your hand, and shove it down and across toward me." *Action:* "Ready! Open your hand, and shove it."

Suggested Techniques. Abrupt stretch and resistance.

B. Middle Range

Commands. "Straighten your elbow! Shove it."
Suggested Technique. Sustained resistance.

C. Shortened Range

Commands. "Shove it! All the way! Hold it!" ("Let go!" or "Reverse!")

Suggested Techniques. Resistance; approximation at command to hold; reversal; or hold – relax active motion.

REVERSAL OF THRUST: FLEXION – ABDUCTION –
EXTERNAL ROTATION (D2 fl), LEFT

With eyes regarding therapist, who stands near subject's right hip, head and neck rotated slightly toward right. Right hand grips table edge.

Resisted. Hand closes to the ulnar side as wrist flexes toward ulnar side and forearm pronates; elbow flexes as shoulder flexes in external rotation and abducts.

A. Lengthened Range

Commands. Preparatory: "You are to close your hand and pull it toward your ear." *Action:* "Ready! Close your hand! And pull!"

Suggested Techniques. Stretch and resistance.

B. Middle Range

Commands. "Pull up! Bend your elbow! Keep pulling all the way!"

Suggested Techniques. Resistance, repeated contractions for emphasis.

C. Shortened Range

Command. "Keep pulling all the way!"
Suggested Technique. Resistance.

Related Patterns

Unilateral Upper Extremity. Fig. 1-54: D2 ex, elbow extension. Hand closes toward ulnar side. In D2 ex thrust, hand is closed toward ulnar side (*A*) and opens toward radial side (*B*).

Upper Trunk Flexion with Rotation to Right. Fig. 1-36: D2 ex of left, D1 ex of right (therapist may use left hand on subject's right wrist, and right hand on subject's left wrist). On initiation, both elbows are flexed. Then, in effect, subject will use D2 ex thrust to push right arm down to complete extension. Transpose components for thrusting on left.

Total (Mat Activities). Fig. 1-174: Creeping backward toward right. Bearing weight on hands and pushing backward is based on thrusting with counterrotation of shoulder and forearm.

Upper Extremity Thrusting Variations

Emphasis on Elbow Extensor Thrust and Reversal
Position of Therapist: Less Than Optimal

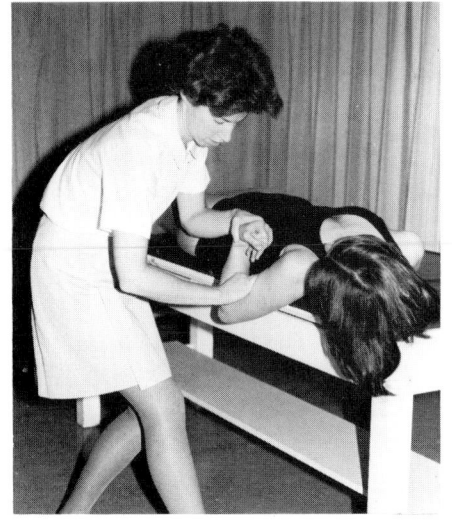 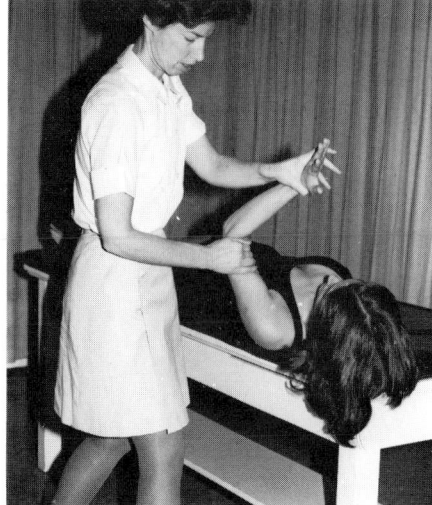 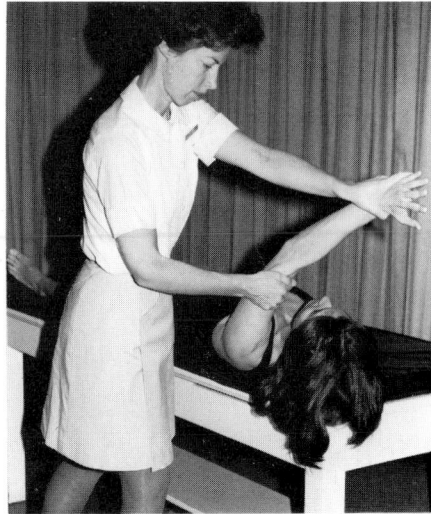

A
THRUST: D1 fl

B

C

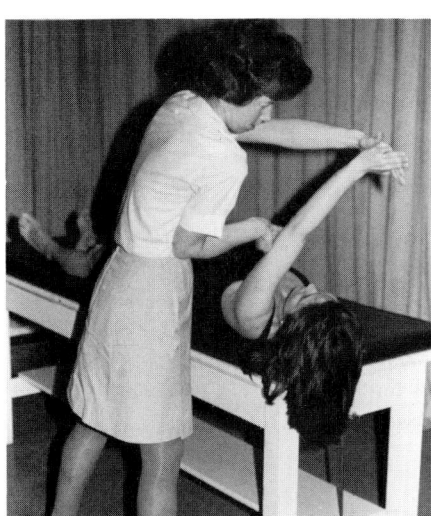 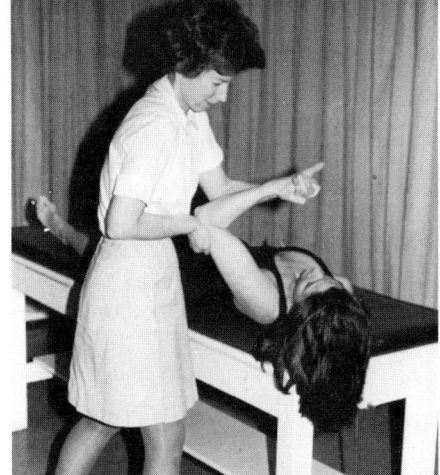 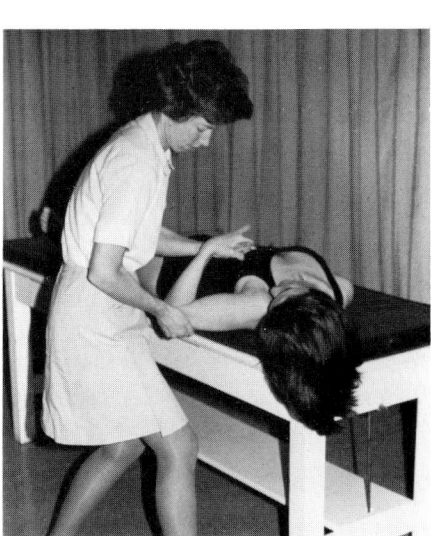

A
REVERSAL: D1 ex

B

C

FIG. 1-62. Ulnar extensor thrust and reversal.

Commands for Thrust (D1 fl)

A. "Ready."
B. "Open your hand."
C. "Shove it up across your face!"

Commands for Reversal (D1 ex)

A. "Ready."
B. "Squeeze my hand and pull down toward me."
C. "Bend your elbow."

Emphasis on Elbow Extensor Thrust and Reversal
Position of Therapist: Less Than Optimal

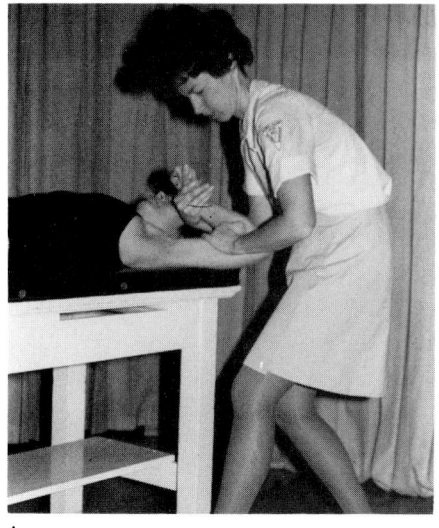 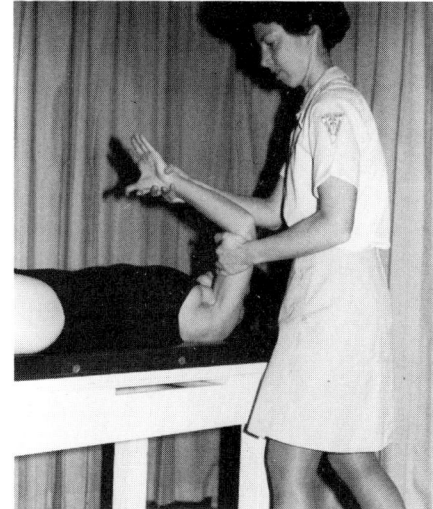 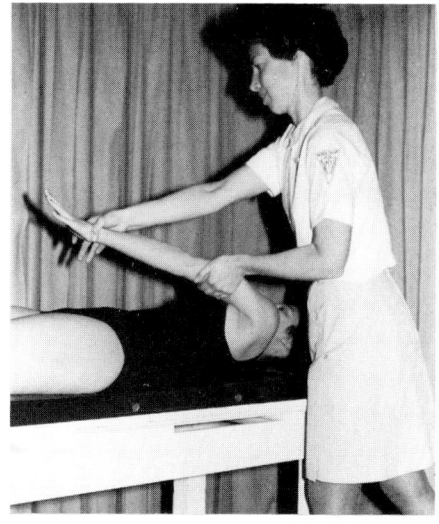

A.   B.   C.
THRUST: D2 ex

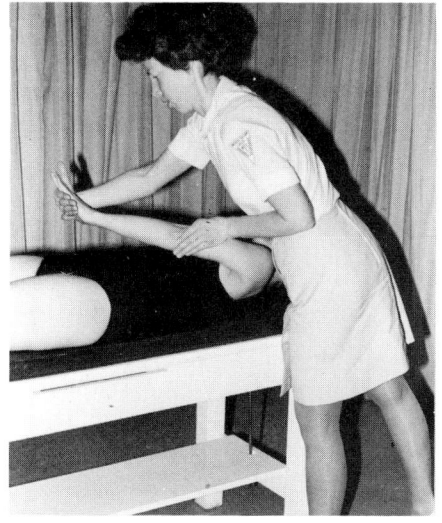 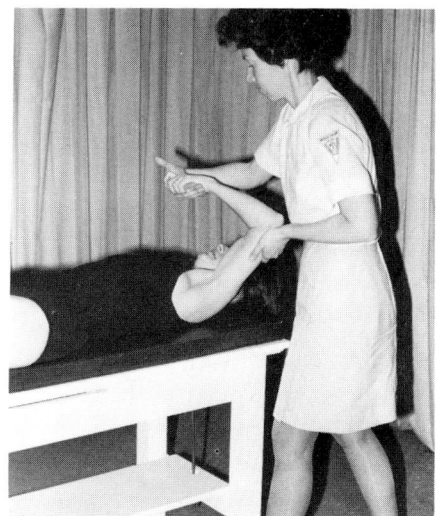 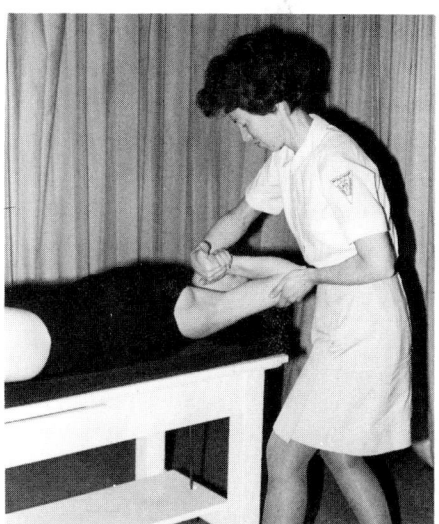

A.   B.   C.
REVERSAL: D2 fl

FIG. 1-63.   Radial extensor thrust and reversal.

Commands for Thrust (D2 ex)

A. "Ready."
B. "Open your hand."
C. "Shove it down and across toward your right hip!"

Commands for Reversal (D2 fl)

A. "Ready."
B. "Squeeze my hand and lift up toward me."
C. Bend your elbow."

Flexion – Adduction – External Rotation (D1 fl)

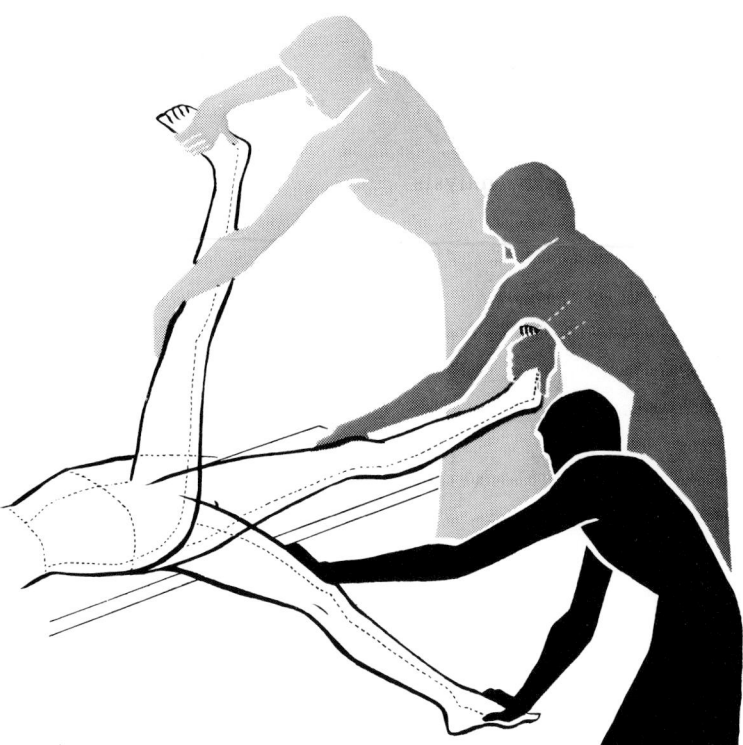

FIG. 1-64. With knee straight.

Antagonistic Pattern

Extension – abduction – internal rotation (with knee straight) pattern (Fig. 1-67).

Components of Motion

Toes extend and abduct (medial toes more than lateral) toward tibial side; foot and ankle dorsiflex with inversion; knee remains straight; hip flexes, adducts, and externally rotates.

Normal Timing

Action is from distal to proximal, that is, action occurs first at toes, then at foot and ankle, then at hip.

Timing for Emphasis

Hip. Allow beginning rotation to occur at toes, foot and ankle, and hip, but do not allow full range of toe extension with abduction, and foot and ankle dorsiflexion and inversion to occur, until hip begins to flex and adduct with external rotation.

NOTE: If normal timing is prevented by excessive resistance to weaker distal components, action cannot occur proximally. Resist stronger distal components, but guide weaker distal components through their optimal range of motion in accordance with normal timing.

Ankle and Foot. Allow beginning rotation to occur at toes, foot and ankle, and hip, but do not allow full range of toe extension with abduction and hip

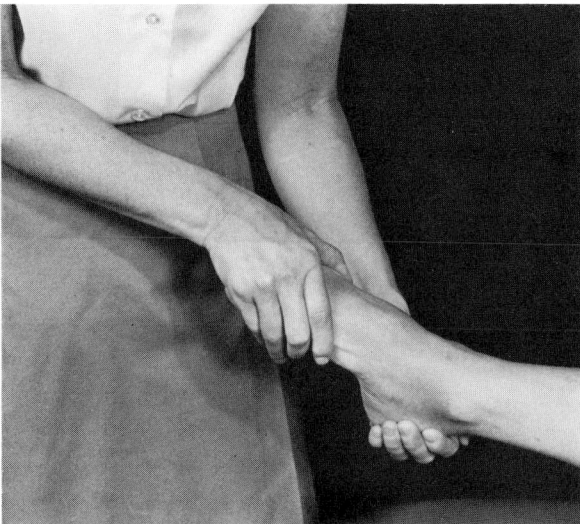

A. Le-R

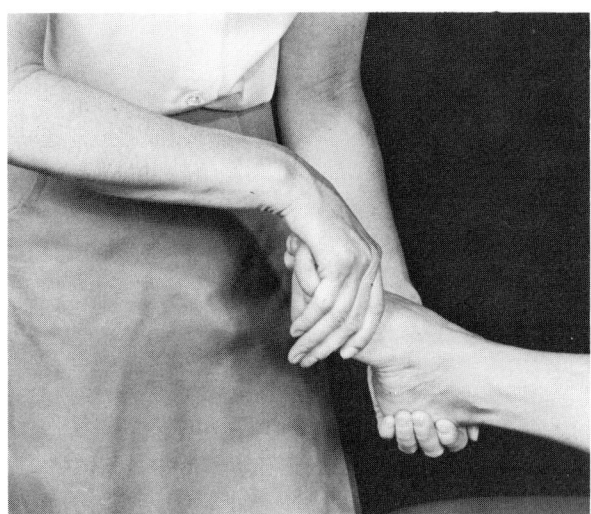

B. Mid-R

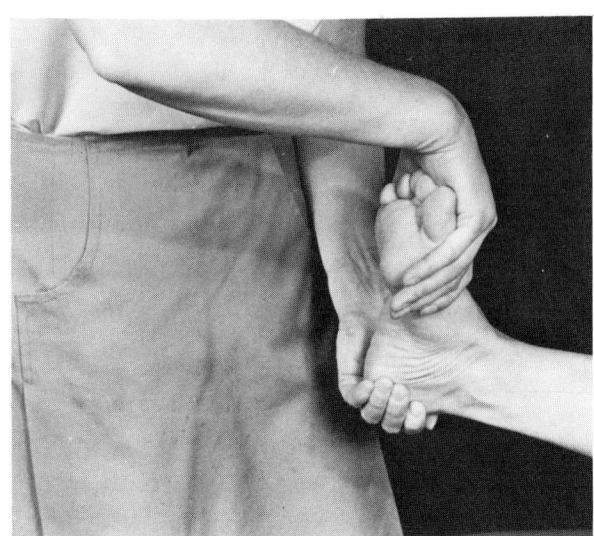

C. Sh-R

FOOT AND ANKLE (D1 fl)

flexion – adduction to occur, until foot and ankle begin to dorsiflex and invert.

NOTE: Resist stronger proximal and distal components, but guide weaker distal components through their optimal range of motion in accordance with normal timing.

Toes. Allow beginning rotation to occur at toes, foot and ankle, and hip, but do not allow full range of foot and ankle dorsiflexion with inversion and hip flexion – adduction to occur, until toes begin to extend and abduct toward tibial side.

NOTE: Resist stronger proximal components. Emphasis may be placed on metatarsal – phalangeal joints, or interphalangeal joints, or on a specific joint of a single toe.

Manual Contacts

Patient Is Able to Work Through Full Range of Pattern. Right hand: Pressure of palmar surface of hand on medial aspect of dorsal surface of foot, as far distal as a firm grip will permit. Avoid pressure on plantar surface of foot (Fig. 1-64). *Left hand:* Pressure of palmar surface of hand or with fingers in close approximation on anterior – medial aspect of thigh proximal to patella (Fig. 1-64).

Patient Has Difficulty in Initiating Motion. Right hand: As above. *Left hand:* Pressure of palmar surface of hand or with fingers in close approximation on the posterior – medial aspect of thigh proximal to popliteal space; or pressure of fingers in close approximation on medial aspect of right heel.

Commands

Preparatory. "You are to turn your heel in, and pull your foot up and across your body."
Action. "Pull! Pull your foot in and up! Pull it up and away from me!"

Pattern Analysis

Hip. *Motion components:* Flexion, adduction, and external rotation. *Major muscle components:* Psoas minor, psoas major, iliacus, obturator externus, pectineus, gracilis, adductor brevis, adductor longus, sartorius (hip flexion component), rectus femoris (medial portion, hip flexion component).
Knee. Straight (no motion).
Ankle, Foot, and Toes. *Motion components:* Dorsiflexion, inversion of ankle and foot, toe extension with abduction toward tibial side. *Major muscle components:* Tibialis anterior, extensor digitorum longus, extensor hallucis longus, extensor digitorum brevis, abductor hallucis, dorsal interossei, lumbricales.

Range-Limiting Factors

Tension or contracture of any muscles of extension – abduction – internal rotation (with knee straight) pattern (Fig. 1-67).

Flexion–Adduction–External Rotation (D1 fl)

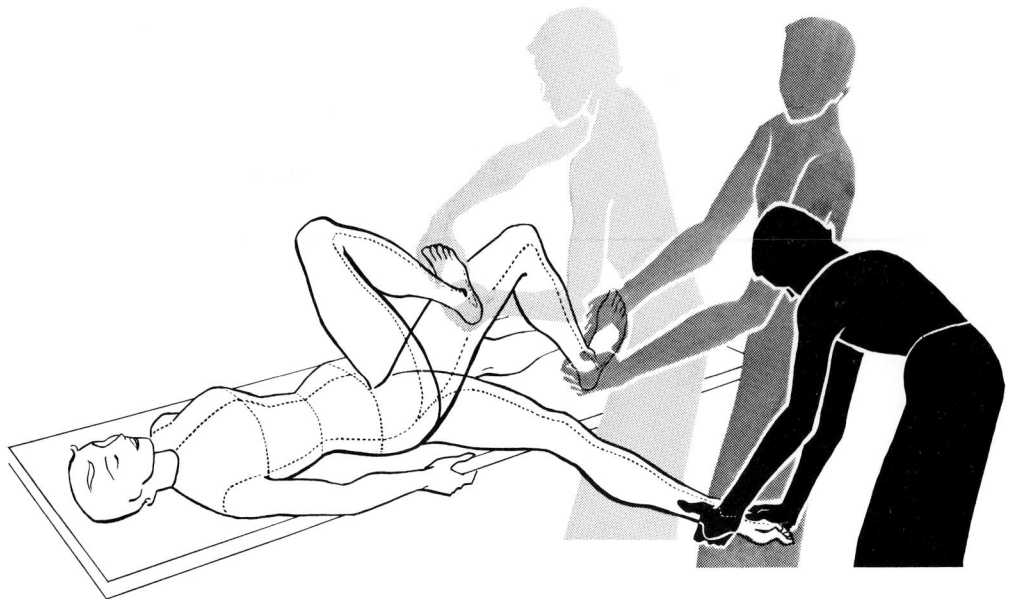

FIG. 1-65. With knee flexion.

Antagonistic Pattern

Extension–abduction–internal rotation (with knee extension) pattern (Fig. 1-68).

Components of Motion

Toes extend and abduct (medial toes more than lateral) toward tibial side; foot and ankle dorsiflex and invert; knee flexes with tibia externally rotating on femur; hip flexes, adducts, and externally rotates.

Normal Timing

Action is from distal to proximal, that is, action occurs first at toes, then foot and ankle, then at knee, then at hip.

Timing for Emphasis

Hip. Allow beginning rotation to occur at toes, foot and ankle, knee, and hip, but do not allow full range of toe extension with abduction, foot and ankle dorsiflexion with inversion, and knee flexion to occur, until hip begins to flex and adduct with external rotation.

NOTE: If normal timing is prevented by excessive resistance to weaker distal components, action cannot occur proximally. Resist stronger distal components, but guide weaker distal components through their optimal range of motion in accordance with normal timing.

Knee. Allow beginning rotation to occur at toes, foot and ankle, knee, and hip, but do not allow full range of toe extension with abduction, foot and ankle

dorsiflexion with inversion, and hip flexion–adduction to occur, until knee begins to flex with external rotation of tibia on femur.

NOTE: Resist stronger proximal and distal components, but guide weaker distal components through their optimal range of motion in accordance with normal timing.

Ankle and Foot. Allow beginning rotation to occur at toes, foot and ankle, knee, and hip, but do not allow full range of toe extension with abduction, knee flexion, and hip flexion–adduction to occur, until foot and ankle begin to dorsiflex and invert.

NOTE: Resist stronger proximal and distal components, but guide weaker distal components through their optimal range of motion in accordance with normal timing.

Toes. Allow beginning rotation to occur at toes, foot and ankle, knee, and hip, but do not allow full range of toe extension with abduction, foot and ankle dorsiflexion with inversion, knee flexion, and hip flexion–adduction to occur, until toes begin to extend and abduct toward tibial side.

NOTE: Resist stronger proximal components. Emphasis may be placed on metatarsal–phalangeal joints or interphalangeal joints, or a specific joint of a single toe.

Manual Contacts

Patient Is Able to Work Through Full Range of Pattern. Right hand: Apply pressure of palmar surface of hand on medial aspect of dorsal surface of foot, as far distal as a firm grip will permit. Avoid pressure on plantar surface of foot (Fig. 1-65). *Left hand:* Apply pressure of palmar surface of hand or with fingers in close approximation on anterior – medial aspect of thigh proximal to patella, or pressure of fingers in close approximation on medial aspect of heel (Fig. 1-65).

Patient Has Difficulty in Initiating Motion. *Right hand:* As above. *Left hand:* Apply pressure of palmar surface of hand or with fingers in close approximation on posterior – medial aspect of thigh proximal to popliteal space.

Commands

Preparatory. "You are to turn your heel, pull your foot up and across your body, and bend your knee."

Action. "Pull! Pull your foot in and up! Bend your knee! Pull it up and away from me!"

Pattern Analysis

Hip. *Motion components:* Flexion, adduction, and external rotation. *Major muscle components:* Psoas minor, psoas major, iliacus, obturator externus, pectineus, gracilis, adductor brevis, adductor longus, sartorius (hip flexion component).

Knee. *Motion components:* Flexion with tibia externally rotating on femur. *Major muscle components:* Semitendinosus, semimembranosus, sartorius, gracilis (knee flexion component).

Ankle, Foot, and Toes. See flexion – adduction – external rotation (with knee straight) pattern (Fig. 1-64).

Range-Limiting Factors

Tension or contracture of any muscles of extension – abduction – internal rotation (with knee extension) pattern (Fig. 1-68).

Flexion–Adduction–External Rotation (D1 fl)

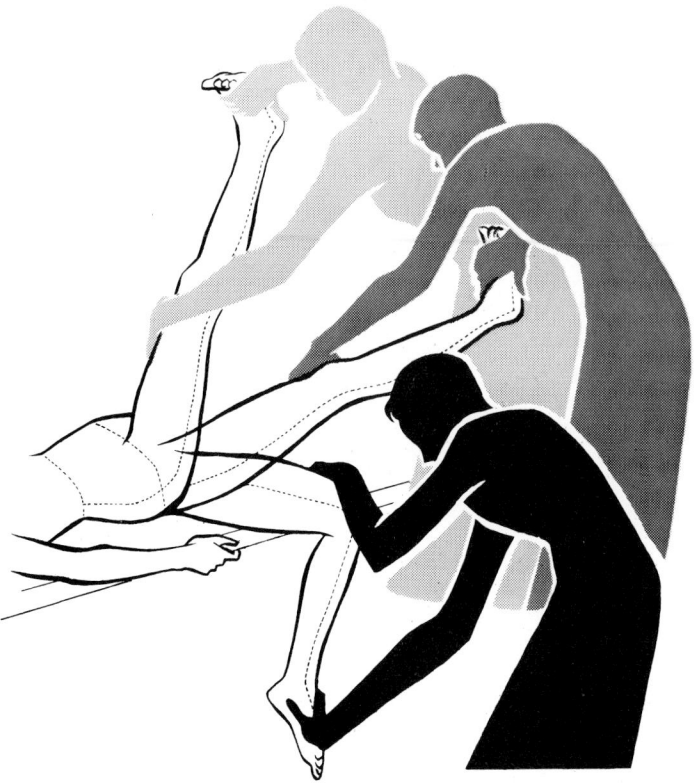

FIG. 1-66. With knee extension.

Antagonistic Pattern

Extension–abduction–internal rotation (with knee flexion) (Fig. 1-69).

Components of Motion

Toes extend and abduct (medial toes more than lateral) toward tibial side, foot and ankle dorsiflex with inversion, knee extends with tibia externally rotating on femur, hip flexes, adducts, and externally rotates.

Normal Timing

Action is from distal to proximal, that is, action occurs first at toes, then foot and ankle, then at knee, then at hip.

Timing for Emphasis

Hip. Allow beginning rotation to occur at toes, foot and ankle, knee, and hip, but do not allow full range of toe extension with abduction, foot and ankle dorsiflexion with inversion, and knee extension to occur, until hip begins to flex and adduct with external rotation.

NOTE: If normal timing is prevented by excessive resistance to weaker distal components, action cannot occur proximally. Resist stronger distal components, but guide weaker distal components through their optimal range of motion in accordance with normal timing.

Knee. Allow beginning rotation to occur at toes, foot and ankle, knee, and hip, but do not allow full range of toe extension with abduction, foot and ankle dorsiflexion with inversion, and hip flexion–adduction to occur until knee begins to extend with external rotation of tibia on femur.

NOTE: Resist stronger proximal and distal components, but guide weaker distal components through their optimal range of motion in accordance with normal timing.

Ankle and Foot. Allow beginning rotation to occur at toes, foot and ankle, knee, and hip, but do not allow full range of toe extension with abduction, knee extension, and hip flexion–adduction to occur, until foot and ankle begin to dorsiflex and invert.

NOTE: Resist stronger proximal and distal components, but guide weaker distal components through their optimal range of motion in accordance with normal timing.

Toes. Allow beginning rotation to occur at toes, foot and ankle, knee, and hip, but do not allow full range of foot and ankle dorsiflexion with inversion, knee extension, and hip-flexion – adduction to occur, until toes begin to extend and abduct toward tibial side.

NOTE: Resist stronger proximal components. Emphasis may be placed on metatarsal-phalangeal joints, or interphalangeal joints, or a specific joint of a single toe.

Manual Contacts

Patient Is Able to Work Through Full Range of Pattern. *Right hand:* Pressure of palmar surface of hand on medial aspect of dorsal surface of foot, as far distal as a firm grip will permit. Avoid pressure on plantar surface of foot (Fig. 1-66). *Left hand:* Pressure of palmar surface of hand, or with fingers in close approximation, on anterior-medial aspect of thigh proximal to patella (Fig. 1-66).

Patient Has Difficulty in Initiating Motion. *Right hand:* As above. Fingers may be used to grip foot in order to guide motion. *Left hand:* Pressure of palmar surface of hand or with fingers in close approximation on posterior – medial surface of thigh proximal to popliteal space; or pressure of fingers in close approximation, on medial aspect of heel.

Commands

Preparatory. "You are to kick your foot up and in across your body, and straighten your knee." *Action.* "Kick!"

Pattern Analysis

Hip. *Motion components:* Flexion, adduction, external rotation. *Major muscle components:* Psoas minor, psoas major, iliacus, obturator externus, pectineus, gracilis, adductor brevis, adductor longus, rectus femoris (medial portion, hip flexion component).

Knee. *Motion components:* Extension with tibia externally rotating on femur. *Major muscle components:* Rectus femoris (medial portion), vastus medialis, articularis genu.

Ankle, Foot, and Toes. See flexion – adduction – external rotation (with knee straight) pattern (Fig. 1-64).

Range-Limiting Factors

Tension or contracture of any muscles of extension – abduction – internal rotation (with knee flexion) pattern (Fig. 1-69).

Extension – Abduction – Internal Rotation (D1 ex)

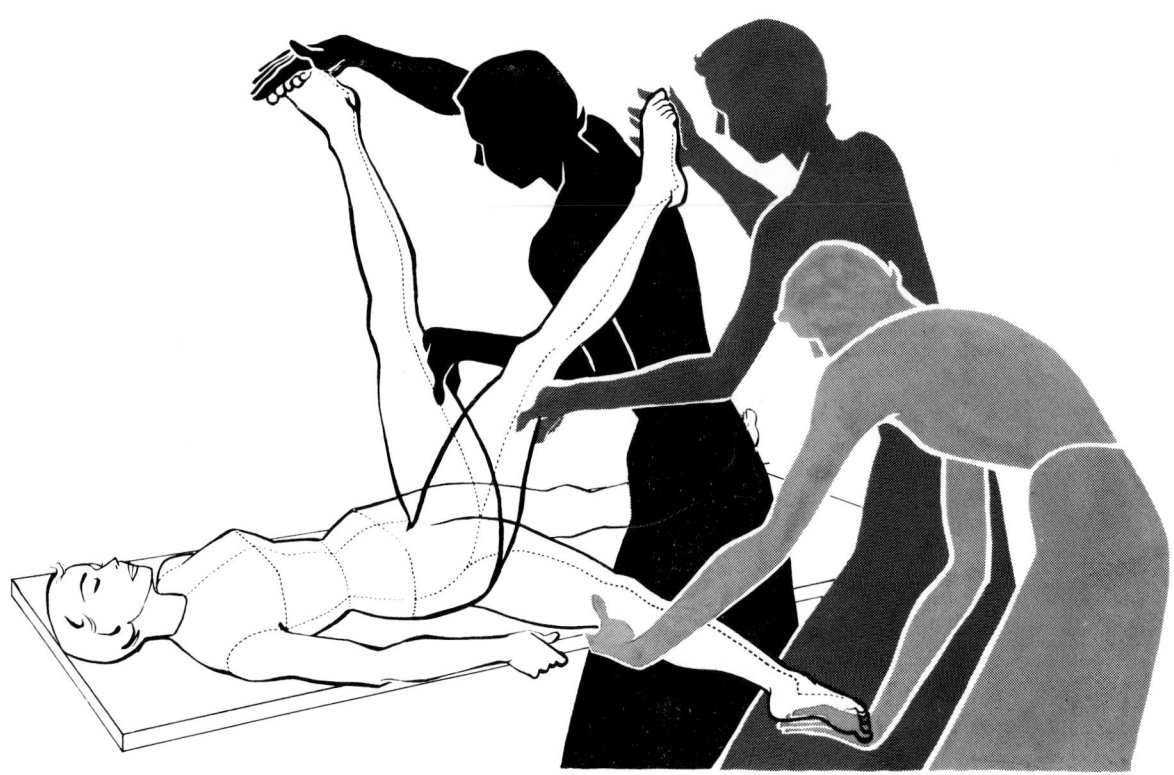

FIG. 1-67.   With knee straight.

Antagonistic Pattern

Flexion – adduction – external rotation (with knee straight) pattern (Fig. 1-64).

Components of Motion

Toes flex and adduct (lateral toes more than medial) toward fibular side; foot and ankle plantar flex with eversion; knee remains straight; hip extends, abducts, and internally rotates.

Normal Timing

Action is from distal to proximal, that is, action occurs first at toes, then at foot and ankle, then at hip.

Timing for Emphasis

Hip.   Allow beginning rotation to occur at toes, foot and ankle, and hip, but do not allow full range of toe flexion with adduction, and foot and ankle plantar flexion with eversion to occur, until hip begins to extend and abduct with internal rotation.

NOTE: If normal timing is prevented by excessive resistance to weaker distal components, action cannot occur proximally. Resist stronger distal components, but guide weaker distal components through their optimal range of motion in accordance with normal timing.

Ankle and Foot.   Allow beginning rotation to occur at toes, foot and ankle, and hip, but do not allow full range of toe flexion with adduction and hip extension – abduction to occur, until foot and ankle begin to plantar flex and evert.

NOTE: Resist stronger proximal and distal components, but guide weaker distal components through their optimal range of motion in accordance with normal timing.

Toes.   Allow beginning rotation to occur at toes, foot and ankle, and hip, but do not allow full range of foot and ankle plantar flexion with eversion to occur, until toes begin to flex and adduct toward fibular side.

NOTE: Resist stronger proximal components. Emphasis may be placed on metatarsal – phalangeal joints, or interphalangeal joints, or on a specific joint of a single toe.

Manual Contacts

Patient Is Able to Work Through Full Range of Pattern.   *Right hand:* Apply pressure of palmar surface of hand and fingers on lateral aspect of plantar surface of foot and toes (Fig. 1-67). *Left hand:* Apply pressure of palmar surface or with fingers in close approximation   on   posterior – lateral   aspect   of   thigh

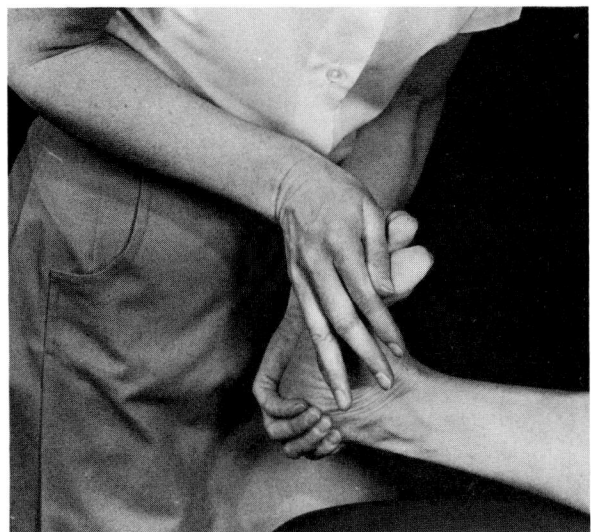

A. Le-R

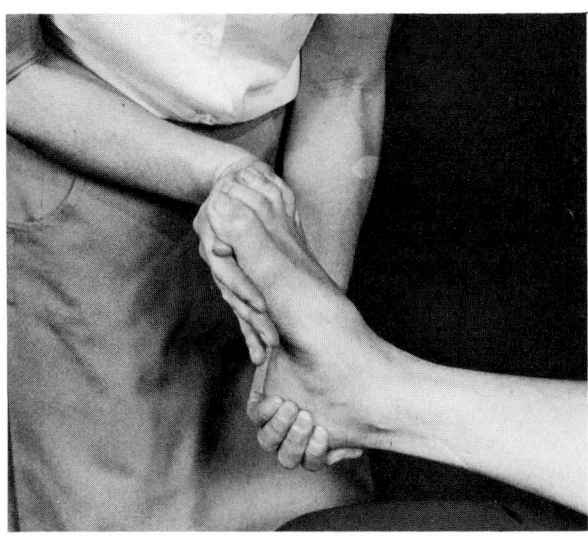

B. Mid-R

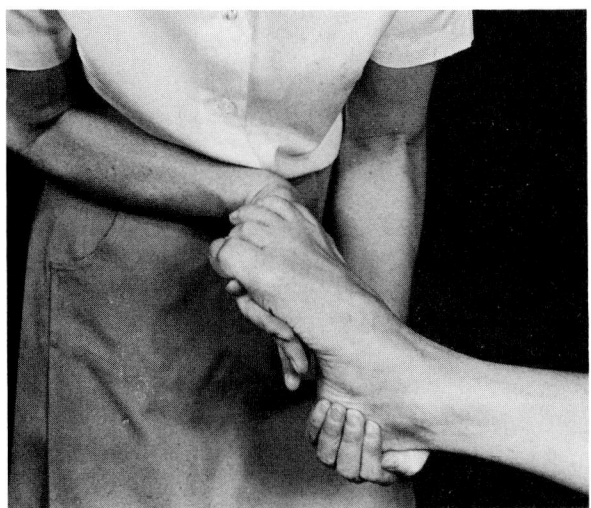

C. Sh-R

FOOT AND ANKLE (D1 ex)

FIG. 1-67, *continued*

proximal to popliteal space (Fig. 1-67).

Patient Has Difficulty in Initiating Motion. *Right hand:* As above. *Left hand:* As above, or with pressure applied by palmar surface with fingers free of contact on lateral aspect of heel.

Commands

Preparatory. "You are to turn your heel, and push your foot down and out toward me."

Action. "Push! Push your foot down and out! Keep your knee straight. Push down at the hip, toward me!"

Pattern Analysis

Hip. *Motion components:* Extension, abduction, internal rotation. *Major muscle components:* Gluteus medius, gluteus minimus, biceps femoris (hip extension component).

Knee. Straight (no motion).

Ankle, Foot, and Toes. *Motion components:* Plantar flexion, eversion of ankle and foot, flexion with adduction of toes toward fibular side. *Major muscle components:* Gastrocnemius (lateral head), soleus (lateral portion), peroneus longus, flexor digitorum longus, flexor digitorum brevis, flexor hallucis brevis, adductor hallucis, flexor digiti quinti brevis, quadratus plantae, plantar interossei, lumbricales.

Range-Limiting Factors

Tension or contracture of any muscles of flexion – adduction – external rotation (with knee straight) pattern (Fig. 1-64).

Extension–Abduction–Internal Rotation (D1 ex)

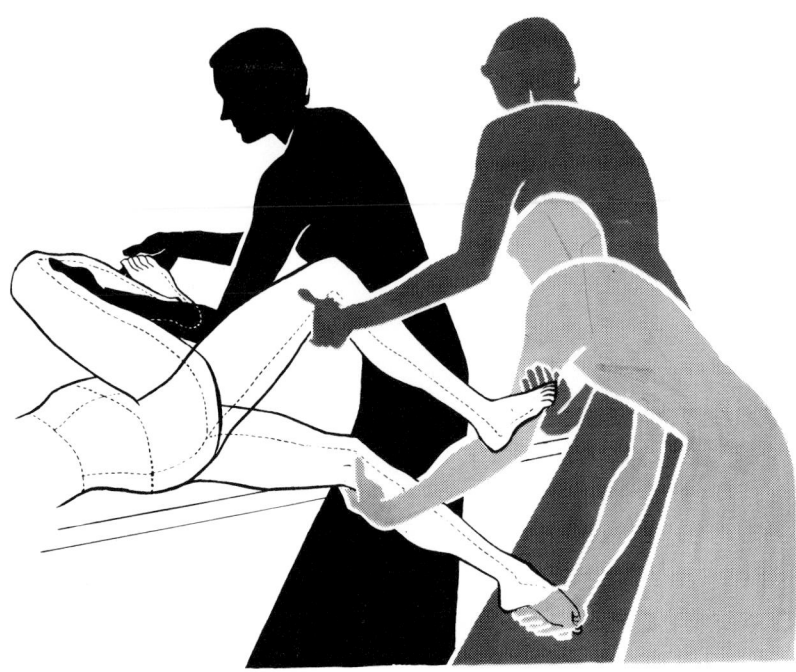

FIG. 1-68. With knee extension.

Antagonistic Pattern

Flexion–adduction–external rotation (with knee flexion) pattern (Fig. 1-65).

Components of Motion

Toes flex and adduct (lateral toes more than medial) toward fibular side; foot and ankle plantar flex with eversion; knee extends with tibia internally rotating on femur; hip extends, abducts, and internally rotates.

Normal Timing

Action is from distal to proximal, that is, action occurs first at toes, then foot and ankle, then knee, then hip.

Timing for Emphasis

Hip. Allow beginning rotation to occur at toes, foot and ankle, knee, and hip, but do not allow full range of flexion with adduction of toes, foot and ankle plantar flexion with eversion, and knee extension to occur, until hip begins to extend and abduct with internal rotation.

NOTE: If normal timing is prevented by excessive resistance to weaker distal components, action cannot occur proximally. Resist stronger distal components, but guide weaker distal components through their optimal range of motion in accordance with normal timing.

Knee. Allow beginning rotation to occur at toes, foot and ankle, knee, and hip, but do not allow full range of toe flexion with adduction, foot and ankle plantar flexion with eversion, and hip extension–abduction to occur, until knee begins to extend with internal rotation of tibia on femur.

NOTE: Resist stronger proximal and distal components, but guide weaker distal components through their optimal range of motion in accordance with normal timing.

Ankle and Foot. Allow beginning rotation to occur at toes, foot and ankle, knee, and hip, but do not allow full range of toe flexion with adduction, knee extension, and hip extension–abduction to occur, until foot and ankle begin to plantar flex and evert.

NOTE: Resist stronger proximal and distal components, but guide weaker distal components through their optimal range of motion in accordance with normal timing.

Toes. Allow beginning rotation to occur at toes, foot and ankle, knee, and hip, but do not allow full range of foot and ankle plantar flexion with eversion, knee extension, and hip extension–abduction to occur, until toes begin to flex and adduct toward fibular side.

NOTE: Resist stronger proximal components. Emphasis may be placed on metatarsal–phalangeal joints or interphalangeal joints, or on a specific joint of a single toe.

Manual Contacts

Patient Is Able to Work Through Full Range of Pattern. *Right hand:* Apply pressure of palmar surface of hand and fingers on lateral aspect of plantar surface of toes and foot (Fig. 1-68). *Left hand:* Apply pressure of palmar surface or with fingers in close approximation on posterior–lateral aspect of thigh proximal to popliteal space (Fig. 1-68).

Patient Has Difficulty in Initiating Motion. *Right hand:* As above. *Left hand:* As above, or with pressure applied by palmar surface with fingers free of contact on lateral aspect of heel.

Commands

Preparatory. "You are to turn your heel, and push your foot down and out toward me, and straighten your knee."

Action. "Push! Push your foot down and out! Push down at the hip and knee, toward me!"

Pattern Analysis

Hip. *Motion components:* Extension, abduction, internal rotation. *Major muscle components:* Gluteus medius, gluteus minimus.

Knee. *Motion components:* Extension with tibia internally rotating on femur. *Major muscle components:* Vastus intermedius, vastus lateralis, articularis genu.

Ankle, Foot, and Toes. See extension–abduction–internal rotation (with knee straight) pattern.

Range-Limiting Factors

Tension or contracture of any muscles of flexion–adduction–external rotation (with knee flexion) pattern (Fig. 1-65).

Extension – Abduction – Internal Rotation (D1 ex)

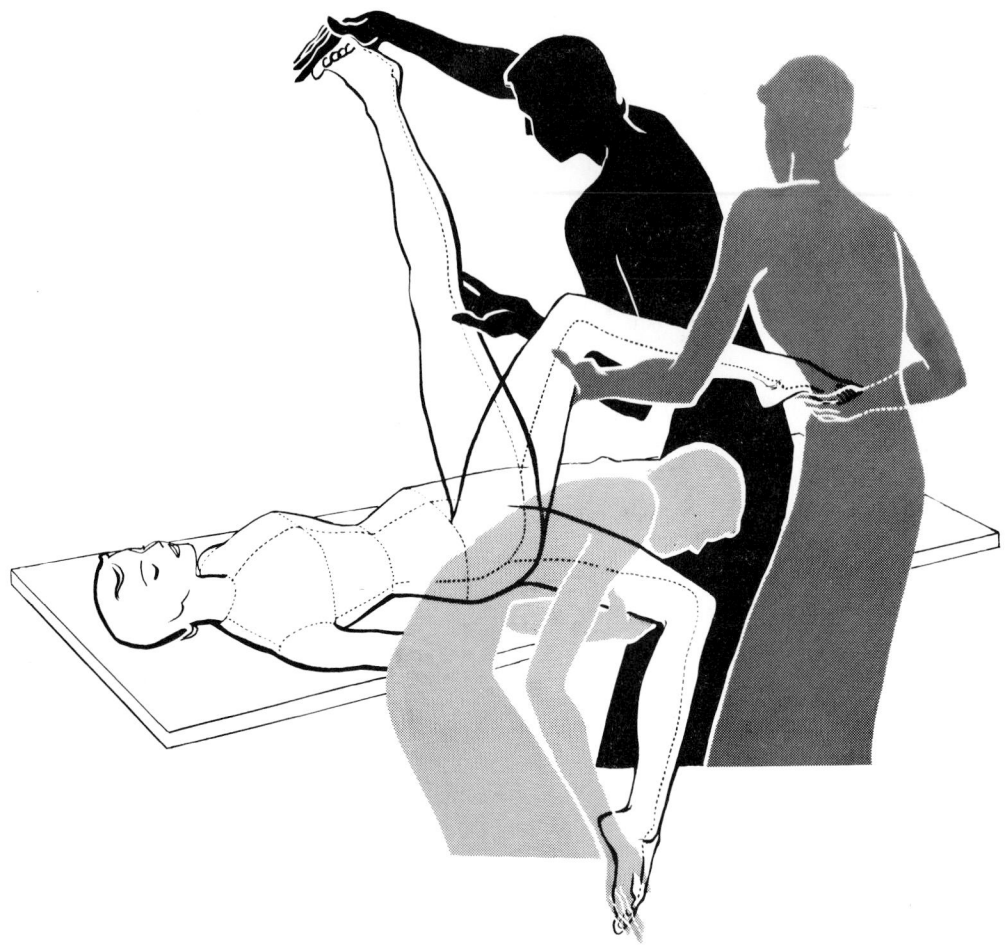

FIG. 1-69. With knee flexion.

Antagonistic Pattern

Flexion – adduction – external rotation (with knee extension) pattern (Fig. 1-66).

Components of Motion

Toes flex and adduct (lateral toes more than medial) toward fibular side; foot and ankle plantar flex with eversion; knee flexes with tibia internally rotating on femur; hip extends, abducts, and internally rotates.

Normal Timing

Action is from distal to proximal, that is, action occurs first at toes, then at foot and ankle, then at knee, then at hip.

Timing for Emphasis

Hip. Allow beginning rotation to occur at toes, foot and ankle, knee, and hip, but do not allow full range of toe flexion with adduction, foot and ankle plantar flexion with eversion, and knee flexion to occur, until hip begins to extend and abduct with internal rotation.

NOTE: If normal timing is prevented by excessive resistance to weaker distal components, action cannot occur proximally. Resist stronger distal components, but guide weaker distal components through their optimal range of motion in accordance with normal timing.

Knee. Allow beginning rotation to occur at toes, foot and ankle, knee, and hip, but do not allow full range of toe flexion with adduction, foot and ankle plantar flexion with eversion, and hip extension – abduction to occur, until knee begins to flex with internal rotation of tibia on femur.

NOTE: Resist stronger proximal and distal components, but guide weaker distal components through their optimal range of motion in accordance with normal timing.

Ankle and Foot. Allow beginning rotation to occur at toes, foot and ankle, knee, and hip, but do not allow full range of toe flexion with adduction, knee flexion, and hip extension – abduction to occur, until foot and ankle begin to plantar flex and evert.

NOTE: Resist stronger proximal and distal components, but guide weaker distal components through their optimal range of motion in accordance with normal timing.

Toes. Allow beginning rotation to occur at toes, foot and ankle, knee, and hip, but do not allow full range of foot and ankle plantar flexion with eversion, knee flexion, and hip extension – abduction to occur, until toes begin to flex and adduct toward fibular side.

NOTE: Resist stronger proximal components. Emphasis may be placed on metatarsal – phalangeal joints, or interphalangeal joints, or a specific joint of a single toe.

Manual Contacts

Patient Is Able to Work Through Full Range of Pattern. *Right hand:* Apply pressure of palmar surface of hand and fingers on lateral aspect of plantar surface of foot and toes (Fig. 1-69). *Left hand:* Apply pressure of palmar surface of hand or with fingers in close approximation on posterior – lateral aspect of thigh proximal to popliteal space (Fig. 1-69).

Patient Has Difficulty in Initiating Motion.

Right hand and left hand same as above.

Commands

Preparatory. "You are to turn your heel, and push your foot down and out toward me, and bend your knee."

Action. "Push! Push your toes down and out! Bend your knee! Push down at the hip, toward me!"

Pattern Analysis

Hip. *Motion components:* Extension, abduction, internal rotation. *Major muscle components:* Gluteus medius, gluteus minimus, biceps femoris (hip extension component).

Knee. *Motion components:* Flexion with internal rotation of tibia on femur. *Major muscle components:* Biceps femoris, popliteus, gastrocnemius (lateral head).

Ankle, Foot, and Toes. See extension – abduction – internal rotation (with knee straight) pattern.

Range-Limiting Factors

Tension or contracture of any muscles of flexion – adduction – external rotation (with knee extension) pattern (Fig. 1-66).

Flexion–Abduction–Internal Rotation (D2 fl)

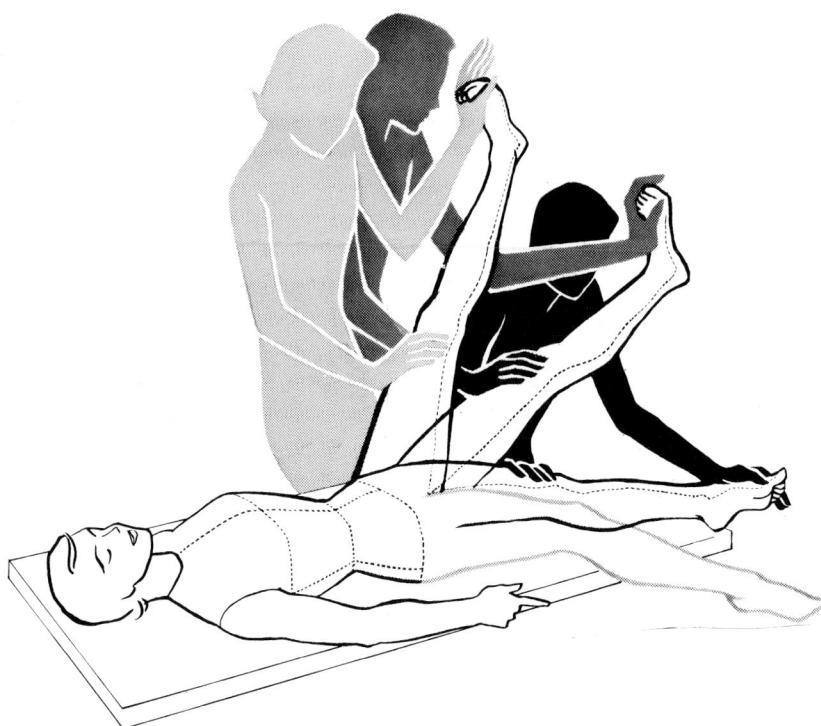

FIG. 1-70. With knee straight.

Antagonistic Pattern

Extension–adduction–external rotation (with knee straight) pattern (Fig. 1-73).

Components of Motion

Toes extend and abduct (lateral toes more than medial) toward the fibular side; foot and ankle dorsiflex with eversion; knee remains straight; hip flexes, abducts, and internally rotates.

Normal Timing

Action is from distal to proximal, that is, action occurs first at toes, then at foot and ankle, then at hip.

Timing for Emphasis

Hip. Allow beginning rotation to occur at toes and at foot and ankle, but do not allow full range of toe extension with abduction, and foot and ankle dorsiflexion with eversion to occur, until hip begins to flex and abduct with internal rotation.

NOTE: If normal timing is prevented by excessive resistance to weaker distal components, action cannot occur proximally. Resist stronger distal components, but guide weaker distal components through their optimal range of motion in accordance with normal timing.

Ankle and Foot. Allow beginning rotation to occur at toes, foot and ankle, and hip, but do not allow full range of toe extension with abduction and hip flexion–abduction to occur, until foot and ankle begin to dorsiflex and evert.

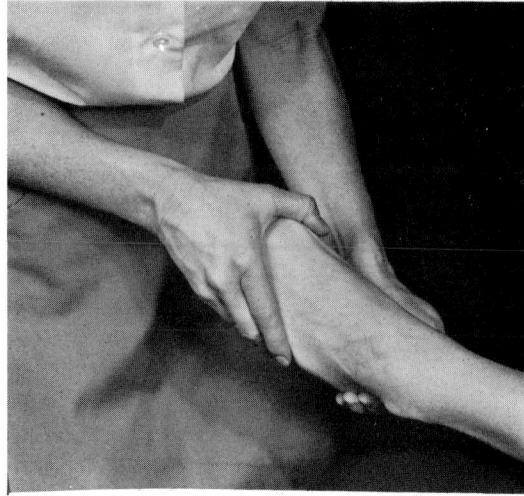

A. Le-R

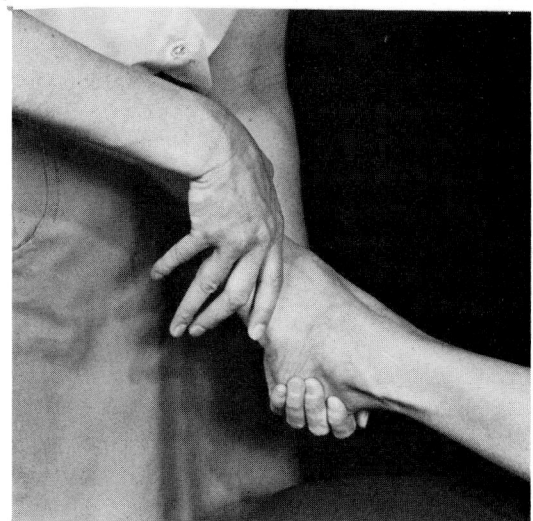

B. Mid-R

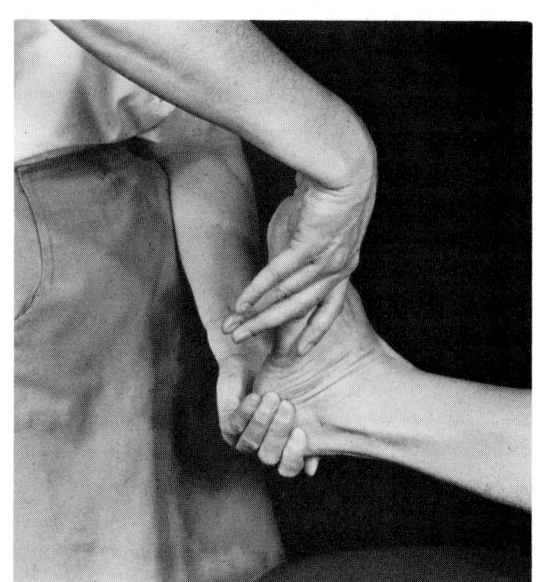

C. Sh-R

FOOT AND ANKLE (D2 fl)

NOTE: Resist stronger proximal and distal components, but guide weaker distal components through their optimal range of motion in accordance with normal timing.

Toes. Allow beginning rotation to occur at toes, foot and ankle, and hip, but do not allow full range of foot and ankle dorsiflexion with eversion and hip flexion – abduction to occur, until toes begin to extend and abduct toward fibular side.

NOTE: Resist stronger proximal components. Emphasis may be placed on metatarsal – phalangeal joints, or interphalangeal joints, or on a specific joint of a single toe.

Manual Contacts

Patient Is Able to Work Through Full Range of Pattern. Left hand: Apply pressure of palmar surface of hand on lateral aspect of dorsal surface of foot as far distal as a firm grip will permit. Avoid pressure on plantar surface of foot (Fig. 1-70). *Right hand:* Apply pressure of palmar surface of hand or with fingers in close approximation on anterior – lateral aspect of thigh proximal to patella (Fig. 1-70).

Patient Has Difficulty in Initiating Motion. Left hand: As above. *Right hand:* Apply pressure of palmar surface of hand or with fingers in close approximation on posterior – lateral aspect of thigh proximal to popliteal space; or pressure of palmar surface of hand on lateral aspect of heel.

Commands

Preparatory. "You are to turn your heel, and pull your foot up and out as far as possible."
Action. "Pull! Pull your foot up and out! Lift it up toward me!"

Pattern Analysis

Hip. Motion components: Flexion, abduction, internal rotation. *Major muscle components:* Tensor fasciae latae, rectus femoris (lateral portion, hip flexion component).
Knee. Straight (no motion).
Ankle, Foot, and Toes. Motion components: Dorsiflexion, eversion of ankle and foot, toe extension with abduction toward fibular side. *Major muscle components:* extensor digitorum longus, extensor hallucis longus, peroneus brevis, peroneus tertius, extensor digitorum brevis, abductor digiti quinti, dorsal interossei, lumbricales.

Range-Limiting Factors

Tension or contracture of any muscles of extension – adduction – external rotation (with knee straight) pattern (Fig. 1-73).

Flexion–Abduction–Internal Rotation (D2 fl)

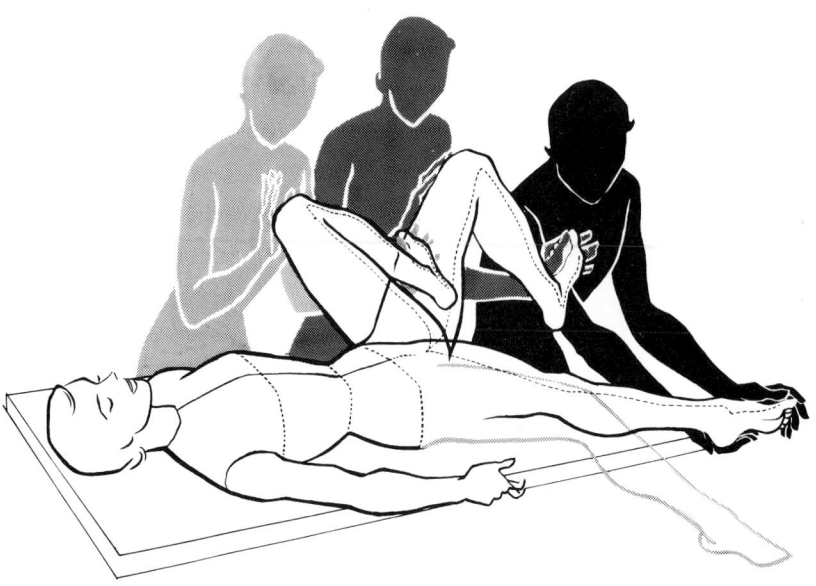

FIG. 1-71. With knee flexion.

Antagonistic Pattern

Extension–adduction–external rotation (with knee extension) pattern (Fig. 1-74).

Components of Motion

Toes extend and abduct (lateral toes more than medial) toward fibular side; foot and ankle dorsiflex with eversion; knee flexes with tibia internally rotating on femur; hip flexes, abducts, and internally rotates.

Normal Timing

Action is from distal to proximal, that is, action occurs first at toes, then at foot and ankle, then at knee, then at hip.

Timing for Emphasis

Hip. Allow beginning rotation to occur at toes, foot and ankle, knee, and hip, but do not allow full range of toe extension with abduction, foot and ankle dorsiflexion with eversion, and knee flexion to occur, until hip begins to flex and abduct with internal rotation.

NOTE: If normal timing is prevented by excessive resistance to weaker distal components, action cannot occur proximally. Resist stronger distal components, but guide weaker distal components through their optimal range of motion in accordance with normal timing.

Knee. Allow beginning rotation to occur at toes, foot and ankle, knee, and hip, but do not allow full range of toe extension with abduction, foot and ankle dorsiflexion with eversion, and hip flexion–abduction to occur, until knee begins to flex with internal rotation of tibia on femur.

NOTE: Resist stronger proximal and distal components, but guide weaker distal components through their optimal range of motion in accordance with normal timing.

Ankle and Foot. Allow beginning rotation to occur at toes, foot and ankle, knee, and hip, but do not allow full range of toe extension with abduction, knee flexion, and hip flexion–abduction to occur, until foot and ankle begin to dorsiflex and evert.

NOTE: Resist stronger proximal and distal components, but guide weaker distal components through their optimal range of motion in accordance with normal timing.

Toes. Allow beginning rotation to occur at toes, foot and ankle, knee, and hip, but do not allow full range of foot and ankle dorsiflexion with eversion, knee flexion, and hip flexion–abduction to occur, until toes begin to extend and abduct toward fibular side.

NOTE: Resist stronger proximal components. Emphasis may be placed on metatarsal–phalangeal joints, or interphalangeal joints, or a specific joint of a single toe.

Manual Contacts

Patient Is Able to Work Through Full Range of Pattern. *Left hand:* Apply pressure of palmar surface of hand on lateral aspect of dorsal surface of foot as far distal as a firm grip will permit. Avoid pressure on plantar surface of foot (Fig. 1-71). *Right hand:* Apply pressure of palmar surface of hand or with four fingers in close approximation on anterior–lateral aspect of thigh proximal to patella (*illustrated:* middle and shortened ranges).

Patient Has Difficulty in Initiating Motion. Left hand: As above. *Right hand:* Apply pressure of palmar surface of hand on posterior–lateral surface of thigh proximal to popliteal space, or pressure of palmar surface on lateral aspect of heel (Fig. 1-71, lengthened range).

Commands

Preparatory. "You are to turn your heel, and pull your foot up and out, and bend your knee."

Action. "Pull! Pull your foot up and out! Bend your knee! Pull up at the hip—toward me!"

Pattern Analysis

Hip. Motion components: Flexion, abduction, internal rotation. *Major muscle components:* Tensor fasciae latae.

Knee. Motion components: Flexion with tibia internally rotating on femur. *Major muscle components:* Biceps femoris, popliteus.

Ankle, Foot, and Toes. See flexion–abduction–internal rotation (with knee straight) pattern.

Range-Limiting Factors

Tension or contracture of any muscles of extension–adduction–external rotation (with knee extension) pattern (Fig. 1-74).

Flexion – Abduction – Internal Rotation (D2 fl)

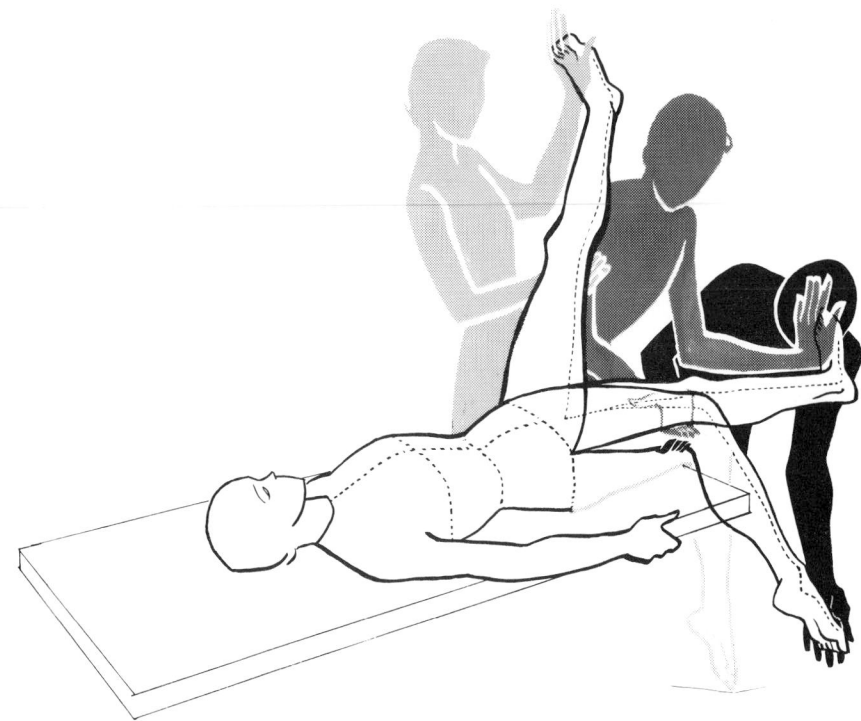

FIG. 1-72. With knee extension.

Antagonistic Pattern

Extension – adduction – external rotation (with knee flexion) pattern (Fig. 1-75).

Components of Motion

Toes extend and abduct (lateral toes more than medial) toward fibular side; foot and ankle dorsiflex with eversion; knee extends with tibia internally rotating on femur; hip flexes, abducts, and internally rotates.

Normal Timing

Action is from distal to proximal, that is, action occurs at toes, then foot and ankle, then at knee, and then at hip.

Timing for Emphasis

Hip. Allow beginning rotation to occur at toes, foot and ankle, knee, and hip, but do not allow full range of toe extension with abduction, foot and ankle dorsiflexion with eversion, and extension of knee to occur, until hip begins to flex and abduct with internal rotation.

NOTE: If normal timing is prevented by excessive resistance to weaker distal components, action cannot occur proximally. Resist stronger distal components, but guide weaker distal components through their optimal range of motion in accordance with normal timing.

Knee. Allow beginning rotation to occur at toes, foot and ankle, knee, and hip, but do not allow full range of toe extension with abduction, foot and ankle dorsiflexion with eversion, and hip flexion – abduction to occur, until knee begins to extend with internal rotation of tibia on femur.

NOTE: Resist stronger proximal and distal components, but guide weaker distal components through their optimal range of motion in accordance with normal timing.

Toes. Allow beginning rotation to occur at toes, foot and ankle, knee, and hip, but do not allow full range of foot and ankle dorsiflexion with inversion, knee extension, and hip flexion – abduction to occur, until toes begin to extend and abduct toward fibular side.

NOTE: Resist stronger proximal components. Emphasis may be placed on metatarsal – phalangeal joints, or interphalangeal joints, or on a specific joint of a single toe.

Manual Contacts

Patient Is Able to Work Through Full Range of Pattern. *Left hand:* Apply pressure of palmar surface of hand on lateral aspect of dorsal surface of foot as far distal as a firm grip will permit. Avoid pressure on plantar surface of foot (Fig. 1-72). *Right hand:* Apply pressure of palmar surface of hand or with fingers in close approximation on anterior–lateral surface of thigh proximal to patella.

Patient Has Difficulty in Initiating Motion. Left hand: As above. Fingers may be used to grip foot in order to guide motion. *Right hand:* Apply pressure of palmar surface of hand or with fingers in close approximation on posterior–lateral aspect of thigh proximal to popliteal space (Fig. 1-72).

Commands

Preparatory. "You are to turn your heel, and kick your foot up and out, and straighten your knee."

Action. "Kick! Pull your foot up and out! Kick it up here! Pull up at the hip toward me!"

Pattern Analysis

Hip. Motion components: Flexion, abduction, internal rotation. *Major muscle components:* Tensor fasciae latae, rectus femoris (lateral portion, hip flexion component).

Knee. Motion components: Extension with tibia internally rotating on femur. *Major muscle components:* Vastus intermedius, vastus lateralis, rectus femoris (lateral portion, articularis genu).

Ankle, Foot, and Toes. See flexion–abduction–internal rotation (with knee straight) pattern.

Range-Limiting Factors

Tension or contracture of any muscle of extension–adduction–external rotation (with knee flexion) pattern (Fig. 1-75).

Extension–Adduction–External Rotation (D2 ex)

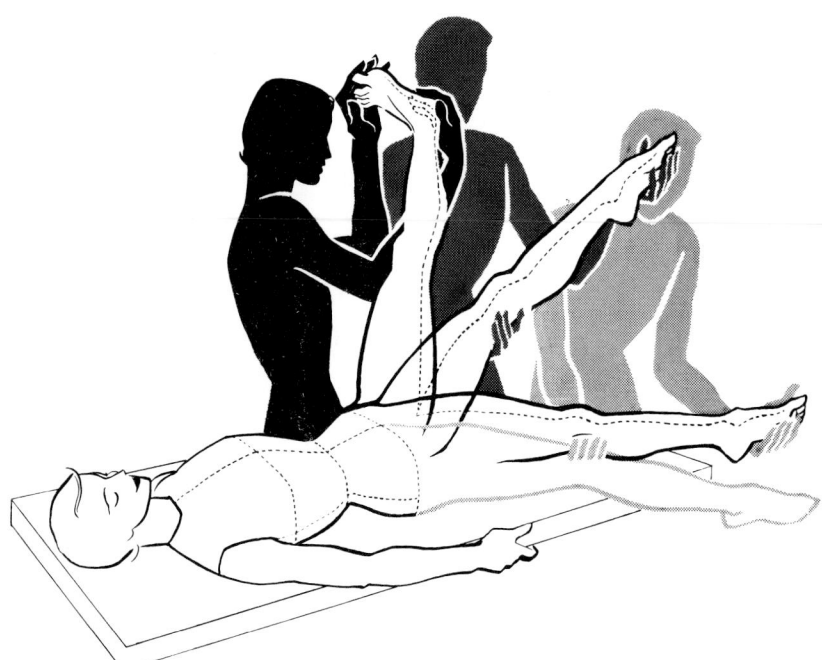

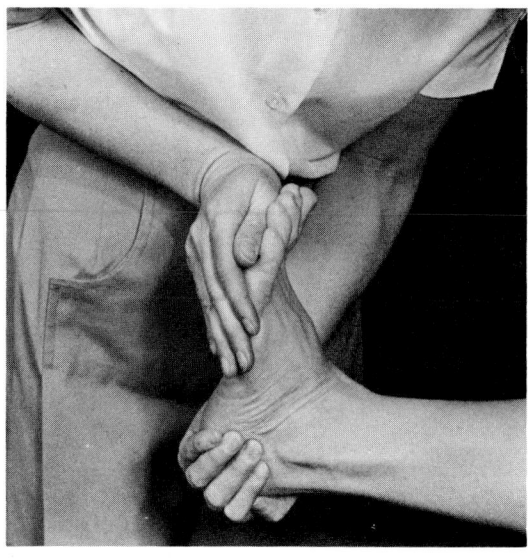

A. Le-R

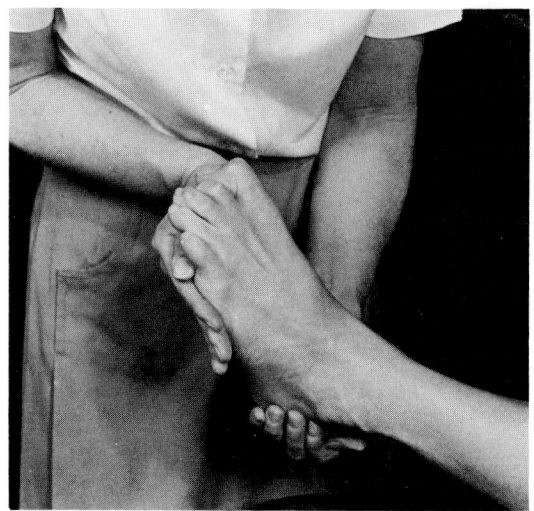

B. Mid-R

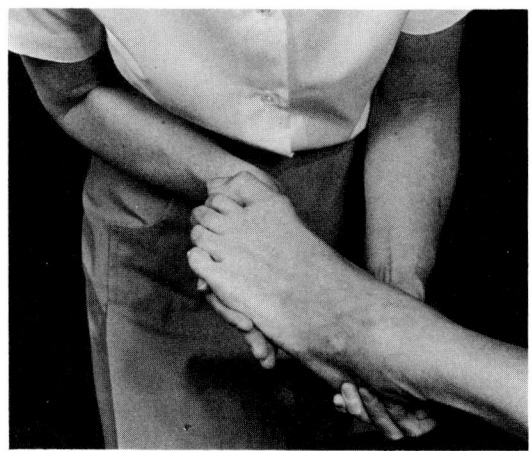

C. Sh-R

FOOT AND ANKLE (D2 ex)

FIG. 1-73. With knee straight.

Antagonistic Pattern

Flexion–abduction–internal rotation (with knee straight) pattern (Fig. 1-70).

Components of Motion

Toes flex and adduct (medial toes more than lateral) toward tibial side; foot and ankle plantar flex with inversion; knee remains straight; hip extends, adducts, and externally rotates.

Normal Timing

Action is from distal to proximal, that is, action occurs first at toes, then at foot and ankle, then at hip.

Timing for Emphasis

Hip. Allow beginning rotation to occur at toes, foot and ankle, and hip, but do not allow full range of toe flexion with adduction, and foot and ankle plantar flexion with inversion to occur, until hip begins to extend and adduct with external rotation.

NOTE: If normal timing is prevented by excessive resistance to weaker distal components, action cannot occur proximally. Resist stronger distal components, but guide weaker distal components through their optimal range of motion in accordance with normal timing.

Ankle and Foot. Allow beginning rotation to occur at toes, foot and ankle, and hip, but do not allow full range of toe flexion with adduction, and extension–adduction of hip to occur, until the foot and ankle begin to plantar flex and invert.

NOTE: Resist stronger proximal and distal components, but guide weaker distal components through their optimal range of motion in accordance with normal timing.

Toes. Allow beginning rotation to occur at toes, foot and ankle, and hip, but do not allow full range of foot and ankle plantar flexion with inversion, and hip extension–adduction to occur, until toes begin to flex and adduct toward tibial side.

NOTE: Resist stronger proximal components. Emphasis may be placed on metatarsal–phalangeal joints, or interphalangeal joints, or on a specific joint of a single toe.

Manual Contacts

Patient Is Able to Work Through Full Range of Pattern. *Left hand:* Apply pressure of palmar surface of hand and fingers on medial aspect of plantar surface of toes and foot (Fig. 1-73). *Right hand:* Apply pressure of palmar surface of hand on posterior–medial aspect of thigh proximal to popliteal space (Fig. 1-73, middle and shortened ranges).

Patient Has Difficulty in Initiating Motion. *Left hand:* As above. *Right hand:* As above, or apply pressure of fingers in close approximation on the medial aspect of heel. (Fig. 1-73, lengthened range; **A, B, C,** left hand).

Commands

Preparatory. "You are to turn your heel, and push your foot down and in, away from me."
Action. "Push! Push your foot down and in! Push down at the hip, away from me!"

Pattern analysis

Hip. *Motion components:* Extension, adduction, external rotation. *Major muscle components:* Gluteus maximus, piriformis, gemellus superior, gemellus inferior, obturator internus, quadratus femoris, adductor magnus, and semimembranosus and semitendinosus (hip extension components).
Knee. Straight (no motion).
Ankle, Foot, and Toes. *Motion components:* Plantar flexion and inversion of ankle and foot, flexion with adduction of toes toward tibial side. *Major muscle components:* Plantaris, gastrocnemius (medial head), soleus (medial portion), tibialis posterior, flexor digitorum longus, flexor hallucis longus, quadratus plantae, flexor digitorum brevis, flexor hallucis brevis, plantar interossei, lumbricales.

Range-Limiting Factors

Tension or contracture of any muscles of flexion–abduction–internal rotation (with knee straight) pattern (Fig. 1-70).

Extension–Adduction–External Rotation (D2 ex)

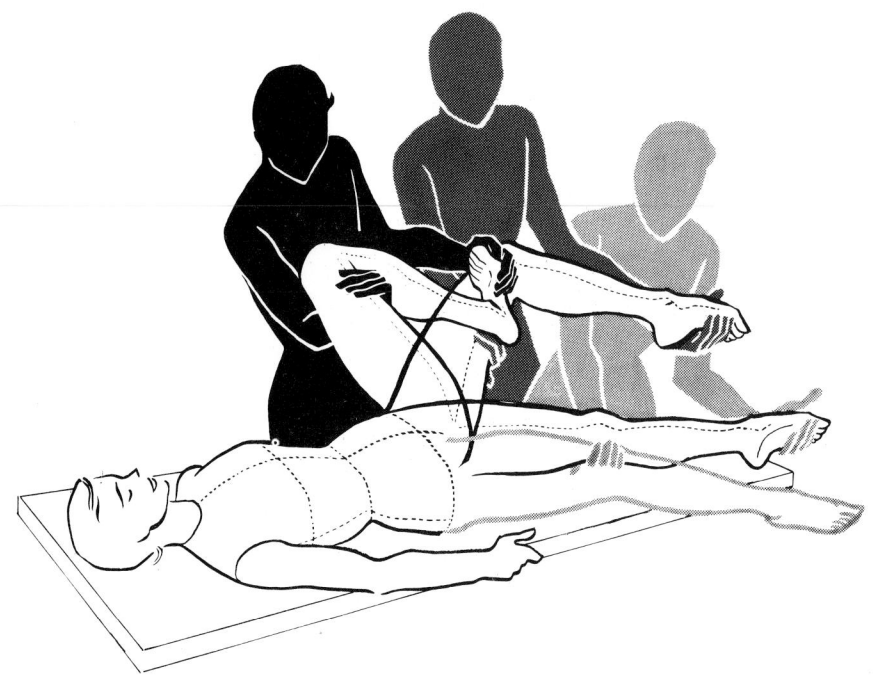

FIG. 1-74. With knee extension.

Antagonistic Pattern

Flexion–abduction–internal rotation (with knee flexion) pattern (Fig. 1-71).

Components of Motion

Toes flex and adduct (medial toes more than lateral) toward tibial side; foot and ankle plantar flex with inversion; knee extends with tibia externally rotating on femur; hip extends, adducts, and externally rotates.

Normal Timing

Action is from distal to proximal, that is, action occurs first at toes, then at foot and ankle, then at knee, and then at hip.

Timing for Emphasis

Hip. Allow beginning rotation to occur at toes, foot and ankle, knee, and hip, but do not allow full range of toe flexion with adduction, foot and ankle plantar flexion with inversion, and knee extension to occur, until hip begins to extend and adduct with external rotation.

NOTE: If normal timing is prevented by excessive resistance to weaker distal components, action cannot occur proximally. Resist stronger distal components, but guide weaker distal components through their optimal range of motion in accordance with normal timing.

Knee. Allow beginning rotation to occur at toes, foot and ankle, knee, and hip, but do not allow full range of toe flexion with adduction, foot and ankle plantar flexion with inversion, and hip extension–adduction to occur, until knee begins to extend with external rotation of tibia on femur.

NOTE: Resist stronger proximal and distal components, but guide weaker distal components through their optimal range of motion in accordance with normal timing.

Ankle and Foot. Allow beginning rotation to occur at toes, foot and ankle, knee, and hip, but do not allow full range of toe flexion with adduction, knee extension, and hip extension–adduction to occur, until foot and ankle begin to plantar flex and invert.

NOTE: Resist stronger proximal and distal components, but guide weaker distal components through their optimal range of motion in accordance with normal timing.

Toes. Allow beginning rotation to occur at toes, foot and ankle, knee, and hip, but do not allow full range of foot and ankle plantar flexion with inversion, knee extension, and hip extension–adduction to occur, until toes begin to flex and adduct toward tibial side.

NOTE: Resist stronger proximal components. Emphasis may be placed on metatarsal–phalangeal joints, or interphalangeal joints, or on a specific joint of a single toe.

Manual Contacts

Patient Is Able to Work Through Full Range of Pattern. *Left hand:* Apply pressure of palmar surface of hand or with fingers in close approximation on medial aspect of plantar surface of toes and foot (Fig. 1-74). *Right hand:* Apply pressure of palmar surface of hand or with fingers in close approximation on posterior–medial aspect of thigh proximal to popliteal space (Fig. 1-74).

Patient Has Difficulty in Initiating Motion. *Left hand:* As above. *Right hand:* As above.

Commands

Preparatory. "You are to turn your heel, and push your foot down and in, and straighten your knee."

Action. "Push! Push your foot down and in! Push down at the knee and hip, away from me!"

Pattern analysis

Hip. *Motion components:* Extension, adduction, external rotation. *Major muscle components:* Gluteus maximus, piriformis, gemellus superior, gemellus inferior, obturator internus, quadratus femoris, adductor magnus.

Knee. *Motion components:* Extension with tibia externally rotating on femur. *Major muscle components:* Vastus medialis, articularis genu.

Ankle, Foot, and Toes. See extension–adduction–external rotation (with knee straight) pattern (Fig. 1-73).

Range-Limiting Factors

Tension or contracture of any muscles of flexion–abduction–internal rotation (with knee flexion) pattern (Fig. 1-71).

Extension – Adduction – External Rotation (D2 ex)

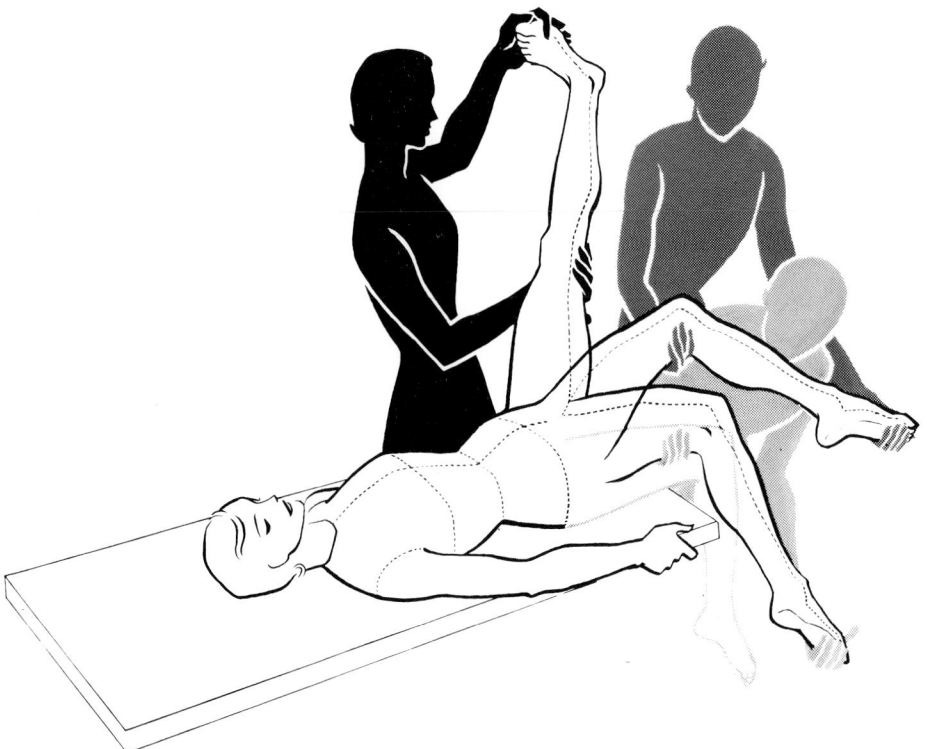

FIG. 1-75. With knee flexion.

Antagonistic Pattern

Flexion – abduction – internal rotation (with knee extension) pattern (Fig. 1-72).

Components of Motion

Toes flex and adduct (medial toes more than lateral) toward tibial side; foot and ankle plantar flex with inversion; knee flexes with tibia externally rotating on femur; hip extends, adducts, and externally rotates.

Normal Timing

Action is from distal to proximal, that is, action occurs first at toes, then at foot and ankle, then at knee, and then at hip.

Timing for Emphasis

Hip. Allow beginning rotation to occur at toes, foot and ankle, knee, and hip, but do not allow full range of toe flexion with adduction, foot and ankle plantar flexion with inversion, and knee flexion to occur, until hip begins to extend and adduct with external rotation.

NOTE: If normal timing is prevented by excessive resistance to weaker distal components, action cannot occur proximally. Resist stronger distal components, but guide weaker distal components through their optimal range of motion in accordance with normal timing.

Knee. Allow beginning rotation to occur at toes, foot and ankle, knee, and hip, but do not allow full range of toe flexion with adduction, foot and ankle plantar flexion with inversion, and hip extension – adduction to occur, until knee begins to flex with external rotation of tibia on femur.

NOTE: Resist stronger proximal and distal components, but guide weaker distal components through their optimal range of motion in accordance with normal timing.

Ankle and Foot. Allow beginning rotation to occur at toes, foot and ankle, knee, and hip, but do not allow full range of toe flexion with adduction, knee flexion, and hip extension – adduction to occur until foot and ankle begin to plantar flex and invert.

NOTE: Resist stronger proximal and distal components, but guide weaker distal components through their optimal range of motion in accordance with normal timing.

Toes. Allow beginning rotation to occur at toes, foot and ankle, knee, and hip, but do not allow full range of foot and ankle plantar flexion with inversion, knee flexion, and hip extension – adduction to occur, until the toes begin to flex and adduct toward tibial side.

NOTE: Resist stronger proximal components. Emphasis may be placed on metatarsal – phalangeal joints, or interphalangeal joints, or on a specific joint of a single toe.

Manual Contacts

Patient Is Able to Work Through Full Range of Pattern. *Left hand:* Apply pressure of palmar surface of hand or with fingers in close approximation on medial aspect of plantar surface of toes and foot (Fig. 1-75). *Right hand:* Apply pressure of palmar surface of hand or with fingers in close approximation on posterior – medial aspect of thigh proximal to popliteal space (Fig. 1-75).

Patient Has Difficulty in Initiating Motion. *Left hand:* As above, or with pressure on posterior – medial aspect of heel. *Right hand:* As above.

Commands

Preparatory. "You are to turn your heel, and push your foot down and in, and bend your knee."

Action. "Push! Push your foot down and in! Push down at the hip, away from me!"

Pattern Analysis

Hip. *Motion components:* Extension, adduction, external rotation. *Major muscle components:* Gluteus maximus, piriformis, gemellus superior, gemellus inferior, obturator internus, quadratus femoris, adductor magnus, and semimembranosus and semitendinosus (hip extension components).

Knee. *Motion components:* Flexion with external rotation of tibia on femur. *Major muscle components:* Semimembranosus, semitendinosus, gastrocnemius (medial head), plantaris.

Ankle, Foot, and Toes. See extension – adduction – external rotation (with knee straight) pattern (Fig. 1-73).

Range-Limiting Factors

Tension or contracture of any muscles of flexion – abduction – internal rotation (with knee extension) pattern (Fig. 1-72).

TIMING FOR EMPHASIS AND RANGE OF MOTION VARIATION

Timing for emphasis of various pivots of action has been presented for each pattern of facilitation. When timing for emphasis is applied as a technique, the range of motion varies according to the pivot emphasized. When a proximal pivot is emphasized, complete range of motion of that pivot is desired. When a distal pivot is emphasized, range of motion of the proximal pivot may be prevented by resistance as a means for stimulating or increasing the responses of the distal pivot. Figures 1-76 through 1-81 show variations in range of motion. The components of motion and the major muscle components are the same as when the pattern is performed with complete range of all pivots

of action. Le-R = lengthened range, Mid-R = middle range, and Sh-R = shortened range.

Selected Bilateral Combinations for Emphasis

Legends include pivots of action or points in range to be emphasized.

Upper Extremities
Shoulders: Figs. 1-83, 1-84, 1-86, and 1-88
Shoulders and Elbows: Figs. 1-94, 1-95, 1-96, and 1-97
Elbows: Figs. 1-99, 1-101, 1-102, and 1-103
Hands and Wrists: Figs. 1-104, 1-105, 1-107, and 1-108

Lower Extremities
Hips: Figs. 1-110, 1-112, 1-113, and 1-115
Hips and Knees: Figs. 1-121, 1-123, 1-125, and 1-126
Knees: Figs. 1-127, 1-128, 1-130, and 1-133
Feet and Ankles: Figs. 1-139, 1-142, 1-146, and 1-147

(Text continues on page 134)

Upper Extremity

Flexion–Abduction–External Rotation (D2 fl)

WITH MASS OPENING OF THE HAND

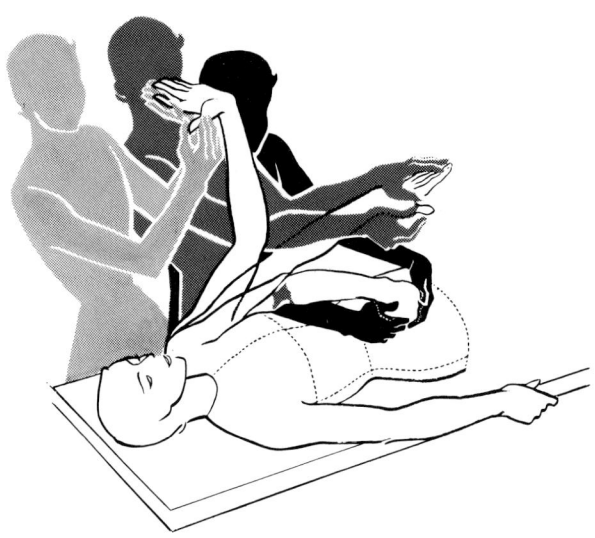

FIG. 1-76. Emphasis of the distal pivots, fingers, and hand prevents complete range of shoulder motion. For complete range of motion see the flexion – abduction – external rotation (with elbow straight) pattern (Fig. 1-50).

D1 fl, Le-R for Closing   REVERSAL: D1 ex, Sh-R for Opening

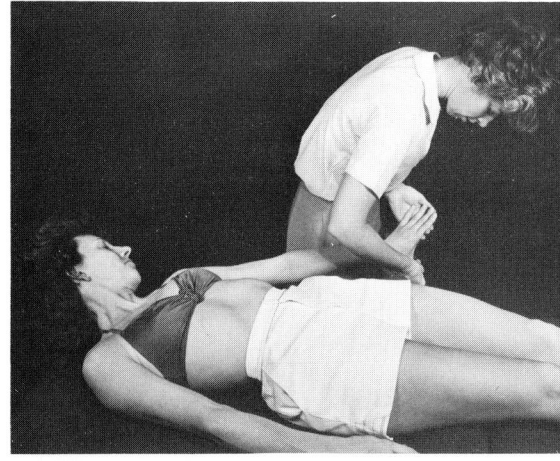

A. Le-R

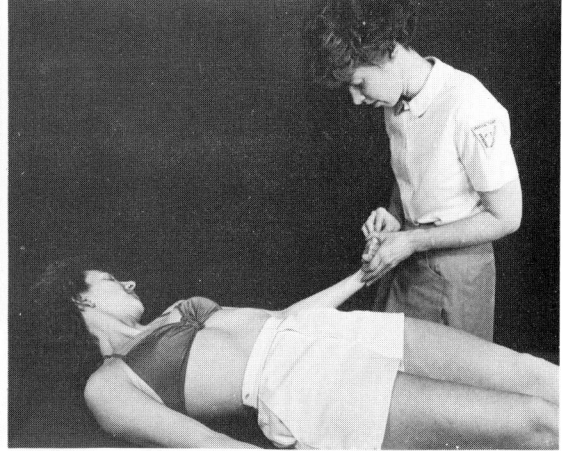

A. Le-R

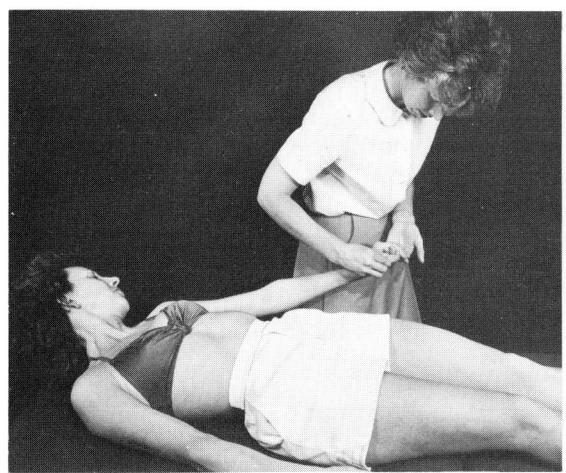

B. Mid-R

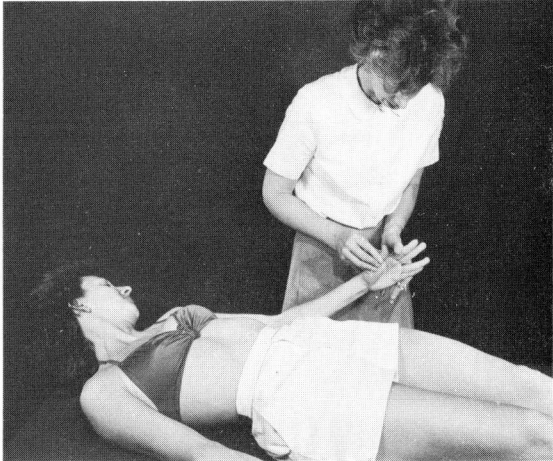

B. Mid-R

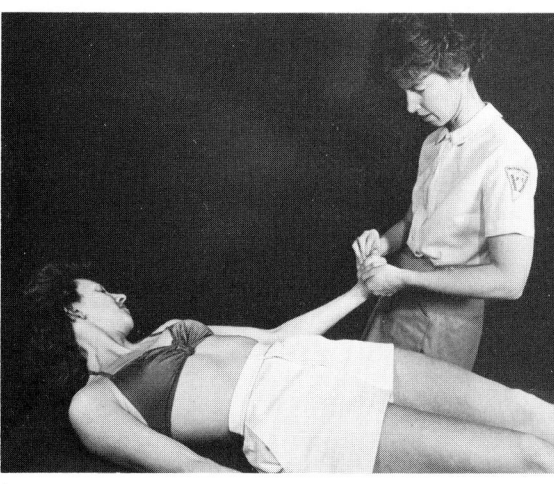

C. Sh-R

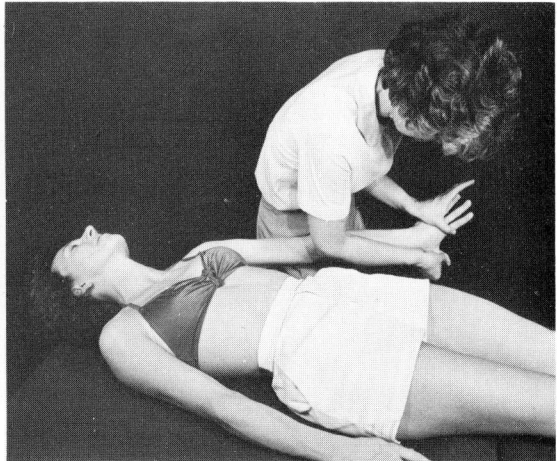

C. Sh-R

FIG. 1-77

D1 ex, Le-R for Opening   REVERSAL: D1 fl, Sh-R for Closing

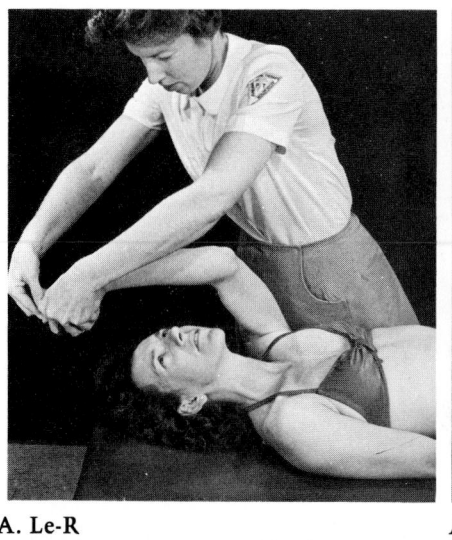 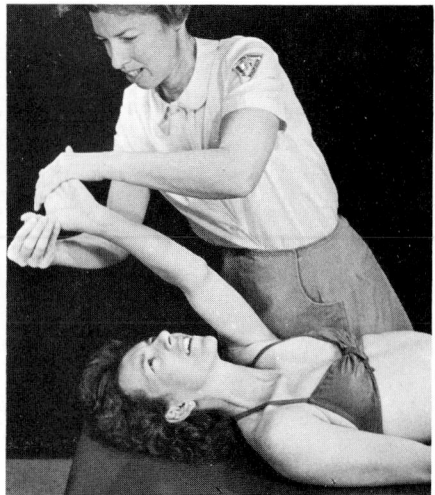

A. Le-R   A. Le-R

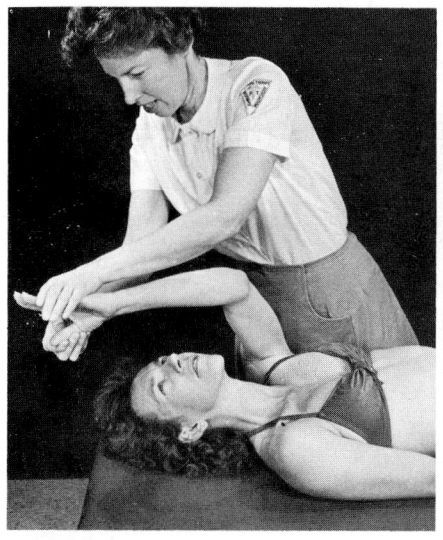 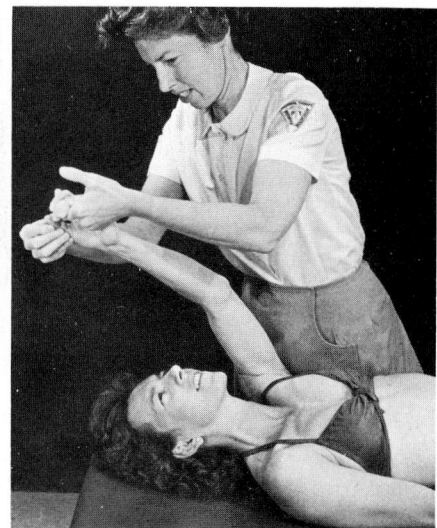

B. Mid-R   B. Mid-R

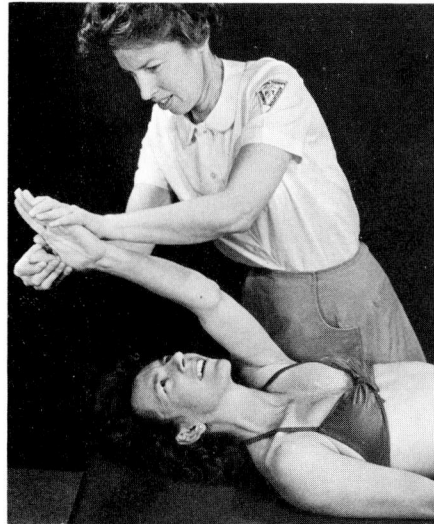 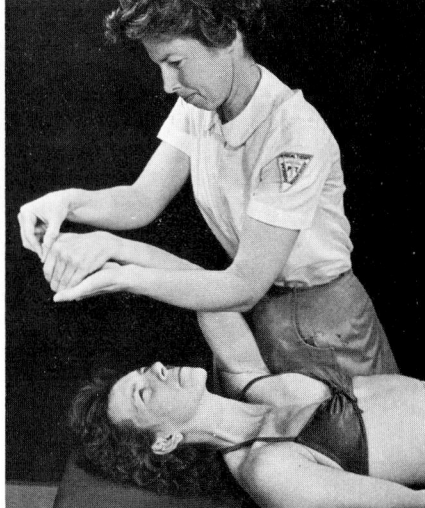

C. Sh-R   C. Sh-R

FIG. 1-78

D2 fl, Le-R for Opening   REVERSAL: D2 ex, Le-R for Closing

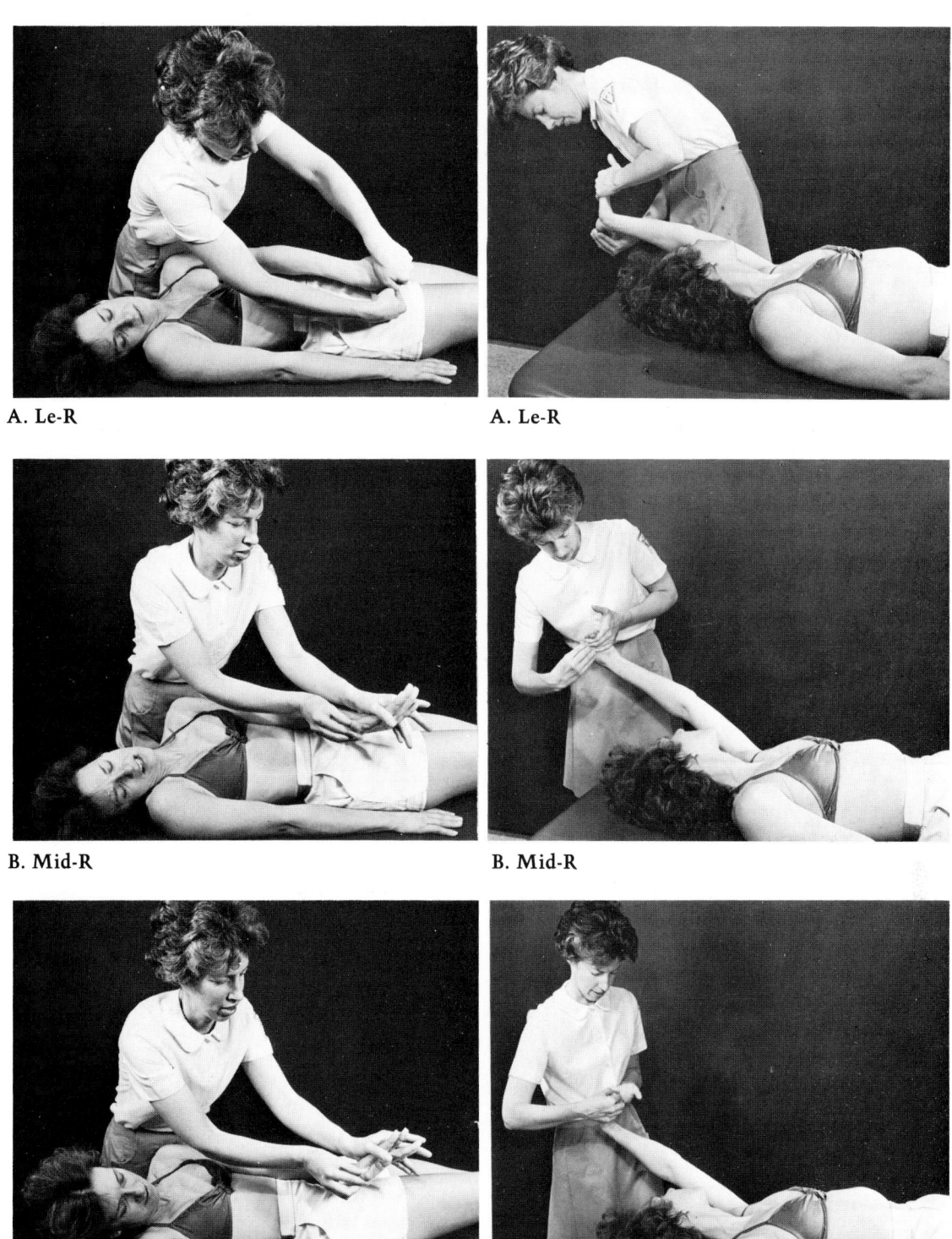

A. Le-R   A. Le-R

B. Mid-R   B. Mid-R

C. Sh-R   C. Sh-R

FIG. 1-79

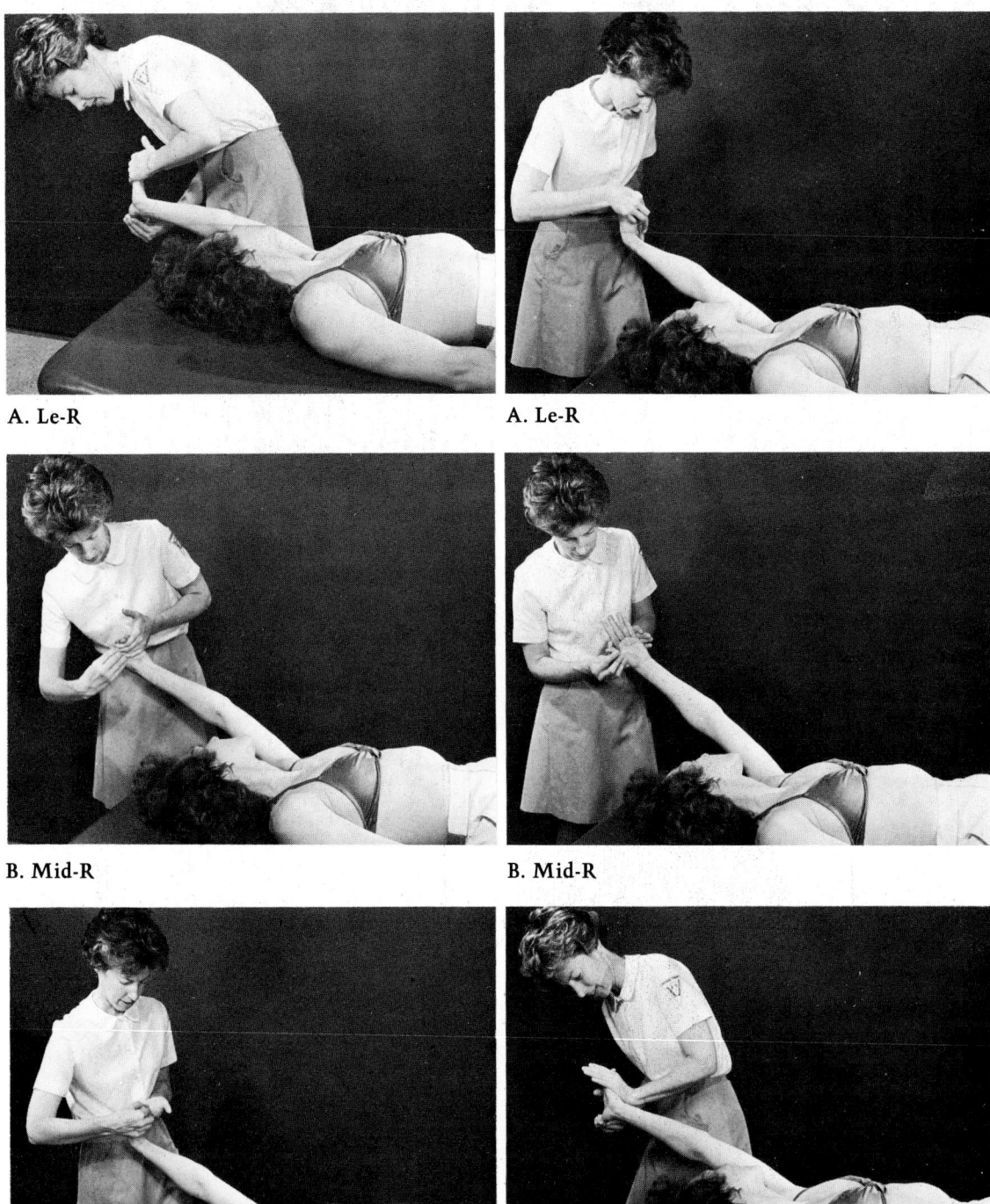

A. Le-R   A. Le-R

B. Mid-R   B. Mid-R

C. Sh-R   C. Sh-R

FIG. 1-80

Lower Extremity

Flexion–Adduction–External Rotation (D1 fl)

WITH DORSIFLEXION AND INVERSION OF THE ANKLE

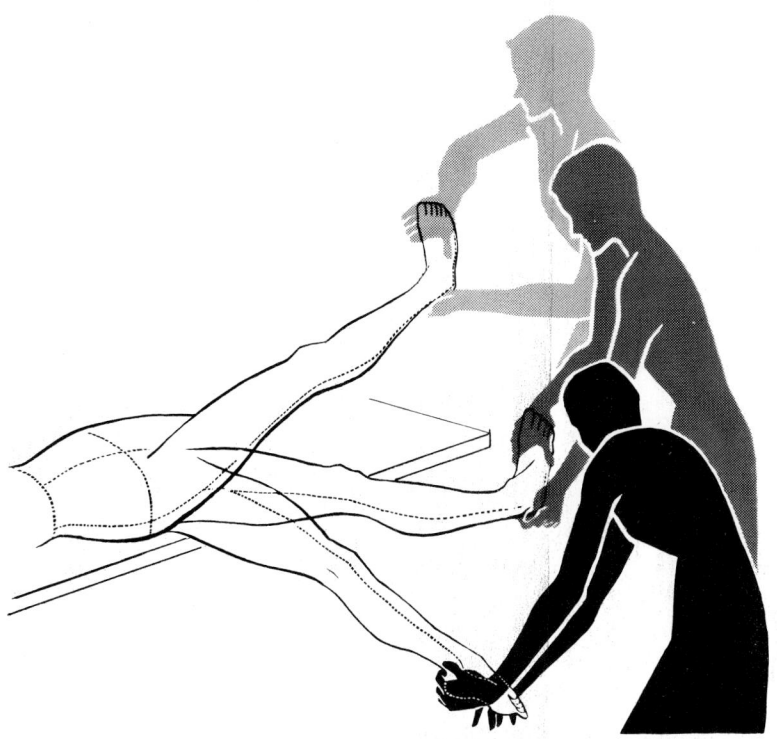

FIG. 1-81. Emphasis of the distal pivots, the foot, and the ankle prevents a complete range of hip motion. For complete range of motion see the flexion – adduction – external rotation (with knee straight) pattern (Fig. 1-64). *Note:* For Manual Contacts, Foot and Ankle, see Figs. 1-64, 1-67, 1-70, and 1-73.

BILATERAL COMBINATIONS FOR REINFORCEMENT

The method of PNF employs reinforcement and irradiation as means of increasing the strength of a response. The major muscle components of a specific pattern augment and reinforce each other in order that the motion may be accomplished. Reinforcement extends beyond the specific pattern when maximal resistance is superimposed.[48] An extremity pattern performed against resistance may demand reinforcement by the neck, trunk, and all other extremities. Combinations of patterns performed against resistance simulate stress situations which call into play the basic reflexes as reinforcement.

Combining Patterns

Normal motor activity requires innumerable combinations of motions. Segments of the body interact in an integrated fashion in order that movement may be coordinated and purposeful (see Table 1-7). This cooperation of various body segments may be termed *reinforcement*, since it is necessary to successful performance. In stress situations or in activities referred to as large muscle activities, such as active sports or manual labor, reinforcement becomes readily evident. Reinforcement in the mature normal subject occurs automatically and in accordance with the demands of the situation. Under stress, irradiation or spread of muscle activity occurs automatically in other body parts to support the desired movement or activity.[17]

Reinforcing motions are acquired in the developmental process and in the learning of functional skills. They become established at the reflex level and include basic reflexes such as the tonic neck and labyrinthine reflexes, the primitive mass flexion and mass extension reflexes, and the postural and righting reflexes. These reflexes play a role in the automaticity of reinforcement in stress situations.

The relationships between vision and movement provide further keys to reinforcement. In normal subjects, vision is important to perception and performance of a motor act.[41] As head and neck and upper trunk patterns are performed, vision leads the movement. Asking the patient to look in the direction of the movement will contribute to his performance. As the upper extremity patterns are done, the eyes may follow the hand, or, again, the patient may be asked to look in the desired direction so that the hand follows the eyes. Children are lured to look and pursue. Adults may require similar stimuli.

The normal subject is capable of performing all combinations of patterns of facilitation, and the potentials for reinforcement are many. Reinforcement is a two-way proposition depending upon the demands of the situation.

The patterns of the neck may reinforce the trunk, or the trunk may reinforce the neck. The neck and trunk may reinforce the unilateral or bilateral extremities, or the extremities may reinforce the neck and trunk. The unilateral upper extremity patterns which reinforce the neck, or are reinforced by the neck, are those in which the eye may readily follow the hand. The extremities may reinforce each other with bilateral symmetrical, bilateral asymmetrical, or bilateral reciprocal combinations. One extremity may reinforce its ipsilateral or contralateral upper or lower extremity. An example of bilateral extremity patterns is charted in Table 1-4. Although the potentials for reinforcement are many, certain combinations of the major components are used. Flexion, extension, or rotation patterns of the neck reinforce the homologous trunk patterns. Flexion of the upper extremities reinforces upper trunk extension. Extension of the upper extremities reinforces upper trunk flexion. Flexion of the lower extremities reinforces lower trunk flexion, and extension of the lower extremities reinforces lower trunk extension. Flexion or extension of one extremity reinforces flexion or extension of the opposite extremity. Flexion of a lower extremity reinforces adduction of an upper extremity. Extension of a lower extremity reinforces abduction of an upper extremity. The pattern combinations for reinforcement are given in Reference Tables 1 to 7.

The deficient neuromuscular mechanism is incapable of meeting the physical demands of life. This does not preclude the reinforcement of weak patterns by stronger patterns. The less the deficiency, the more effective reinforcement will be. The greater the defi-

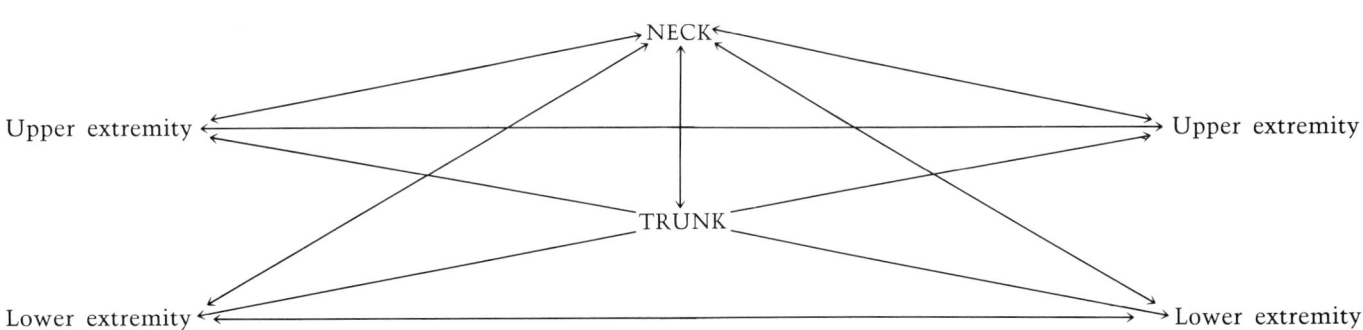

Table 1-4. Sample Bilateral Extremity Patterns

| | Patterns of Opposite Extremity Used as Reinforcement | | | |
| | | | Reciprocal | |
Extremity and pattern to be reinforced	Symmetrical	Asymmetrical	Same diagonal	Opposite diagonal
Lower extremity Flexion– adduction– external rotation	Flexion– adduction– external rotation	Flexion– abduction– internal rotation	Extension– abduction– internal rotation	Extension– adduction– external rotation

ciency, the greater the need for reinforcement.

When selecting pattern combinations for reinforcement, the developmental level of the subject must be considered. The infant who has not reached the level of reciprocal motions cannot be expected to respond to reciprocal patterns. Bilateral symmetrical and asymmetrical patterns must first be established, along with mass flexion and mass extension of neck, trunk, and extremities.

The adult who presents gross deficiency of the neuromuscular mechanism must begin recovery with the same fundamental patterns that he used in infancy. Response in the child and the adult may be stimulated by resisted rolling, pivoting, creeping, and plantigrade walking. Activities such as coming to a sitting position, push-ups, getting to a kneeling position, and getting to a standing position may be resisted in order to accelerate the learning process. Resistance to sitting balance, balancing in the hand–knee position, kneeling balance, and standing balance bring into play the postural and righting reflexes, which augment the strength of response. Other techniques of facilitation including timing for emphasis, reversals, rhythmic stabilization, and repeated contractions may be superimposed.

Whereas the use of developmental activities increases the response of the neuromuscular mechanism, refinement of response and function is dependent upon specific reinforcements. A specific pattern that is deficient is reinforced by a related pattern. The relationship may be functional and topographical. Functional relationship exists between the bilateral patterns of the upper extremities when they are combined with upper trunk flexion or extension in motions such as chopping and lifting. Topographical contiguity exists, for example, between the flexion–abduction–external rotation pattern of the upper extremity and the neck extension with rotation pattern, when this pattern is performed toward the side of the extremity. The trapezius muscle provides their topographical contiguity.

The specific pattern of reinforcement must present greater total ability than the pattern it is to reinforce. For example, the extension–abduction–

internal rotation pattern is a good choice of reinforcement for the flexion–adduction–external rotation pattern of the opposite extremity. However, if it does not enhance the response of the less adequate pattern, a second pattern must be selected.

Decisions about desirable patterns of reinforcement are partially based upon whether they correct or prevent imbalances. Since the potentials for reinforcement are so numerous, it should be possible to prevent increase of imbalances. Wise selection of reinforcements may serve a dual purpose. A reinforcement may strengthen the response in a weaker pattern and may, at the same time, be a desired pivot of emphasis. For example, the flexion–adduction–external rotation pattern of the left upper extremity may be deficient. The extension–abduction–internal rotation pattern of the right upper extremity may provide good reinforcement even though it may be less strong than its antagonistic pattern. Using this reinforcement benefits the reinforcing pattern as well as the reinforced pattern.

The use of various related patterns as reinforcement for a deficient pattern is advisable, since in normal activity many combinations of motion are used. A specific pattern should be reeducated and trained to work in combination with its related patterns. Such a procedure helps to reestablish the automaticity of reinforcing motions.

Reinforcement is comparatively simple. It is necessary to have a meticulous regard for manual contacts, stretch, and traction of the part to be reinforced, and maximal resistance is of paramount importance. The pattern used as a reinforcement, being stronger, may be given slightly less regard. Where great weakness exists, the more skillfully both parts are handled, the more effective reinforcement will be. Both parts may be placed in the lengthened range of the desired patterns. The patient is instructed and commanded to "push" or "pull" while the therapist controls the situation by allowing the stronger pattern to respond first, but resisting it strongly enough to encourage the weaker pattern to respond. The patient's urge is to accomplish the motions, and by resisting the stronger motion, the weaker motion derives stimulation.

Recuperative Motion

Recuperative motion is the use of a new combination of movements to reduce or circumvent fatigue produced by repetitive activity against resistance.[19]

Fatigue resulting from repeated or strenuous physical activity is a well-recognized and accepted phenomenon in normal life. The normal subject recognizes and circumvents the fatigue factor in his performance of physical tasks requiring effort. He knows that if he wants to do something, he does not tire as readily as he does when performing a disliked task. He knows through experience that he can improve his endurance for a certain activity by working to the point of fatigue. He knows that while he may tire of a certain task or tire physically in performing it, he may perform for a longer period by changing the routine procedure of the task itself or by changing to another activity for a brief period of time.

A simple example is that of the normal subject who sets himself the task of waxing a piece of furniture. He wants to do the job, or someone else wants him to do it, to the extent that he is provided with a motive. Having started with determination, he may find that very soon his right arm is tired. If he shifts from short strokes to longer strokes, it seems to help in relieving the fatigue momentarily. If he emphasizes pulling motions rather than pushing motions he may lengthen his period of performance. If he changes the position of his body or reinforces his arm motions with his trunk or other extremities, he may again lengthen his work period. Or he may shift from the use of his right hand to the use of his left hand and find some relief of fatigue. Finally, he may change to a completely different task, and later, returning to the waxing job, find he is again able to perform adequately.

The task described requires many combinations of motions involving many parts of the body. When a certain combination of motions becomes fatiguing, the normal subject shifts the emphasis to another combination that may accomplish the task. He reinforces one combination of motions with other combinations and proceeds to vary his own activity in order to work for a longer period of time. This shifting of emphasis to other combinations of motions amounts to recuperative motion in the normal subject.

Techniques of proprioceptive neuromuscular facilitation employ recuperative motion in order to reverse fatigue factors. The reversal of antagonist techniques may be used as recuperative motion, and the use of several different patterns of reinforcement constitute recuperative motion. When recuperative motion is employed, the patient will be able to work at a specific pattern, which is in need of emphasis, for a longer period of time, thereby improving his strength and endurance in relation to that specific pattern.

A patient having weakness of elbow extension in the extension–abduction–internal rotation pattern of the upper extremity may fatigue readily in the performance of repeated contractions emphasizing elbow extension. Reversing the pattern to flexion–adduction–external rotation with elbow flexion may make it possible for the patient to repeat elbow extension in the initial pattern. If the elbow extension was being performed unilaterally without reinforcement of another stronger pattern, resisting the pattern bilaterally symmetrically, bilaterally asymmetrically, reciprocally in the same diagonal, or reciprocally in the opposite diagonal, or resisting in combination with neck rotation to the same side may enhance the ability to continue repetitions of elbow extension. Further recuperation may be brought about by shifting to another pattern that requires emphasis in the trunk or other extremities, making it possible to again return to the initial pattern emphasizing elbow extension.

By following such a procedure, in view of the many combinations of motion available for reinforcement, it becomes possible to place an intensive demand on a specific, desired combination of motions. It is by such a procedure that the fatigue factor is circumvented.

Illustrations (Figs. 1-82 to 1-150)

The sequence of bilateral combinations of extremity patterns is in keeping with normal development: symmetrical, asymmetrical, and reciprocal. Intermediate joints (elbows and knees) are portrayed in the straight position, or as flexing or extending.

Although the sequence presents 69 figures with 207 photographs, in some respects the sequence is limited. Each figure shows lengthened range (Le-R), middle range (Mid-R), and shortened range (Sh-R) as do figures of unilateral patterns and, in most instances, total patterns. Application of techniques may be made at any point in the range. In treatment, the strongest part of the range of one extremity is used to reinforce the weaker segment at the comparable point of the range.

In general, the eyes follow the hands, or the eyes lead and the hands follow. When possible, eyes may follow or lead feet and ankles in lower extremity patterns. Eyes, and head and neck patterns, may reinforce. If, however, resistance is excessive so that the patient is unable to move when told to do so, he may try to reinforce in another unrelated pattern or, if he is supine, by extending head and neck against the table.

The legends include commands expressed in terms of use of an appropriate technique or sequence of techniques for indication in Le-R, *A* . Shifting to RS may occur at *B*, and a reversal at *C*. Many variations will be noted. A technique of emphasis such as RC may be given two or three repetitions in the legends. In practice or treatment, the number of repetitions depends upon the point of fatigue (see Recuperative Motion, above).

Manual contacts are one of the most important keys to facilitation. In the bilateral sequence, contact with upper extremities is on forearms near the wrists in order to control the movements, especially rotation throughout the patterns. In lower extremities, contact is at heels when knees are straight (again, for control) and on the forefoot when emphasizing knee movements and when resisting foot and ankle patterns. If marked imbalance exists at proximal pivots with lack of control, unilateral patterns or total patterns with two hands in contact may better serve to correct imbalances. Bilateral combinations may be too advanced.

Where the sequence of combinations is incomplete, as in hands and wrists where only BS and BA are shown, BR thrusting may be useful (see Free Active Motion). Bilateral combinations also may be performed sitting or supine.

The manual contacts in some instances may seem unclear in the photographs, or perhaps may not seem to reflect the diagonal direction. During photography the therapist may have adjusted her position to accommodate the position of the camera, or the photographer may have adjusted his position, thus causing distortion in the manual contact and diagonal direction photographs.

The legends identify the antagonistic pattern and, in the majority of instances, the related unilateral patterns and related total patterns. In the combinations where elbows or knees are straight, there is a limited number of total patterns from which to select. In some legends only one pattern of the combination is identified.

Emphasis on Shoulder with Elbow Straight:
Symmetrical (BS)

FLEXION – ADDUCTION – EXTERNAL ROTATION
(D1 fl), LEFT AND RIGHT

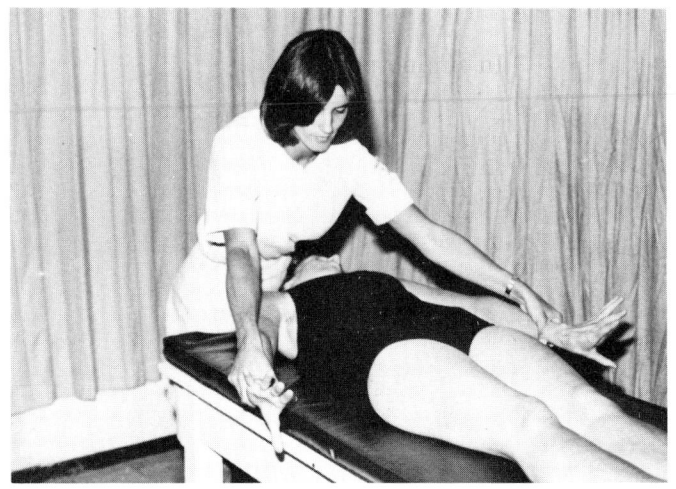

A

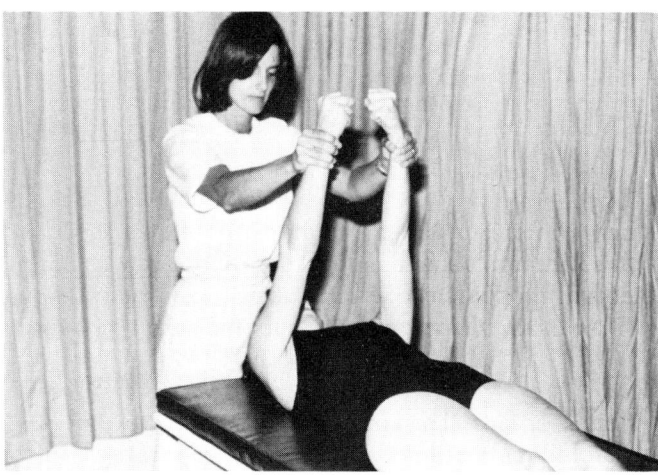

B

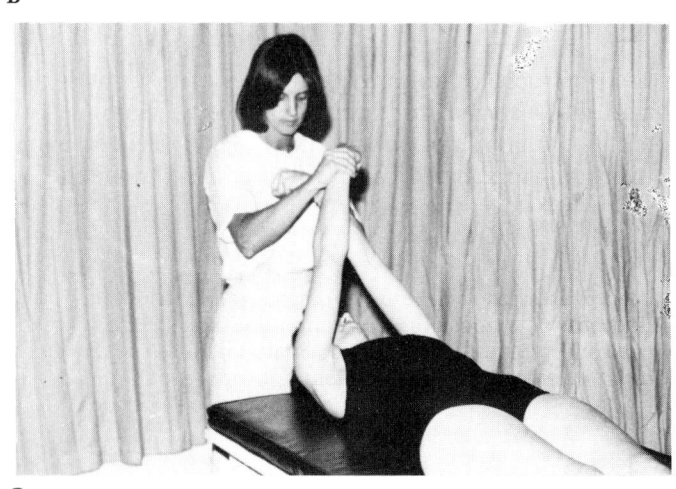

C

FIG. 1-82

Components of Motion

Free. In supine posture, head and neck are at midline. Alternative postures: sitting on bench or stool; standing.

Resisted. Hands close and wrists flex toward radial side and initiate shoulder flexion, adduction, and external rotation bilaterally.

A. Lengthened Range

Commands. Preparatory. "You will close both hands and turn as you lift arms up and toward your nose. Keep your elbows straight!" *Action.* "Close your hands, turn them toward your face, and pull arms up and across. Move! Elbows straight!"

Suggested Techniques. Traction, stretch, resistance.

B. Middle Range

Commands. "Good! Now, hold! and hold! Again, move both arms toward your nose. Hold, and move again! and again. Elbows straight!"

Suggested Techniques. Approximation; rhythmic stabilization followed by repeated contractions for emphasis.

C. Shortened Range

Commands. "Keep your hands closed toward thumb side. Now hold! and hold, and hold. Open your hands and turn them away from your face and push down and out. Hold! And relax." (See Fig. 1-83.)

Suggested Techniques. Rhythmic stabilization, slow reversal, slow reversal – hold, repeated contractions.

Antagonistic Pattern

Extension – abduction – internal rotation (D1 ex), left and right (Fig. 1-83).

Related Pattern

Unilateral upper extremity D1 fl with elbow straight (Fig. 1-44).

Emphasis on Shoulder with Elbow Straight: Symmetrical (BS)

EXTENSION – ABDUCTION – INTERNAL ROTATION
(D1 ex), LEFT AND RIGHT

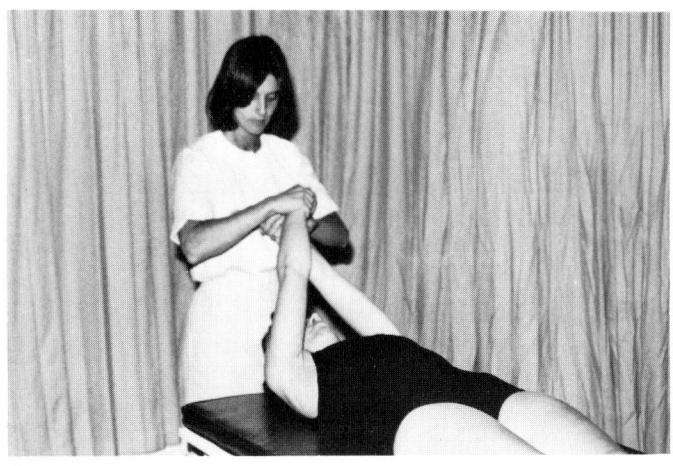

A

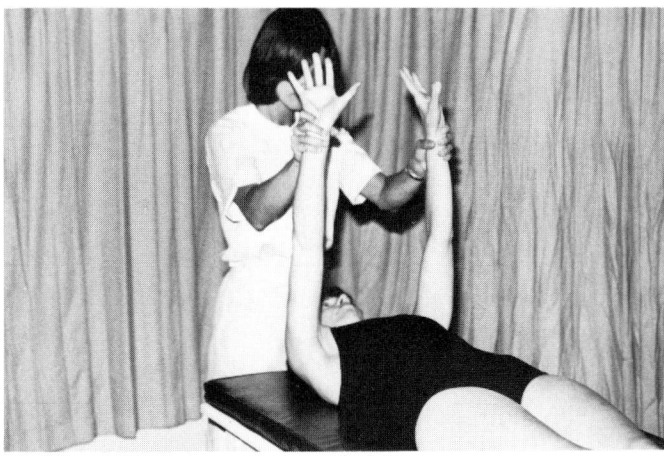

B

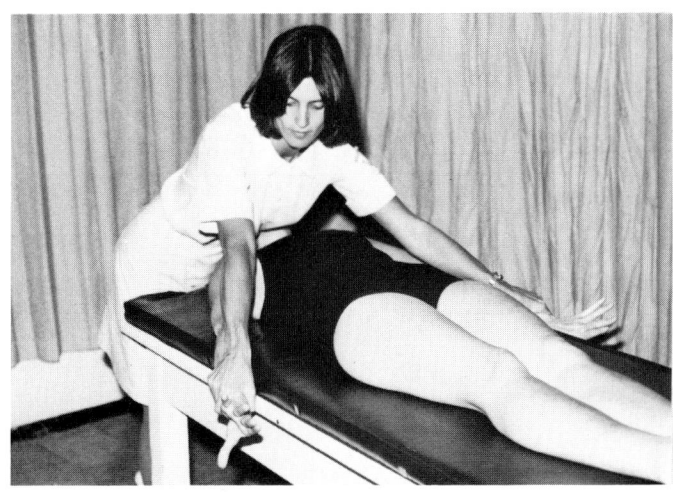

C

FIG. 1-83

Components of Motion

Free. In supine posture, head and neck are at midline. Alternative postures: sitting on bench or stool; standing.

Resisted. Hands open, wrists extend toward ulnar side and initiate shoulder extension, abduction, and internal rotation bilaterally.

A. Lengthened Range

Commands. Preparatory. "You are to open both of your hands and turn (thumbs pointed toward floor) as you push down and away from your face. Keep your elbows straight!" *Action.* "Open your hands, turn, push down and away. Move! Elbows straight!"

Suggested Techniques. Stretch, resistance.

B. Middle Range

Commands. "Good. Now hold! and hold! and hold! Again, push down and away. Hold! and push again, and push. Keep elbows straight!"

Suggested Techniques. Approximation, rhythmic stabilization followed by repeated contractions for emphasis.

C. Shortened Range

Commands. "Keep your fingers straight, thumbs pointed toward floor, wrists up toward little finger side. Now hold! and hold! and hold. Close your hands and turn as you lift your arms up and across your nose. Hold! And relax!" (See Fig. 1-82.)

Suggested Techniques. Approximation, rhythmic stabilization, repeated contractions, slow reversal, slow reversal – hold.

Antagonistic Pattern

Flexion – adduction – external rotation (D1 fl), left and right (Fig. 1-82).

Related Unilateral Pattern

Upper extremity D1 ex with elbow straight (Fig. 1-47).

Related Total Patterns (Mat Activities)

Lower trunk rotation, supine. Upper extremities are placed in bilateral symmetrical D1 ex with elbows straight (Fig. 1-162).

Pelvic elevation, supine. Upper extremities are placed in bilateral symmetrical D1 ex with elbows straight. Upper extremities adjust when lower trunk rotation occurs but remain in a symmetrical posture with pelvic elevation, supine (Fig. 1-163).

Emphasis on Shoulder with Elbows Straight:
Symmetrical (BS)

FLEXION – ABDUCTION – EXTERNAL ROTATION (D2 fl),
LEFT AND RIGHT

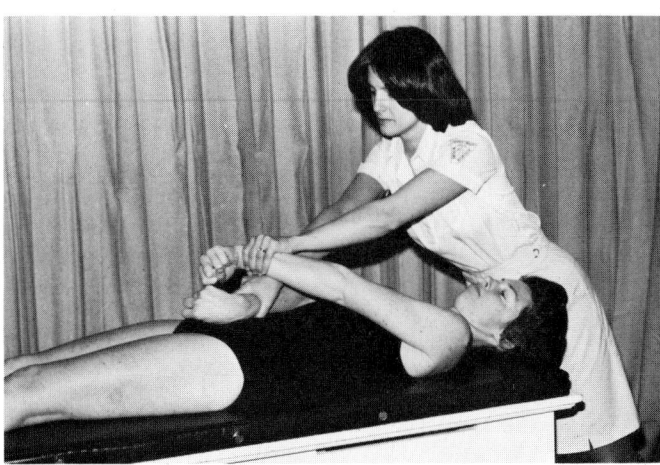

A

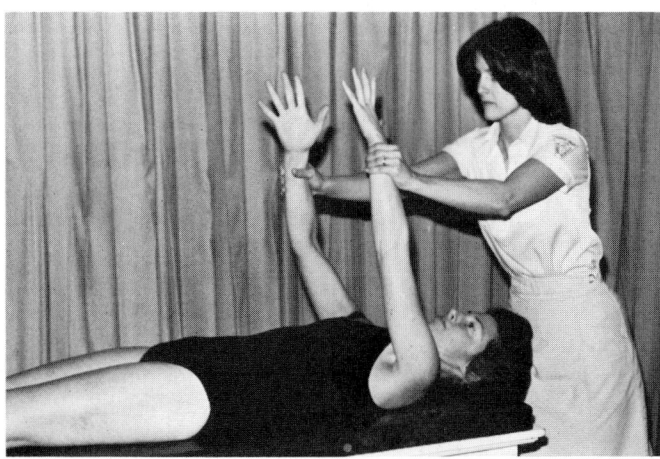

B

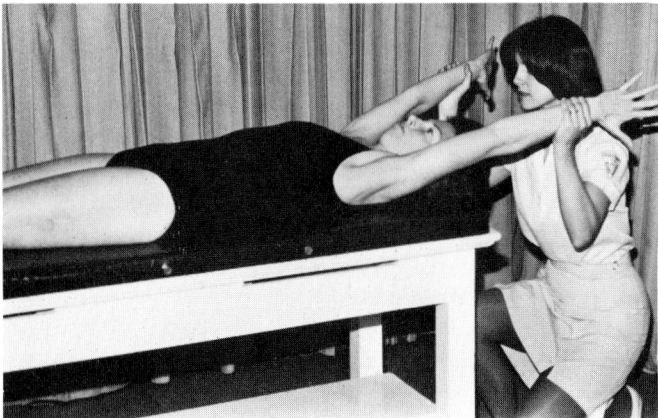

C

FIG. 1-84

Components of Motion

Free. In supine posture, head and neck are at midline. Head and neck may extend as upper extremities flex. Alternative postures: sitting on stool or bench; standing.

Resisted. Left and right hands open; wrists extend to radial side and initiate shoulder flexion, abduction, and external rotation bilaterally.

A. Lengthened Range

Commands. Preparatory. "You are to open your hands toward thumb side, turn as you lift arms up and away. Keep your elbows straight!" *Action.* "Open your hands, turn, lift your arms up and away. Move! Elbows straight!"

Suggested Techniques. Traction, stretch, and resistance.

B. Middle Range

Commands. "Good! Now, hold! and hold! and hold! Now lift up and away. Hold! And push again, and push. Elbows straight!"

Suggested Techniques. Approximation, rhythmic stabilization followed by repeated contractions.

C. Shortened Range

Commands. "Keep your hands open, point thumbs to floor. Now, hold! and hold! and hold! Close your hands, pull down and across toward opposite hip. Hold! And relax!" (See Fig. 1-85.)

Suggested Techniques. Approximation, rhythmic stabilization, slow reversal, slow reversal – hold.

Antagonistic Patterns

Extension – adduction – internal rotation (D2 ex), left and right (Fig. 1-85).

Related Patterns

Unilateral upper extremity D2 fl with elbow straight (Fig. 1-50).

Emphasis on Shoulder with Elbow Straight: Symmetrical (BS)

EXTENSION – ADDUCTION – INTERNAL ROTATION (D2 ex), LEFT AND RIGHT

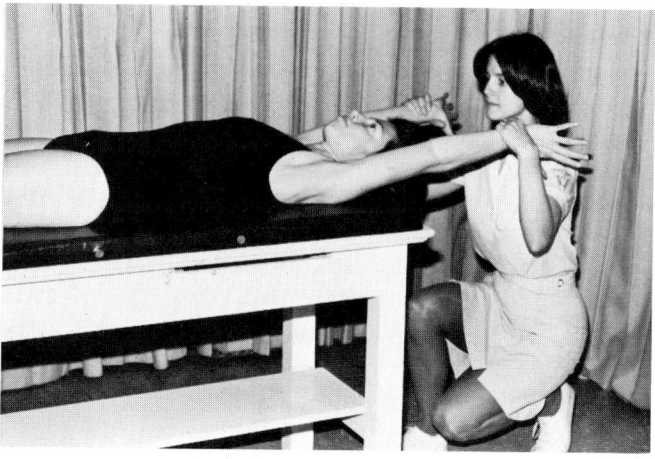

A

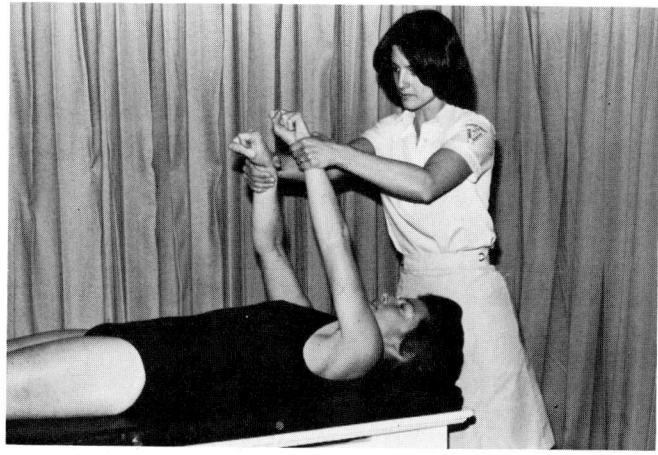

B

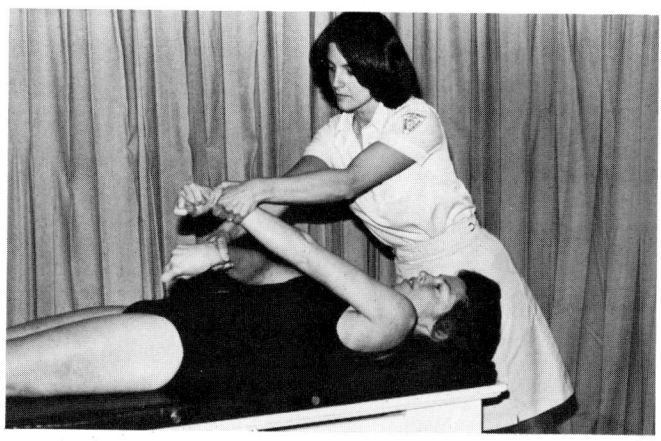

C

FIG. 1-85

Components of Motion

Free. In supine posture head and neck are at midline. Head and neck may flex slightly while staying in midline as shoulders extend. Alternative postures: sitting on bench or stool; standing.

Resisted. Left and right hands close, thumbs move into opposition, and wrists flex to ulnar side and initiate shoulder extension, adduction and internal rotation bilaterally.

A. Lengthened Range

Commands. Preparatory. "You are going to close your hands toward the little finger as you pull your arms down and across toward your opposite hip. Keep your elbows straight." *Action.* "Close your hands and pull your arms down and across toward opposite hips. Move! Elbows straight!"

Suggested Techniques. Stretch, resistance.

B. Middle Range

Commands. "Good! Hold! And hold! And hold. Now move your arms down and across toward the opposite hip. Hold! and pull, and pull, and pull again. Keep elbows straight!"

Suggested Techniques. Approximation, rhythmic stabilization followed by repeated contractions.

C. Shortened Range

Commands. "Keep your hands closed. Bend your wrists toward the little finger side. Elbows straight! Now hold! and hold! and hold. Open your hands, lift up and out. Hold! And relax!" (See Fig. 1-84.)

Suggested Techniques. Approximation, rhythmic stabilization, repeated contractions, slow reversal, slow reversal – hold.

Antagonistic Pattern

Flexion – abduction – external rotation (D2 fl), left and right (Fig. 1-84).

Related Pattern

Unilateral upper extremity D2 ex with elbow straight (Fig. 1-53).

Upper Extremity

Emphasis on Shoulders with Elbow Straight: Asymmetrical (BA)

FLEXION – ADDUCTION – EXTERNAL ROTATION (D1 fl), LEFT; FLEXION – ABDUCTION – EXTERNAL ROTATION (D2 fl), RIGHT

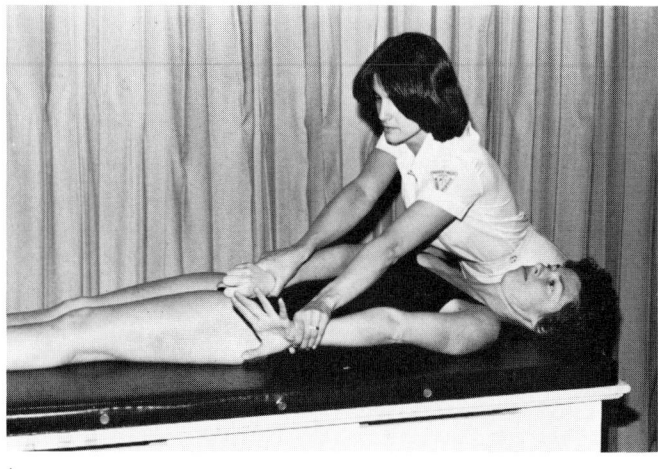

A

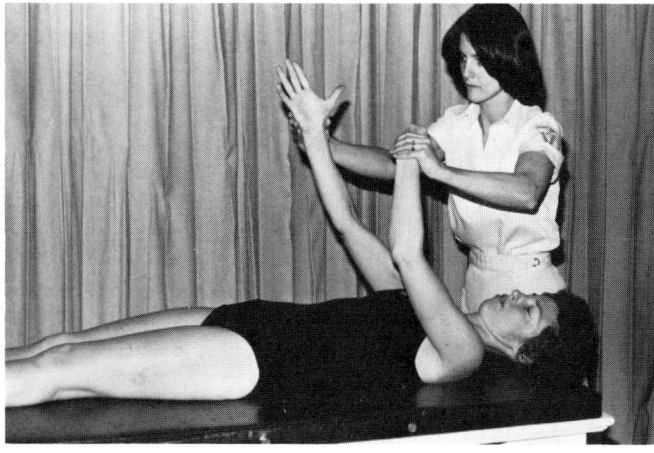

B

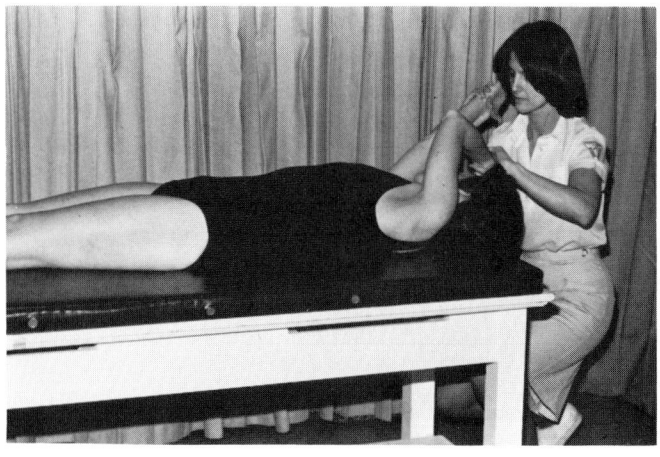

C

FIG. 1-86

Components of Motion

Free. In supine posture, head and neck may flex slightly with rotation to the left as eyes regard hands. Head and neck rotate to right (*C*), in keeping with asymmetric tonic neck reflex (ATNR). Alternative postures: sitting on bench or stool; standing.

Resisted. Left hand closes and wrist flexes to radial side as right hand opens and wrist extends to radial side; each initiates flexion of limbs to the right.

A. Lengthened Range

Commands. *Preparatory.* "You are to close your left hand (D1 fl) and open your right (D2 fl), and lift up and across toward me." *Action.* "Close your left, open your right! Lift up toward me. Lift!"

Suggested Techniques. Traction, stretch, and resistance.

B. Middle Range

Commands. "Good! Now hold! and hold! and hold, again! Now reach toward me, and reach; and again, reach toward me. Elbows straight!"

Suggested Techniques. Approximation, rhythmic stabilization, repeated contractions.

C. Shortened Range

Commands. "Keep your left hand closed and right open. Right thumb toward floor! Now hold! and hold, and hold! Open your left, close your right, and pull your hands down and away from me. Hold! And relax." (See Fig. 1-87.)

Suggested Techniques. Rhythmic stabilization, repeated contractions, slow reversal, slow reversal – hold, hold – relax – active motion for emphasis.

Antagonistic Pattern

(BA): D1 ex, left; D2 ex, right (Fig. 1-87).

Related Unilateral Patterns

Upper extremity with elbows straight: D1 fl, left (Fig. 1-44); D2 fl, right (Fig. 1-50).

Upper trunk extension with rotation to right: see Figure 1-37, extension with rotation to left. D2, fl, left; D1, fl, right, hands in contact (lifting), elbows straight as possible. Transpose for patterns to right.

Related Total Patterns (Mat Activities)

Rolling: prone toward supine: see Figure 1-159. Head and neck extend with rotation toward left while D2 fl of left and D1 fl of right move in asymmetrical flexion toward left (lifting). Transpose for asymmetrical flexion to right with hands free of contact.

Rising to sitting from hyperflexion: see Figure 1-178. Head and neck extend with rotation to right. D1 fl of left, D2 fl of right.

Upper Extremity

Emphasis on Shoulders with Elbow Straight: Asymmetrical (BA)

EXTENSION – ABDUCTION – INTERNAL ROTATION (D1 ex), LEFT; EXTENSION – ADDUCTION – INTERNAL ROTATION (D2 ex), RIGHT

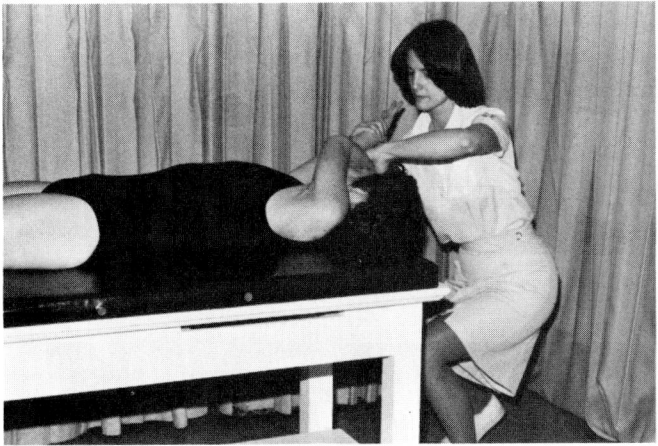

A

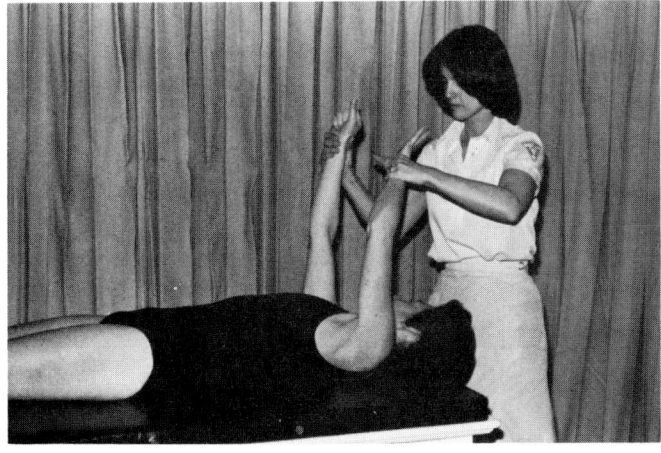

B

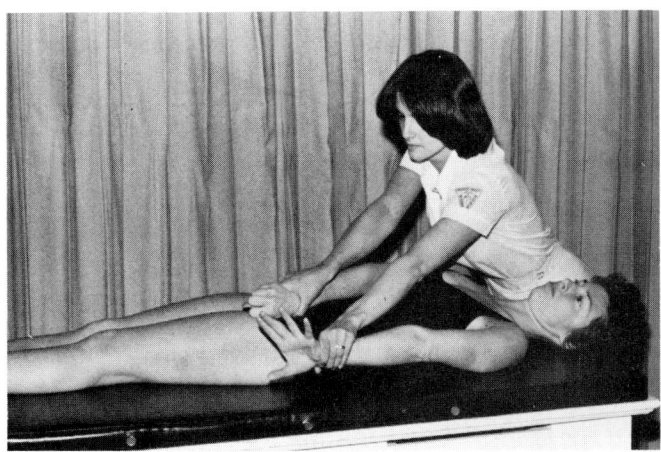

C

FIG. 1-87

Components of Motion

Free. In supine posture, head and neck are slightly extended with rotation to right as eyes regard hands. Head and neck rotate to left in keeping with asymmetric tonic reflex (ATNR). (Head and neck: C, shortened range. Head and neck rotate to left as eyes regard hands and actively reinforce asymmetrical pattern.) Alternative postures: sitting on bench or stool; standing.

Resisted. Left hand opens, wrist extends to ulnar side as right hand closes, and wrist flexes to ulnar side; each initiates extension of limbs to left.

A. Lengthened Range

Commands. Preparatory. "You are to open your left hand (D1 ex) as you close your right (D2 ex) and pull down and away from me." *Action.* "Open your left, close your right, pull down and away. Move!"

Suggested Techniques. Stretch, resistance.

B. Middle Range

Commands. "Good! Now hold! and hold! and hold again! Now pull down and away, and pull, and pull again. Elbows straight!"

Suggested Techniques. Approximation, rhythmic stabilization, repeated contractions for emphasis.

C. Shortened Range

Commands. "Keep your left hand open, thumb toward floor, and right closed. Elbows straight. Now hold! and hold! and hold! Close your left, open your right, lift your limbs up toward me." (See Fig. 1-86.)

Suggested Techniques. Rhythmic stabilization, repeated contractions, slow reversal, slow reversal–hold.

Antagonistic Pattern

(BA): D1 fl, left; D2 fl, right (Fig. 1-86).

Related Unilateral Patterns

Upper extremity with elbow straight: D1 ex, left (Fig. 1-48); D2 ex, right (Fig. 1-53).

Upper trunk flexion with rotation to left. See Figure 1-36, flexion with rotation to right. D2 ex, left; D1 ex, right, hands in contact (chopping to right). Transpose for chopping to left. Elbows as straight as possible.

Related Total Pattern (Mat Activity)

Rolling: supine toward prone (Fig. 1-153). Head and neck flex with rotation to right while left (D2 ex) and right (D1 ex) limbs move in asymmetrical extension toward right (chopping). Transpose for asymmetrical extension to left with hands free of contact.

Upper Extremity

Emphasis on Shoulders with Elbow Straight:
Reciprocal (BR, SD)

EXTENSION – ABDUCTION – INTERNAL ROTATION
(D1 ex), LEFT; FLEXION – ADDUCTION – EXTERNAL
ROTATION (D1 fl), RIGHT

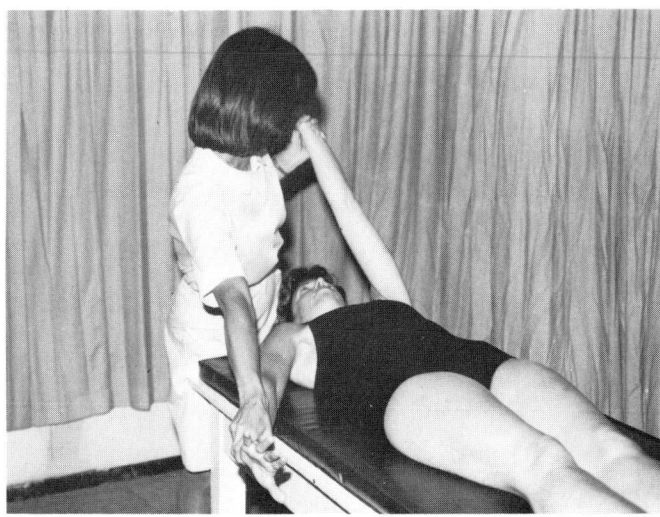

A

B

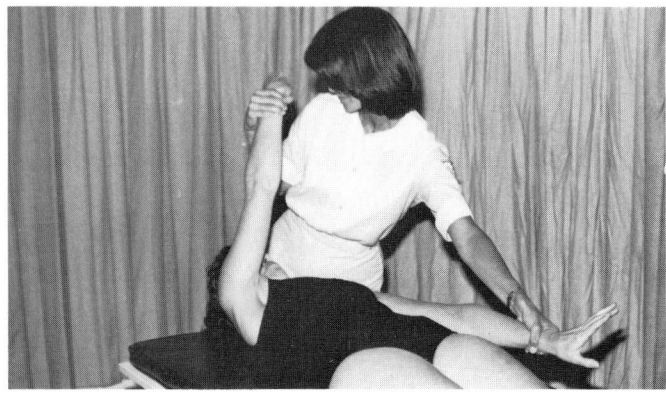

C

FIG. 1-88

Components of Motion

Free. In supine posture, head and neck are at midline. Alternative postures: sitting on bench or stool; standing.

Resisted. Left hand opens; wrist extends to ulnar side and initiates shoulder extension – abduction – internal rotation as right hand closes; wrist flexes to radial side and initiates shoulder flexion – adduction – external rotation.

A. Lengthened Range

Commands. *Preparatory.* "You are to open your left hand and push your left arm down and away from your face as you close your right hand and pull your right arm up and across your nose. Keep your elbows straight." *Action.* "Open your left hand and push your left arm down and away. Close your right and pull up and across your nose. Move! Elbows straight!"

Suggested Techniques. Traction and stretch on the right, stretch on the left, resistance.

B. Middle Range

Commands. "Good! Now hold! And hold! And hold. Elbows straight. Now push down and away with your left arm as you lift up and across your nose with your right arm."

Suggested Techniques. Approximation, rhythmic stabilization.

C. Shortened Range

Commands. "Keep your left hand open, thumb pointing to floor, while you keep your right hand closed. Elbows straight! Now, close your left hand, pull up and across your nose as you open your right, push down and away and change, and change, and change." (See Fig. 1-89.)

Suggested Techniques. Stretch, resistance, traction to flexing extremity, slow reversal.

Antagonistic Pattern

(BR, SD): D1 fl, left; D1 ex, right (Fig. 1-89).

Related Unilateral Patterns

Upper extremity with elbow straight: D1 ex, left (Fig. 1-47); D1 fl, right (Fig. 1-44).

Related Total Pattern (Mat Activity)

Sitting balance (Fig. 1-180, *C*). Transpose for D1 ex of left, D1 fl of right with elbows straight.

Upper Extremity

Emphasis on Shoulders with Elbow Straight:
Reciprocal (BR, SD)

FLEXION – ADDUCTION – EXTERNAL ROTATION
(D1 fl), LEFT; EXTENSION – ABDUCTION – INTERNAL
ROTATION (D1 ex), RIGHT

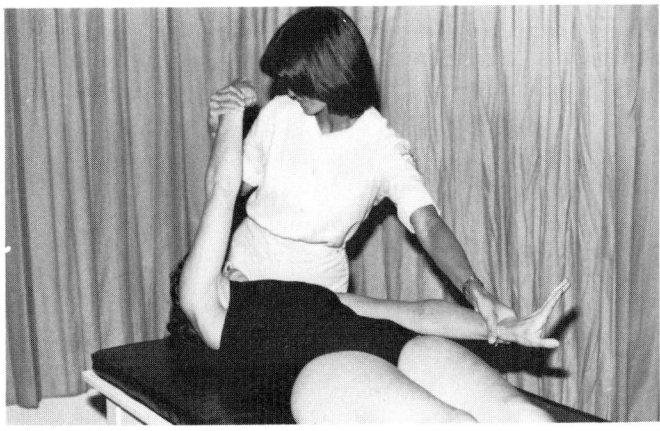

A

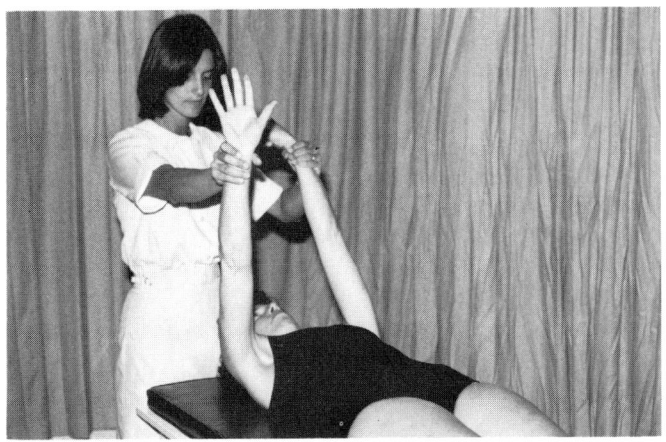

B

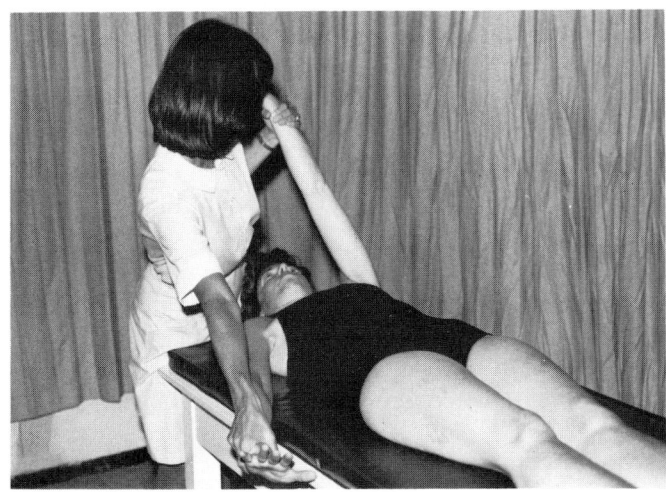

C

FIG. 1-89

Components of Motion

Free. In supine posture, head and neck are at midline. Alternative postures: sitting on bench or stool; standing.

Resisted. Left hand closes to radial side and initiates shoulder flexion – adduction – external rotation, as right hand opens to ulnar side and initiates shoulder extension – abduction – internal rotation.

A. Lengthened Range

Commands. Preparatory. "You are to close your left hand, pull it up and across your nose as you open your right hand, and push it down and away from your face. Keep your elbows straight." *Action.* "Close your left hand, pull up and across; open your right and push down and away. Move! Elbows straight!"

Suggested Techniques. Stretch on the right, traction and stretch on the left, resistance.

B. Middle Range

Commands. "Good! Now hold! And hold! And hold. Keep elbows straight! Now hold your left and push down and away with your right. And push! Again! And relax."

Suggested Techniques. Approximation, rhythmic stabilization, repeated contractions on right for emphasis.

C. Shortened Range

Commands. "Left hand closed and right hand open. Elbows straight. Point your right thumb toward floor! Now, open your left, push down and away. Close your right, pull up and across. Now change, and change, and change." (See Fig. 1-88.)

Suggested Techniques. Stretch, resistance, traction and stretch to flexing extremity, slow reversal.

Antagonistic Pattern

(BR, SD): D1 ex, left; D1 fl, right (Fig. 1-88).

Related Unilateral Patterns

Upper extremity with elbow straight: D1 fl, left (Fig. 1-44); D1 ex, right (Fig. 1-47).

Related Total Pattern (Mat Activity)

Sitting balance (Fig. 1-180, *C*). Reciprocal (SD); left, flexion; right, extension with elbows straight.

Emphasis on Shoulder with Elbow Straight:
Reciprocal (BR, SD)

EXTENSION – ADDUCTION – INTERNAL ROTATION
(D2 ex), LEFT; FLEXION – ABDUCTION – EXTERNAL
ROTATION (D2 fl), RIGHT

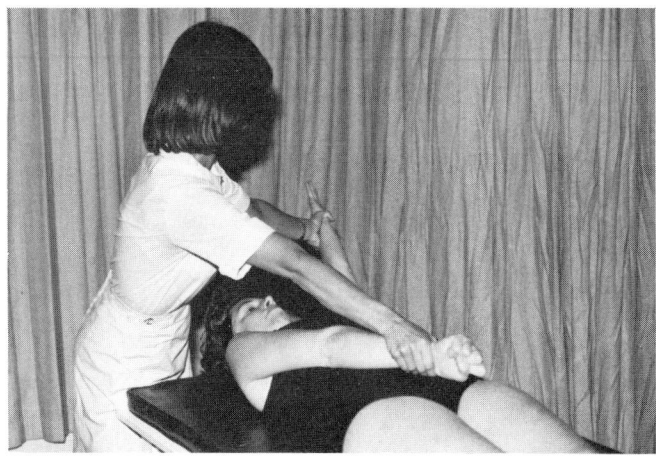

A

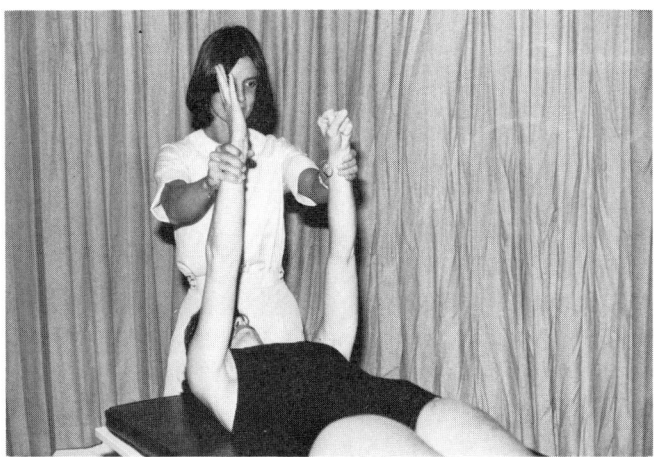

B

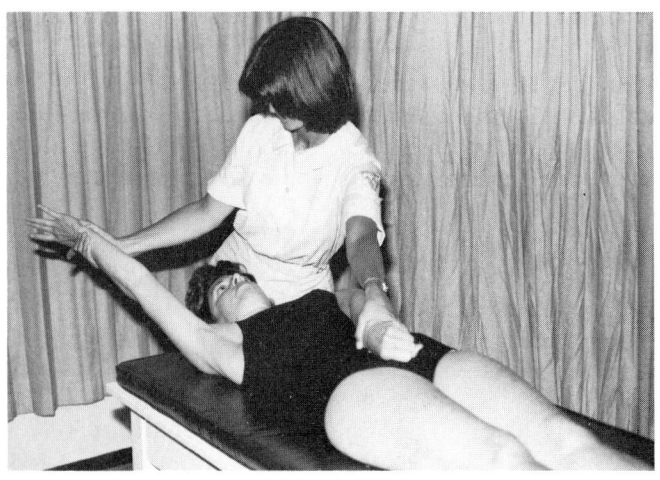

C

FIG. 1-90

Components of Motion

Free. In supine posture, head and neck are at midline. Alternative postures: sitting on bench or stool; standing.

Resisted. Left hand closes to ulnar side and initiates shoulder extension – adduction – internal rotation as right hand opens to radial side and initiates shoulder flexion – abduction – external rotation.

A. Lengthened Range

Commands. *Preparatory.* "You are to close your left hand, pull down and across to your right hip as you open your right and lift it up and away from your head. Keep your elbows straight!" *Action.* "Close your left hand, pull down and across to your opposite hip. Open your right, lift up and away. Move! Elbows straight!"

Suggested Techniques. Traction and stretch on the right, stretch on the left, resistance.

B. Middle Range

Commands. "Good! Now hold! And hold! And hold! Elbows straight! Now pull left arm down and across to right hip as you lift right arm up and away."

Suggested Techniques. Approximation, rhythmic stabilization.

C. Shortened Range

Commands. "Left hand closed and right hand open. Elbows straight. Point your right thumb toward floor! Now open your left, lift up and away. Close your right, pull down and across. Now change, and change, and change." (See Fig. 1-91.)

Suggested Techniques. Stretch, resistance, traction and stretch to flexing extremity, slow reversal.

Antagonistic Pattern

(BR, SD): D2 fl, left; D2 ex, right (Fig. 1-91).

Related Patterns

Unilateral upper extremity with elbow straight: D2 ex, left (Fig. 1-53); D2 fl, right (Fig. 1-50).

Upper Extremity

Emphasis on Shoulder with Elbow Straight:
Reciprocal (BR, SD)

FLEXION – ABDUCTION – EXTERNAL ROTATION (D2 fl),
LEFT; EXTENSION – ADDUCTION – INTERNAL ROTATION
(D2 ex), RIGHT

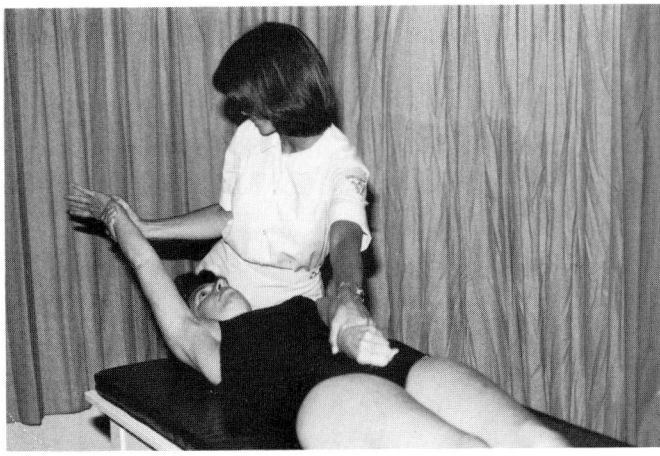

A

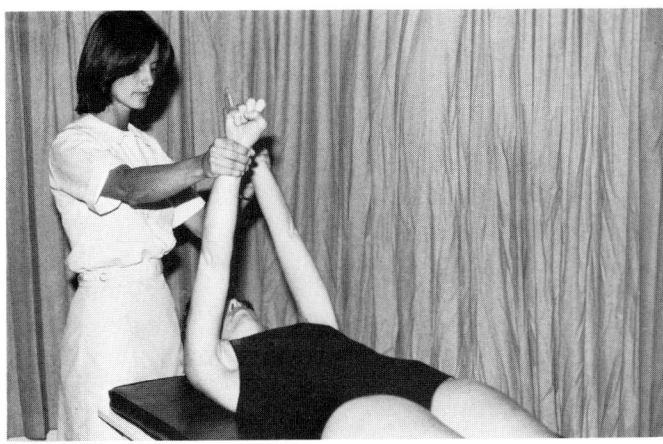

B

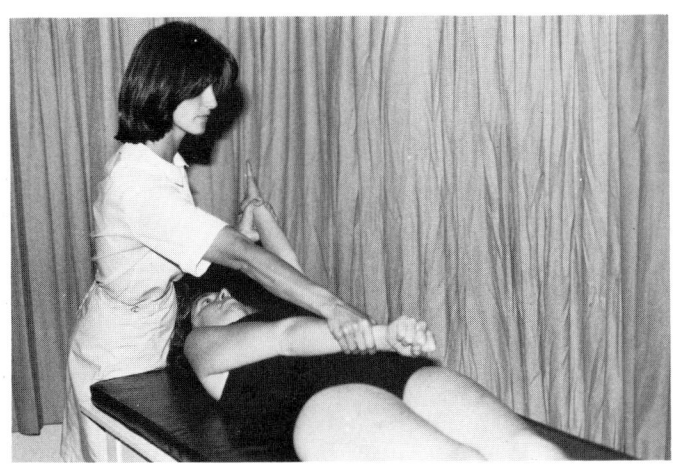

C

FIG. 1-91

Components of Motion

Free. In supine posture, head and neck are at midline. Eyes follow flexing arm. alternative postures: sitting on bench or stool; standing.

Resisted. Left hand opens to radial side and initiates shoulder flexion – abduction – external rotation as right hand closes to ulnar side and initiates shoulder extension – adduction – internal rotation.

A. Lengthened Range

Commands. *Preparatory.* "You are to open your left hand, lift up and away as you close your right hand, pull down and across toward opposite hip. Keep your elbows straight!" *Action.* "Open your left hand, lift up and away. Close your right, pull down and across to opposite hip. Move! Elbows straight!"

Suggested Techniques. Traction and stretch on the left, stretch on the right, resistance.

B. Middle Range

Commands. "Good! Now hold! And hold! And hold! Elbows straight! Now lift your left arm up and away as you pull your right arm down and across toward the opposite hip."

Suggested Techniques. Approximation, rhythmic stabilization.

C. Shortened Range

Commands. "Left hand open, thumb pointed to floor, and right hand closed. Now close your left hand, pull down and across toward the opposite hip. Open your right, lift up and away. Now change, and change, and change." (See Fig. 1-90.)

Suggested Techniques. Stretch, resistance, traction and stretch to flexing extremity, slow reversal.

Antagonistic Pattern

(BR, SD): D2 ex, left; D2 fl, right (Fig. 1-92).

Related Patterns

Unilateral upper extremity with elbow straight: D2 fl, left (Fig. 1-50); D2 ex, right (Fig. 1-53).

Emphasis on Shoulder with Elbow Straight:
Reciprocal (BR, CD)

EXTENSION – ADDUCTION – INTERNAL ROTATION
(D2 ex), LEFT; FLEXION – ADDUCTION – EXTERNAL
ROTATION (D1 fl), RIGHT

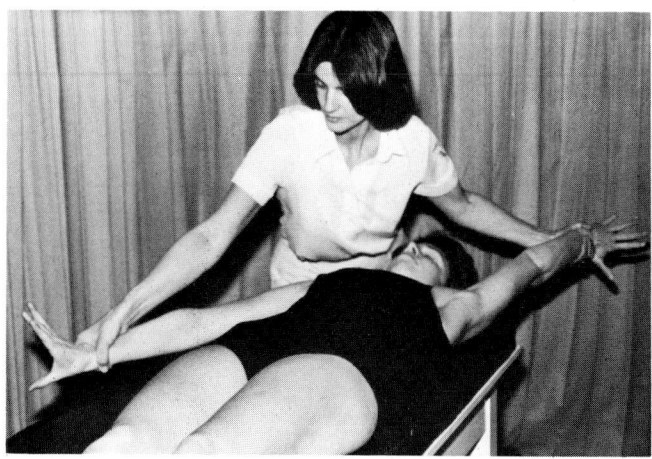

A

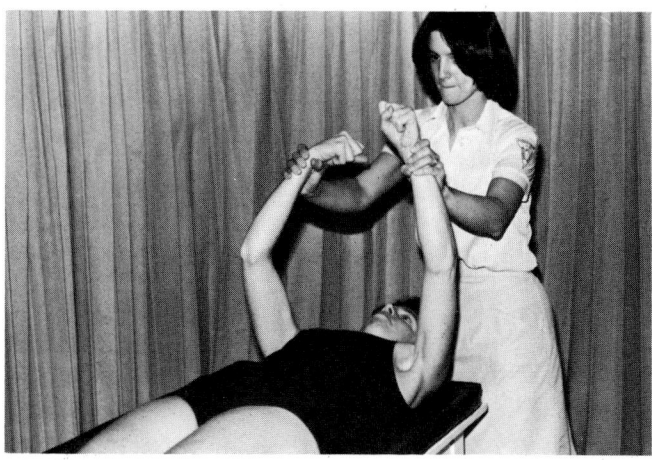

B

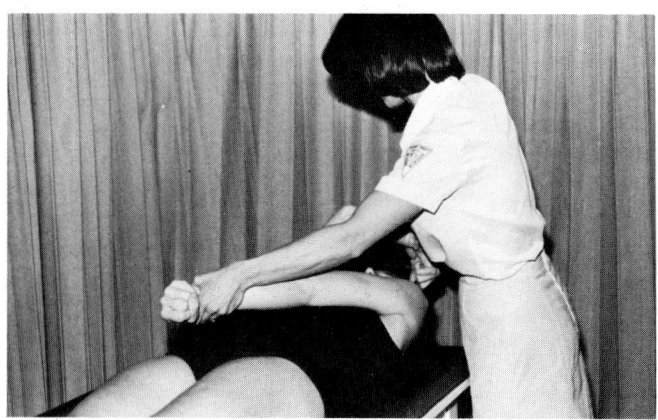

C

FIG. 1-92

Components of Motion

Free. In supine posture, head and neck are at midline. Alternative postures: sitting on bench or stool; standing.

Resisted. Left hand closes to ulnar side and initiates shoulder extension – adduction – internal rotation as right hand closes to radial side and initiates shoulder flexion – adduction – external rotation.

A. Lengthened Range

Commands. Preparatory. "You are to close your hands, pull your left hand down and across toward the opposite hip as you lift your right up and across your nose. Keep your elbows straight!" *Action.* "Close your hands, pull the left down and across toward opposite hip; lift the right up and across your nose. Elbows straight!"

Suggested Techniques. Traction and stretch, right; stretch, left; resistance.

B. Middle Range

Commands. "Good! Now hold! And hold! And hold! Keep elbows straight. Now pull your left down and across and lift your right up and across."

Suggested Techniques. Approximation, rhythmic stabilization.

C. Shortened Range

Commands. "Keep your hands closed and elbows straight. Now hold! And hold! And hold! Open your hands! Lift up and away with your left as you push down and out with your right. And change! Change again! Again! And relax!" (See Fig. 1-93.)

Suggested Techniques. Approximation, rhythmic stabilization, slow reversal, slow reversal – hold. Apply traction to flexing extremity.

Antagonistic Pattern

(BR, CD): D2 fl, left; D1 ex, right (Fig. 1-91).

Related Patterns

Unilateral upper extremity with elbow straight: D2 ex, left (Fig. 1-53); D1 fl, right (Fig. 1-44).

Emphasis on Shoulder with Elbow Straight:
Reciprocal (BR, CD)

FLEXION – ABDUCTION – EXTERNAL ROTATION (D2 fl),
LEFT; EXTENSION – ABDUCTION – INTERNAL
ROTATION (D1 ex), RIGHT

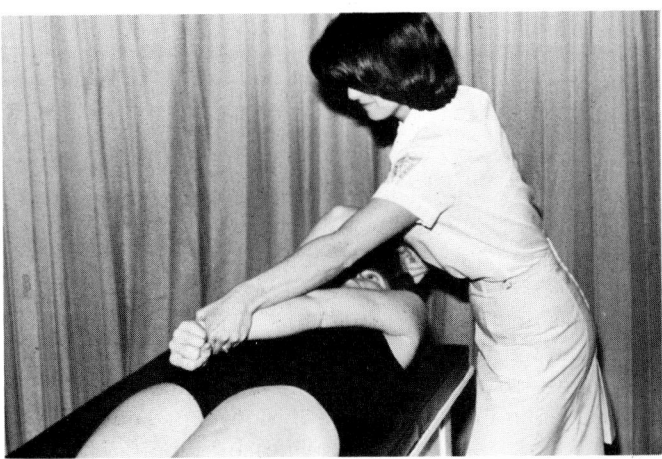

A

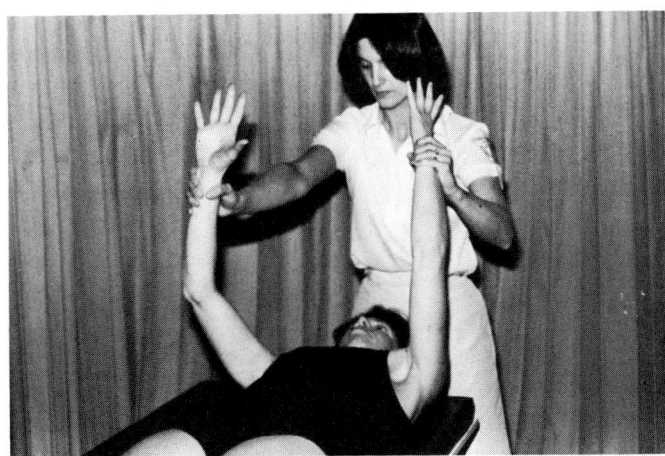

B

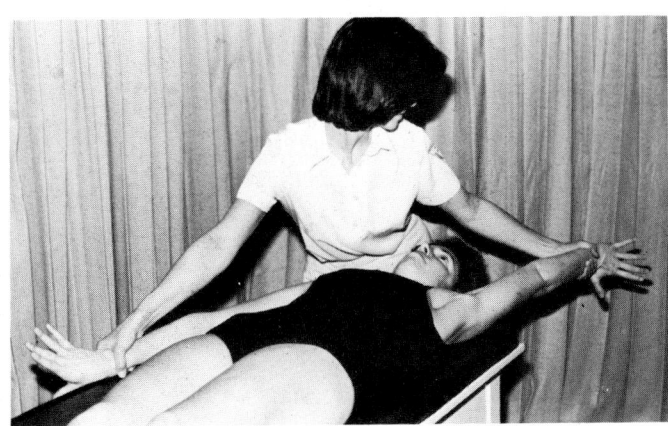

C

FIG. 1-93

Components of Motion

Free. In supine posture, head and neck are at midline. Alternative postures: sitting on bench or stool; standing.

Resisted. Left hand opens to radial side and initiates shoulder flexion – abduction – external rotation as right hand opens to ulnar side and initiates shoulder extension – abduction – internal rotation.

A. Lengthened Range

Commands. Preparatory. "You are to open your hands, lift up and away with your left as you push down and out with your right. Keep your elbows straight!" *Action.* "Open your hands, lift up and away with left; push down and out with right. Elbows straight!"

Suggested Techniques. Traction and stretch, left; stretch, right; resistance.

B. Middle Range

Commands. "Good! Now hold! And hold! And hold! Keep elbows straight. Now lift your left and push with your right."

Suggested Techniques. Approximation, rhythmic stabilization.

C. Shortened Range

Commands. "Keep your hands open and elbows straight. Now hold! And hold! And hold. Close your hands! Pull your left down and across as you lift your right up and across. And change! Change again! Again! And relax!" (See Fig. 1-92.)

Suggested Techniques. Approximation, rhythmic stabilization, slow reversal, slow reversal – hold. Apply traction to flexing extremity.

Antagonistic Pattern

(BR, CD): D2 ex, left; D1 fl, right (Fig. 1-92).

Related Patterns

Unilateral upper extremity with elbow straight: D2 fl, left (Fig. 1-50); D1 ex, right (Fig. 1-47).

Emphasis on Shoulder and Elbow: Symmetrical (BS)

FLEXION – ADDUCTION – EXTERNAL ROTATION (D1 fl)
WITH ELBOW FLEXION, LEFT AND RIGHT

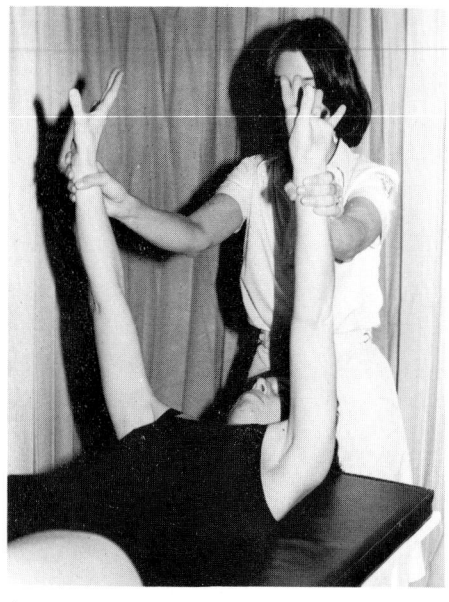 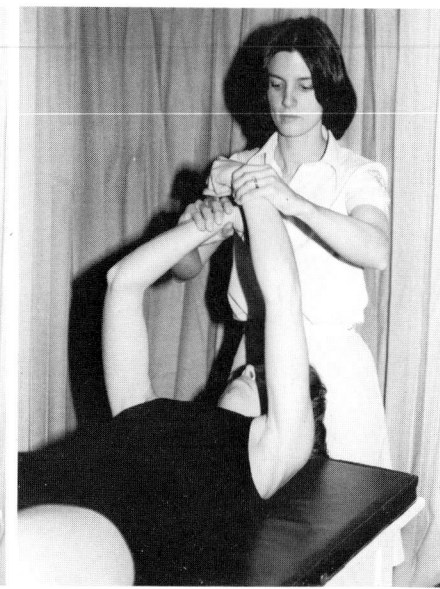 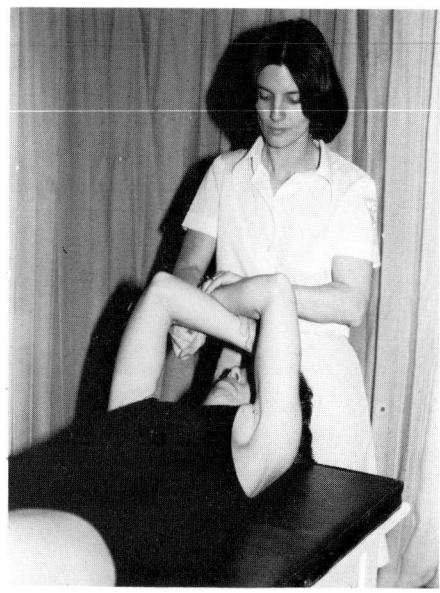

A   B   C

FIG. 1-94

Components of Motion

Free. In supine posture, head and neck may be elevated slightly. Head is in midline. Eyes regard hands. Alternative postures: sitting on bench or stool, or over edge of table for emphasis on elbow flexion.

Resisted. Hands close with wrist flexion toward radial side and initiate forearm supination and external rotation of shoulders as elbows flex, and shoulders flex and adduct.

A. Lengthened Range (Middle Range, Shoulder)

Commands. Preparatory. "You are to close your hands, bend your elbows, and reach down and across your nose and eyes." *Action.* "Close your hands and turn them toward your face! Hold it! And hold! And hold!"

Suggested Techniques. Stretch, resistance, approximation, rhythmic stabilization.

B. Middle Range

Commands. "Bend your elbows! And hold! Now pull down to your face! Now hold on the left and bend your right elbow! And pull! And pull! And relax!"

Suggested Techniques. Resistance to elbow flexors on "hold," followed by resistance to shoulder flexion and adduction. Repeated contractions for emphasis of elbow flexion: left "holds" as right flexes followed by right "holds" as left flexes.

C. Shortened Range

Commands. "Open your hands and push them up and away. Now close your hands and bend your elbows. Hold it! Now pull down and across! And again! And hold! And rest."

Suggested Techniques. Slow reversal, stretch and resistance, repeated contractions.

Antagonistic Pattern

Extension – abduction – internal rotation (D1 ex) with elbow extension, left and right: Figure 1-95.

Related Patterns

Unilateral upper extremity D1 fl with elbow flexion, right (Fig. 1-45).

Total (Mat Activity): Rolling: supine to prone (Fig. 1-155): D1 fl with elbow flexion, left.

Emphasis on Shoulder and Elbow: Symmetrical (BS)

EXTENSION – ABDUCTION – INTERNAL ROTATION
(D1 ex) WITH ELBOW EXTENSION, LEFT AND RIGHT

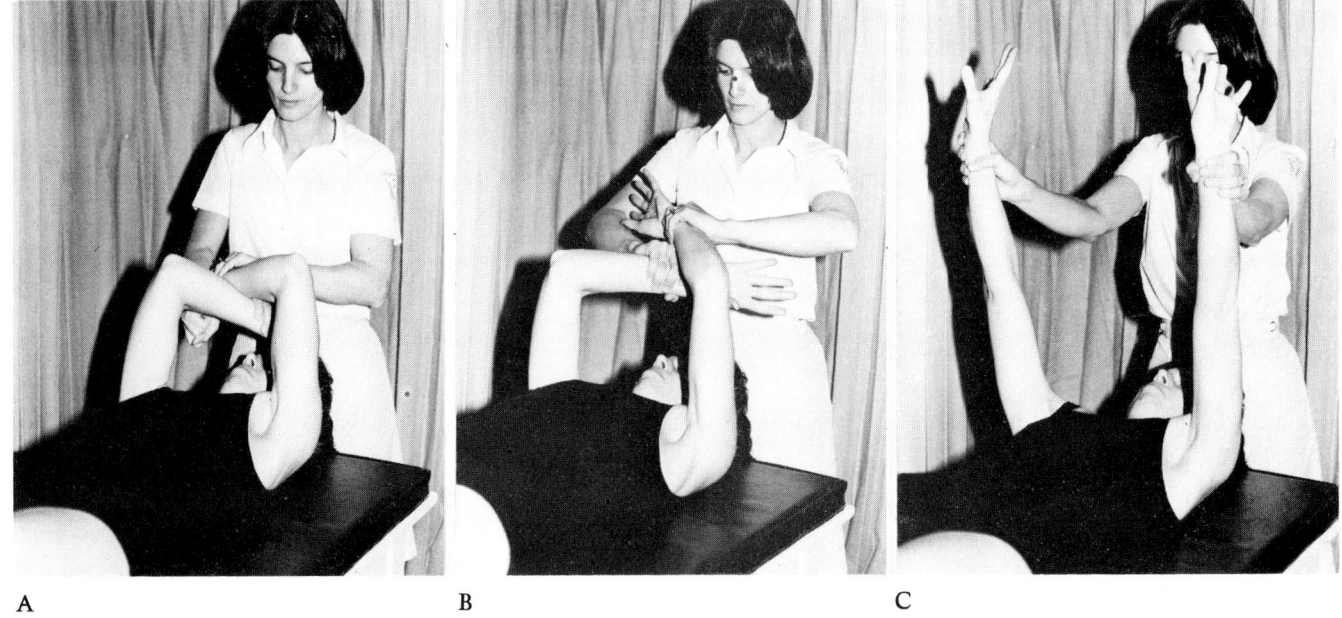

A   B   C

FIG. 1-95

Components of Motion

Free. In supine posture, head and neck may be elevated slightly. Head is in midline. Eyes regard hands. Alternative postures: sitting on bench or stool, or over the edge of table for emphasis on elbow extension.

Resisted. Hands open with wrist extension toward ulnar side and initiate forearm pronation and internal rotation of shoulders as elbows extend, and shoulders extend and abduct.

A. Lengthened Range

Commands. Preparatory. "You are to open your hands, straighten your elbows, and push them down and away toward the floor." *Action.* "Open your hands! Turn them away from your face!"

Suggested Techniques. Traction, stretch, and resistance.

B. Middle Range

Commands. "Straighten your elbows! And hold! Now hold on the right and straighten the left! And push! And push! And hold! Now hold on the left and straighten the right! And push! And push! And hold! And relax!"

Suggested Techniques. Resistance to elbow extensors on "hold" followed by resistance to shoulders, extension, and abduction. Repeated contractions for emphasis of elbow extension: right "holds" as left extends followed by left "holds" as right extends.

C. Shortened Range (Middle Range, Shoulder)

Commands. "Now hold! And hold! And hold! Now close your hands and pull them down and across your face! Now open your hands and push away from your face! Hold it! Push down and away! And again! And hold! And rest."

Suggested Techniques. Approximation, rhythmic stabilization, stretch, slow reversal, resistance, repeated contractions.

Antagonistic Pattern

Flexion – adduction – external rotation (D1 fl) with elbow flexion, left and right (Fig. 1-94).

Related Unilateral Pattern

Upper extremity D1 ex with elbow extension, right (Fig. 1-48).

Related Total Patterns (Mat Activities)

Rolling: prone toward supine: D1 ex with elbow extension, left (Fig. 1-158).

Rising to hands and knees from prone (Fig. 1-168).

Rising to sitting from prone (Fig. 1-177).

From chair to standing to bed: D1 ex with elbow extension of right used in rising to stand (Fig. 1-199).

Emphasis on Shoulder and Elbow: Symmetrical (BS)

FLEXION – ABDUCTION – EXTERNAL ROTATION (D2 fl)
WITH ELBOW FLEXION, LEFT AND RIGHT

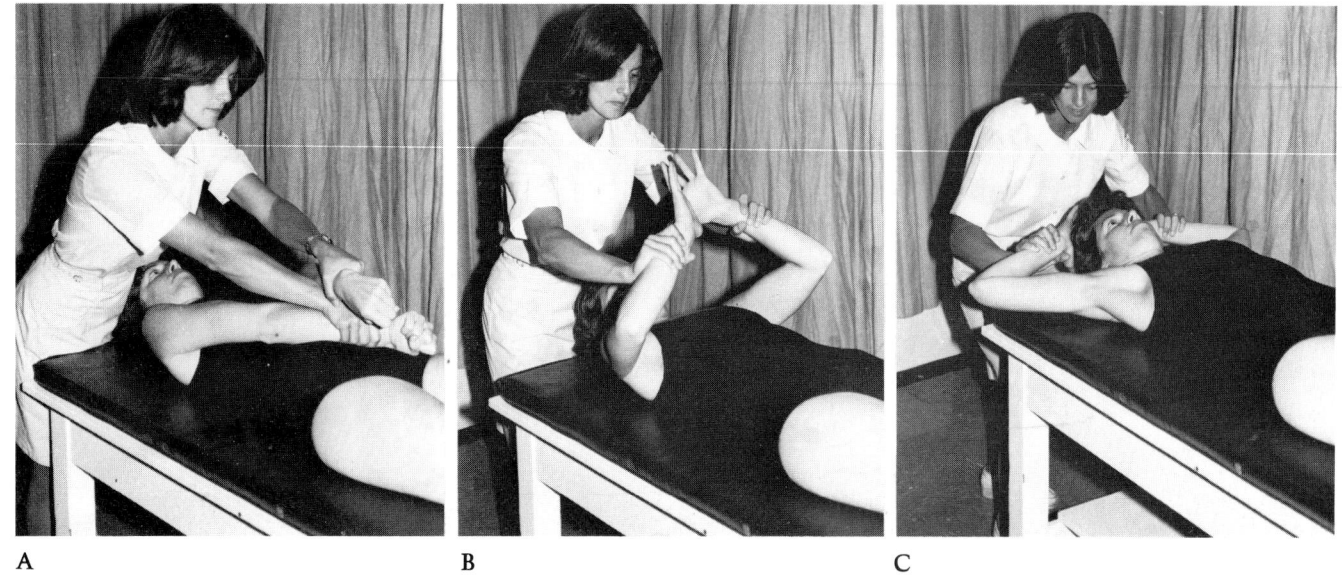

A   B   C

FIG. 1-96

Components of Motion

Free. In supine posture, head and neck may be elevated slightly. Head is in midline. Eyes regard hands. Alternative postures: sitting on bench or stool, or over edge of table for emphasis on elbow flexion.

Resisted. Hands open with wrist extension toward radial side and initiate forearm supination and external rotation of shoulders as elbows flex, and shoulders flex and abduct.

A. Lengthened Range

Commands. *Preparatory.* "You are to open your hands, bend your elbows, and pull up and out behind your ears." *Action.* "Open your hands! Thumbs up!"

Suggested Techniques. Traction, stretch, and resistance.

B. Middle Range

Commands. "Bend your elbows! And hold! Now pull up and out toward your ears! Now hold on the right, and bend your left elbow! And pull! And pull! And relax."

Suggested Techniques. Resistance to elbow flexors on "hold," followed by resistance to shoulders, flexion, and abduction. Repeated contractions for emphasis of elbow flexion: left "holds" as right flexes, followed by right "holds" as left flexes.

C. Shortened Range

Commands. "Close your hands and push them down toward the opposite hip [A]." "Now open your hands and bend your elbows [B]. Hold it! Now reach toward your ears [C]. Again, and hold! And elbows back to the table! And rest!"

Suggested Techniques. Slow reversal, stretch and resistance, repeated contractions.

Antagonistic Pattern

Extension – adduction – internal rotation (D2 ex) with elbow extension, left and right (Fig. 1-97).

Related Patterns

Unilateral upper extremity D2 fl with elbow flexion (Fig. 1-51).

Total (Mat Activity): Crawling forward on elbows (Fig. 1-164): D2 fl with elbows flexion is used alternately, left and right.

Emphasis on Shoulder and Elbow: Symmetrical (BS)

EXTENSION – ADDUCTION – INTERNAL ROTATION
(D2 ex) WITH ELBOW EXTENSION, LEFT AND RIGHT

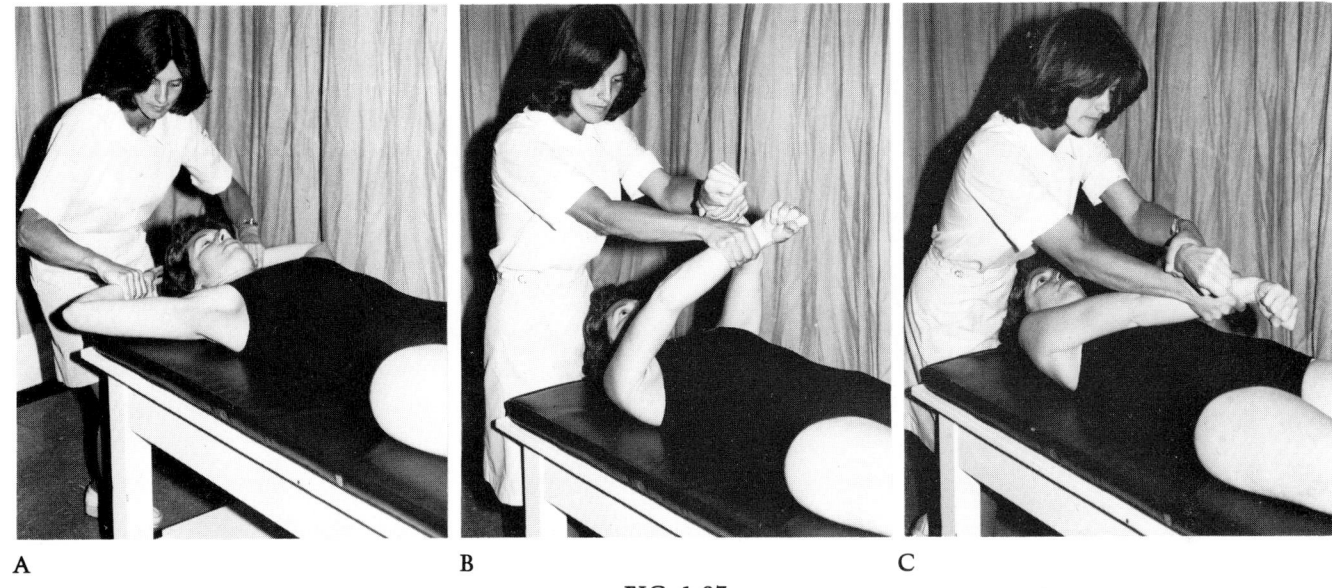

A B C

FIG. 1-97

Components of Motion

Free. In supine posture, head and neck may be elevated slightly. Head is in midline. Eyes regard hands. Alternative postures: sitting on bench or stool, or over edge of table for emphasis on elbow extension.

Resisted. Hands close with wrist flexion toward ulnar side and initiate forearm pronation and internal rotation of shoulders as elbows extend, and shoulders extend and adduct.

A. Lengthened Range

Commands. *Preparatory:* "You are to close your hands, straighten your elbows, and reach down and across towards your hips." *Action.* "Close your hands! Turn them away from your face!"

Suggested Techniques. Traction, stretch, and resistance.

B. Middle Range

Commands. "Straighten your elbows! And hold! Now push down and across toward your hips! Hold on the left, and straighten your right elbow! And push down! And push! And relax."

Suggested Techniques. Resistance to elbow extensors on "hold," followed by resistance to shoulders, extension, and adduction. Repeated contractions for emphasis of elbow extension; left "holds" as right extends, followed by right "holds" as left extends.

C. Shortened Range

Commands. "Open your hands and pull them up and back to your ears. Now close your hands and straighten your elbows. Hold it! Now reach toward your hips! And reach! And reach! And hold! And hold! And hold! And relax."

Suggested Techniques. Slow reversal, stretch, resistance, repeated contractions, approximation, and rhythmic stabilization.

Antagonistic Pattern

Flexion – abduction – external rotation (D2 fl) with elbow flexion, left and right (Fig. 1-96).

Related Unilateral Pattern

Upper extremity D2 ex with elbow extension (Fig. 1-54).

Related Total Patterns (Mat Activities)

Rolling: supine to prone (Figs. 1-151 and 1-152): D2 ex with elbow extension, left.

Use of handbrake (Fig. 1-196): D2 ex with elbow extension, left.

Emphasis on Shoulder and Elbow: Symmetrical (BS)

FLEXION – ADDUCTION – EXTERNAL ROTATION (D1 fl)
WITH ELBOW EXTENSION, LEFT AND RIGHT

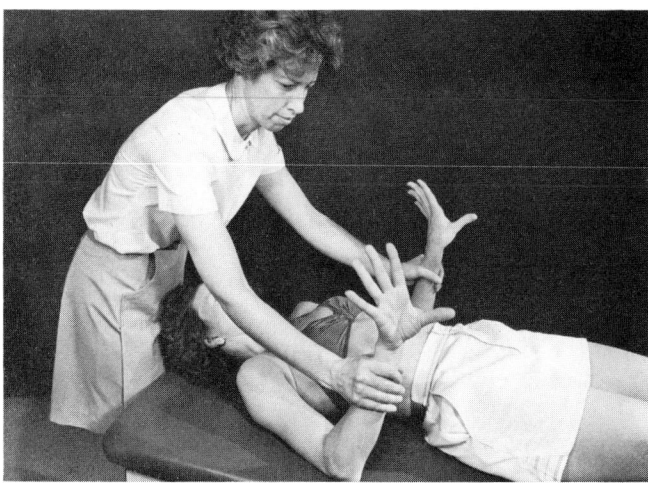

A

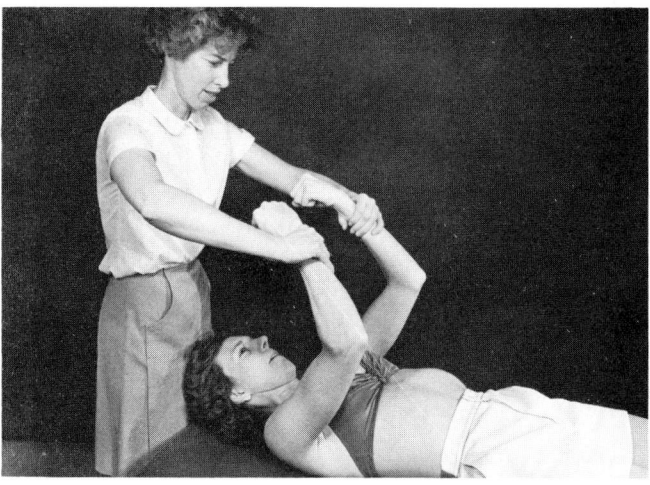

B

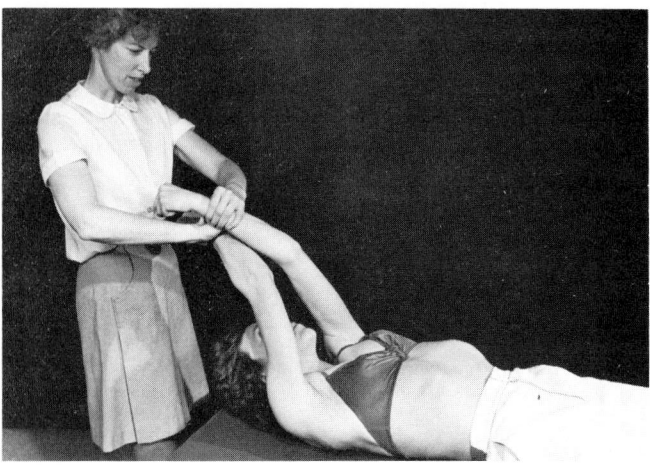

C

FIG. 1-98

Components of Motion

Free. In supine posture, head and neck may be elevated slightly. Head is in midline. Hands follow eyes. Alternative postures: sitting on bench or stool, or over edge of table for emphasis on elbow extension.

Resisted. Hands close with wrist flexion toward radial side and initiate forearm supination and external rotation of shoulders as elbows extend, and shoulders flex and adduct.

A. Lengthened Range

Commands. Preparatory. "You are to close your hands, straighten your elbows, and pull your arms up and across." *Action.* "Close your hands! Turn them toward your face!"

Suggested Techniques. Traction, stretch, and resistance.

B. Middle Range

Commands. "Straighten your elbows and pull your arms up and across! And hold! Now push them up straight! And push! And hold! And relax."

Suggested Techniques. Stretch and resistance to elbow extensors followed by approximation and resistance to shoulders, flexion, and adduction on "hold"! Repeated contractions for emphasis of elbow extension: bilateral symmetrical.

C. Shortened Range

Commands. "Now hold! And hold! And hold! Now open your hands and pull them down and away. Close your hands and turn them toward your face. And hold! Now straighten your elbows! And again! And hold! And rest."

Suggested Techniques. Approximation, rhythmic stabilization, stretch, resistance, slow reversal, repeated contractions.

Antagonistic Pattern

Extension – abduction – internal rotation (D1 ex) with elbow flexion, left and right (Fig. 1-99).

Related Unilateral Patterns

Upper extremity D1 fl with elbow extension (Fig. 1-46). Dressing in bed, inferior region (Fig. 1-202): D1 fl with elbow extension in reaching for pants on chair.

Emphasis on shoulder and Elbow: Symmetrical (BS)

EXTENSION – ABDUCTION – INTERNAL ROTATION
(D1 ex) WITH ELBOW FLEXION, LEFT AND RIGHT

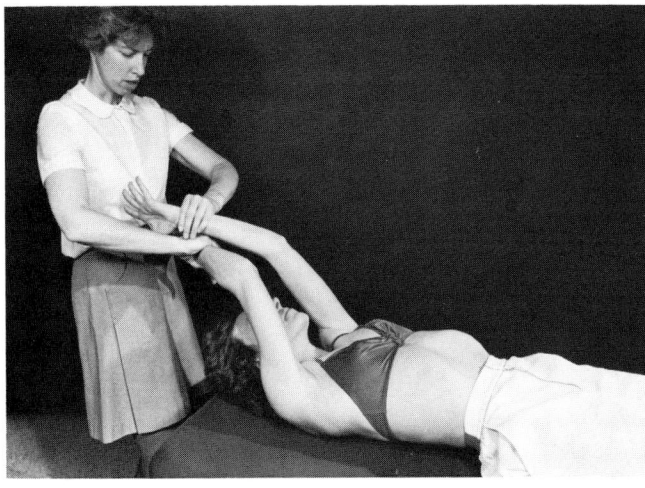

A

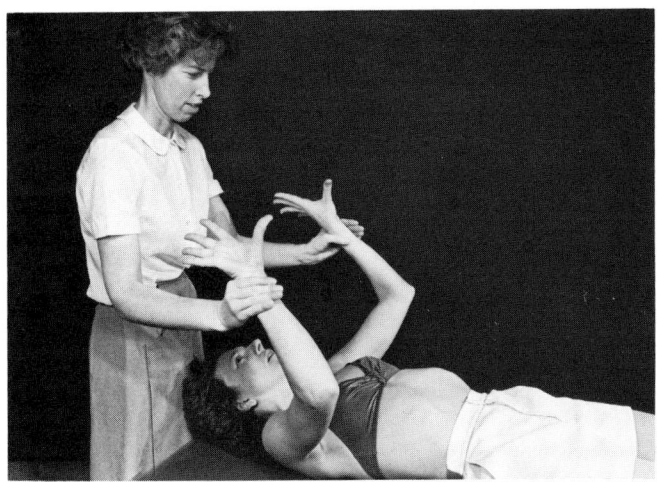

B

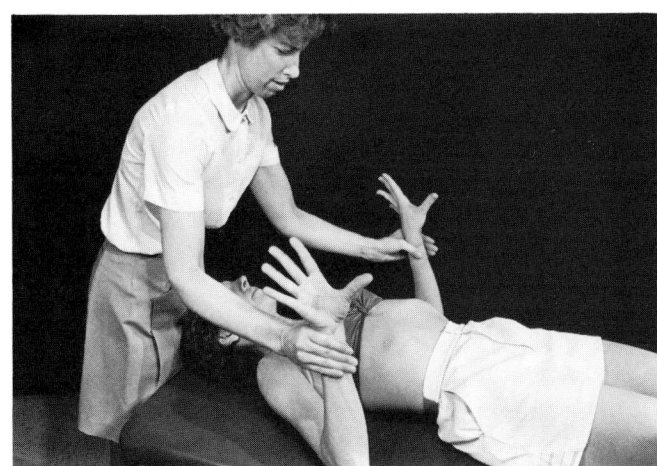

C

FIG. 1-99

Components of Motion

Free. In supine posture, head and neck may be elevated slightly. Head is in midline. Eyes regard hands. Alternative postures: sitting on bench or stool, or over edge of table for emphasis on elbow flexion.

Resisted. Hands open with wrist extension to ulnar side and initiate forearm pronation and internal rotation of shoulders as elbows flex, and shoulders extend and abduct.

A. Lengthened Range

Commands. Preparatory. "You are to open your hands, bend your elbows, and pull your arms down and away." *Action.* "Open your hands! Turn them away from your face!"

Suggested Techniques. Traction, stretch, and resistance.

B. Middle Range

Commands. "Bend your elbows! And hold! Now hold on the right and pull the left arm down and away! And pull! And hold! And rest!"

Suggested Techniques. Stretch and resistance to elbow flexors followed by resistance to shoulders, extension, and abduction. Repeated contractions for emphasis of elbow flexion on the left.

C. Shortened Range

Commands. "Now close your hands and push your arms up and across. Open your hands and bend your elbows. And hold! Now bend! And again! And relax."

Suggested Techniques. Slow reversal, stretch, resistance, repeated contractions.

Antagonistic Pattern

Flexion – adduction – external rotation (D1 fl) with extension, left and right (Fig. 1-98).

Related Unilateral Pattern

Upper extremity D1 ex with elbow flexion (Fig. 1-49).

Related Total Patterns (Mat Activities)

Pulling to standing, stall bars (Fig. 1-185): D1 fl with elbow flexion in middle range of rising to stand.

Crawling forward on elbows (Fig. 1-164): arms move from D2 fl with elbow flexion to D1 ex with elbow flexion in preparation for pulling lower limbs forward.

Emphasis on Shoulder and Elbow: Symmetrical (BS)

FLEXION – ABDUCTION – EXTERNAL ROTATION (D2 fl)
WITH ELBOW EXTENSION, LEFT AND RIGHT

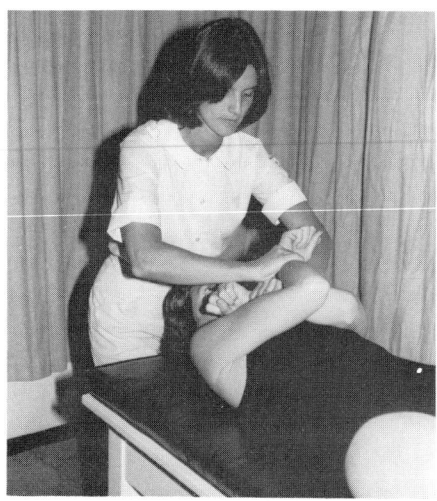

A

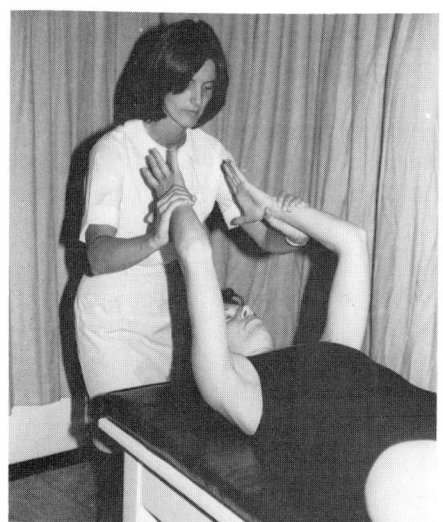

B

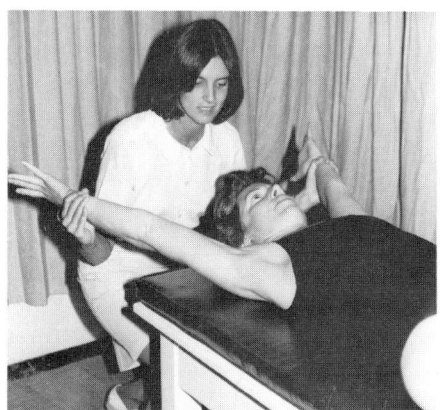

C

FIG. 1-100

Components of Motion

Free. In supine posture, head and neck may be elevated slightly. Head is in midline. Alternative postures: sitting on bench, stool, or armless chair.

Resisted. Hands open with wrist extension to radial side and initiate forearm supination and external rotation of shoulders as elbows extend, and shoulders flex and abduct.

A. Lengthened Range

Commands. *Preparatory.* "You are to open your hands, straighten your elbows, and push your arms up and away." *Action.* "Open your hands! Thumbs pointing back!"

Suggested Techniques. Stretch and resistance.

B. Middle Range

Commands. "Straighten your elbows! And hold! Now hold on the left and push your right elbow straight! And push! And hold! And relax."

Suggested Techniques. Stretch and resistance to elbow extensors followed by resistance to shoulders, flexion, and abduction. Repeated contractions for emphasis of elbow extension on the right.

C. Shortened Range

Commands. "Close your hands and pull your arms down and across. Now open your hands and straighten your elbows. And hold! Push back and out! And again! And rest."

Suggested Techniques. Slow reversal, approximation, resistance, repeated contractions.

Antagonistic Pattern

Extension – adduction – internal rotation (D2 ex) with elbow flexion, right and left (Fig. 1-101).

Related Pattern

Unilateral upper extremity D2 fl with elbow extension (Fig. 1-52).

Emphasis on Shoulder and Elbow: Symmetrical (BS)

EXTENSION – ADDUCTION – INTERNAL ROTATION
(D2 ex) WITH ELBOW FLEXION, LEFT AND RIGHT

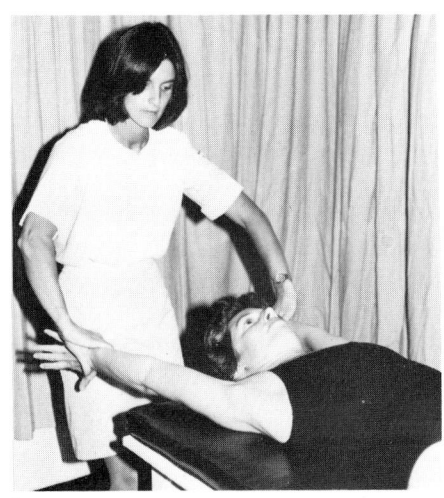

A

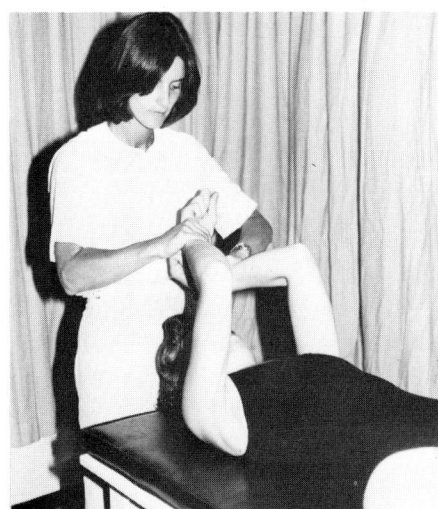

B

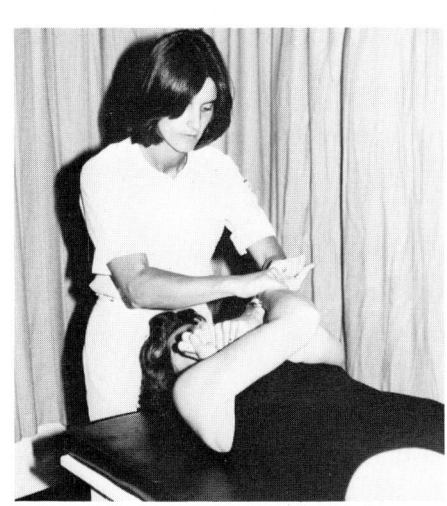

C

FIG. 1-101

Components of Motion

Free. In supine position, head and neck may be elevated slightly. Head is in midline. Alternative postures: sitting on bench, stool, or armless chair.

Resisted. Hands close with wrist flexion to ulnar side and initiate forearm pronation and internal rotation of shoulders as elbows flex, and shoulders extend and adduct.

A. Lengthened Range

Commands. *Preparatory.* "You are to close your hands, bend your elbows, and pull down and across." *Action.* "Close your hands! Turn your hands away from your face!"

Suggested Techniques.. Traction, stretch, and resistance.

B. Middle Range

Commands. "Hold it! Don't let me move you! And hold! And hold! Now pull your left hand down to your right shoulder! And again! Now hold on the left and pull the right hand down and across! And pull! And relax."

Suggested Techniques. Rhythmic stabilization. Stretch and resistance to elbow flexors followed by resistance to shoulder, extension, and adduction. Repeated contractions for emphasis of elbow flexion, alternately left, then right.

C. Shortened Range

Commands. "Open your hands and turn them toward your face. Push your arms up and out. And hold! Now close your hands! Turn them away from your face! And hold! And pull them down to your shoulders! And pull! And hold! And relax."

Suggested Techniques. Slow reversal hold, stretch, resistance, and repeated contractions.

Antagonistic Pattern

Flexion – abduction – external rotation (D2 fl), elbow extension, left and right (Fig. 1-100).

Related Pattern

Unilateral upper extremity D2 ex with elbow flexion (Fig. 1-55).

Emphasis on Shoulder and Elbow: Asymmetrical (BA)

FLEXION – ABDUCTION – EXTERNAL ROTATION (D2 fl)
WITH ELBOW FLEXION, LEFT; FLEXION – ADDUCTION –
EXTERNAL ROTATION (D1 fl) WITH
ELBOW FLEXION, RIGHT

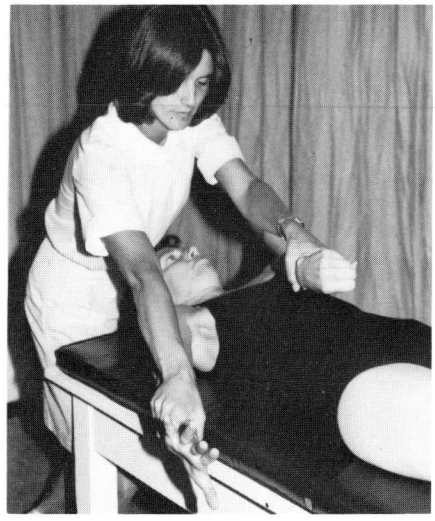

A

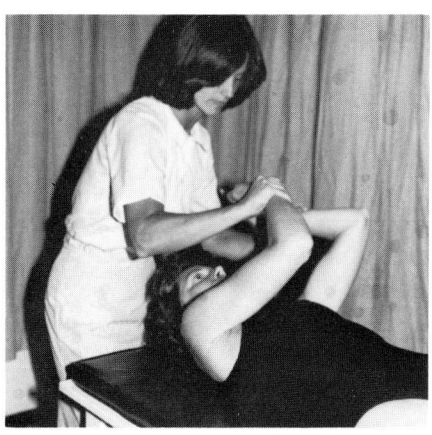

B

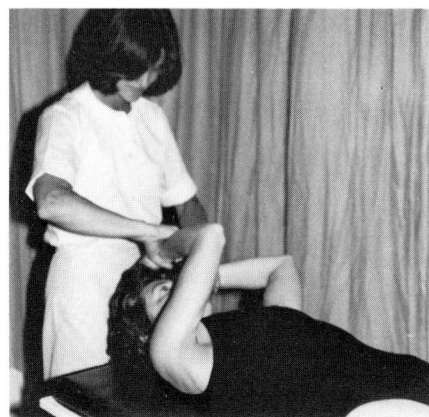

C

FIG. 1-102

Components of Motion

Free. In supine position, head and neck may be elevated slightly. Head is in midline, but may rotate to left as eyes regard hands. Alternative postures: sitting on bench, stool, or armless chair.

Resisted. Left hand opens with wrist extension to radial side as right hand closes with wrist flexion to radial side. Each initiates forearm supination and external rotation of shoulders. Elbows flex and shoulders flex, the left abducting as the right adducts.

A. Lengthened Range

Commands. Preparatory. "You are to open your left hand and close your right. Turn your hands toward your face and pull them up toward the left." *Action.* "Open your left! Close your right! Turn your hands toward your face!"

Suggested Techniques. Traction, stretch, and resistance.

B. Middle Range

Commands. "Pull your hands up toward me! Hold! Now hold the right and bend your left elbow! And bend some more! Now hold on the left and bend your right elbow! And again! And hold! And relax."

Suggested Techniques. Repeated contractions for emphasis, alternately left and right.

C. Shortened Range

Commands. "Open your right hand and close your left! Pull down and away from me! And hold! Now close your right and open your left! Turn your hands toward your face and pull to me! And hold! Now bend your elbows! And bend again! And again! And rest."

Suggested Techniques. Slow reversal-hold, stretch, resistance, repeated contractions.

Antagonistic Pattern

Extension – adduction – internal rotation (D2 ex) with elbow extension, left; extension – abduction – internal rotation (D1 ex) with elbow extension, right (Fig. 1-103).

Related Patterns

Unilateral upper extremity: D2 fl with elbow flexion, left (Fig. 1-51); D1 fl with elbow flexion, right (Fig. 1-45).

Upper Extremity

Emphasis on Shoulder and Elbow: Asymmetrical (BA)

EXTENSION – ADDUCTION – INTERNAL ROTATION (D2 ex) WITH ELBOW EXTENSION, LEFT; EXTENSION – ABDUCTION – INTERNAL ROTATION (D1 ex) WITH ELBOW EXTENSION, RIGHT

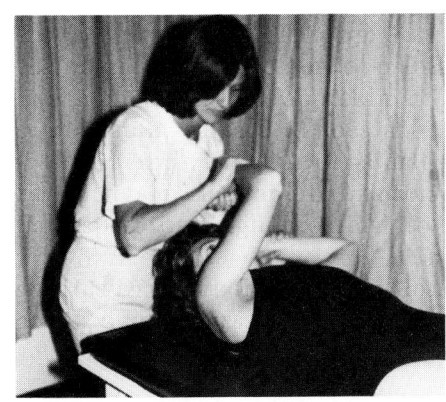

A

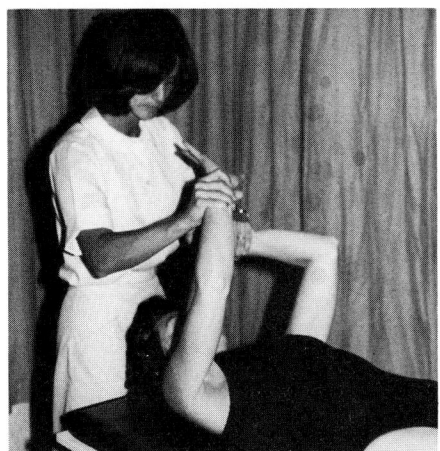

B

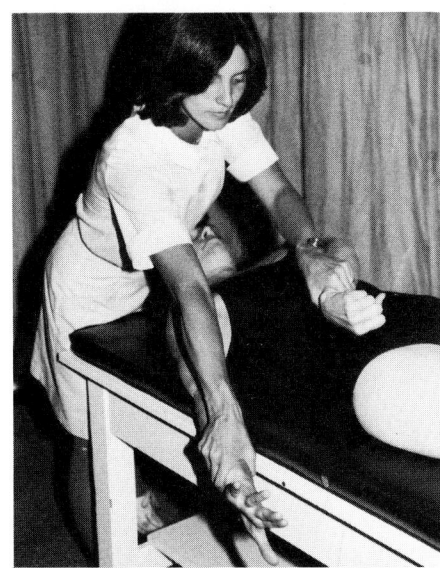

C

FIG. 1-103

Components of Motion

Free. In supine position, head and neck may be elevated slightly. Head is in midline, but may rotate as eyes regard hands. Alternative postures: sitting on bench, stool, or armless chair.

Resisted. Left hand closes with wrist flexion to ulnar side, as right hand opens with wrist extension to ulnar side. Each initiates forearm pronation and internal rotation of shoulders. Elbows extend and shoulders extend, the left adducting as the right abducts.

A. Lengthened Range

Commands. *Preparatory.* "You are to close your left hand and open your right. Turn your hands away from your face and push them away from me." *Action.* "Close your left hand! Open your right! Turn your hands away from your face!"

Suggested Techniques. Stretch and resistance.

B. Middle Range

Commands. "Straighten your arms! Hold it! Now hold on the left and straighten the right! And push! Now hold on the right and straighten the left! And push! And hold! Don't let me move you! And hold! And hold! And relax."

Suggested Techniques. Stretch and resistance to elbow extension, followed by repeated contractions, alternately right and left. Rhythmic stabilization with elbow extension, shoulder in middle range.

C. Shortened Range

Commands. "Open your left and close your right! Turn your hands toward me! Lift your hands to the left! Hold! Now close the left and open the right and push down to the right! Hold! And push! And push! And rest."

Suggested Techniques. Slow reversal – hold, stretch, resistance, repeated contractions.

Antagonistic Pattern

Flexion – abduction – external rotation (D2 fl) with elbow flexion, left; flexion – adduction – external rotation (D1 fl) with elbow flexion, right (Fig. 1-102).

Related Patterns

Unilateral upper extremity: D2 ex with elbow extension (Fig. 1-54); D1 ex with elbow extension (Fig. 1-48).

Total (Mat Activity): Rolling: supine toward prone (Fig. 1-153): D2 ex with elbow extension, left; D1 ex with elbow extension, right. Arms are in contact, as in reverse of the lift, for emphasis on trunk.

Emphasis on Hand and Wrist: Symmetrical (BS)

EXTENSION – ABDUCTION – INTERNAL ROTATION
(D1 ex), HANDS OPEN, LEFT AND RIGHT

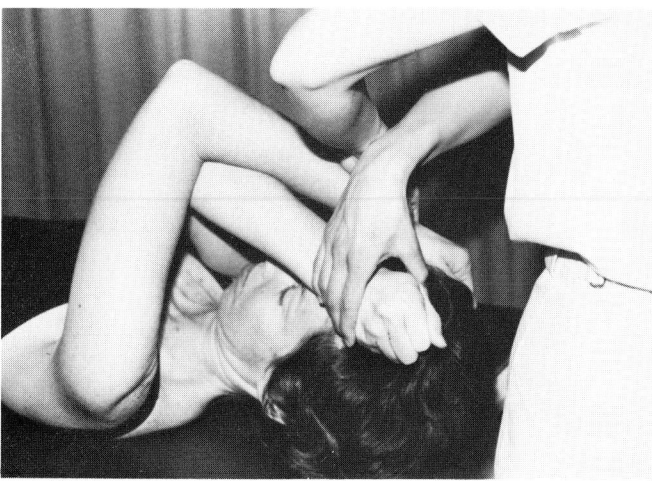

A

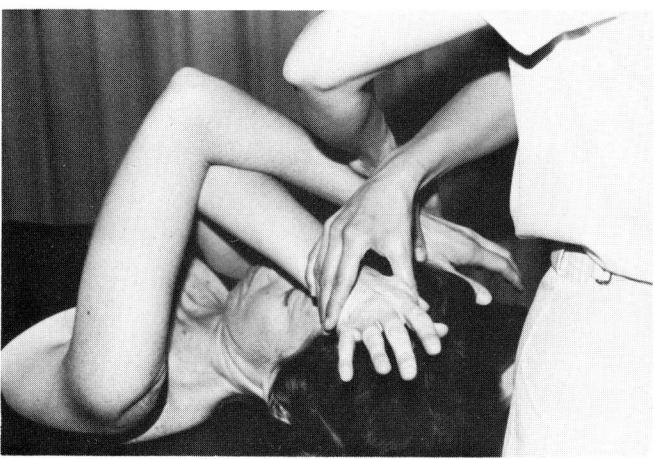

B

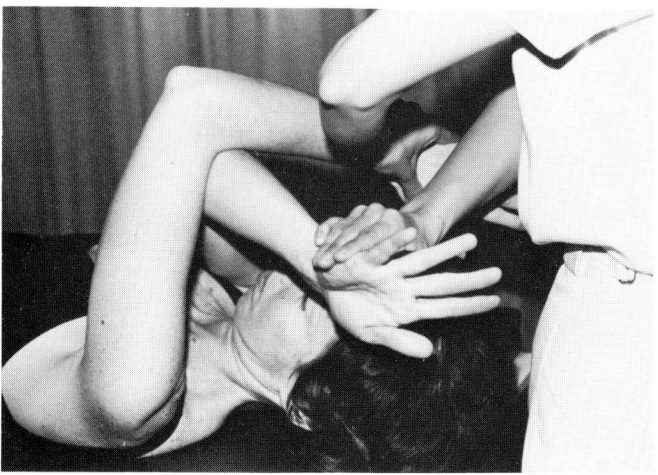

C

FIG. 1-104

Components of Motion

Free. In supine posture, head and neck may be elevated slightly. Head is in midline. Alternative postures: sitting on bench, stool, or armless chair.

Resisted. Hands open with wrist extension toward ulnar side and initiate forearm pronation and internal rotation of shoulders as elbows extend.

A. Lengthened Range

Commands. *Preparatory.* "You are to open your hands and push them down and away from your face." *Action.* "Open your hands! Thumbs down!"

Suggested Techniques. Traction, stretch, and resistance.

B. Middle Range

Commands. "Hold everything! Hold on the right! Push the left away from your face! And push! Now hold on the left! Push away with the right! And push! And relax."

Suggested Technique. Repeated contractions for emphasis, alternately left and right.

C. Shortened Range

Commands. "Close your hands toward your face! and hold! Now open your hands! Turn them away from your face! And hold! Now push the wrists back! Back some more! And relax."

Suggested Techniques. Slow reversal – hold, stretch, resistance, and repeated contractions with emphasis on ulnar wrist extension.

Antagonistic Pattern

Flexion – adduction – external rotation (D1 fl), hands close, left and right (Fig. 1-105).

Related Patterns

Unilateral upper extremity D1 ex with elbow extension, right (Fig. 1-48).

Emphasis on Hand and Wrist: Symmetrical (BS)

FLEXION – ADDUCTION – EXTERNAL ROTATION (D1 fl)
HANDS CLOSE, LEFT AND RIGHT

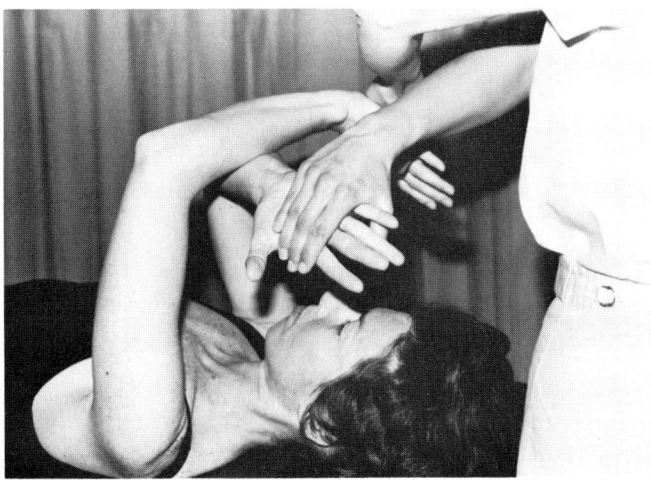

A

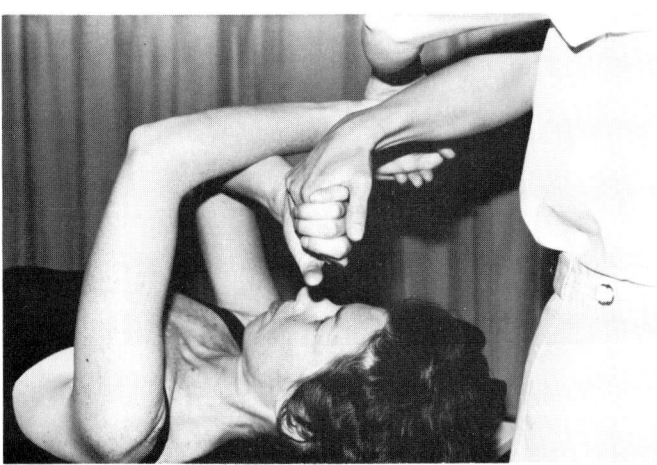

B

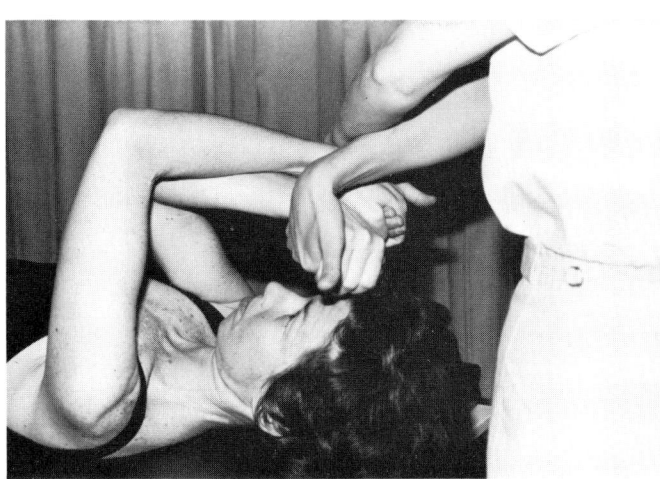

C

FIG. 1-105

Components of Motion

Free. In supine posture, head and neck may be elevated slightly and may flex in midline. Eyes regard hands. Alternative postures: sitting on bench, stool, or armless chair.

Resisted. Hands close with wrist flexion toward radial side and initiate forearm supination and external rotation of shoulders as elbows flex.

A. Lengthened Range

Commands. *Preparatory.* "You are to close your hands toward your face." *Action.* "Close your hands toward your face!"

Suggested Techniques. Stretch and resistance.

B. Middle Range

Commands. "Hold everything! Hold on the left! Turn your right hand toward your face and bend your wrists! And turn some more! Now hold on the right and turn the left hand! And turn! And bend your wrist! And rest!"

Suggested Techniques. Repeated contractions for emphasis, alternately left and right.

C. Shortened Range

Commands. "Open your hands away from your face! [Therapist must shift manual contacts to dorsal surface.] Now close your hands again and toward your face! And hold! Now pull them down and out toward your ears! And pull! And pull! And relax!"

Suggested Techniques

Slow reversal, stretch, resistance, repeated contractions.

Antagonistic Pattern

Extension – abduction – internal rotation (D1 ex), hands open, left and right (Fig. 1-104).

Related Patterns

Unilateral upper extremity D1 fl with elbow flexion, right (Fig. 1-45).

Emphasis on Hand and Wrist: Symmetrical (BS)

FLEXION – ABDUCTION – EXTERNAL ROTATION (D2 fl),
HANDS OPEN, LEFT AND RIGHT

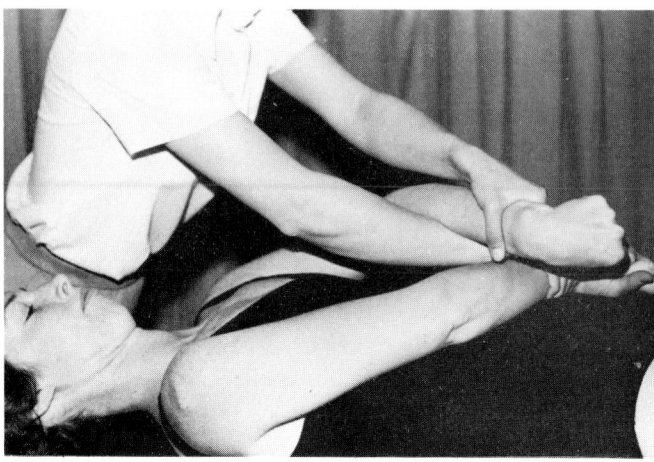

A

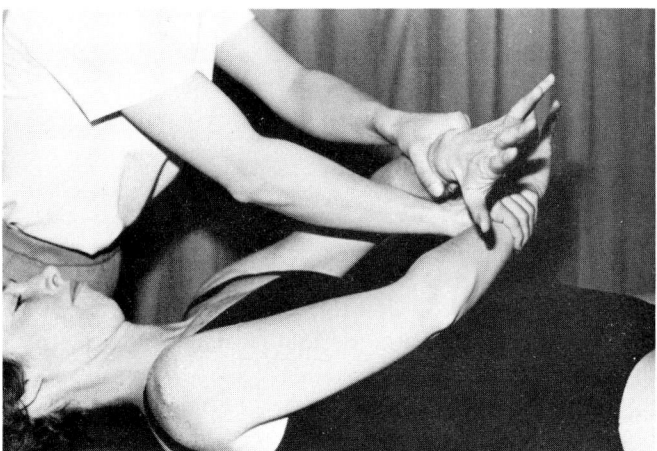

B

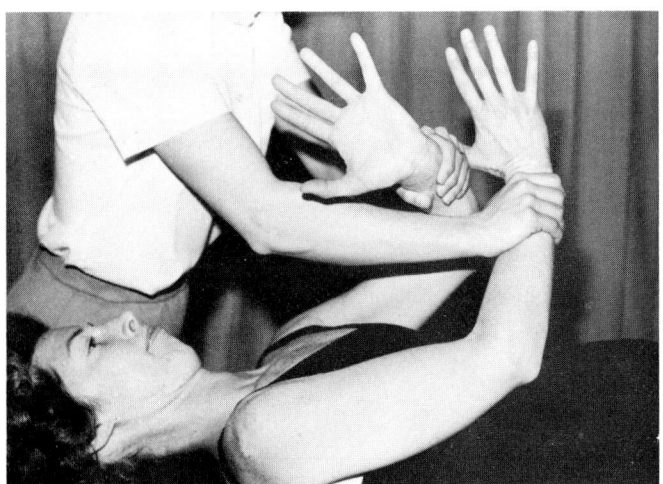

C

FIG. 1-106

Components of Motion

Free. In supine posture, head and neck may be elevated slightly. Head is in midline position. Eyes regard hands. Alternative postures: sitting on bench, stool, or armless chair.

Resisted. Hands open with wrist extension toward radial side and initiate forearm supination and external rotation of shoulders as elbows flex.

A. Lengthened Range

Commands. *Preparatory.* "You are to open your hands and pull them toward your face." *Action.* "Open your hands! Point your thumbs toward me!"

Suggested Techniques. Traction, stretch, and resistance.

B. Middle Range

Commands. "Hold everything! Hold on the right! Pull up and out with the left! And pull! Now hold on the left! Pull up and out with the right! And pull! And relax!"

Suggested Techniques. Repeated contractions for emphasis, alternately left and right.

C. Shortened Range

Commands. "Close your hands and push down and across! Straighten your elbows! Now open your hands and pull them up and out! And hold! Now get those thumbs back! And again! And again! And relax!"

Suggested Techniques. Slow reversal, stretch, resistance, and repeated contractions with emphasis on radial wrist extension.

Antagonistic Pattern

Extension – adduction – internal rotation (D2 ex), hands close, left and right (Fig. 1-107).

Related Patterns

Unilateral upper extremity D2 fl with elbow flexion, left (Fig. 1-51).

Total (Mat Activity): Crawling forward on elbows (Fig. 1-164). Open hand contacts floor.

Upper Extremity

Emphasis on Hand and Wrist: Symmetrical (BS)

EXTENSION – ADDUCTION – INTERNAL ROTATION
(D2 ex), HANDS CLOSE, LEFT AND RIGHT

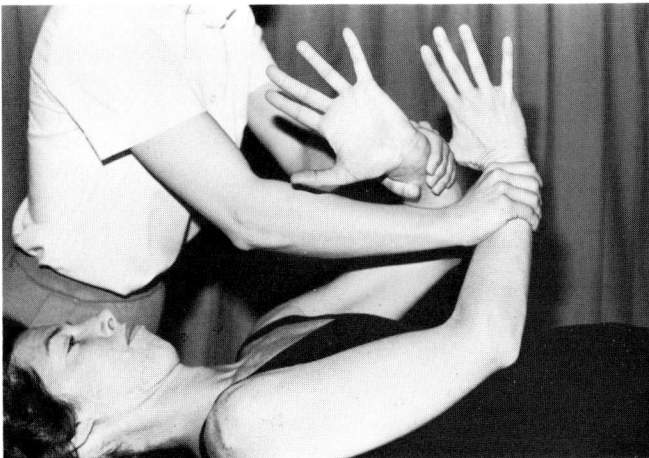

A

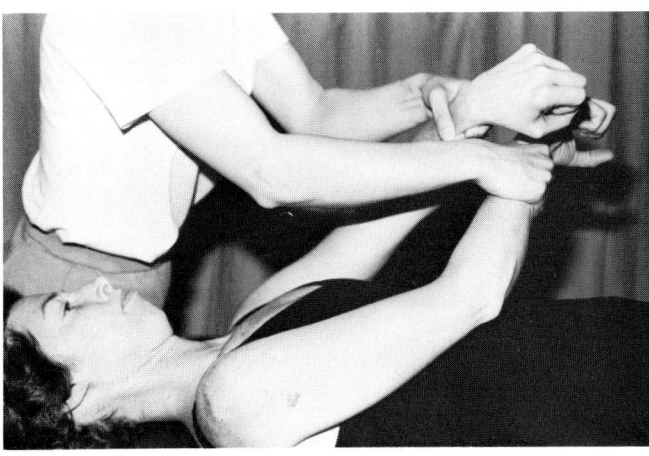

B

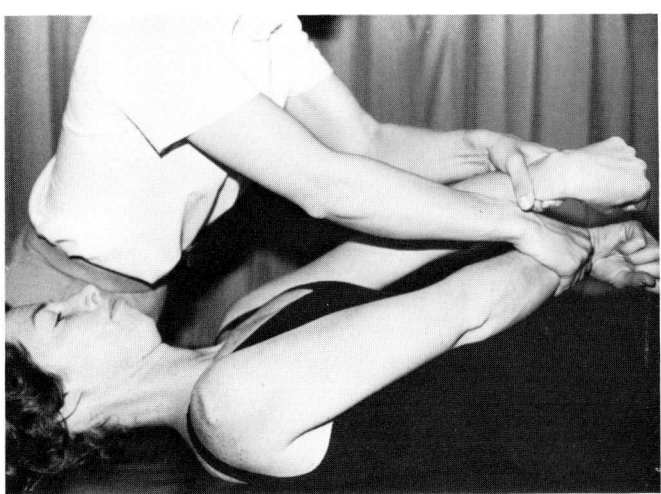

C

FIG. 1-107

Components of Motion

Free. In supine posture, head and neck may be elevated slightly. Head is in midline. Eyes regard hands. Alternative postures: sitting on bench, stool, or armless chair.

Resisted. Hands close with wrist flexion toward ulnar side and initiate forearm pronation and internal rotation of shoulders as elbows extend.

A. Lengthened Range

Commands. *Preparatory.* "You are to close your hands and push them down and across toward your hips." *Action.* "Close your hands! Turn and push across!"

Suggested Techniques. Stretch and resistance.

B. Middle Range

Commands. "Hold everything! Hold on the left! Push down and across with the right! And push! Now hold on the right and push down and across with the left! And push! And relax!"

Suggested Techniques. Repeated contractions for emphasis, alternately right and left.

C. Shortened Range

Commands. "Hold! Don't let me move you! And hold! And hold! Now cross your arms and push hands toward hips! And hold! And relax!"

Suggested Techniques. Approximation, rhythmic stabilization, stretch, and resistance.

Antagonistic Pattern

Flexion – abduction – external rotation (D2 fl), hands open, left and right (Fig. 1-106).

Related Unilateral Pattern

Upper extremity D2 ex with elbow extension, left (Fig. 1-54).

Upper Extremity

Emphasis on Hand and Wrist: Asymmetrical (BA)

FLEXION – ADDUCTION – EXTERNAL ROTATION (D1 fl), HAND CLOSES, RIGHT; FLEXION – ABDUCTION – EXTERNAL ROTATION (D2 fl), HAND OPENS, LEFT

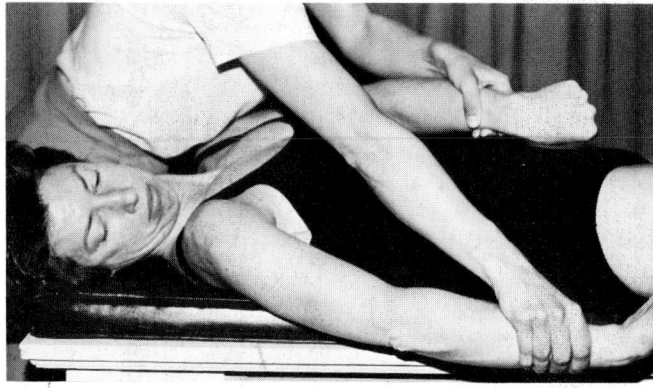

A

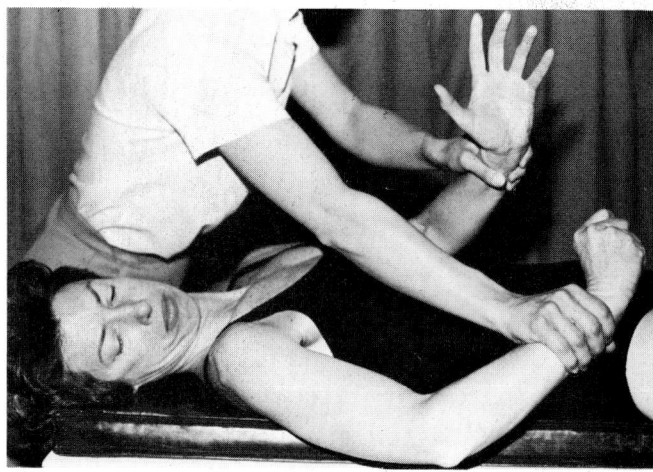

B

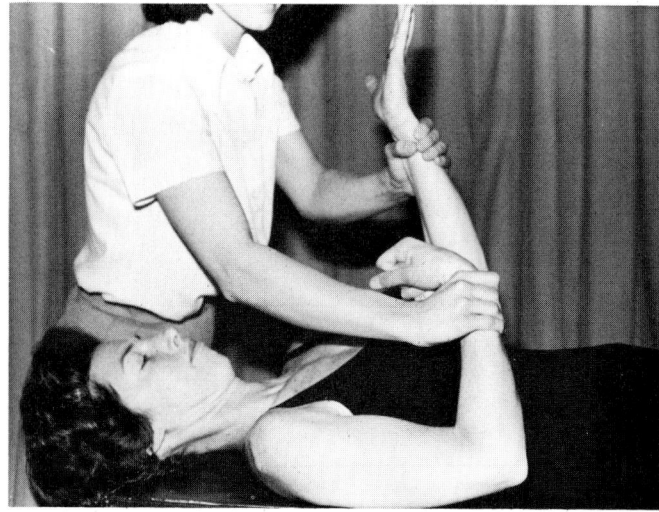

C

FIG. 1-108

Components of Motion

Free. In supine posture, head and neck may be elevated slightly. Eyes regard right hand with head to right. Then eyes follow hands, and head assumes position in midline. Alternative postures: sitting on bench, stool, or armless chair.

Resisted. Left hand opens with wrist extension toward radial side, as right closes with wrist flexion toward radial side. Each initiates forearm supination and external rotation of shoulders as elbows flex.

A. Lengthened Range

Commands. *Preparatory.* "You are to open your left hand [D2 fl] and close your right [D1 fl], and pull them up and out toward me." *Action.* "Open your left! Close your right! Pull up and out to me!"

Suggested Techniques. Stretch and resistance.

B. Middle Range

Commands. "Hold everything! Hold on the right! Pull up and out with the left! And pull! And pull! Now hold on the left! Pull up and across with the right! And pull! And relax!"

Suggested Techniques. Repeated contractions for emphasis, alternately left and right.

C. Shortened Range

Commands. "Hold your hands up toward me! Turn your left wrist and point your thumb toward me! Hold! Don't let me turn it; thumb toward me! Relax!"

Suggested Techniques. Guided resistance to pronation to reduce excessive supination of left forearm, repeated contractions.

Antagonistic Pattern

Extension – adduction – internal rotation (D2 ex), hand closes, left; extension – abduction – internal rotation (D1 ex), hands open, right (Fig. 1-109).

Related Unilateral Patterns

Upper extremity D2 fl with elbow flexion, left (Fig. 1-51); D1 fl with elbow flexion, right (Fig. 1-45).

Upper trunk extension with rotation to the left (Fig. 1-37): D2 fl of left, D1 fl of right, hands in contact (lifting). Emphasis on trunk, therefore elbows are straight.

Related Total Pattern (Mat Activity)

Rolling: prone toward supine (Fig. 1-159): D2 fl of left with elbow extension, D1 fl of right. Hands in contact as in lifting. Head rotates to left.

Upper Extremity

Emphasis on Hand and Wrist: Asymmetrical (BA)

EXTENSION – ADDUCTION – INTERNAL ROTATION (D2 ex), HAND CLOSES, LEFT; EXTENSION – ABDUCTION – INTERNAL ROTATION (D1 ex), HAND OPENS, RIGHT

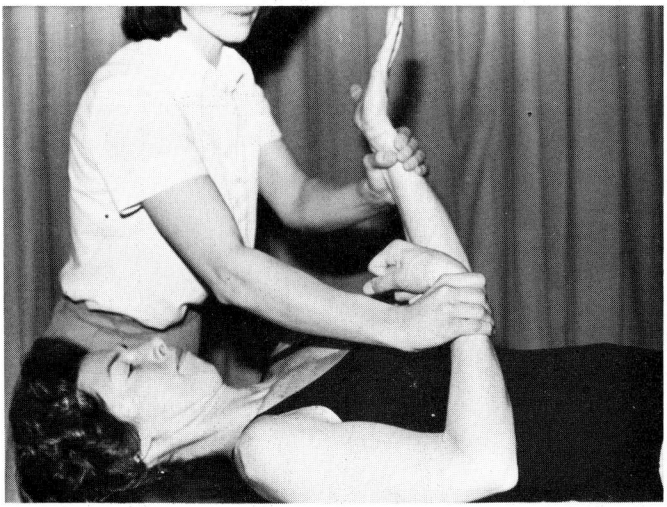

A

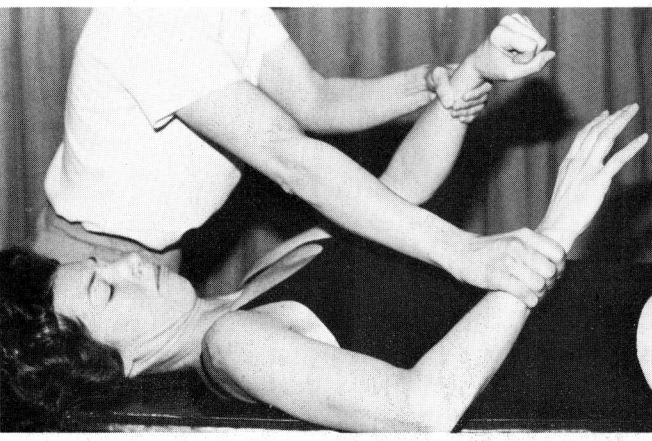

B

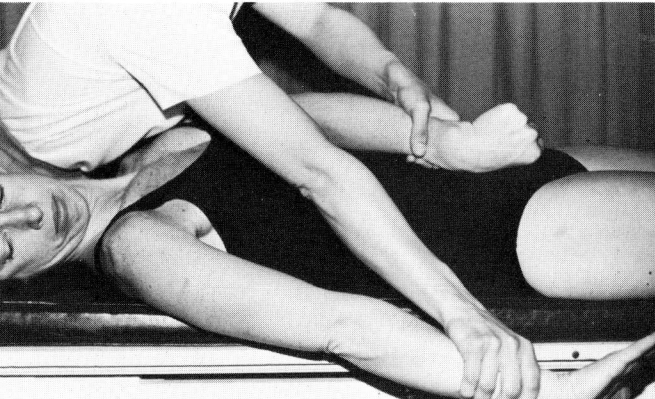

C

FIG. 1-109

Components of Motion

Free. In supine posture, head and neck may be elevated slightly. Eyes follow hands. Head rotates toward right. Alternative postures: sitting on bench, stool, or armless chair.

Resisted. Left hand closes toward ulnar side as right opens toward ulnar side. Each initiates forearm pronation and internal rotation of shoulder as elbows extend, and shoulders extend in shortened range with left adducting as right abducts.

A. Lengthened Range

Commands. *Preparatory.* "You are to close your left hand (D2 ex) and open your right (D1 ex), and push them down and away; left hand toward your right hip; right hand toward the floor." *Action.* "Close your left! Open your right! Push down and away!"

Suggested Techniques. Stretch and resistance.

B. Middle Range

Commands. "Hold everything! Hold the right! Reach across with the left! And push! Now hold on the left! Push down with the right! And push! And relax!"

Suggested Techniques. Repeated contractions for emphasis, alternately left and right.

C. Shortened Range

Commands. "Hold your arms down and away from me! Turn your right wrist; point your right thumb toward the floor! Hold! Don't let me turn it; thumb down! Relax."

Suggested Techniques. Emphasis on right forearm, wrist, and hand with repeated contractions.

Antagonistic Pattern

Flexion – abduction – external rotation (D2 fl), hand opens, left; flexion – adduction – external rotation (D1 fl), hand closes, right (Fig. 1-108).

Related Unilateral Patterns

Upper extremity D2 ex with elbow extension, left (Fig. 1-54); D1 ex with elbow extension, right (Fig. 1-48).

Upper trunk flexion with rotation to right (Fig. 1-36): D2 ex of left, D1 ex of right, hands in contact (chopping). Emphasis on trunk, therefore elbows are straight.

Related Total Pattern (Mat Activity)

Rolling supine toward prone (Fig. 1-151): D2 ex of left, elbow straight; D1 ex of right, open hand contacts mat.

Emphasis on Hip with Knee Straight: Symmetrical (BS)

FLEXION – ADDUCTION – EXTERNAL ROTATION
(D1 fl), LEFT AND RIGHT

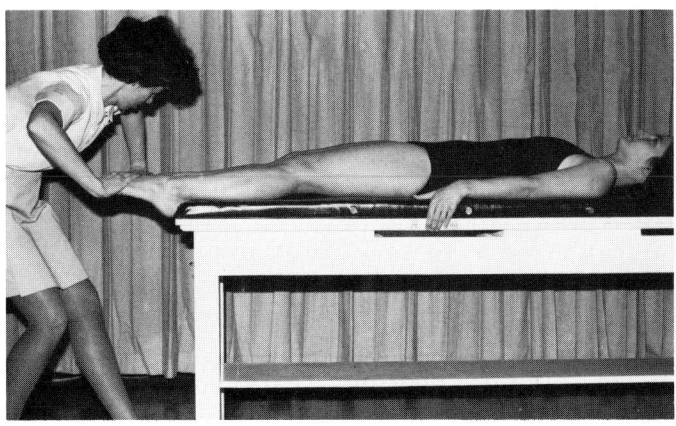

A

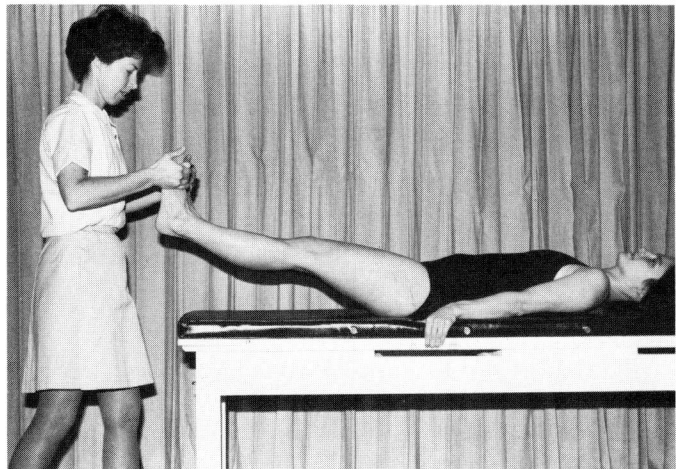

B

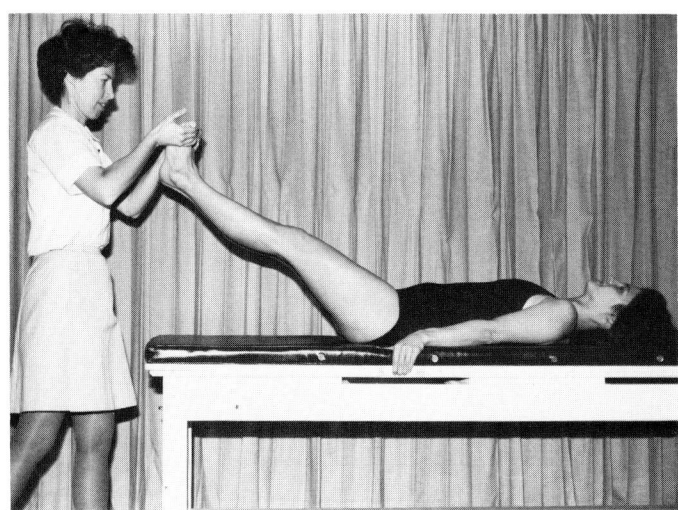

C

FIG. 1-110

Components of Motion

Free. In supine posture, patient's head and shoulders may be elevated slightly. Head maintains midline position. Hands grip table edges for stability and reinforcement. Alternative posture: prone with hips extended over end of table.

Resisted. Feet and ankles dorsiflex and invert, and initiate hip flexion, adduction, and external rotation, bilaterally.

A. Lengthened Range

Commands. Preparatory. "You will pull your feet up and in. Toes up! Turn your heels in, and lift your limbs up and together as high as possible. Keep your knees straight." (D1 fl bilaterally. Limbs are free of contact.) *Action.* "Now pull your toes toward your nose! Feet up and in! And lift up and in!"

Suggested Techniques. Traction, stretch, and resistance.

B. Middle Range

Commands. "Hold! Now hold with the right and lift the left! Lift! Again! And hold! Now lift with the right! Lift! And again! And relax."

Suggested Techniques. Maximally resisted hold, followed by repeated contractions for emphasis. Left limb, then right.

C. Shortened Range

Commands. "Now hold! Hold both feet still! And hold! Hold! And relax."

Suggested Techniques. Rhythmic stabilization, repeated contractions for emphasis, slow reversal, slow reversal–hold.

Antagonistic Pattern

D1 ex with straight knee, left and right (Fig. 1-111).

Related Unilateral Patterns

Lower extremity D1 fl with straight knee. (Fig. 1-64).

Lower trunk flexion with rotation to the left (Fig. 1-38); D1 fl with straight knee, right. Limbs in contact.

Related Total Patterns (Mat Activities)

Rising to plantigrade (Fig. 1-175, *C*): bilateral symmetrical posture.

Lower trunk rocking backwards, limbs in contact, D1 fl bilaterally (Fig. 1-181, *B*).

Inferior region balance (patient on crutches; Fig. 1-192).

Emphasis on Hip with Knee Straight: Symmetrical (BS)

EXTENSION – ABDUCTION – INTERNAL ROTATION
(D1 ex) LEFT AND RIGHT

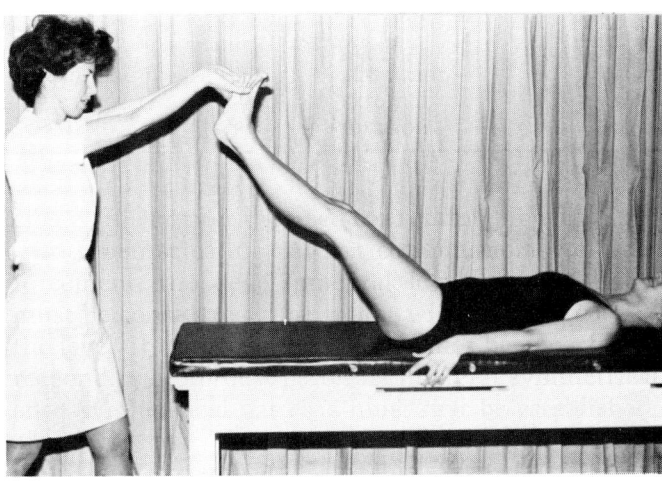

A

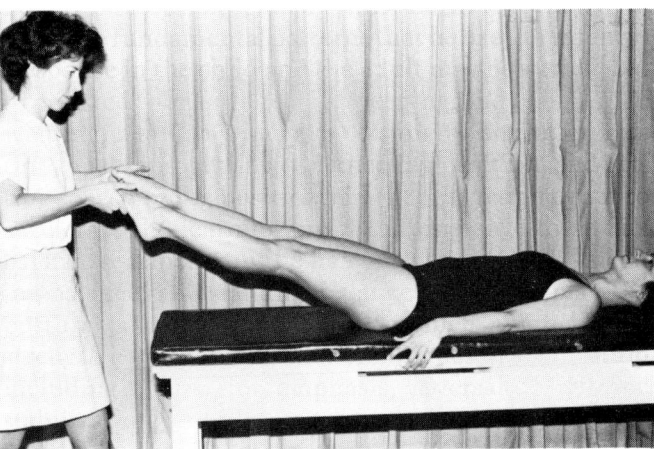

B

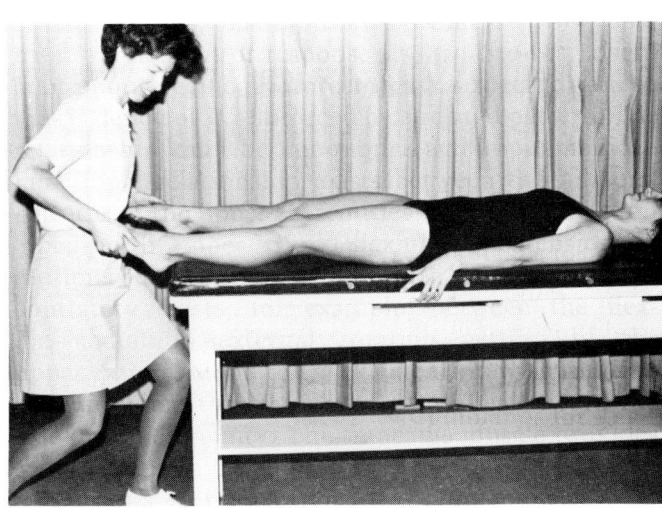

C

FIG. 1-111

Components of Motion

Free. In supine posture, head and shoulders may be elevated slightly. Head maintains midline position. Hands grip table edges for stability and reinforcement. Alternative posture: prone with hips extended over end of table.

Resisted. Feet and ankles plantar flex and evert, and initiate hip extension, abduction, and internal rotation, bilaterally.

A. Lengthened Range

Commands. Preparatory. "You are to push your feet down and out, turn your heels out, and push your limbs down and out. Keep your knees straight." (D1 ex bilaterally.) *Action.* "Toes and feet down and out! And push down and out!"

Suggested Techniques. Approximation, stretch, and resistance.

B. Middle Range

Commands. "Hold everything! Now hold the right still and push the left down and out! Push again! Push! And hold! Now hold the left! And push the right down and out! Push again! And push! And rest."

Suggested Techniques. Maximal "hold" with one limb, and repeated contractions to emphasize the other.

C. Shortened Range

Commands. "Now hold both feet still! And hold! Hold! And relax."

Suggested Techniques. Rhythmic stabilization, repeated contractions for emphasis, slow reversal, slow reversal–hold.

Antagonistic Pattern

Flexion–adduction–external rotation (D1 fl), left and right (Fig. 1-110).

Related Unilateral Patterns

Lower extremity D1 ex with knee straight (Fig. 1-67).

Lower trunk extension with rotation to the left (Fig. 1-41): D1 ex with straight knees, right. Limbs in contact.

Related Total Patterns (Mat Activities)

Rolling toward prone, hip and knee extension, D1 ex (Fig. 1-156).

Inferior region balance, patient on crutches (Fig. 1-192, *B*).

Emphasis on Hip with Knee Straight: Symmetrical (BS)

FLEXION – ABDUCTION – INTERNAL ROTATION (D2 fl),
LEFT AND RIGHT

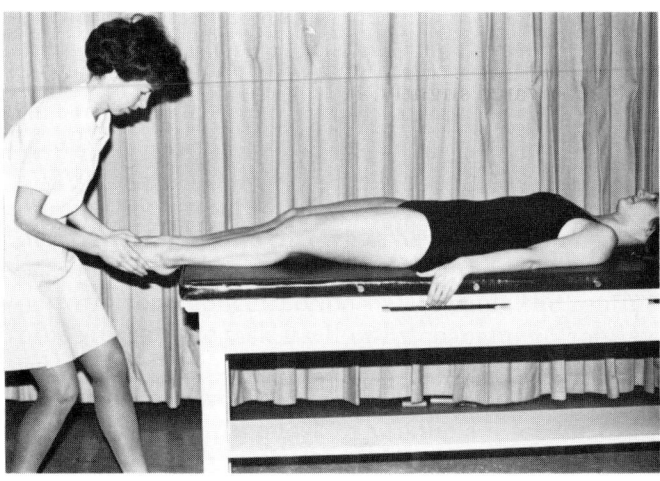

A

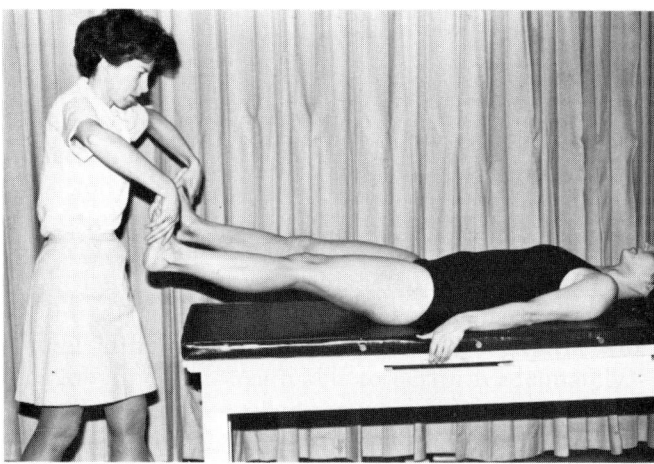

B

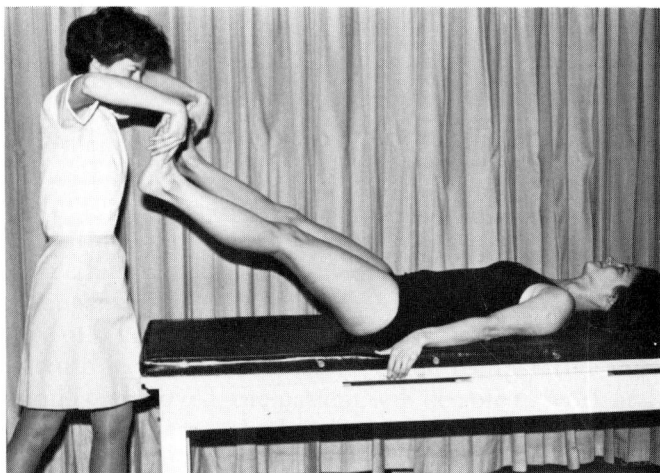

C

FIG. 1-112

Components of Motion

Free. In supine posture, head and shoulders may be elevated slightly. Head maintains midline position. Hands grip table edges for stability and reinforcement. Alternative posture: prone with hips flexed over end of table.

Resisted. Feet and ankles dorsiflex and evert, and initiate hip flexion, abduction, and internal rotation, bilaterally.

A. Lengthened Range

Commands. Preparatory. "You are to pull your feet up and out, turn your heels out, and lift your limbs up and out. Keep your knees straight." (D2 fl bilaterally.) *Action.* "Pull your toes and feet up towards your hands! Pull your limbs up and out!"

Suggested Techniques. Traction, stretch, and resistance.

B. Middle Range

Commands. "Hold! Now hold the right still! And lift the left up and out! Lift again! And hold! Now hold the left still! And lift the right! And again! Again! And rest."

Suggested Techniques. Repeated contractions on the left, as the right holds. Emphasize left limb, then hold the left still, and emphasize the right.

C. Shortened Range

Commands. "Now hold! Hold both feet still! And hold! And hold! And relax."

Suggested Techniques. Rhythmic stabilization, repeated contractions for emphasis, slow reversal, slow reversal – hold.

Antagonistic Pattern

BS, extension – adduction – external rotation (D2 ex), left and right (Fig. 1-113).

Related Unilateral Patterns

Lower extremity D2 fl with straight knee (Fig. 1-70).

Lower trunk flexion with rotation to the left (Fig. 1-38): D2 fl with knees straight, to left. Limbs in contact. Repeat right side.

Related Total Patterns (Mat Activities)

Rising to plantigrade, bilateral symmetrical posture (Fig. 1-175, *C*).

Inferior region balance, patient on crutches (Fig. 1-192).

Emphasis on Hip with Knee Straight: Symmetrical (BS)

EXTENSION – ADDUCTION – EXTERNAL ROTATION
(D2 ex), LEFT AND RIGHT

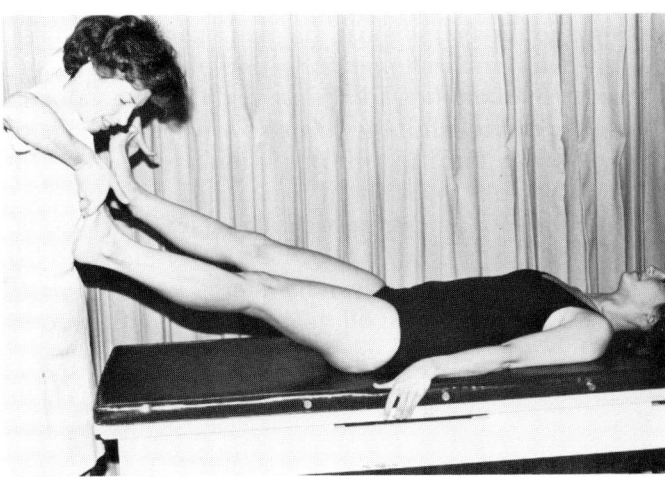

A

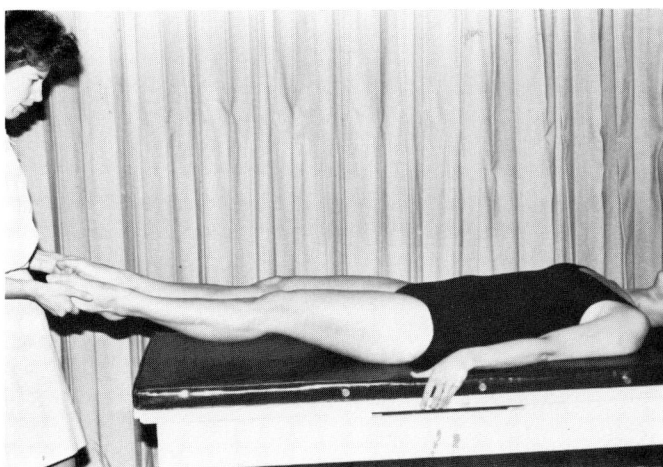

B

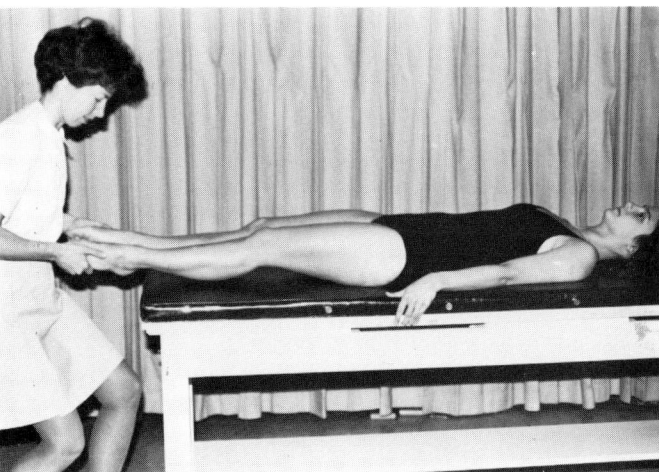

C

FIG. 1-113

Components of Motion

Free. In supine posture, head and shoulders may be elevated slightly. Head maintains midline position. Hands grip table edges for stability and reinforcement. Alternative posture: prone with hips flexed over end of table.

Resisted. Feet and ankles plantar flex and invert, and initiate hip extension, adduction, and external rotation, bilaterally.

A. Lengthened Range

Commands. Preparatory. "You are to push your feet down and in, turn your heels in, and push your limbs down and in. Keep your knees straight." (D2 ex bilaterally.) *Action.* "Toes and feet down and in! Push down and in!"

Suggested Techniques. Approximation, stretch, resistance.

B. Middle Range

Commands. "Hold! Now hold with the right! And push down and in with the left! Again! And push! And hold the left still! Now push down and in with the right! And again! Push! And rest."

Suggested Techniques. Repeated contractions on the left, as right holds. Emphasize left, then hold with left, and emphasize right.

C. Shortened Range

Commands. "Now hold both feet still! Hold! And hold! And relax."

Suggested Techniques. Rhythmic stabilization, repeated contractions for emphasis, slow reversal, slow reversal – hold.

Antagonistic Pattern

Flexion – abduction – internal rotation (D2 fl), left and right (Fig. 1-112).

Related Unilateral Patterns

Lower extremity D2 ex with straight knee (Fig. 1-73).

Lower trunk extension with rotation to the left (Fig. 1-41): D2 extension left, with knees straight. Limbs in contact. Repeat right side.

Related Total Pattern (Mat Activities)

Inferior region balance, patient on crutches (Fig. 1-192, B).

Lower Extremity

Emphasis on Hip with Knee Straight:
Asymmetrical (BA)

FLEXION TO RIGHT: FLEXION – ABDUCTION –
INTERNAL ROTATION (D2 fl), RIGHT, AND FLEXION –
ADDUCTION – EXTERNAL ROTATION (D1 fl), LEFT

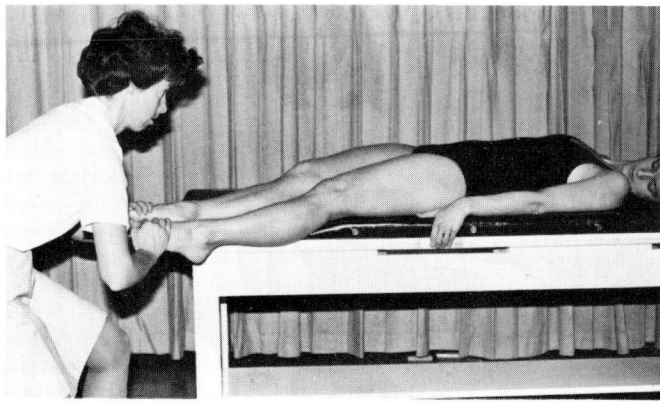

A

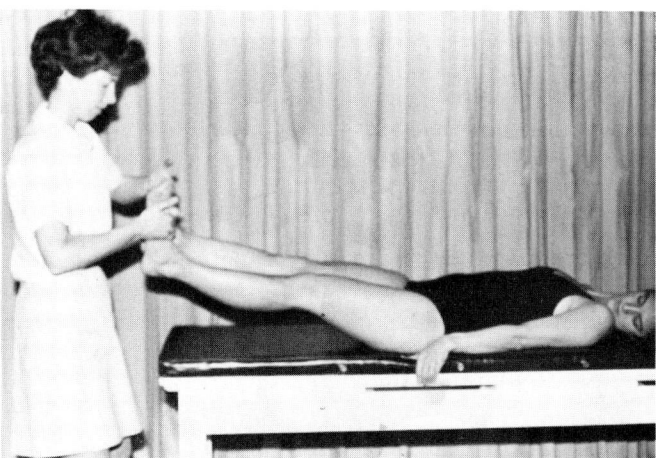

B

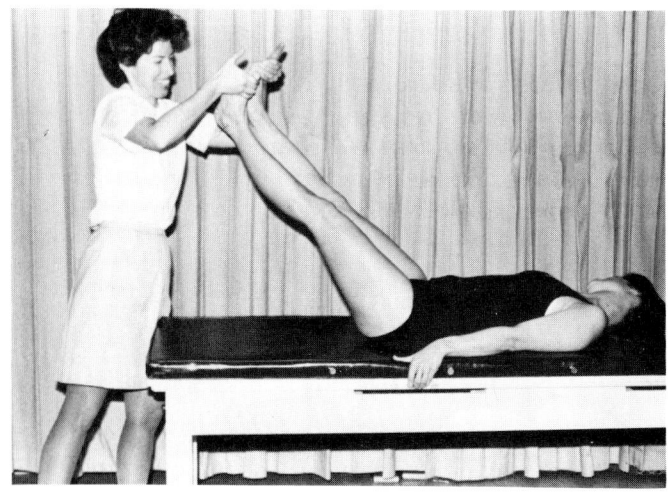

C

FIG. 1-114

Components of Motion

Free. In supine position, the patient's head and shoulders may be elevated slightly. Head rotates to left, then to right. Hands grip the table edges for stability and to reinforce the motion. Alternate posture: prone with hips flexed over end of table.

Resisted. Right foot and ankle dorsiflex and evert as the left foot and ankle dorsiflex and invert, to initiate BA flexion (D2 and D1) up and out to the right.

A. Lengthened Range

Commands. Preparatory. "You are to lift your feet up and out toward your right side, turn your heels out to the right, keep your knees straight, and lift both limbs up the right side." *Action.* "Lift your feet up and out to the right! Toes up! Pull up and over."

Suggested Techniques. Stretch, traction, resistance.

B. Middle Range

Commands. "Hold! Keep your knees straight! Lift up and out! Lift! And lift! And rest."

Suggested Techniques. Repeated contractions.

C. Shortened Range

Commands. "Now hold! Look at your feet! Hold them still! Hold! Hold! And rest."

Suggested Techniques. Rhythmic stabilization, repeated contractions for emphasis.

Antagonistic Pattern

BA extension to left: D2 ex, right; D1 ex, left (Fig. 1-115).

Related Unilateral Patterns

Lower extremity D2 fl, right (Fig. 1-70); D1 fl, left (Fig. 1-64). Knees kept straight.

Lower trunk flexion with rotation to right (Fig. 1-38): D2 fl with knees straight, right. Extremities in contact.

NOTE: Consider patient's abilities and needs before choosing this difficult-to-perform pattern.

Emphasis on Hip with Knee Straight: Asymmetrical (BA)

EXTENSION TO LEFT: EXTENSION – ABDUCTION –
INTERNAL ROTATION (D1 ex), LEFT; EXTENSION –
ADDUCTION – EXTERNAL ROTATION (D2 ex), RIGHT

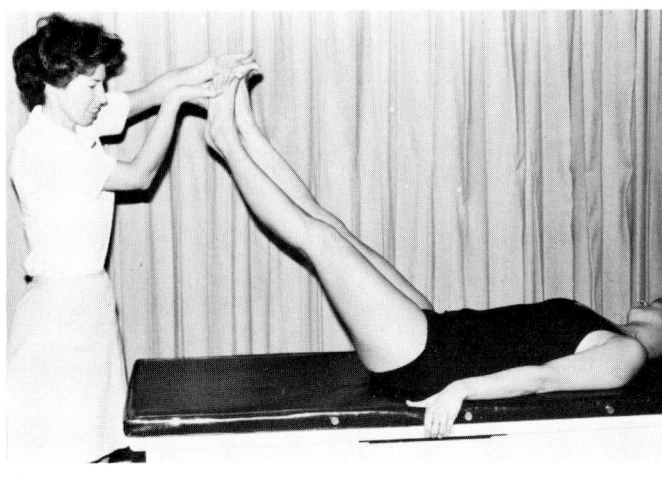

A

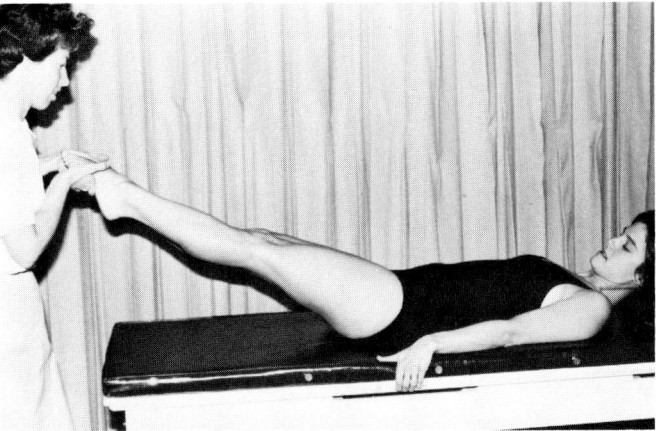

B

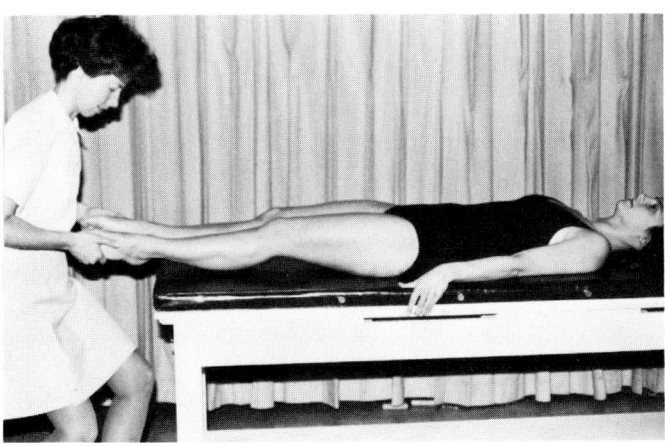

C

FIG. 1-115

Components of Motion

Free. In supine position, the head and shoulders may be elevated slightly. Eyes engage feet, head and neck flex, then assume position in midline. Hands grip the table edges for stability and reinforcement. Alternative posture: prone with hips flexed over end of table.

Resisted. Feet and ankles plantar flex with eversion of left, and inversion of right, to initiate extension of limbs downward to the left.

A. Lengthened Range

Commands. *Preparatory.* "You are to turn your heels to the left, and push your feet down and out to the table edge." (D1 ex, left, D2 ex, right). *Action.* "Push your feet down to the left! Keep your knees straight! All the way! Down and out to the left!"

Suggested Techniques. Approximation, stretch, and resistance.

B. Middle Range

Commands. "Hold! Keep your knees straight! Now push! Push again! And rest."

Suggested Techniques. Maximally resist "hold," repeated contractions for emphasis.

C. Shortened Range

Commands. "Now hold! Look at your feet! Hold everything still! Hold! Hold again! And rest."

Suggested Techniques. Rhythmic stabilization, repeated contractions for emphasis.

Antagonistic Pattern

BA flexion to right: D1 fl, left; D2 fl, right (Fig. 1-114).

Related Unilateral Patterns

Lower extremity D1 ex, left (Fig. 1-67), and D2 ex, right (Fig. 1-73), knees straight.

Lower trunk extension to the left (Fig. 1-41): bilateral extension (D1, left and D2, right) to the left. Extremities in contact.

Lower Extremity

Emphasis on Hip with Knee Straight: Reciprocal (BR, SD)

FLEXION – ADDUCTION – EXTERNAL ROTATION (D1 fl), LEFT; EXTENSION – ABDUCTION – INTERNAL ROTATION (D1 ex), RIGHT

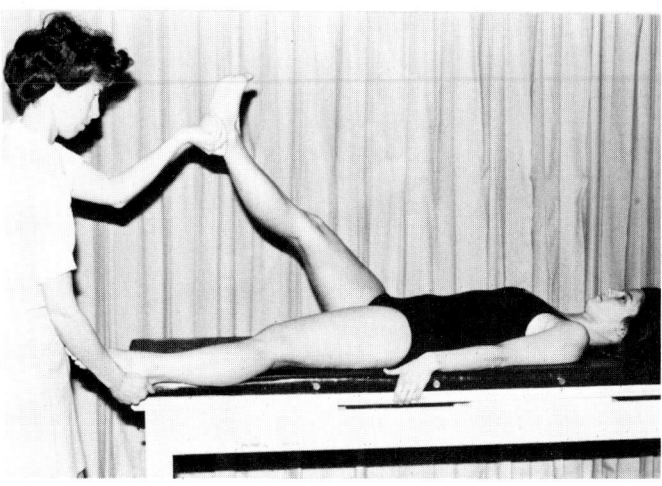

A

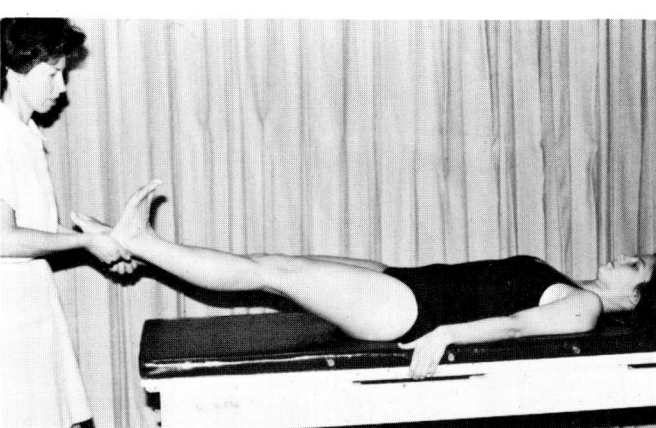

B

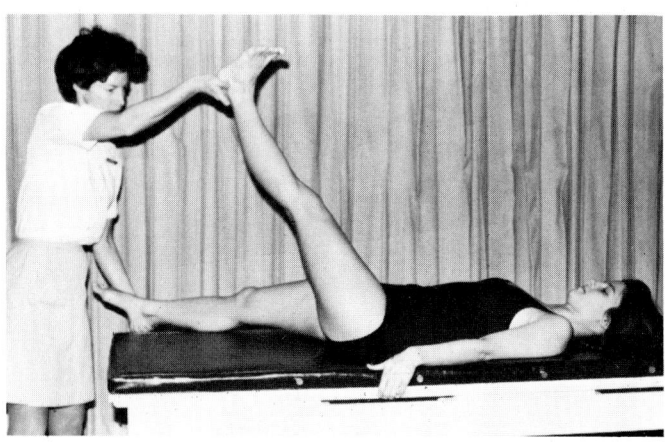

C

FIG. 1-116

Components of Motion

Free. In supine posture, head and shoulders may be elevated slightly. Eyes regard foot of flexing limb. Hands grip table edges for stability and reinforcement. (Manual contacts are on heels for good control. Toes and foot initiate limb action by active motion.) Alternative posture: prone with hips flexed over end of table.

Resisted. Left foot and ankle dorsiflex and invert and initiate hip flexion, adduction, and external rotation, as the right foot and ankle plantar flexes and everts, and initiates hip extension, abduction, and internal rotation.

A. Lengthened Range

Commands. Preparatory. "You are to pull your left foot up and in, and lift your limb up and in, and push your right foot and limb down and out." *Action.* "Pull in and up with your left limb! Push down and out with the right! Hold everything! Now hold with the right and pull up with the left! Pull again! Pull! And relax."

Suggested Techniques. Stretch on the right, traction and stretch on the left; resistance.

B. Middle Range

Commands. "Hold everything! Now pull your left limb towards your right shoulder! Pull! Pull again! And rest!"

Suggested Techniques. Maximal resistance for "hold" on the right; repeated contractions on the left for emphasis. Slow reversal – hold, then repeated contractions at various points in the range, *A* to *C*.

C. Shortened Range

Commands. "Hold everything! Now hold! And hold! And hold! Now push down and out with your right! Push again! Once more! And relax."

Suggested Techniques. Rhythmic stabilization; repeated contractions on right for emphasis. Slow reversal – hold to middle range, then to shortened range followed by repeated contractions.

Antagonistic Pattern

(BR, SD): D1 ex, left; D1 fl, right (Fig. 1-117).

Related Unilateral Patterns

Lower extremity D1 fl with knee flexion (Fig. 1-65); D1 ex with knee extension, antagonistic pattern (Fig. 1-68).

Lower trunk flexion and extension: D1 fl with knee flexion, left (Fig. 1-39); D1 ex with knee extension, right (Fig. 1-41). Limbs in contact.

Lower Extremity

Emphasis on Hip with Knee Straight: Reciprocal (BR, SD)

EXTENSION – ABDUCTION – INTERNAL ROTATION (D1 ex), LEFT; FLEXION – ADDUCTION – EXTERNAL ROTATION (D1 fl), RIGHT

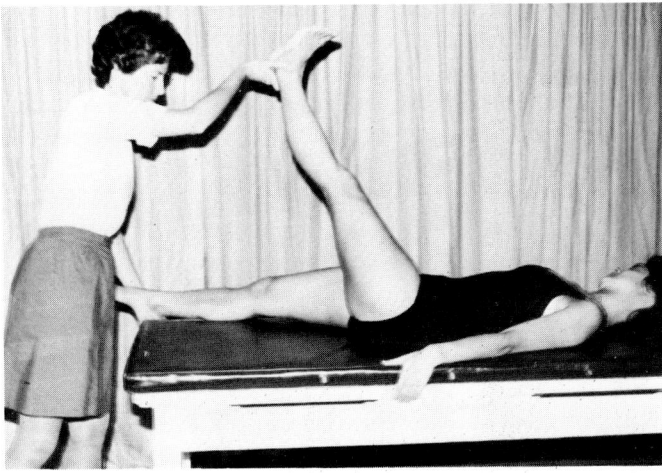

A

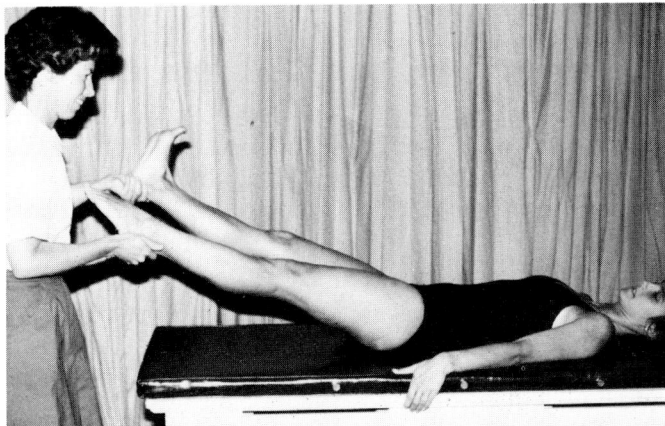

B

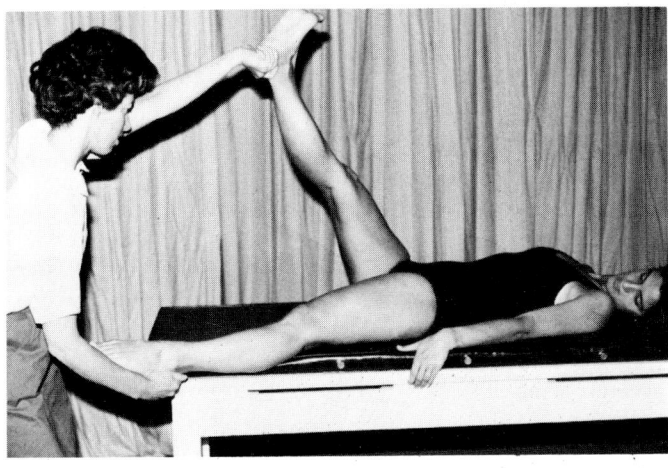

C

FIG. 1-117

Components of Motion

Free. In supine posture, head and shoulders may be elevated slightly. Head rotates as eyes regard foot of extending limb. Hands grip table edges for stability and reinforcement. (Manual contacts are on heels for good control. Toe and foot initiate limb action by active motion.) Alternative posture: prone with hips flexed over end of table.

Resisted. Left foot and ankle plantar flex and evert, and initiate hip extension, abduction, and internal rotation, as the right foot dorsiflexes and inverts, and initiates hip flexion, adduction, and external rotation.

A. Lengthened Range

Commands. *Preparatory.* "You are to push your left foot down and out, and push your limb down and out, and lift your right foot up and in, and pull the limb up and in. Keep your knees straight." *Action.* "Push your left foot and limb down and out! Pull in and up with the right! Hold everything! Now hold the left, and pull up with the right! Pull in and up! Pull! And relax."

Suggested Techniques. Stretch on the left, traction and stretch on the right; resistance and repeated contractions.

B. Middle Range

Commands. "Hold everything! Keep your knees straight! Now pull the right limb up and in! Pull again! Pull! And rest."

Suggested Techniques. Maximal resistance for the "hold" on left, repeated contractions on right for emphasis. Slow reversal – hold, then repeated contractions at various points in the range, *A* to *C*.

C. Shortened Range

Commands. "Hold everything! Hold! And hold! And hold! Now push down and out with your left! And push! Again! And again! And relax."

Suggested Techniques. Rhythmic stabilization, repeated contractions on left for emphasis. Slow reversal – hold to middle range, then to shortened range, followed by repeated contractions on left.

Antagonistic Pattern

(BR, SD): D1fl, left; D1 ex, right (Fig. 1-116).

Related Unilateral Patterns

Lower extremities D1 fl with straight knee (Fig. 1-64); D1 ex with straight knee, antagonistic pattern (Fig. 1-67).

Lower trunk flexion and extension: D1 ex with straight knee, left (Fig. 1-41); D1 fl with straight knee, right (Fig. 1-38). Extremities in contact.

Lower Extremity

Emphasis on Hip with Knee Straight: Reciprocal (BR, SD)

FLEXION – ABDUCTION – INTERNAL ROTATION (D2 fl), LEFT; EXTENSION – ADDUCTION – EXTERNAL ROTATION (D2 ex), RIGHT

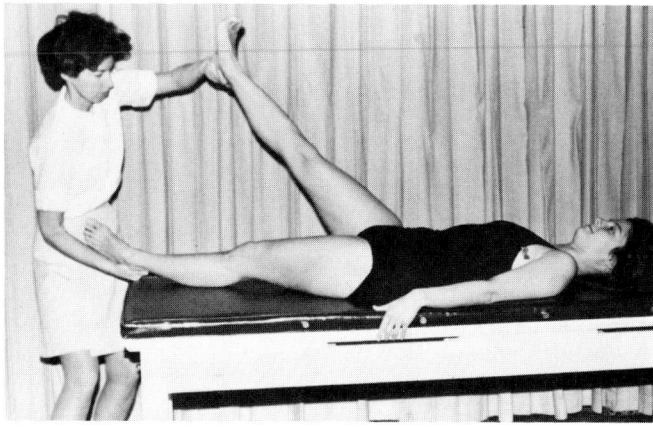

A

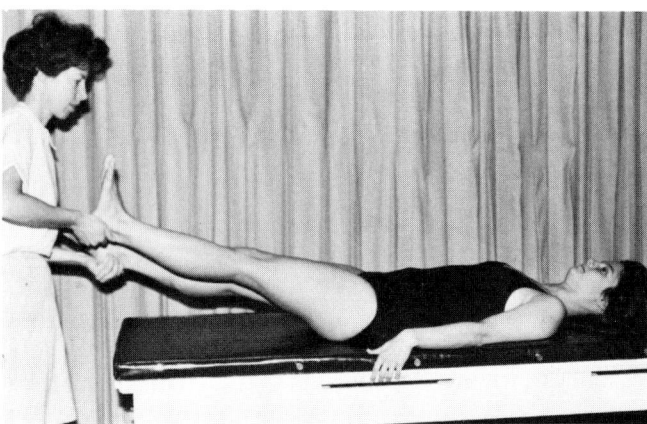

B

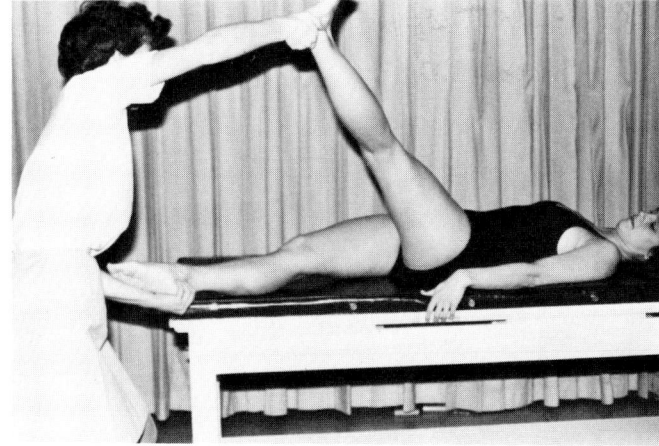

C

FIG. 1-118

Components of Motion

Free. In supine posture, head and shoulders may be elevated slightly. Head rotates as eyes regard foot of flexed limb. Hands grip table edges for stability and reinforcement. (Manual contacts are on heels for good control. Toes and foot move actively to initiate limb action.) Alternative posture: prone with hips flexed over end of table.

Resisted. Left foot and ankle dorsiflex and evert, and initiate hip flexion, abduction, and internal rotation, as right foot and ankle plantar flex and invert, and initiate hip extension, adduction, and external rotation.

A. Lengthened Range

Commands. Preparatory. "You are to lift your left foot up and out, and pull your limb up and out (D2 fl), and push your right foot down and in and push the limb down and in (D2 ex). Keep your knees straight." *Action.* "Lift up and out with your left limb! Pull down and in with the right! Hold everything! Now hold with the right and pull up with the left! Pull! And again! And relax."

Suggested Techniques. Stretch on the right, traction and stretch on the left; resistance and repeated contractions.

B. Middle Range

Commands. "Hold everything! Now pull your left limb up and out! Pull again! Pull! And rest."

Suggested Techniques. Maximal resistance for "hold" on the right, repeated contractions on the left for emphasis. Slow reversal–hold, then repeated contractions at various points in the range, *A* to *C*.

C. Shortened Range

Commands. "Hold everything! Hold! And hold, and hold! Pull up and out with your left! And pull! Pull! And again! And relax."

Suggested Techniques. Rhythmic stabilization, repeated contractions on left for emphasis. Slow reversal–hold to middle range, then to shortened range, followed by repeated contractions on left.

Antagonistic Pattern

(BR, SD): D2 ex, left; D2 fl, right (Fig. 1-119).

Related Patterns

Lower extremity D2 fl with straight knee (Fig. 1-70); D2 ex with straight knee, antagonistic pattern (Fig. 1-73).

Lower trunk flexion and extension: D2 fl with straight knee, left (Fig. 1-38); D2 ex with straight knee, left (Fig. 1-41). Extremities in contact.

Lower Extremity

Emphasis on Hip with Knee Straight: Reciprocal (BR, SD)

EXTENSION – ADDUCTION – EXTERNAL ROTATION (D2 ex), LEFT; FLEXION – ABDUCTION – INTERNAL ROTATION (D2 fl), RIGHT

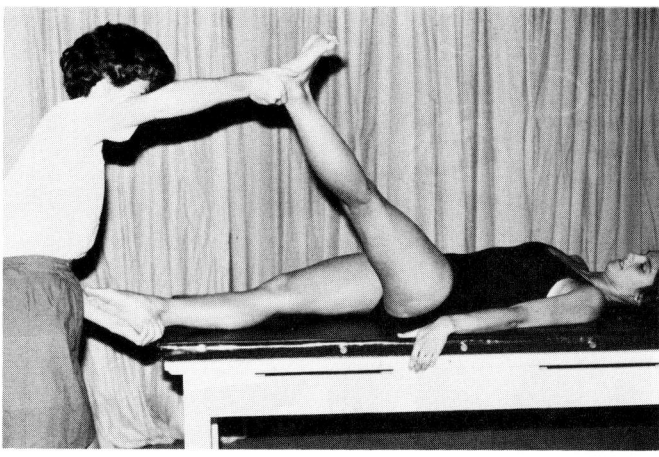

A

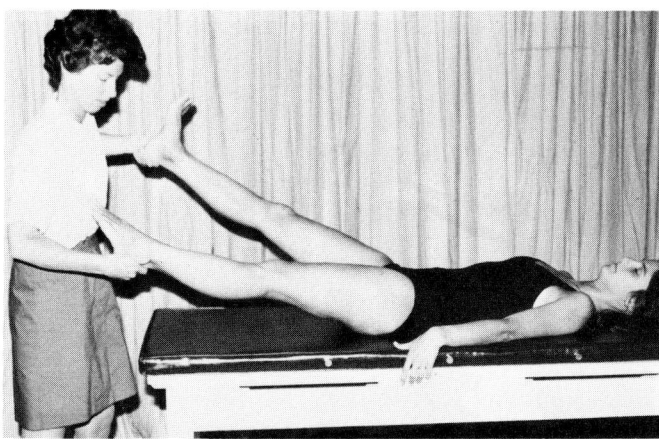

B

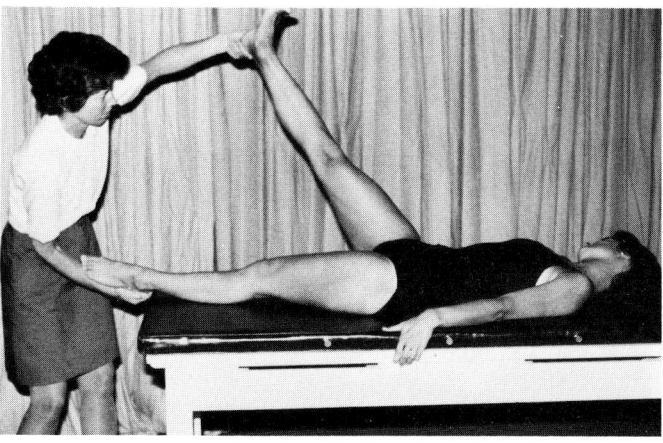

C

FIG. 1-119

Components of Motion

Free. In supine posture, head and shoulders may be elevated slightly. Head rotates as eyes regard foot of flexed limb. Hands grip table edges for stability and reinforcement. (Manual contacts are on heels for good control. Toes and foot initiate limb action by active motion.) Alternative posture: prone with hips flexed over end of table.

Resisted. Left foot and ankle plantar flex and invert, and initiate hip extension, adduction, and external rotation, as the right foot and ankle dorsiflex and evert, and initiate hip flexion abduction, and internal rotation.

A. Lengthened Range

Commands. *Preparatory.* "You are to push your left foot down and in, and push your limb down and in (D2 ex), and pull your right foot up and out, and pull the limb up and out (D2 fl). Keep the knees straight." *Action.* "Push down and in with your left! Pull up and out with your right! Hold everything! Now hold with the left and pull up and out with the right! Pull! Again! And relax."

Suggested Techniques. Stretch on the left, stretch and traction on the right; resistance and repeated contractions.

B. Middle Range

Commands. "Hold everything! Now pull up and out with the right! Pull again! Pull! And rest."

Suggested Techniques. Maximal resistance for hold on left; repeated contractions on right for emphasis. Slow reversal – hold, then repeated contractions at various points in the range, *A* to *C*.

C. Shortened Range

Commands. "Hold everything! Now hold! And hold! And hold! Now pull up and out with your right! And pull! Again! And again! And relax."

Suggested Techniques. Rhythmic stabilization; repeated contractions on right for emphasis. Slow reversal – hold to middle range, then to shortened range, followed by repeated contractions on right.

Antagonistic Pattern

(BR, SD); D2 fl, left; D2 ex, right (Fig. 1-118).

Related Unilateral Patterns

Lower extremity D2 fl with straight knee (Fig. 1-70); D2 ex with straight knee, antagonistic pattern (Fig. 1-73).

Lower trunk flexion and extension: D2 fl with straight knee, right (Fig. 1-38); D2 ex with straight knee, right (Fig. 1-41). Extremities in contact.

Lower Extremity

Emphasis on Hip with Knee Straight: Reciprocal (BR, CD)

FLEXION – ABDUCTION – INTERNAL ROTATION (D2 fl), RIGHT; EXTENSION – ABDUCTION – INTERNAL ROTATION (D1 ex), LEFT

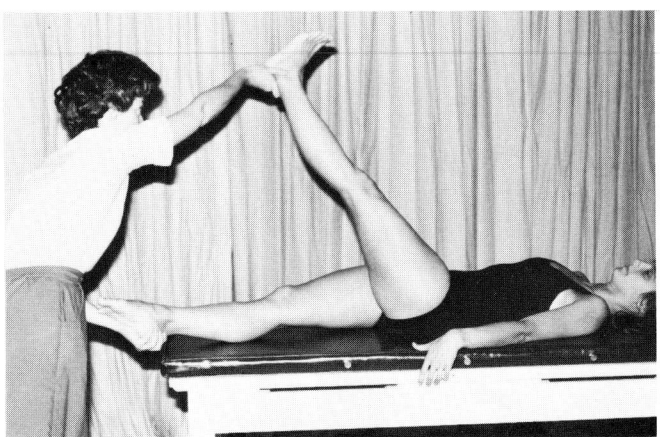

A

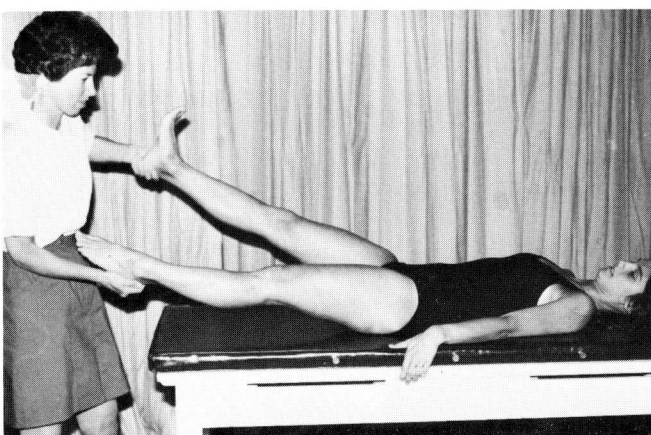

B

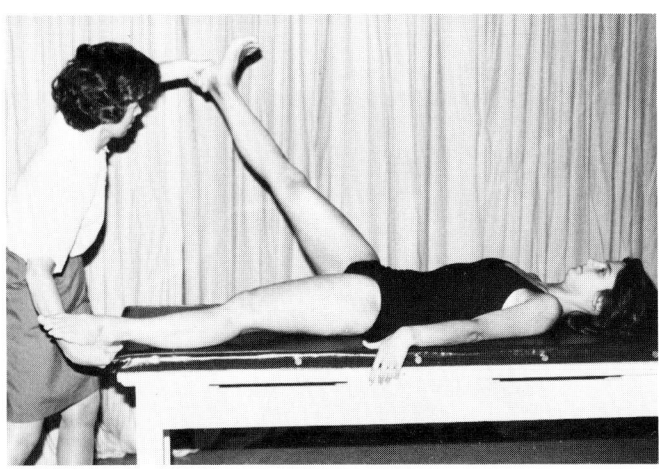

C

FIG. 1-120

Components of Motion

Free. In supine posture, head and shoulders may be elevated slightly. Head maintains midline position. Hands grip table edges for stability and reinforcement. (Manual contacts on heels for control of action. Toes and foot initiate limb action by active motion.) Alternative posture: prone with hips flexed over end of table.

Resisted. Right foot and ankle move up and out to right, and initiate hip flexion, abduction, and internal rotation. At the same time, the left foot and ankle push down and out, and initiate hip extension, abduction, and internal rotation.

A. Lengthened Range

Commands. Preparatory. "You are to lift your right foot up and out, turn your heel outward, and lift the limb up and out; and, at the same time, push your left foot down and out, turn your heel outward, and push down and out. Keep the knees straight." *Action.* "Lift your right foot up and out! And pull up and out! And push your left foot down and out! Push down and out! Move!"

Suggested Techniques. Stretch and traction, right, stretch left limb; resistance.

B. Middle Range

Commands. "And hold! Keep your right limb still! Push the left down and out! Push! Push again! And rest."

Suggested Techniques. Repeated contractions for emphasis.

C. Shortened Range

Commands. "And hold! Hold both limbs still! And rest."

Suggested Techniques. Rhythmic stabilization; repeated contractions for emphasis.

Antagonistic Pattern

(BR, CD): D2 ex, right; D1 fl, left.

Related Unilateral Patterns

Lower extremity D2 fl with straight knee, right (Fig. 1-70). D1 ex with straight knee, left (Fig. 1-67).

Lower trunk flexion and extension with rotation: D2 fl with straight knees, right (Fig. 1-38); D1 ex with straight knees, left (Fig. 1-41). Extremities in contact.

Related Total Pattern (Mat Activities)

Plantigrade walking forward to right, D2 fl, right; D1 fl, left (Fig. 1-176).

Lower Extremity

Emphasis on Hip and Knee: Reciprocal (BR, SD)

FLEXION – ADDUCTION – EXTERNAL ROTATION (D1 fl), WITH KNEE FLEXION, RIGHT; EXTENSION – ABDUCTION – INTERNAL ROTATION (D1 ex), WITH KNEE EXTENSION, LEFT

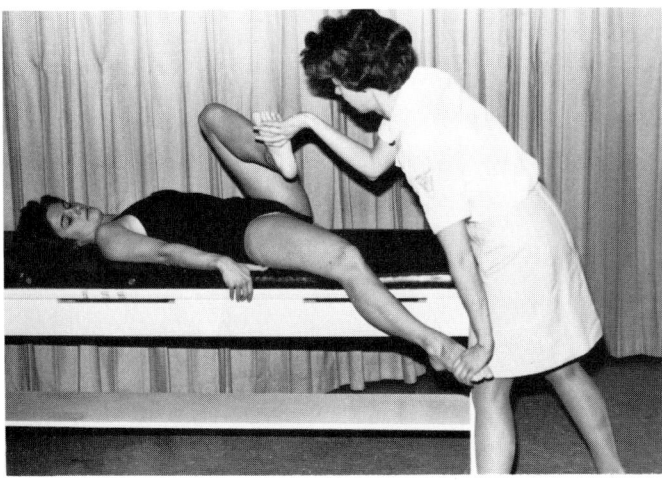

A

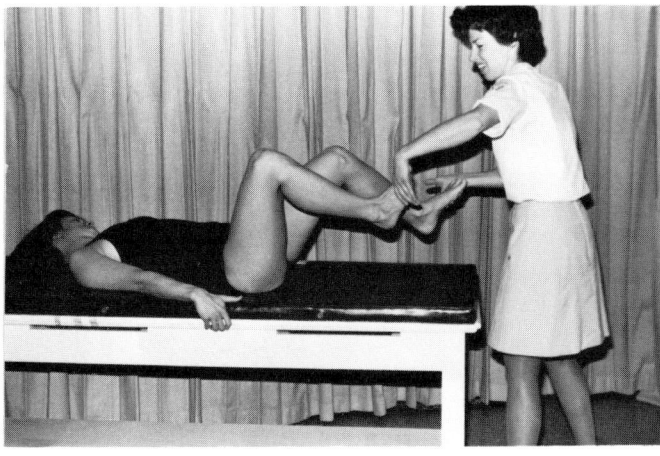

B

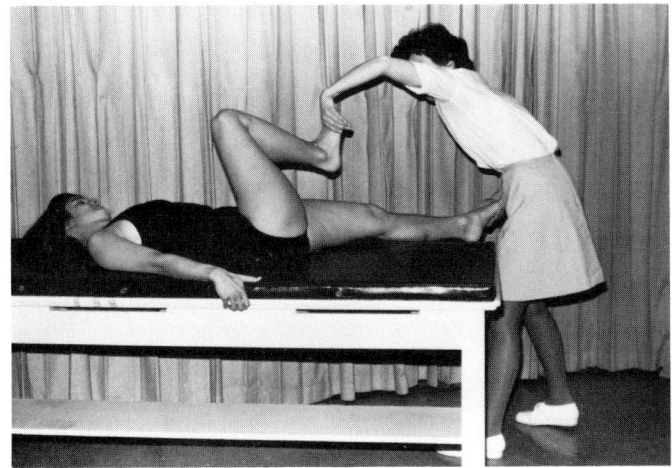

C

FIG. 1-121

Components of Motion

Free. In supine posture, head and shoulders may be elevated slightly. Eyes follow left foot, then right. Hands grip table edges for stability and reinforcement. Alternative posture: prone with hips flexed over end of table.

Resisted. Right foot and ankle dorsiflex and invert, and initiate hip flexion, adduction, and external rotation, as the left foot and ankle plantar flex and evert, and initiate hip extension, abduction, and internal rotation, and knee extension.

A. Lengthened Range

Commands. Preparatory. "You are to pull your right foot up and in, and bend your hip and knee (D1 fl), and push your left foot down and out, and straighten your hip and knee (D1 ex)." *Action.* "Pull in and up with your right! Push down and out with your left! Hold everything! Now hold with the left and pull up with the right! Again! And again, and relax."

Suggested Techniques. Stretch on the right, traction and stretch on the left; resistance and repeated contractions.

B. Middle Range

Commands. "Hold everything! Now pull with the right! Pull your knee toward your left shoulder! Pull again! Pull! And rest!"

Suggested Techniques. Maximal resistance for "hold" on the left; repeated contractions on the right for emphasis. Slow reversal – hold, then repeated contractions at various points in the range, *A* to *C*.

C. Shortened Range

Commands. "Hold everything! Now hold, and hold, and hold! Pull up and in with your right! And pull! Again, and again, and relax."

Suggested Techniques. Rhythmic stabilization; repeated contractions on right for emphasis. Slow reversal – hold to middle range, then to shortened range, followed by repeated contractions on right.

Antagonistic Pattern

(BR, SD): D1 fl with knee flexion, left; D1 ex with knee extension, right (Fig. 1-122).

Related Unilateral Patterns

Lower extremity D1 fl with knee flexion, right (Fig. 1-65). D1 ex with knee extension, antagonistic pattern (Fig. 1-68).

Lower trunk flexion and extension: D1 fl with knee flexion, right (Fig. 1-39); D1 ex with knee extension, right (Fig. 1-42). Extremities in contact.

Related Total Patterns (Mat Activities)

Rolling toward prone, D1 fl with hip and knee flexion (Fig. 1-155).

Rolling toward prone, D1 ex with hip and knee extension (Fig. 1-156).

Lower Extremity

Emphasis on Hip and Knee: Reciprocal (BR, SD)

FLEXION – ADDUCTION – EXTERNAL ROTATION (D1 fl), WITH KNEE FLEXION, LEFT; EXTENSION – ABDUCTION – INTERNAL ROTATION (D1 ex), WITH KNEE EXTENSION, RIGHT

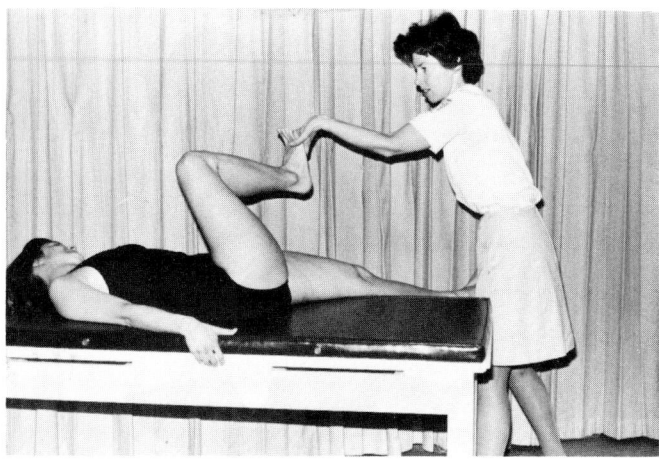

A

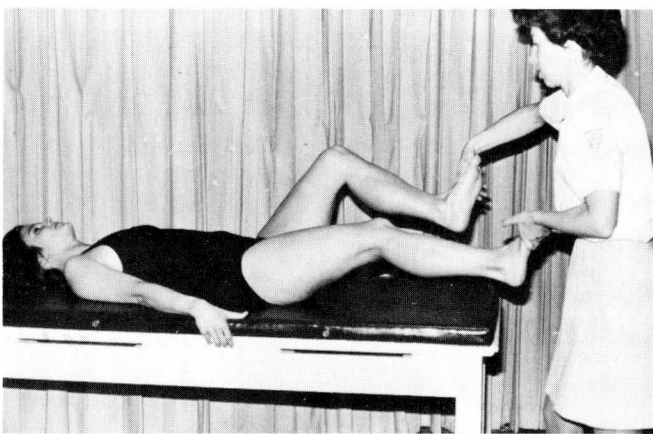

B

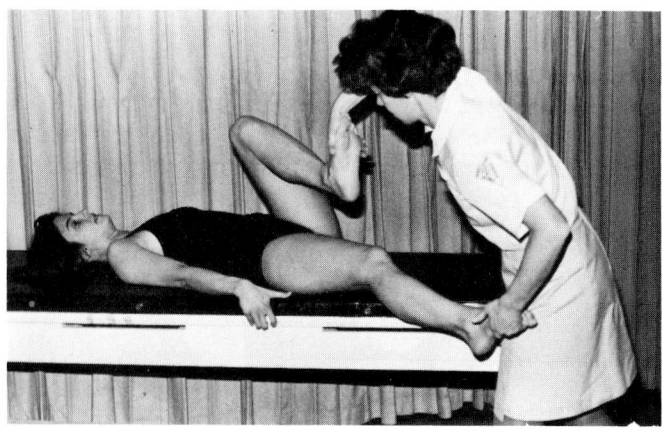

C

FIG. 1-122

Components of Motion

Free. In supine posture, head and shoulders may be elevated slightly. Eyes engage right foot, then disregard movements. Hands grip table edges for stability and reinforcement. Alternative posture: prone with hips flexed over end of table.

Resisted. Left foot and ankle dorsiflex and invert, and initiate hip flexion, adduction, external rotation, and knee flexion as the right foot and ankle plantar flex and evert, and initiate hip extension, abduction, internal rotation, and knee extension.

A. Lengthened Range

Commands. *Preparatory.* "You are to pull your left foot up and in, and bend your hip and knee (D1 fl), and push your right foot down and out, and straighten your hip and knee (D1 ex)." *Action.* "Pull in and up with the left! Push down and out with your right! Hold everything! Now hold with the right and pull up and in with the left! Pull! Again! And relax."

Suggested Techniques. Stretch on the right, traction and stretch on the left; resistance and repeated contractions.

B. Middle Range

Commands. "Hold everything! Now pull with the left! Pull your knee toward your right shoulder! Pull again! And again, and rest."

Suggested Techniques. Maximal resistance for hold on the right, repeated contractions on the left for emphasis. Slow reversal – hold, then repeated contractions at various points in the range, *A* to *C*.

C. Shortened Range

Commands. "Hold everything! Now hold! And hold! And hold! Push down and out with your left! And push! Again, and again, and relax." (See Fig. 1-121.)

Suggested Techniques. Rhythmic stabilization, repeated contractions on left for emphasis. Slow reversal – hold to middle range, then to shortened range, followed by repeated contractions on right.

Antagonistic Pattern

(BR, SD): D1 fl with knee flexion, right; D1 ex with knee extension, left (Fig. 1-121).

Related Unilateral Patterns

Lower extremity D1 fl with knee flexion (Fig. 1-65); D1 ex with knee extension, antagonistic pattern (Fig. 1-68).

Lower trunk flexion and extension: D1 fl with knee flexion, left (Fig. 1-39); D1 ex with knee extension, right (Fig. 1-42): extremities in contact.

Related Total Patterns (Mat Activities)

Rolling toward prone, D1 fl with hip and knee flexion (Fig. 1-155); and D1 ex with hip and knee extension (Fig. 1-156).

Lower Extremity

Emphasis on Hip and Knee: Reciprocal (BR, SD)

FLEXION – ABDUCTION – INTERNAL ROTATION (D2 fl), WITH KNEE FLEXION, RIGHT; EXTENSION – ADDUCTION – EXTERNAL ROTATION (D2 ex), WITH KNEE EXTENSION, LEFT

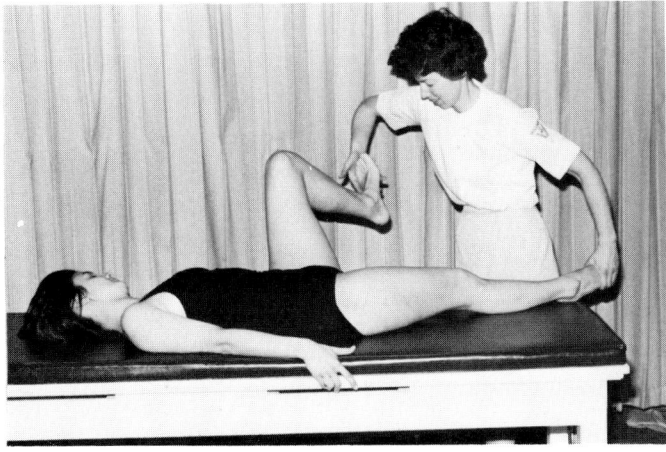

A

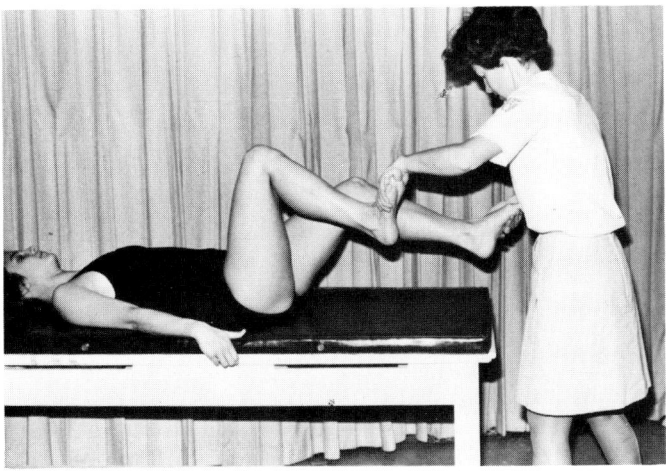

B

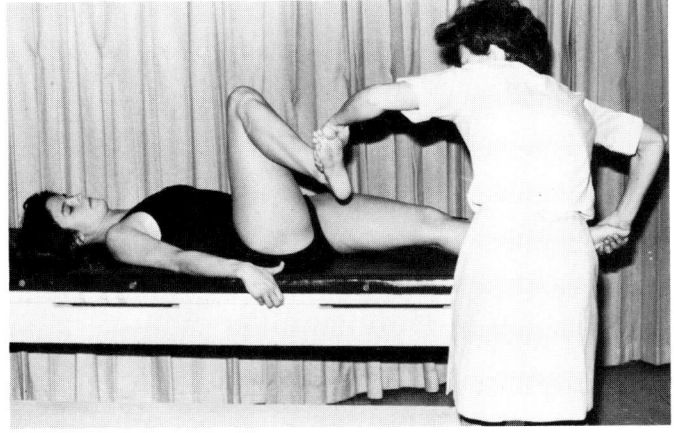

C

FIG. 1-123

Components of Motion

Free. In supine posture, head and shoulders may be elevated slightly. Eyes engage left foot, then head assumes midline position. Hands grip table edges for stability and reinforcement. Alternative posture: prone with hips flexed over end of table.

Resisted. Right foot and ankle dorsiflex and evert, and initiate hip flexion, abduction, and internal rotation, and knee flexion, as the left foot and ankle plantar flex and invert, and initiate hip extension, adduction, and external rotation, and knee extension.

A. Lengthened Range

Commands. Preparatory. "You are to pull your right foot up and out, and bend your hip and knee (D2 fl), and push your left foot down and in, and straighten your hip and knee (D2 ex)." *Action.* "Pull up and out with your right! Push down and in with the left! Hold everything! Now hold with the left, and pull up with the right! Pull! And again, and relax."

Suggested Techniques. Stretch on the left, traction and stretch on the right; resistance and repeated contractions.

B. Middle Range

Commands. "Hold everything! Now pull your right knee up and out! Pull again! Pull! And rest."

Suggested Techniques. Maximal resistance for "hold" on left, repeated contractions on right for emphasis. Slow reversal – hold, then repeated contractions at various points in the range, *A* to *C.*

C. Shortened Range

Commands. "Hold everything! Now hold, and hold, and hold! Push down and in with your right! And relax."

Suggested Techniques. Rhythmic stabilization, and repeated contractions on right for emphasis. Slow reversal – hold to middle range, then to shortened range, followed by repeated contractions on right.

Antagonistic Pattern

(BR, SD): D2 fl with knee flexion, left; D2 ex with knee extension, right (Fig. 1-124).

Related Unilateral Patterns

Lower extremity D2 fl with knee flexion (Fig. 1-71); D2 ex with knee extension, antagonistic pattern (Fig. 1-74).

Lower trunk flexion and extension: D2 with knee flexion, left (Fig. 1-39); D2 ex with knee extension, right (Fig. 1-42): extremities in contact.

Related Total Patterns (Mat Activities)

Crawling forward on elbows, D2 with hip and knee flexion (Fig. 1-164).

Lower Extremity

Emphasis on Hip and Knee: Reciprocal (BR, SD)

FLEXION – ABDUCTION – INTERNAL ROTATION
(D2 fl), WITH KNEE FLEXION, LEFT; EXTENSION –
ADDUCTION – EXTERNAL ROTATION (D2 ex), WITH
KNEE EXTENSION, RIGHT

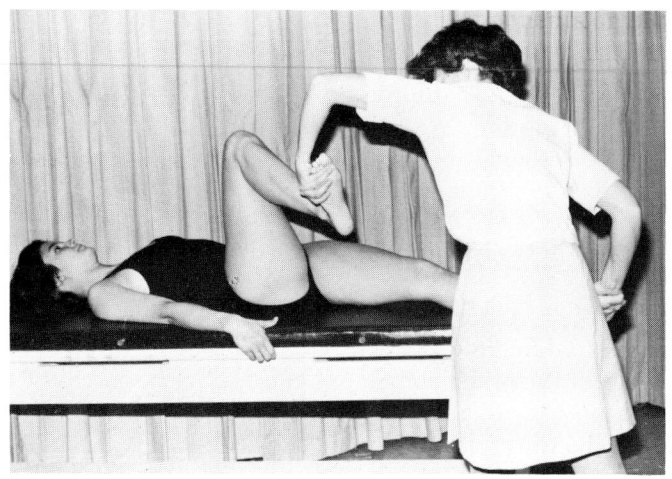

A

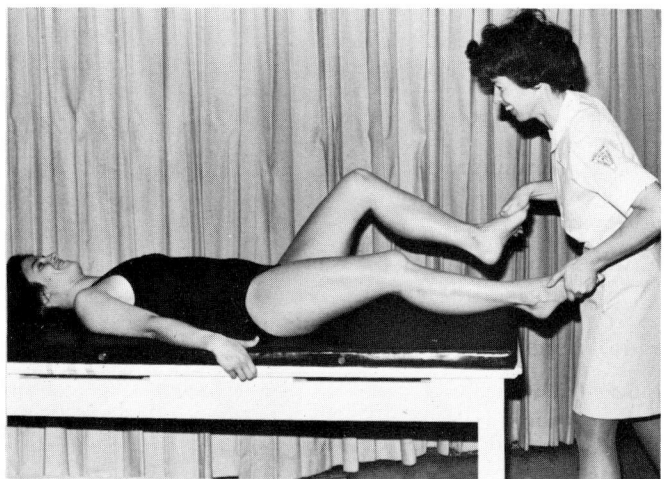

B

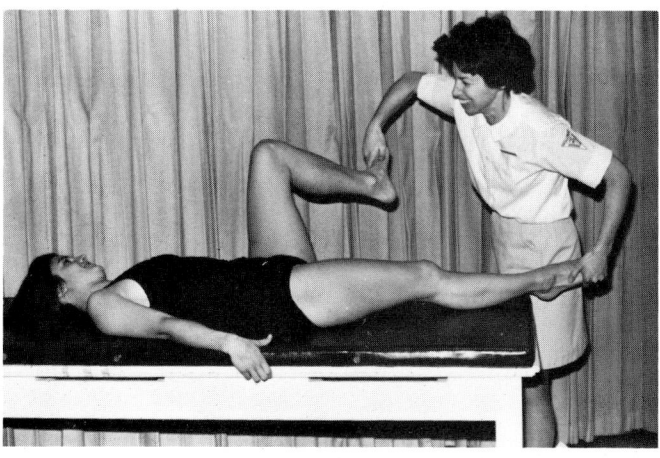

C

FIG. 1-124

Components of Motion

Free. In supine posture, head and shoulders may be elevated slightly. Head maintains midline position. Hands grip table edges for stability and reinforcement. Alternative posture: prone with hips flexed over end of table.

Resisted. Left foot and ankle dorsiflex and evert, and initiate hip flexion, abduction, and internal rotation, and knee flexion, as the right foot and ankle plantar flex and invert, and initiate hip extension, adduction, and external rotation, and knee extension.

A. Lengthened Range

Commands. Preparatory. "You are to pull your left foot up and out, and bend your hip and knee [D2 fl], and push your right down and in, and straighten your hip and knee [D2 ex]." *Action.* "Pull up and out with the left! And push down and in with your right! Hold everything! Now hold with the right and pull up and out with the left! Pull! And pull! And relax."

Suggested Techniques. Stretch on the right, traction and stretch on the left; resistance and repeated contractions.

B. Middle Range

Commands. "Hold everything! Now pull your left knee up and out! Pull again! Pull! And rest."

Suggested Techniques. Maximal resistance for "hold" on the right; repeated contractions on the left for emphasis. Slow reversal – hold, then repeated contractions at various points in the range, *A* to *C*.

C. Shortened Range

Commands. "Hold everything! Now hold! And hold! And hold! And hold! Now push down and in with your left! And push! Push! And relax."

Suggested Techniques. Rhythmic stabilization, and repeated contractions on the left for emphasis. Slow reversal – hold to middle range, then to shortened range, followed by repeated contractions on left.

Antagonistic Pattern

(BR, SD): D2 fl with knee flexion, right; D2 ex with knee extension, left (Fig. 1-123).

Related Unilateral Patterns

Lower extremity D2 fl with knee flexion (Fig. 1-71); D2 ex with knee extension, antagonistic pattern (Fig. 1-74).

Lower trunk flexion and extension: D2 fl with knee flexion (Fig. 1-39); D2 ex with knee extension (Fig. 1-42): limbs in contact.

Related Total Patterns (Mat Activities)

Crawling forward on elbows, hip and knee flexion (D2). (See Fig. 1-164.)

Emphasis on Hip and Knee: Reciprocal (BR, CD)

EXTENSION – ADDUCTION – EXTERNAL ROTATION (D2 ex), WITH KNEE EXTENSION, RIGHT; FLEXION – ADDUCTION – EXTERNAL ROTATION (D1 fl), WITH KNEE FLEXION, LEFT

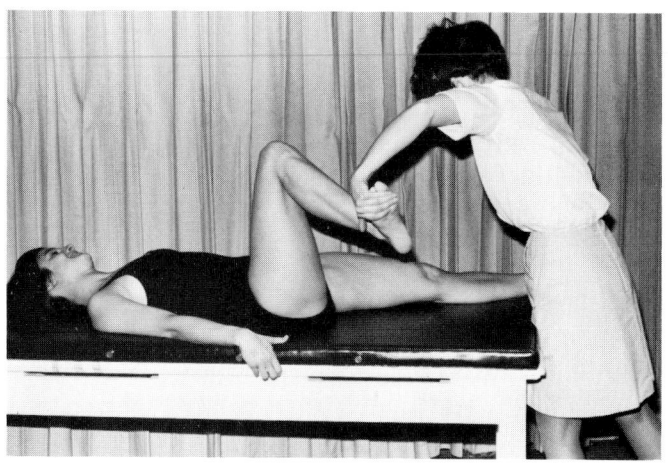

A

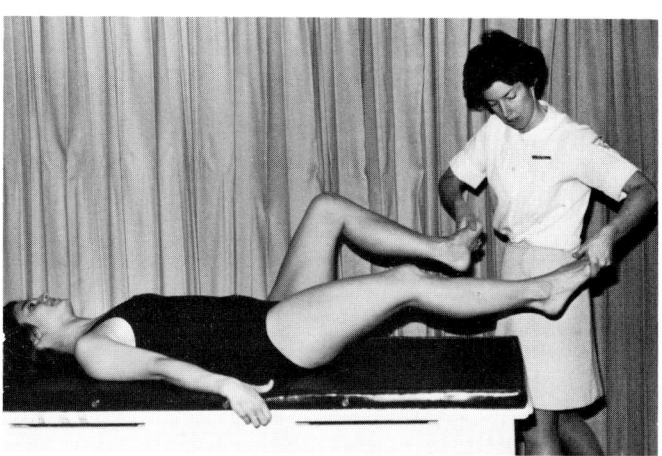

B

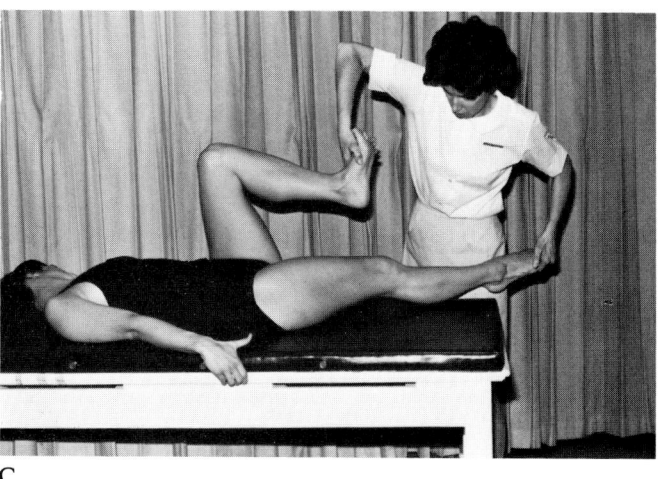

C

FIG. 1-125

Components of Motion

Free. In supine posture, head and shoulders may be elevated slightly. Head is in midline, then rotates to left. Hands grip table edges for stability and reinforcement. Alternative posture: prone with hips flexed over end of table.

Resisted. Right foot and ankle plantar flex and invert, and initiate hip extension, adduction, and external rotation, and knee extension, as the left foot and ankle dorsiflex and invert, and initiate hip flexion, adduction, and external rotation, and knee flexion.

A. Lengthened Range

Commands. *Preparatory.* "You are to push your right foot down and in, and straighten your hip and knee (D2 ex), and pull your left foot up and in, and bend the hip and knee (D1 fl)." *Action.* "Push down and in with your right! And pull in and up with the left! Hold everything! Now hold with the right! And pull up and in with the left! Pull! Pull again! And relax."

Suggested Techniques. Stretch on the right, traction and stretch on the left; resistance and repeated contractions.

B. Middle Range

Commands. "Hold everything! Now pull your left knee toward your right shoulder! Pull again! Pull hard! And rest."

Suggested Techniques. Maximal resistance for "hold" on the right, repeated contractions on left for emphasis. Slow reversal – hold, then repeated contractions at various points in the range, *A* to *C*.

C. Shortened Range

Commands. "Hold everything! Now hold! And hold! Hold! Now pull up and in with your left! And pull! Pull! Pull again! And relax."

Suggested Techniques. Rhythmic stabilization, repeated contractions for emphasis. Slow reversal – hold to middle range, then to shortened range, followed by repeated contractions on left.

Antagonistic Pattern

(BR, CD): D2 fl with knee flexion, right; D1 ex with knee extension, left (Fig. 1-126).

Related Unilateral Patterns

Lower extremity D2 ex with knee extension (Fig. 1-74); D2 fl with knee flexion, antagonistic pattern (Fig. 1-71); D1 fl with hip and knee flexion (Fig. 1-65).

Lower trunk flexion and extension: D2 ex with knee extension, right (Fig. 1-42); D1 fl with knee flexion, right (Fig. 1-39): extremities in contact.

Related Total Patterns (Mat Activities)

Rolling toward prone, D1 fl with hip and knee flexion (Fig. 1-155).

Creeping forward to right, D1 fl with hip and knee flexion, left (Fig. 1-172).

Creeping backward to left, D2 ex with hip and knee extension, right (Fig. 1-174).

Plantigrade walking forward to right, D1 fl, left (Fig. 1-176); plantigrade walking backward to left, D2 ex, right.

Lower Extremity

Emphasis on Hip and Knee: Reciprocal (BR, CD)

FLEXION – ABDUCTION – INTERNAL ROTATION (D2 fl),
WITH KNEE FLEXION, RIGHT; EXTENSION –
ABDUCTION – INTERNAL ROTATION (D1 ex), WITH
KNEE EXTENSION, LEFT

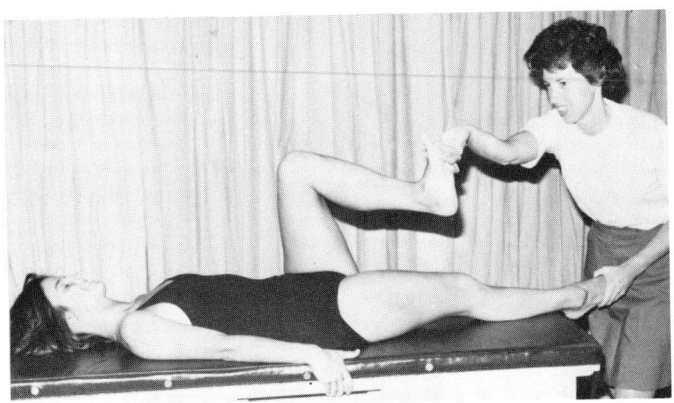

A

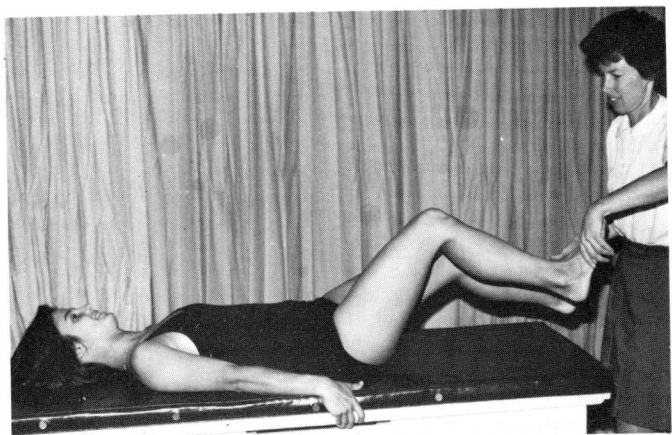

B

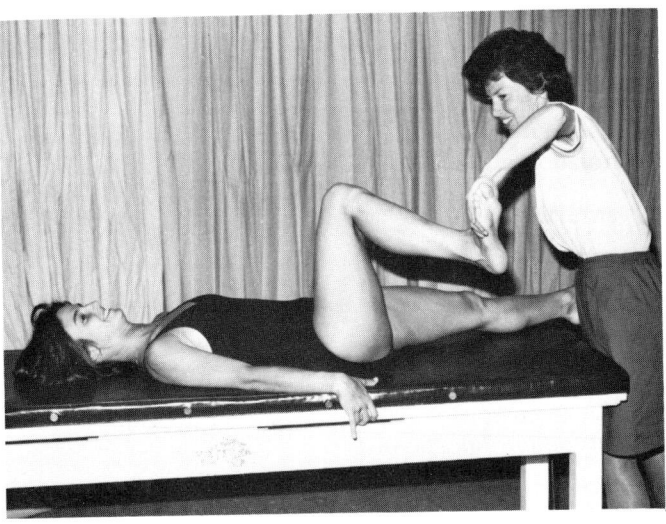

C

FIG. 1-126

Components of Motion

Free. In supine posture, head and shoulders may be elevated slightly. Head maintains midline position. Hands grip table edges for stability and reinforcement. Alternative posture: prone with hips flexed over end of table.

Resisted. Right foot and ankle dorsiflex and evert, and initiate hip flexion, abduction, and internal rotation, and knee flexion, as the left foot plantar flexes and everts, and initiates hip extension, abduction, and internal rotation, and knee extension.

A. Lengthened Range

Commands. Preparatory. "You are to pull your right foot up and out, turn your heel out, and bend your hip and knee [D2 fl], and push your left foot down and out, turn your heel out, and straighten your hip and knee [D1 ex]." *Action.* "Pull up and out with your right! Push down and out with your left! Hold everything! Now hold the left! And pull up and out with the right! Pull! And pull! And relax."

Suggested Techniques. Stretch on the left, traction and stretch on the right; resistance and repeated contractions.

B. Middle Range

Commands. "Hold everything! Now pull your right knee up and out! Pull again! Pull! And rest."

Suggested Techniques. Maximal resistance for the "hold" contraction on left, repeated contractions on right for emphasis. Slow reversal–hold, then repeated contractions at various points in range, *A* to *C.*

C. Shortened Range

Commands. "Hold everything! Now hold! And hold! And hold! Now pull up and out with your right! And pull! Pull! Pull again! And relax."

Suggested Techniques. Rhythmic stabilization, repeated contractions on right for emphasis. Slow reversal–hold to middle range, then to shortened range, followed by repeated contractions on right. Eccentric contractions.

Antagonistic Pattern

(BR, CD): D2 ex with knee extension, right; D1 fl with knee flexion, left (Fig. 1-125).

Related Unilateral Patterns

Lower extremity D2 with knee flexion (Fig. 1-71); D1 ex with knee extension (Fig. 1-68).

Lower trunk flexion and extension: D2 fl with knee flexion, right (Fig. 1-39); D1 ex with knee extension, left (Fig. 1-42): extremities in contact.

Related Total Patterns (Mat Activities)

Creeping forward to right, D2 fl with hip and knee flexion, right (Fig. 1-172).

Creeping backward to left, D1 ex with hip and knee extension, left (Fig. 1-174).

Plantigrade walking forward to right, D2 with hip and knee flexion, right (Fig. 1-176).

Emphasis on Knee: Symmetrical (BS)

FLEXION – ADDUCTION – EXTERNAL ROTATION
(D1 fl), WITH KNEE EXTENSION, LEFT AND RIGHT

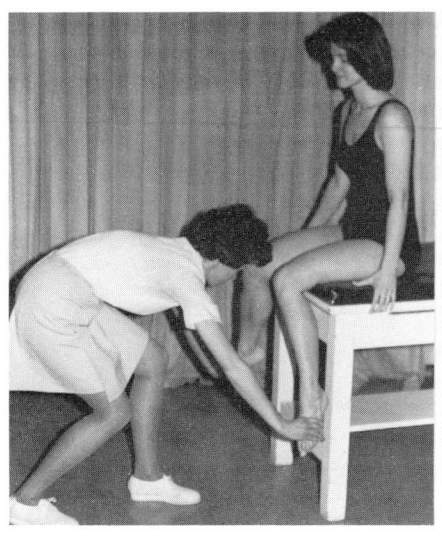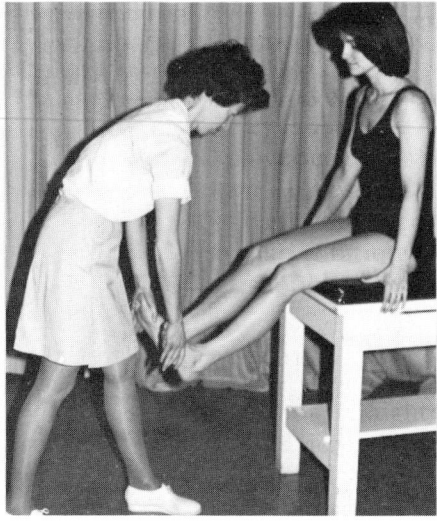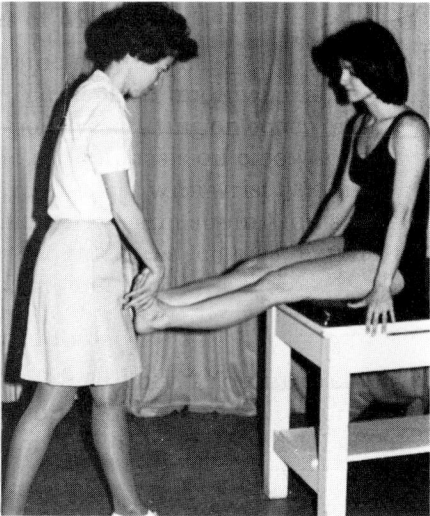

A   B   C

FIG. 1-127

Components of Motion

Free. In sitting posture, eyes regard foot and ankle movements. Head, neck, and trunk are slightly flexed with hands gripping table edge for stability and reinforcement. Alternative posture: supine, knees flexed over table edge.

Resisted. Left and right feet and ankles dorsiflex, invert, and initiate knee extension with external rotation.

A. Lengthened Range

Commands. *Preparatory.* "You are to kick your feet up and in as you straighten your knees, bringing your heels together (D1 fl)." *Action.* "Lift your toes! Kick your feet in and up! Straighten your knees!"

Suggested Techniques. Traction, stretch, and resistance.

B. Middle Range

Commands. "Hold with your right! And straighten your left knee! More! Again! And again! And relax."

Suggested Techniques. Maximal resistance for "hold" on right; repeated contractions on left. Repeated contractions may be preceded or followed by rhythmic stabilization. Slow reversals may follow with above sequence of techniques performed at various points in range, A through C.

C. Shortened Range

Commands. "Hold it! Don't let me move you. And hold, and hold, and hold it! And relax!"

Suggested Techniques. Rhythmic stabilization followed by relaxation.

Antagonistic Pattern

BS: D1 ex, with knee flexion, left and right (Fig. 1-128).

Related Unilateral Patterns

Lower extremity D1 fl with knee extension (Fig. 1-72).

Lower trunk flexion with rotation to the left: D1 fl with knee extension, right (Fig. 1-40).

Related Total Patterns (Mat Activities)

Sitting: lower trunk rocking, backward (Fig. 1-181, A and B): D1 fl in knee extension.

Balance on hands and knees (Fig. 1-170): symmetrical position for rhythmic stabilization.

Emphasis on Knee: Symmetrical (BS)

EXTENSION – ABDUCTION – INTERNAL ROTATION
(D1 ex), WITH KNEE FLEXION, LEFT AND RIGHT

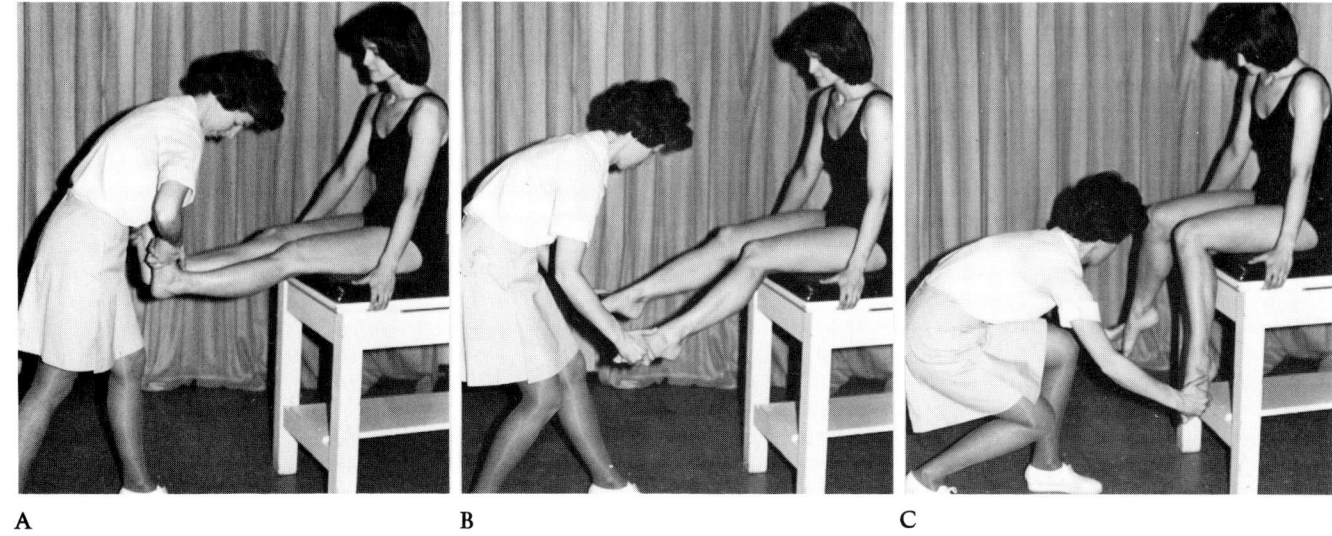

A   B   C

FIG. 1-128

Components of Motion

Free. In sitting posture, eyes regard foot and ankle movements. Head, neck, and trunk are slightly flexed with hands gripping table edge for stability and reinforcement. Alternative posture: supine, knees flexed over table edge.

Resisted. Left and right feet and ankles plantar flex, evert, and initiate knee flexion with internal rotation.

A. Lengthened Range

Commands. Preparatory. "You are to push your feet down and out, and bend your knees (D1 ex)." *Action.* "Bend your toes, turn your feet down and out. Now pull your heels down and out!"

Suggested Techniques. Stretch and resistance; slow reversal.

B. Middle Range

Commands. "Hold it! Don't let me move you. And hold, and hold, and hold it! And now pull down and out."

Suggested Techniques. Rhythmic stabilization followed by stretch and resistance to shortened range.

Appropriate techniques include combinations of repeated contractions, and slow reversals.

C. Shortened Range

Commands. "Now hold the right; and bend your left knee! More! Again! And again! And relax."

Suggested Techniques. Maximal resistance for "hold" on right; repeated contractions on left. Other appropriate techniques include rhythmic stabilization and slow reversal – hold.

Antagonistic Pattern

BS: D1 fl, with knee extension, left and right (Fig. 1-127).

Related Patterns

Lower extremity D1 ex with knee flexion (Fig. 1-69).

Lower trunk flexion and extension: D1 ex with knee flexion, right (Fig. 1-43).

Related Total Patterns (Mat Activities)

Pelvic elevation, supine (Fig. 1-163): D1 ex with heels placed apart.

Emphasis on Knee: Symmetrical (BS)

FLEXION – ABDUCTION – INTERNAL ROTATION (D2 fl), WITH KNEE EXTENSION, LEFT AND RIGHT

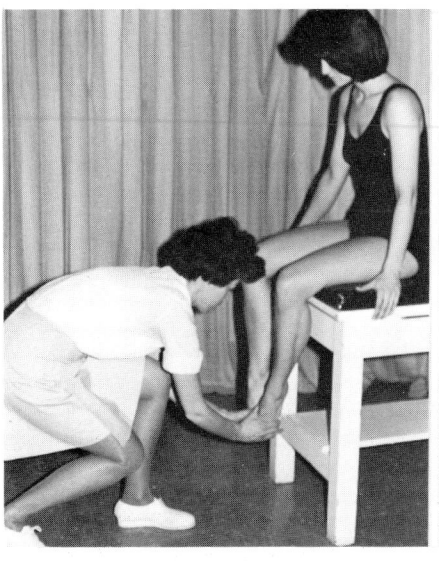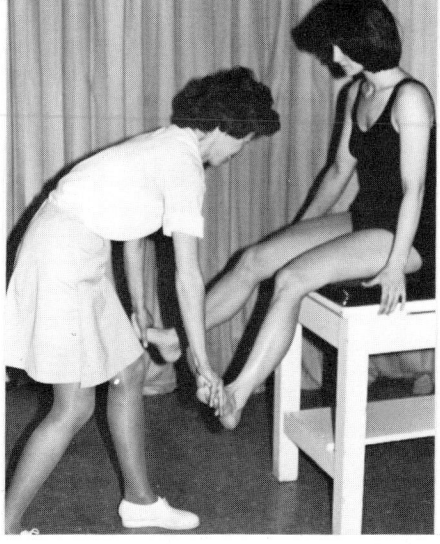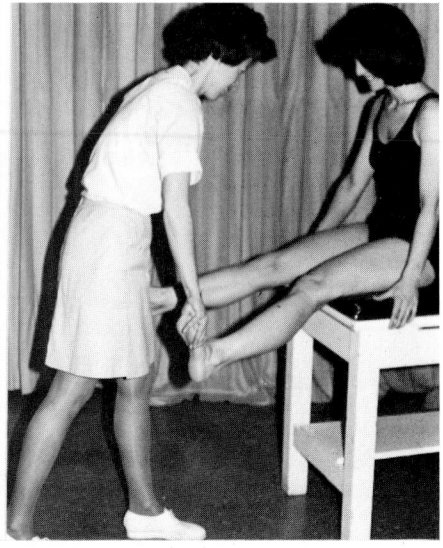

A   B   C

FIG. 1-129

Components of Motion

Free. In sitting posture, eyes regard foot and ankle movements. Head, neck, and trunk are slightly flexed with hands gripping table edge for stability and reinforcement. Alternative posture: supine, knees flexed over table edge.

Resisted. Feet and ankles dorsiflex, evert, and initiate knee extension with internal rotation.

A. Lengthened Range

Commands. Preparatory. "You are to lift your feet up and out and as you straighten your knees, turn the heels outward (D2 fl)." *Action.* "Lift your toes up and out! Kick your heels up and out! Straighten your knees!"

Suggested Techniques. Traction, stretch, and resistance.

B. Middle Range

Commands. "Hold it! And hold, and hold, and hold! Now kick all the way, up and out to me!"

Suggested Techniques. Rhythmic stabilization followed by stretch, then active resisted movement to shortened range.

C. Shortened Range

Commands. "Hold! [At limit of range, change manual contact to plantar surface. See antagonistic pattern.] Now pull your heels down and in! Hold! [Reverse hand position as in A.] Now kick your heels up and out! Hold! And relax."

Suggested Techniques. Slow reversal–hold (see details of Antagonistic Pattern).

Antagonistic Pattern

BS: D2 ex with knee flexion, left and right (Fig. 1-130).

Related Unilateral Patterns

Lower extremity D2 fl with knee extension (Fig. 1-72).

Lower trunk flexion and extension: D2 fl with knee extension, left (Fig. 1-40).

Related Total Pattern (Mat Activity)

Rising to plantigrade (Fig. 1-175, *C*); with feet positioned in slight internal rotation, BS, D2 fl, knee extension can be challenged by activities of balance, rocking, and rhythmic stabilization.

Lower Extremity

Emphasis on Knee: Symmetrical (BS)

EXTENSION – ADDUCTION – EXTERNAL ROTATION
(D2 ex), WITH KNEE FLEXION, LEFT AND RIGHT

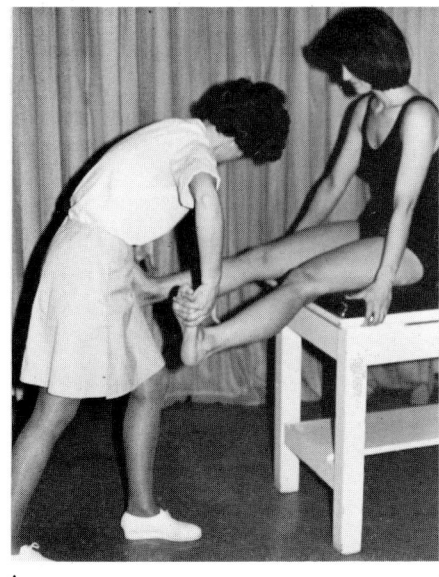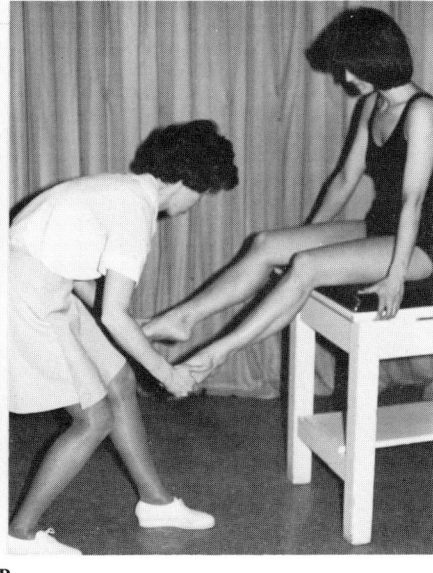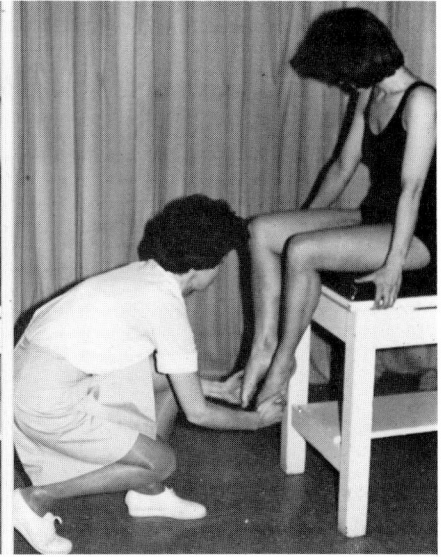

A   B   C

FIG. 1-130

Components of Motion

Free. In sitting posture, eyes regard foot and ankle movements. Head, neck, and trunk are slightly flexed with hands gripping table edge for stability and reinforcement. Alternative posture: supine, knees flexed over table edge.

Resisted. Feet and ankles plantar flex, invert, and initiate knee flexion with external rotation bilaterally.

A. Lengthened Range

Commands. Preparatory. "You are to push your feet down and in, bringing the heels together as you bend your knees (D2 ex)." *Action.* "Bend your toes! Push your feet down and in! Bend your knees!"

Suggested Techniques. Stretch and resistance.

B. Middle Range

Commands. "Hold everything! Now continue to hold on the right while you pull your left foot down and in! More! Again! And again! And relax."

Suggested Techniques. Repeated contractions on the left with facilitation from a hold on the right.

C. Shortened Range

Commands. "Hold it! Now don't let me move your feet! Don't let me move them! Hold! Now hold the right and don't let me push the left back! Hold! And now, relax."

Suggested Techniques. Rhythmic stabilization followed by an isometric hold on the right and a hold–relax on the left.

Antagonistic Pattern

BS: D2 fl, with knee extension, left and right (Fig. 1-129).

Related Unilateral Patterns

Lower extremity D2 ex with knee flexion (Fig. 1-75).

Lower trunk flexion and extension: D2 ex with knee flexion, left (Fig. 1-43).

Related Total Patterns (Mat Activities)

Pelvic elevation, supine (Fig. 1-163): D2 ex when heels are placed together.

Kneeling balance (Fig. 1-183): hips extended while knees are flexed.

Emphasis on Knee: Asymmetrical (BA)

FLEXION – ADDUCTION – EXTERNAL ROTATION (D1 fl), WITH KNEE EXTENSION, RIGHT; FLEXION – ABDUCTION – INTERNAL ROTATION (D2 fl), WITH KNEE EXTENSION, LEFT

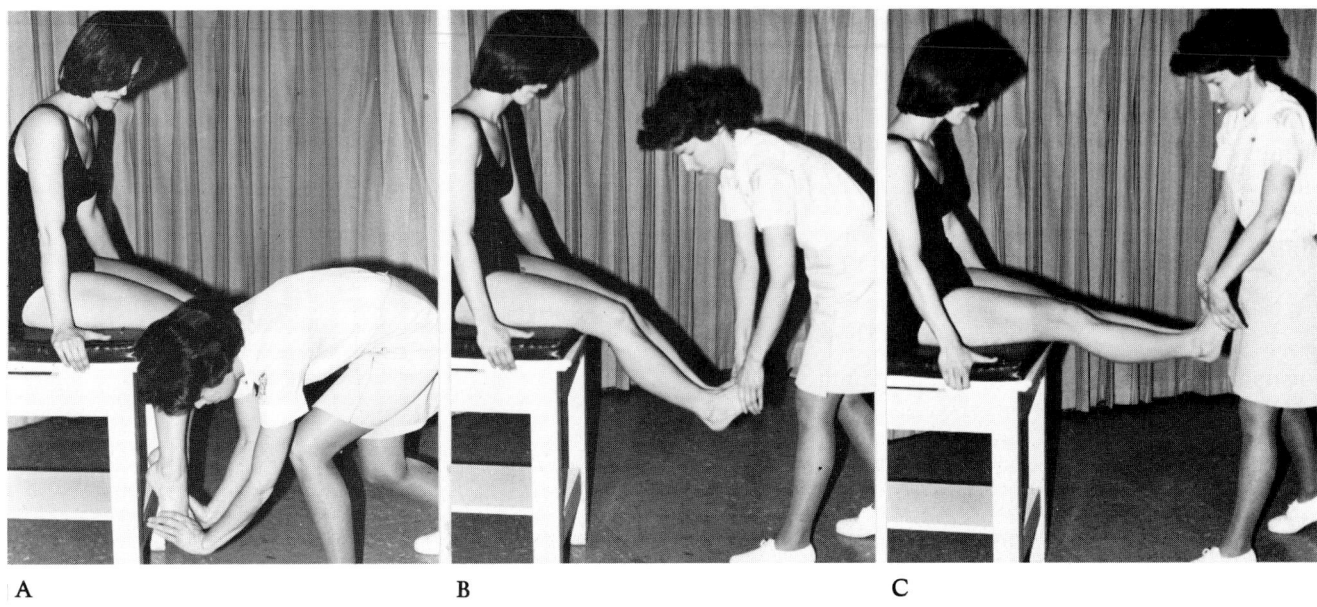

A   B   C

FIG. 1-131

Components of Motion

Free. In sitting posture, eyes regard foot and ankle movements. Head, neck, and trunk are slightly flexed with hands gripping table edge for stability and reinforcement. Alternative posture: supine, knees flexed over table edge.

Resisted. Right foot and ankle dorsiflex and invert, and initiate knee extension with external rotation, as left foot and ankle dorsiflex and evert, and initiate knee extension with internal rotation.

A. Lengthened Range

Commands. *Preparatory.* "You are to lift your feet up and to the left and, as you straighten your knees, turn your heels to the left." *Action.* "Lift your toes! Kick your heels up and out to me! Straighten your knees!"

Suggested Techniques. Traction, stretch, and resistance.

B. Middle Range

Commands. "Hold! Now, kick up to me! Again! More! Again! And again!"

Suggested Technique. Repeated contractions.

C. Shortened Range

Commands. "Kick, up and out! Pull, down and in! Kick up! Pull down! And kick up! Hold! and relax!"

Suggested Techniques. Quick reversals of this and its antagonistic pattern, ending with a hold to emphasize knee extension.

Antagonistic Pattern

BA extension to the right: D1 ex, with knee flexion, right, and D2 ex, with knee flexion, left (Fig. 1-132).

Related Unilateral Patterns

Lower extremity D1 fl with knee extension (Fig. 1-66). D2 fl with knee extension (Fig. 1-72).

Lower trunk flexion and extension: D1 fl with knee extension, right and D2 fl with knee extension, left (Fig. 1-40).

Related Total Pattern (Mat Activity)

Rocking on hands and knees (Fig. 1-169). Rocking backward to the right would produce a bilateral lower extremity asymmetrical flexion to the left.

Emphasis on Knee: Asymmetrical (BA)

EXTENSION – ABDUCTION – INTERNAL ROTATION
(D1 ex), WITH KNEE FLEXION, RIGHT; EXTENSION –
ADDUCTION – EXTERNAL ROTATION (D2 ex), WITH
KNEE FLEXION, LEFT

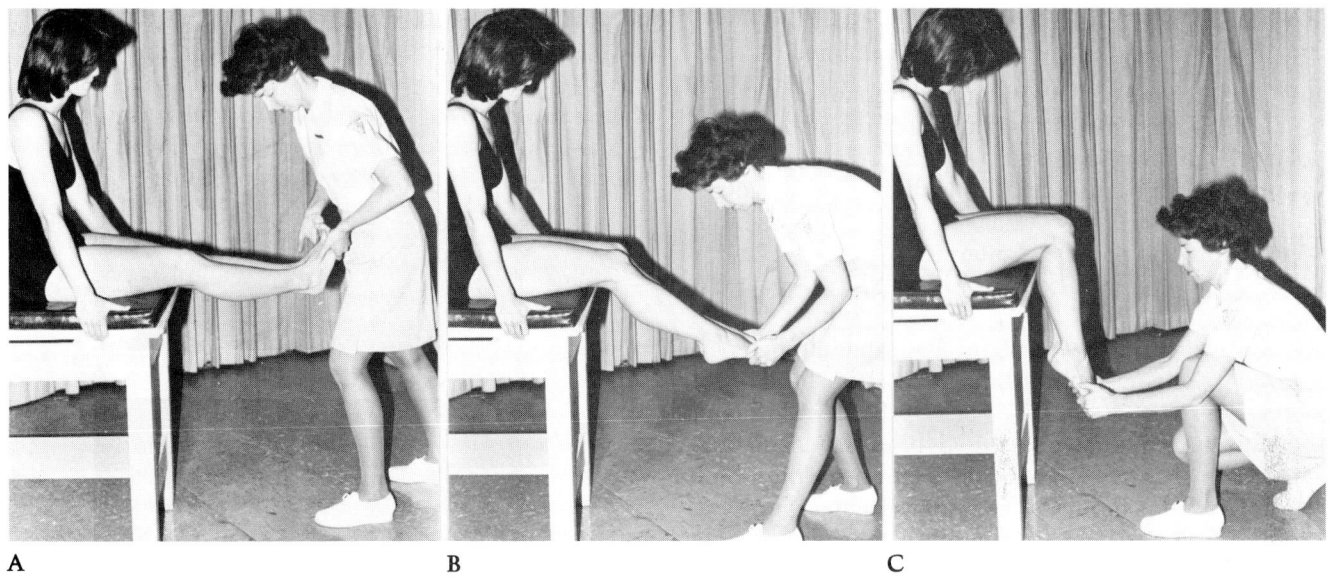

A   B   C

FIG. 1-132

Components of Motion

Free. In sitting posture, eyes regard foot and ankle movements. Head, neck, and trunk are slightly flexed with hands gripping table edge for stability and reinforcement. Alternative posture: supine, knees flexed over table edge.

Resisted. Feet and ankles plantar flex with eversion of right, and inversion of left to initiate bilateral knee flexion to the right.

A. Lengthened Range

Commands. Preparatory. "You are to push your feet down and to the right, and, as you bend your knees, turn your heels to the right. *Action.* "Bend your toes! Pull your heels down and to the right."

Suggested Techniques. Stretch and resistance.

B. Middle Range

Commands. "Hold it! And hold, and hold, and hold it! Now, change! Kick your heels up and out to me!" At lengthened range: "Hold again, and hold! And relax."

Suggested Techniques. Rhythmic stabilization followed by a reversal to lengthened range and completed with rhythmic stabilization in the lengthened range.

C. Shortened Range

Commands. "Now hold! Hold both feet still, and hold, and hold! And relax."

Suggested Techniques. Rhythmic stabilization. Rhythmic stabilization can effectively be followed by repeated contractions progressing to slow reversals through this and its antagonistic pattern.

Antagonistic Pattern

BA flexion to the left: D1 fl, with knee extension, right, and D2 fl, with knee extension, left (Fig. 1-131).

Related Unilateral Patterns

Lower extremity D1 ex with knee flexion (Fig. 1-69); D2 ex with knee flexion (Fig. 1-75).

Lower trunk flexion and extension: D1 ex with knee flexion, right, and D2 ex with knee flexion, left (Fig. 1-43).

Related Total Patterns (Mat Activities)

Rocking on hands and knees (Fig. 1-169). Rocking forward to the right (A and C) causes a bilateral lower extremity asymmetrical extension to the left.

Rising to kneeling toward left (Fig. 1-182); results in bilateral lower extremity asymmetrical extension to the right.

Emphasis on Knee: Reciprocal (BR, SD)

EXTENSION–ABDUCTION–INTERNAL ROTATION
(D1 ex), WITH KNEE FLEXION, LEFT; FLEXION–
ADDUCTION–EXTERNAL ROTATION (D1 fl), WITH
KNEE EXTENSION, RIGHT

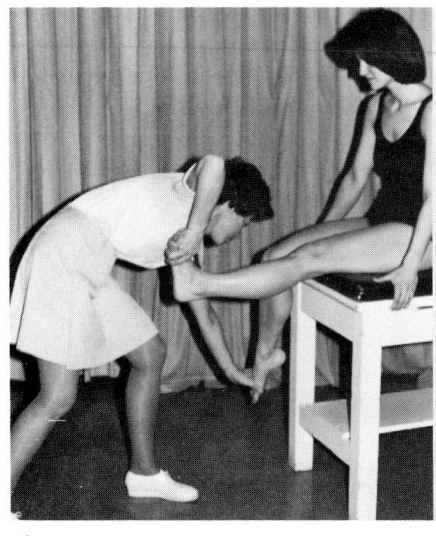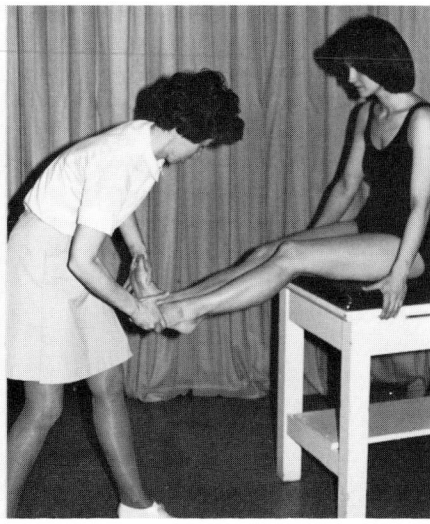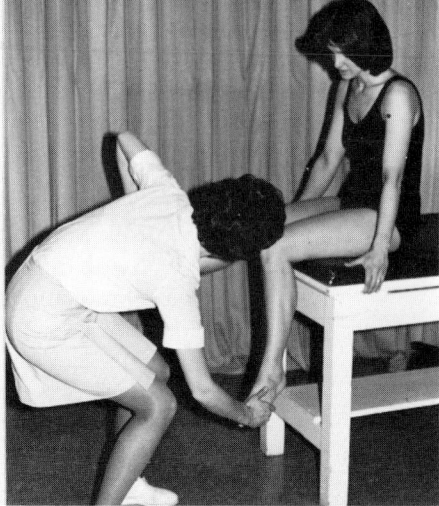

A   B   C

FIG. 1-133

Components of Motion

Free. In sitting posture, eyes regard foot and ankle movements. Head, neck, and trunk are slightly flexed with hands gripping table edge for stability and reinforcement. Alternative posture: supine, knees flexed over table edge.

Resisted. Left foot and ankle plantar flex, evert, and initiate knee flexion with internal rotation, as right foot and ankle dorsiflex, invert, and initiate knee extension with external rotation.

A. Lengthened Range

Commands. *Preparatory.* "You are to kick your right foot up and in, and straighten your knee [D1 fl], and push your left down and out, and bend your knee [D1 ex]." *Action.* "Kick in and up with your right! Straighten your knee! Push down with your left! Bend your knee! And relax."

Suggested Techniques. Stretch and resistance; slow reversal.

B. Middle Range

Left near lengthened, right near shortened.
Commands. "Hold with your right! Bend your left knee! More! Again! And again! And relax."

Suggested Techniques. Maximal resistance for "hold" on right; repeated contractions on left; rhythmic stabilization followed by repeated contractions on left. Reverse and repeat sequence at various points in the range, *A* to *C*.

C. Shortened Range

Commands. "Hold everything! And hold, and hold, and hold it! Now change! Kick with your left and bend your right knee!" At midrange: "Hold again, and hold! And relax."

Suggested Techniques. Rhythmic stabilization followed by reversal to mid range, followed by stabilization.

Antagonistic Pattern

BR: D1 fl, with knee extension, left; D1 ex, with knee flexion, right (Fig. 1-134).

Related Unilateral Patterns

Lower extremity D1 fl with knee extension (Fig. 1-66); D1 ex with knee flexion (Fig. 1-69).

Lower trunk flexion and extension: D1 fl with knee extension, right (Fig. 1-40); D1 ex with knee flexion, right (Fig. 1-43).

Emphasis on Knee: Reciprocal (BR, SD)

FLEXION–ADDUCTION–EXTERNAL ROTATION
(D1 fl), WITH KNEE EXTENSION, LEFT; EXTENSION–
ABDUCTION–INTERNAL ROTATION (D1 ex), WITH
KNEE FLEXION, RIGHT

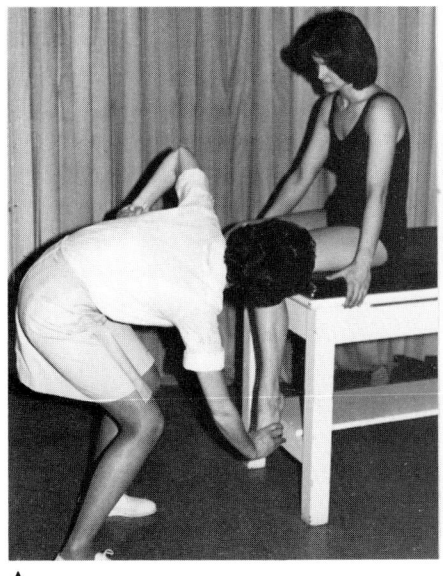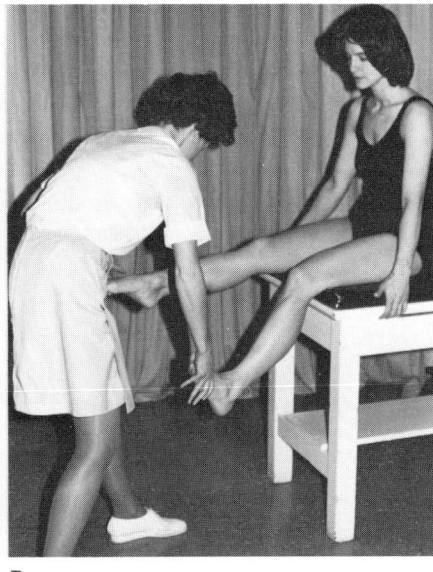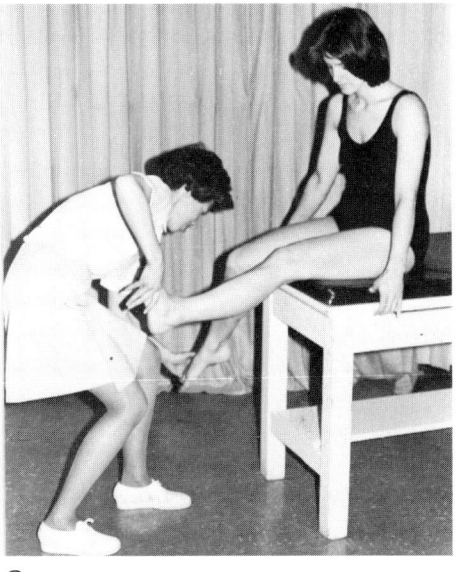

A   B   C

FIG. 1-134

Components of Motion

Free. In sitting posture, eyes regard foot and ankle movements. Head, neck, and trunk are slightly flexed with hands gripping table edge for stability and reinforcement. Alternative posture: supine, knees flexed over table edge.

Resisted. Left foot and ankle dorsiflex, invert, and initiate knee extension with external rotation, as right foot and ankle plantar flex, evert, and initiate knee flexion with internal rotation.

A. Lengthened Range

Commands. Preparatory. "You are to kick your left foot in and up as you straighten your knee (D1 fl), and push your right foot down and out as you bend your knee (D1 ex). Heel to the center when you kick up; heel to the outside when you pull down." *Action.* "Lift your toes! Kick in and up with the left! And bend your toes! Pull the right foot down and out! Straighten the left knee! Bend the right!"

Suggested Techniques. Stretch and resistance.

B. Middle Range

Commands. "Hold everything! Now keep the hold on the right! Straighten the left knee! More! Again! And again! And relax."

Suggested Techniques. Maximal resistance for "hold" on right to facilitate repeated contractions of the left knee extensors from midrange to shortened. Rhythmic stabilization may be effectively added.

C. Shortened Range

Commands. "Hold it! Now change; kick your right foot up and in and the left down and out! Hold! Now change; right down and out left up and in! Hold! Now change! Hold! And change! Hold! Now hold the right and kick the left in and up! Again! Again! And again! Hold everything! And hold! And hold! And hold! And hold! And relax."

Suggested Techniques. Slow reversal–hold, *A* through *C*, followed by repeated contractions on left knee extension in shortened range, ending with rhythmic stabilization.

Antagonistic Pattern

BR: D1 ex, with knee flexion, left; D1 fl, with knee extension, right (Fig. 1-133).

Related Unilateral Patterns

Lower extremity D1 fl with knee extension (Fig. 1-66); D1 ex with knee flexion (Fig. 1-69).

Lower trunk flexion and extension: D1 fl with knee extension, right (Fig. 1-40); D1 ex with knee flexion, right (Fig. 1-43).

Emphasis on Knee: Reciprocal (BR, SD)

FLEXION – ABDUCTION – INTERNAL ROTATION (D2 fl),
WITH KNEE EXTENSION, LEFT; EXTENSION –
ADDUCTION – EXTERNAL ROTATION (D2 ex), WITH
KNEE FLEXION, RIGHT

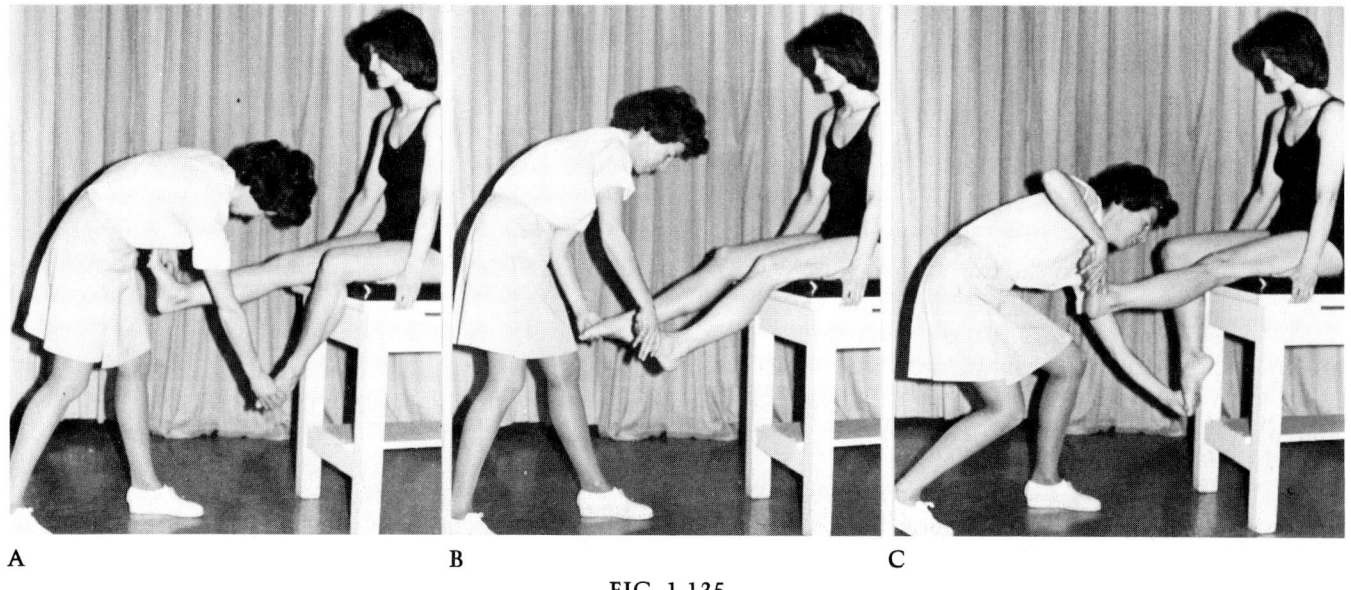

A   B   C

FIG. 1-135

Components of Motion

Free. In sitting posture, eyes regard foot and ankle movements. Head, neck, and trunk are slightly flexed with hands gripping table edge for stability and reinforcement. Alternative posture: supine, knees flexed over table edge.

Resisted. Left foot and ankle dorsiflex, evert, and initiate knee extension with internal rotation, as right foot and ankle plantar flex, invert, and initiate knee flexion with external rotation.

A. Lengthened Range

Commands. Preparatory. "You are to kick your left foot up and out as you straighten your knee (D2 fl); and pull your right foot down and in as you bend your knee (D2 ex). Heels out when up and in when down."
Action. "Lift your toes and turn your left heel out! And straighten your knee! Bend your toes and pull your right heel down and in ! Bend your left knee!"
Suggested Techniques. Stretch and resistance.

B. Middle Range

Commands. "Hold everything! And hold! And hold! And hold! And hold! And relax!"

Suggested Techniques. Rhythmic stabilization at various points through middle range.

C. Shortened Range

Commands. "Hold everything! And hold! And hold! Now keep the hold on the left and try to kick your right foot up and out! Come on, try! Relax the right. Now pull it down and in! Again! And again! And relax."
Suggested Techniques. Rhythmic stabilization, followed by contract – relax for increased right knee flexion, followed by repeated contractions of right knee flexion.

Antagonistic Pattern

BR, SD: D2 ex, with knee flexion, left and D2 fl, with knee extension, right (Fig. 1-136).

Related Unilateral Patterns

Lower extremity D2 fl with knee extension (Fig. 1-72); D2 ex with knee flexion (Fig. 1-75).

Lower trunk flexion and extension: D2 fl with knee extension, left (Fig. 1-40); D2 ex with knee flexion, left (Fig. 1-43).

Lower Extremity

Emphasis on Knee: Reciprocal (BR, SD)

EXTENSION – ADDUCTION – EXTERNAL ROTATION
(D2 ex), WITH KNEE FLEXION, LEFT; FLEXION –
ABDUCTION – INTERNAL ROTATION (D2 fl), WITH
KNEE EXTENSION, RIGHT

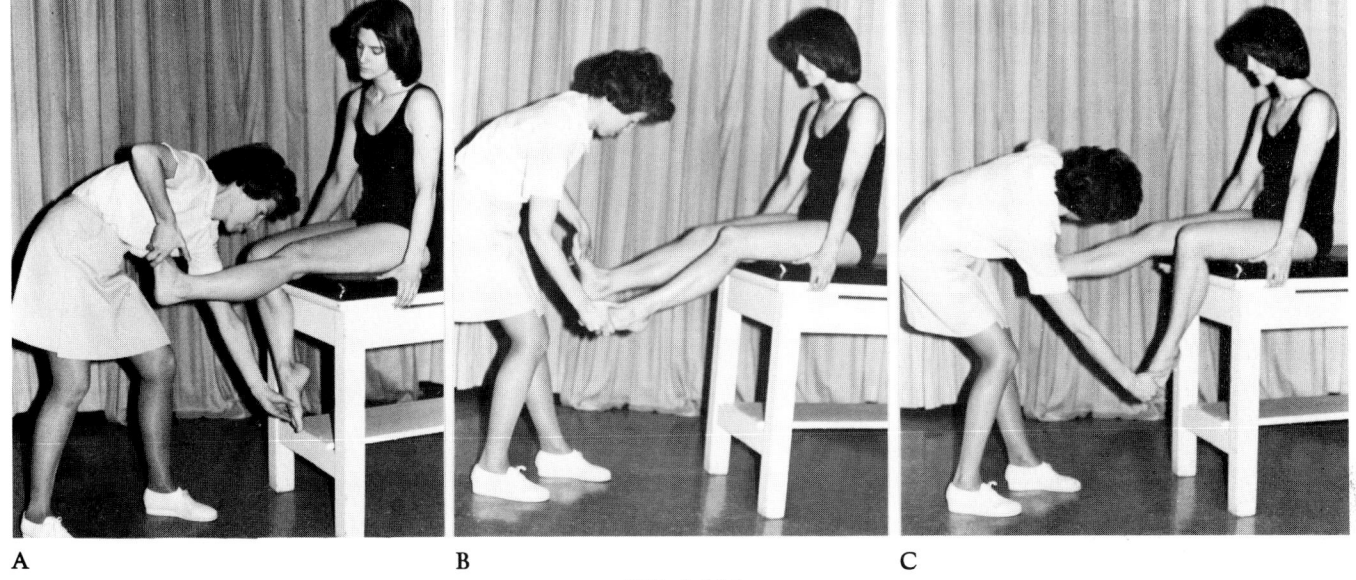

A   B   C

FIG. 1-136

Components of Motion

Free. In sitting posture, eyes regard foot and ankle movements. Head, neck, and trunk are slightly flexed with hands gripping table edge for stability and reinforcement. Alternative posture: supine, knees flexed over table edge.

Resisted. Left foot and ankle plantar flex, invert, and initiate knee flexion with external rotation, as right foot and ankle dorsiflex, evert, and initiate knee extension with internal rotation.

A. Lengthened Range

Commands. Preparatory. "You are to pull your left foot down and in as you bend your knee (D2 ex), and kick your right foot up and out as you straighten your knee (D2 fl). Heels out when up and in when down." *Action.* "Bend your toes and pull your left heel down and in! Bend your left knee! Lift your toes and turn your right heel out! And straighten your right knee!"

Suggested Techniques. Stretch and resistance.

B. Middle Range

Commands. "Hold! Now kick up and out with the left and pull down and in with the right. Hold! And change! Hold! Change! Hold! Change! Hold! And relax."

Suggested Techniques. Slow reversal – hold to various points in midrange.

C. Shortened Range

Commands. "Now hold the left! Don't let me move it! Kick the right foot up and out! Kick it up! Again! And again! Now hold it! Pull the left foot down and in! Get it down! Again! And again! Hold everything! Now kick the left up and out and the right down and in. Hold! Reverse! Hold! And relax."

Suggested Techniques. Repeated contractions for right knee extension with hold on left, followed by repeated contractions for left knee flexion with hold on the right, ending the sequence with slow reversal – hold.

Antagonistic Pattern

(BR, SD): D2 fl, with knee extension, left, and D2 ex, with knee flexion, right (Fig. 1-135).

Related Unilateral Patterns

Lower extremity D2 fl with knee extension (Fig. 1-72); D2 ex with knee flexion (Fig. 1-75).

Lower trunk flexion and extension; D2 fl with knee extension, left (Fig. 1-40); D2 ex with knee flexion, left (Fig. 1-43).

Lower Extremity

Emphasis on Knee: Reciprocal, in Crossed Diagonals
(BR, CD)

EXTENSION – ABDUCTION – INTERNAL ROTATION
(D1 ex), WITH KNEE FLEXION, LEFT; FLEXION – ABDUCTION –
INTERNAL ROTATION (D2 fl), WITH KNEE EXTENSION, RIGHT

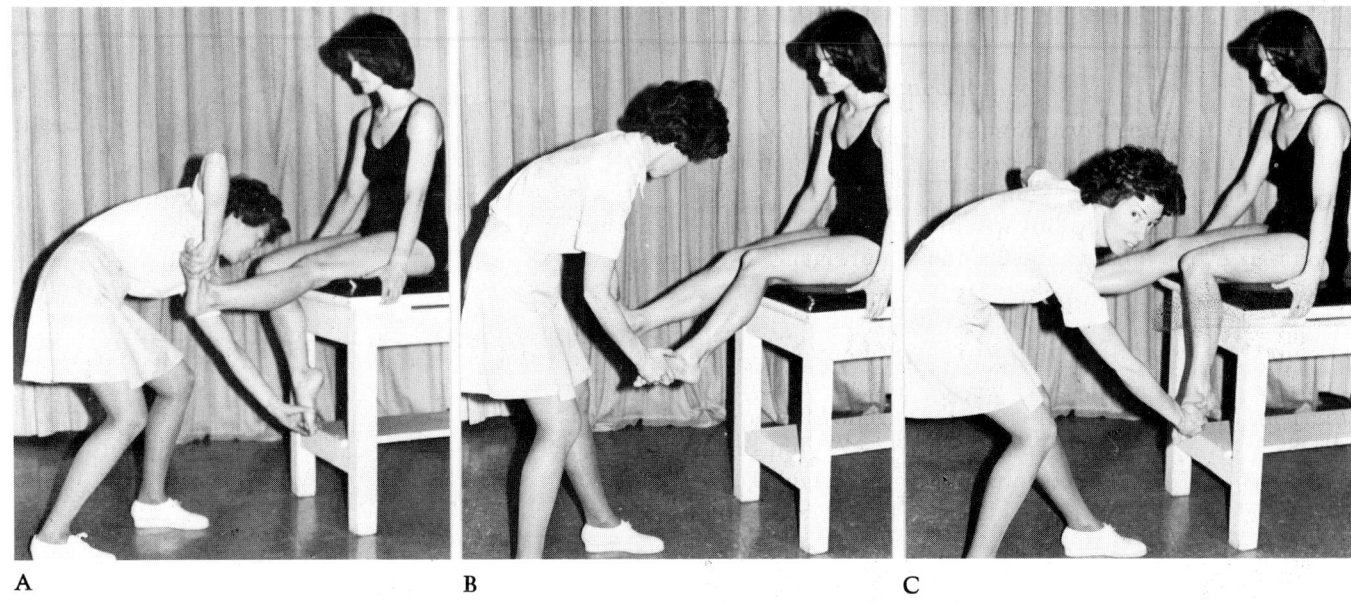

A   B   C

FIG. 1-137

Components of Motion

Free. In sitting posture, eyes regard foot and ankle movements. Head, neck, and trunk are slightly flexed with hands gripping table edge for stability and reinforcement. Alternative posture: supine, knees flexed over table edge.

Resisted. Left foot and ankle plantar flex, evert, and initiate knee flexion with internal rotation, as right foot and ankle dorsiflex, evert, and initiate knee extension with internal rotation.

A. Lengthened Range

Commands. *Preparatory.* "You are to push your left foot down and out as you bend your knee (D1 ex), and kick your right foot up and out as you straighten your knee (D2 fl)." *Action.* "Bend your toes! Pull the left foot down and out! Bend the knee. Lift your toes and turn your right heel out! Straighten your knee!"

Suggested Techniques. Stretch and resistance.

B. Middle Range

Commands. "Hold! Now hold with the right and pull down with the left! Again! And pull! And hold! Now kick out with the right! And again! Hold the left! Straighten the right! And rest!"

Suggested Techniques. Repeated contractions on left as right holds. Emphasize left, then hold with left and emphasize right.

C. Shortened Range

Commands. "Now hold! Hold both feet still, and hold, and hold! And relax."

Suggested Techniques. Rhythmic stabilization. May be followed by repeated contractions for emphasis, or slow reversal, slow reversal – hold.

Antagonistic Pattern

(BR, CD): D1 fl, with knee extension, left, and D2 ex, with knee flexion, right.

Related Unilateral Patterns

Lower extremity D1 ex with knee flexion (Fig. 1-69); D2 fl with knee extension (Fig. 1-72).

Lower trunk flexion and extension: D1 ex with knee flexion, right (Fig. 1-43); D2 fl with knee extension, left (Fig. 1-40).

Related Total Pattern (Mat Activity)

Bipedal walking forward to right (Fig. 1-188):* during swing of the right leg in D2 fl, with knee flexion progressing to extension, while the left stance leg is in D1 ex, progressing from knee flexion to extension.

---

* Patterns of the lower extremities can be changed by changing the direction of the diagonal progression. Flexion and extension phases can be reversed by reversing the direction of movement.

Emphasis on Knee: Reciprocal, Crossed Diagonals
(BR, CD)

FLEXION – ABDUCTION – INTERNAL ROTATION (D2 fl),
WITH KNEE EXTENSION, LEFT; EXTENSION – ABDUCTION –
INTERNAL ROTATION (D1 ex), WITH KNEE FLEXION, RIGHT

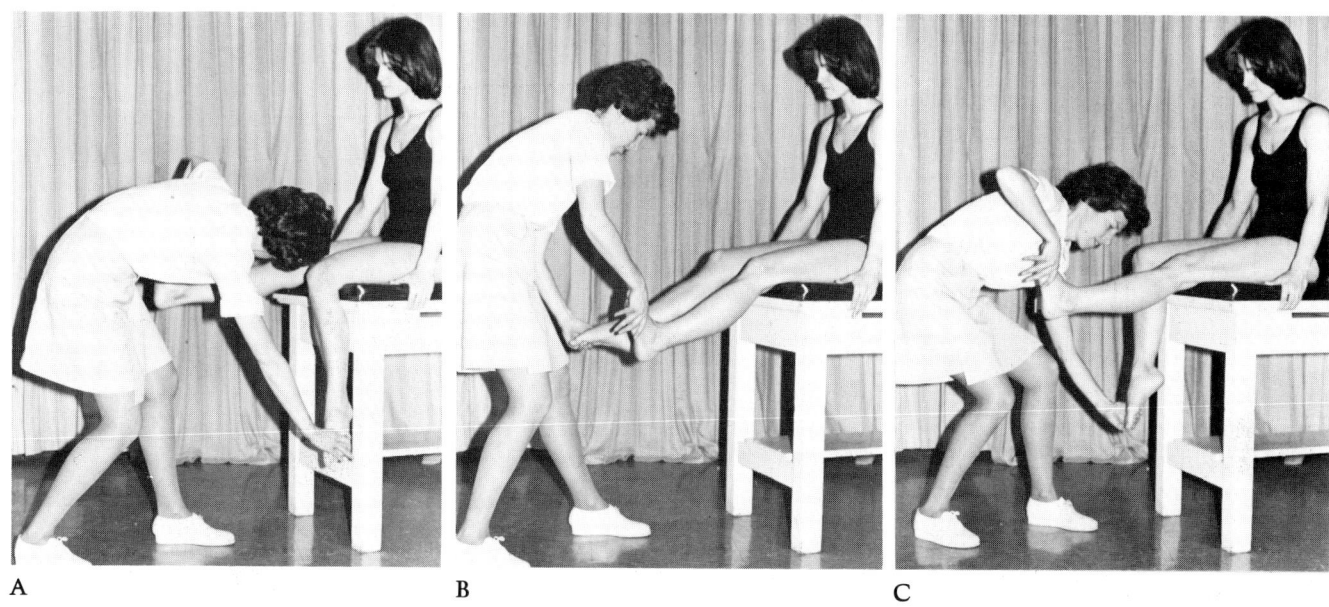

A B C

FIG. 1-138

Components of Motion

Free. In sitting posture, eyes regard foot and ankle movements. Head, neck, and trunk are slightly flexed with hands gripping table edge for stability and reinforcement. Alternative posture: supine, knees flexed over table edge.

Resisted. Left foot and ankle dorsiflex, evert, and initiate knee extension with internal rotation, as right foot and ankle plantar flex, evert, and initiate knee flexion with internal rotation.

A. Lengthened Range

Commands. Preparatory. "You are to kick your left foot up and out as you straighten your knee (D2 fl); and push your right foot down and out as you bend your knee (D1 ex). Turn your heels apart." *Action.* "Lift your toes! Kick your foot up and out as you straighten your knee! Bend your toes! Pull the right foot down and out! Bend the knee!"

Suggested Techniques. Stretch and resistance.

B. Middle Range

Commands. "Hold with your right! And straighten your left knee! More! Again! And again! And relax."

Suggested Techniques. Maximal resistance for "hold" on right; repeated contractions for left knee extension. Repeated contractions may be preceded or followed by rhythmic stabilization. Slow reversals may follow with this sequence of techniques performed at various points in the range.

C. Shortened Range

Commands. "Hold it! And hold! And hold! Now keep the hold on the left and don't let me move your right knee! Come on, hold it! Relax the right. Now pull it down and in! Again! And again! And relax."

Suggested Techniques. Rhythmic stabilization, followed by hold – relax for increased right knee flexion, followed by repeated contractions of right knee flexion.

Antagonistic Pattern

(BR, CD): D2 ex, with knee flexion, left, and D1 fl, with knee extension, right.

Related Unilateral Patterns

Lower extremity D1 ex with knee flexion (Fig. 1-69); D2 fl with knee extension (Fig. 1-72).

Lower trunk flexion and extension: D1 ex with knee flexion, right (Fig. 1-43); D2 fl with knee extension, left (Fig. 1-40).

Related Total Pattern (Mat Activity)

Plantigrade walking forward to left (Fig. 1-176):* during swing of the left leg in D2 fl, with knee flexion progressing to extension, while the right stance leg is in D1 ex, progressing from knee flexion to extension.

* Patterns of the lower extremities can be changed by changing the direction of the diagonal progression. Flexion and extension phases can be reversed by reversing the direction of movement.

Emphasis on Foot and Ankle: Symmetrical (BS)

FLEXION – ADDUCTION – EXTERNAL ROTATION
(D1 fl), LEFT AND RIGHT

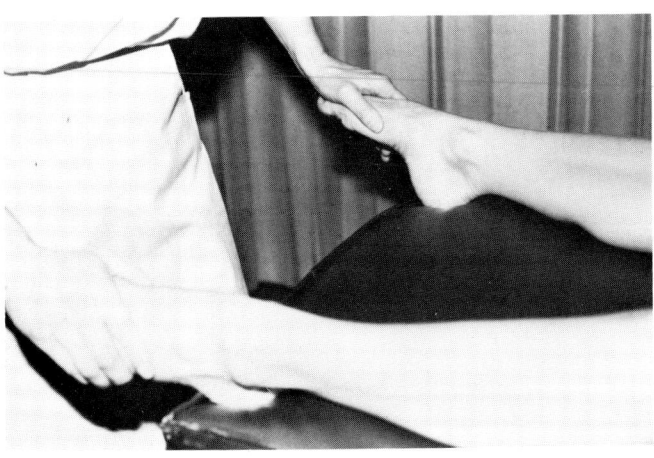

A

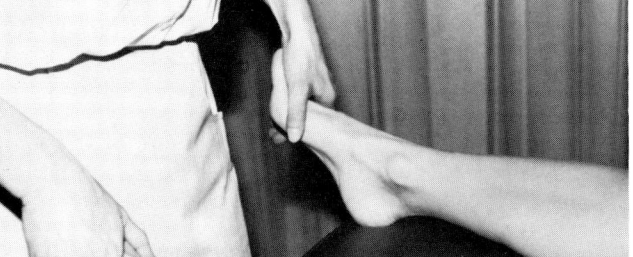

B

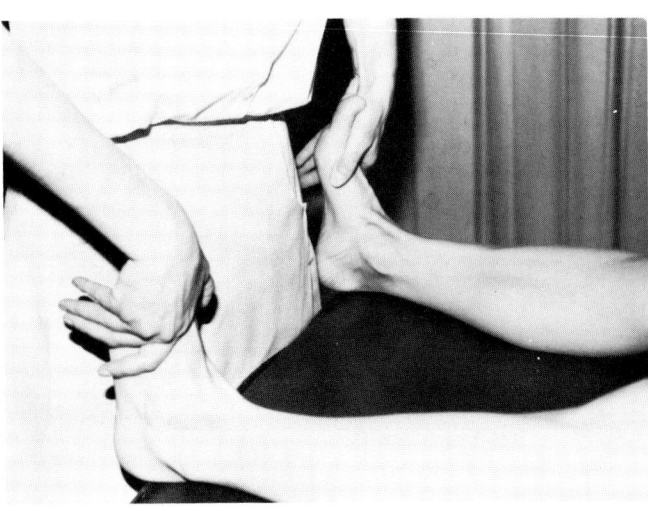

C

FIG. 1-139

Components of Motion

Free. In supine posture, head and shoulders may be elevated slightly so that eyes may follow foot and ankle movements. Hands may grip table edges for stability and reinforcement. Alternative postures: supine or sitting, knees flexed over table edge.

Resisted. Feet and ankles dorsiflex and invert with extremity external rotation.

A. Lengthened Range

Commands. *Preparatory.* "You are to pull your feet in and up as you turn your heels together (D1 fl)." *Action.* "Lift your toes! Pull your feet in and up!"

Suggested Techniques. Traction, stretch and resistance; slow reversal.

B. Middle Range

Commands. "Hold it! Don't let me move you. And hold, and hold, and hold it! And now, pull in and up."

Suggested Techniques. Rhythmic stabilization followed by stretch and resistance to shortened range. Appropriate techniques include combinations of repeated contractions and slow reversals.

C. Shortened Range

Commands. "Now hold the right; and pull the left in and up! More! Again! And again! And relax."

Suggested Techniques. Maximal resistance for "hold" on right; repeated contractions on left. Other appropriate techniques include rhythmic stabilization and slow reversal – hold.

Antagonistic Pattern

(BS): D1 ex, left and right (Fig. 1-140).

Related Unilateral Patterns

Lower extremity D1 fl with knee straight (Fig. 1-64).

Lower trunk flexion and extension: D1 fl of right foot and ankle (Figs. 1-38, 1-39, and 1-40).

Related Total Patterns (Mat Activities)

Rolling: supine toward prone (Figs. 1-151 to 1-155): left foot and ankle D1 fl.

Sitting: lower trunk rocking (Fig. 1-181, *A* and *B*). BS, D1 fl of foot and ankle is challenged.

Emphasis on Foot and Ankle: Symmetrical (BS)

EXTENSION – ABDUCTION – INTERNAL ROTATION
(D1 ex), LEFT AND RIGHT

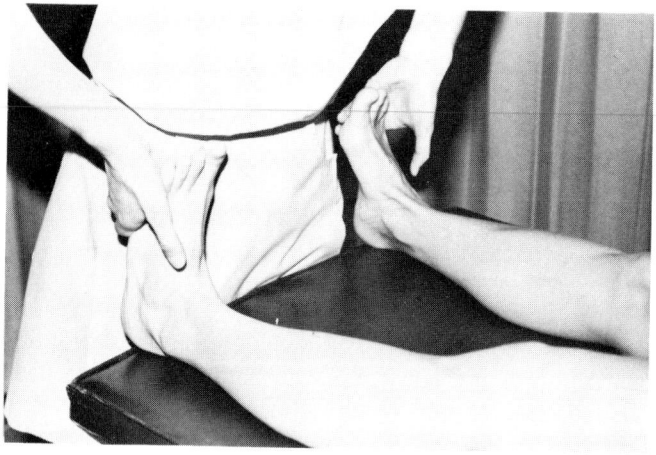

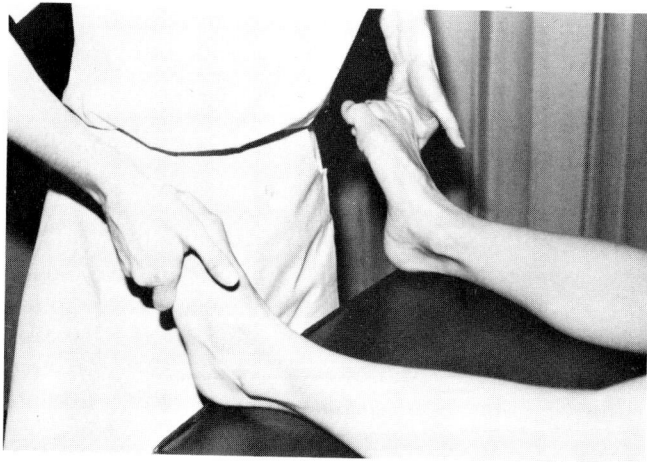

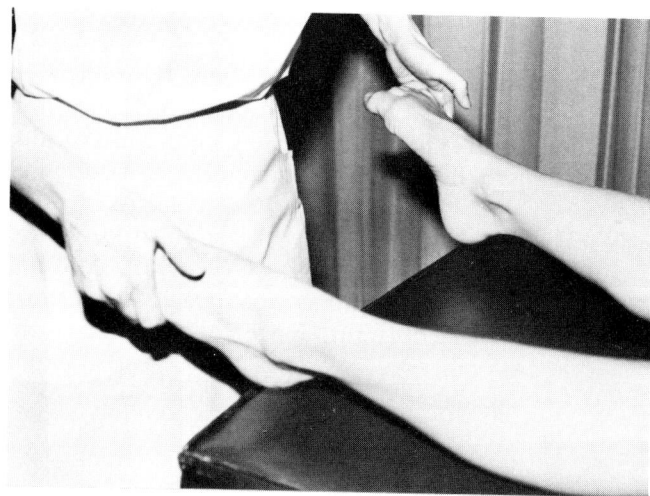

C

FIG. 1-140

Components of Motion

Free. In supine posture, head and shoulders may be elevated slightly so the eyes may follow foot and ankle movements. Hands may grip table edges for stability and reinforcement. Alternative postures: supine or sitting, knees flexed over table edge.

Resisted. Feet and ankles plantar flex and evert with extremity internal rotation.

A. Lengthened Range

Commands. Preparatory. "You are to push your feet down and out (D1 ex)." Action. "Bend your toes, push your feet down and out!"

Suggested Techniques. Stretch and resistance; slow reversal.

B. Middle Range

Commands. "Hold everything! Now continue to hold on the right while you push your left foot down and out! More! Again! And again! And relax."

Suggested Techniques. Repeated contractions on the left with facilitation from an isometric hold on the right.

C. Shortened Range

Commands. "Hold it! Now, don't let me move your feet up and in! Don't let me move them down and out! Hold, don't let me move them! And, hold! Now hold the right and don't let me move the left! Hold! And now, relax."

Suggested Techniques. Rhythmic stabilization followed by an isometric hold on the right and a hold – relax on the left.

Antagonistic Pattern

(BS): D1 fl, left and right (Fig. 1-139).

Related Unilateral Patterns

Lower extremity D1 ex with knee straight (Fig. 1-67).

Lower trunk flexion and extension: D1 ex of right foot and ankle (Figs. 1-41, 1-42, and 1-43).

Related Total Patterns (Mat Activities)

Rolling: prone toward supine (Figs. 1-158 to 1-161): left foot and ankle D1 ex.

Sitting: lower trunk rocking (Fig. 1-181, *C*). BS, D1 ex of foot and ankle is challenged.

Emphasis on Foot and Ankle: Symmetrical (BS)

FLEXION – ABDUCTION – INTERNAL ROTATION (D2 fl),
LEFT AND RIGHT

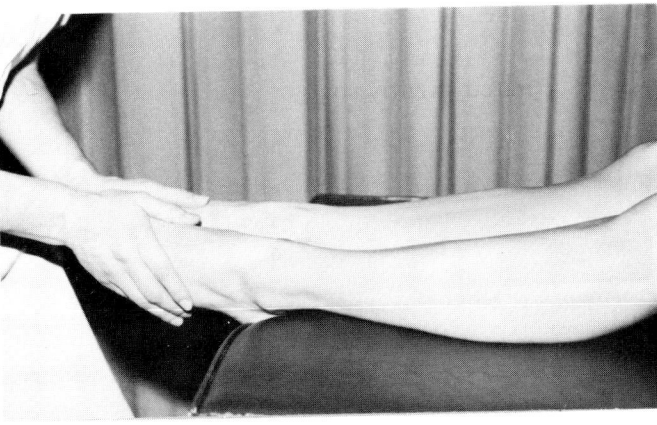

A

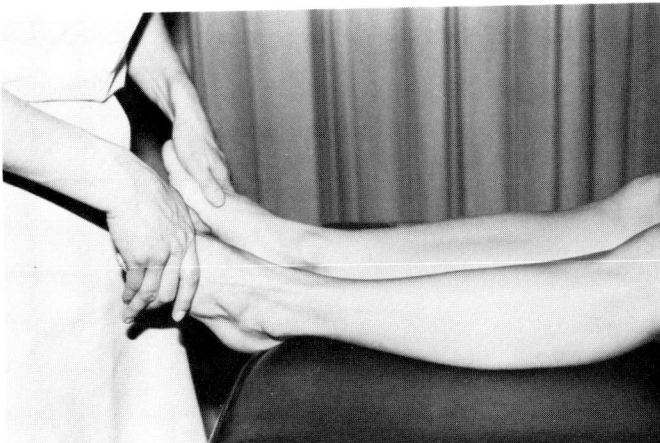

B

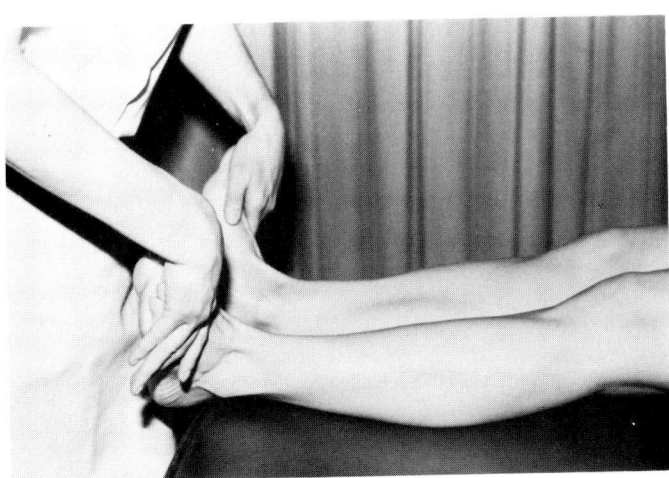

C

FIG. 1-141

Components of Motion

Free. In supine posture, head and shoulders may be elevated slightly so that eyes may follow foot and ankle movements. Hands may grip table edges for stability and reinforcement. Alternative postures: supine or sitting, knees flexed over table edge.

Resisted. Feet and ankles dorsiflex and evert with extremity internal rotation.

A. Lengthened Range

Commands. Preparatory. "You are to lift your feet up and out and turn your heels apart [D2 fl]." *Action.* "Lift your toes up and out!"

Suggested Techniques. Stretch and resistance; slow reversal.

B. Middle Range

Commands. "Hold it! And hold, and hold, and hold! Now pull all the way, up and out!"

Suggested Techniques. Rhythmic stabilization followed by stretch, then active resisted movement to shortened range.

C. Shortened Range

Commands. "Hold! [At limit of range, change manual contacts for antagonistic pattern.] Now push down and in! Hold! [Reverse hand position.] Now pull up and out! Hold! And relax."

Suggested Techniques. Slow reversal – hold.

Antagonistic Pattern

(BS): D2 ex, left and right (Fig. 1-142).

Related Unilateral Patterns

Lower extremity D2 fl with knee straight (Fig. 1-70).

Lower trunk flexion and extension: D2 fl of left foot and ankle (Figs. 1-38, 1-39, and 1-40).

Related Total Pattern (Mat Activity)

Crawling forward on elbows (Fig. 1-164). With manual contacts on dorsum of feet, D2 fl of foot and ankle is emphasized.

Emphasis on Foot and Ankle: Symmetrical (BS)

EXTENSION – ADDUCTION – EXTERNAL ROTATION (D2 ex), LEFT AND RIGHT

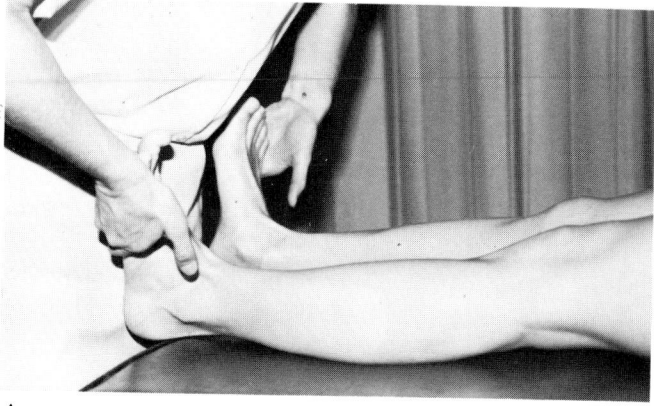

A

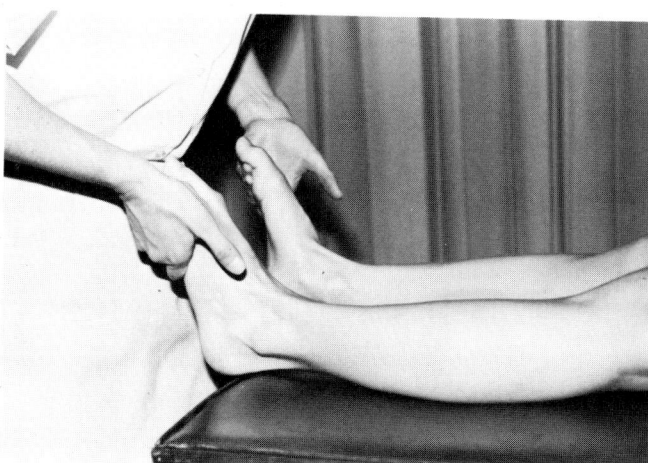

B

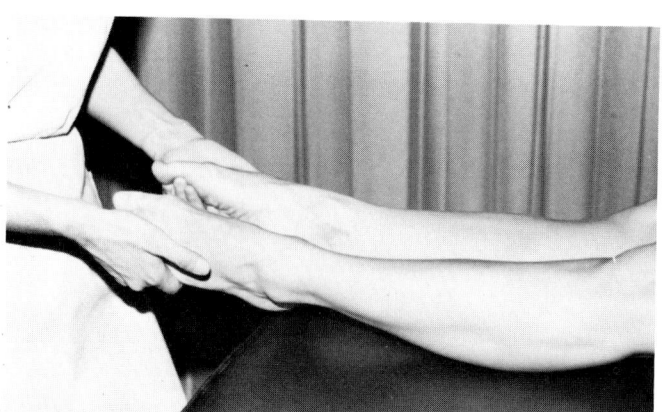

C

FIG. 1-142

Components of Motion

Free. In supine posture, head and shoulders may be elevated slightly so that eyes may follow foot and ankle movements. Hands may grip table edges for stability and reinforcement. Alternative postures: supine or sitting, knees flexed over table edge.

Resisted. Feet and ankles plantar flex and invert with extremity external rotation.

A. Lengthened Range

Commands. Preparatory. "You are to push your feet down and in as you turn your heel together [D2 ex]." *Action.* "Bend your toes! Push your feet down and in!"

Suggested Techniques. Stretch and resistance; slow reversal.

B. Middle Range

Commands. "Hold with your right! And push down and in with your left! More! Again! And again! And relax."

Suggested Techniques. Maximal resistance for "hold" on right; repeated contractions on left. Repeated contractions may be preceded or followed by rhythmic stabilization.

C. Shortened Range

Commands. "Hold it! Don't let me move you. And hold, and hold, and hold it! And relax."

Suggested Techniques. Rhythmic stabilization followed by relaxation.

Antagonistic Pattern

(BS): D2 fl, left and right (Fig. 1-141).

Related Unilateral Patterns

Lower extremity D2 ex with knee straight (Fig. 1-73).

Lower trunk flexion and extension: D2 ex of left foot and ankle (Figs. 1-41, 1-42, and 1-43).

Related Total Pattern (Mat Activity)

Crawling backward on elbows (Fig. 1-165): with manual contacts on plantar surface of feet. D2 ex of foot and ankle is emphasized.

Lower Extremity

Emphasis on Foot and Ankle: Asymmetrical (BA) Flexion, Left

FLEXION – ABDUCTION – INTERNAL ROTATION (D2 fl), LEFT; FLEXION – ADDUCTION – EXTERNAL ROTATION (D1 fl), RIGHT

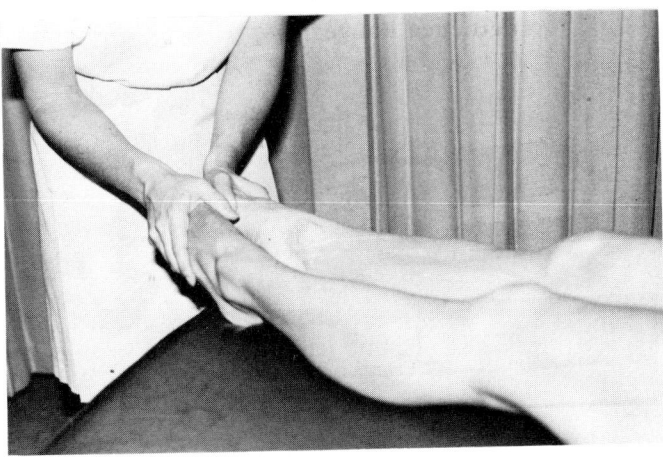

A

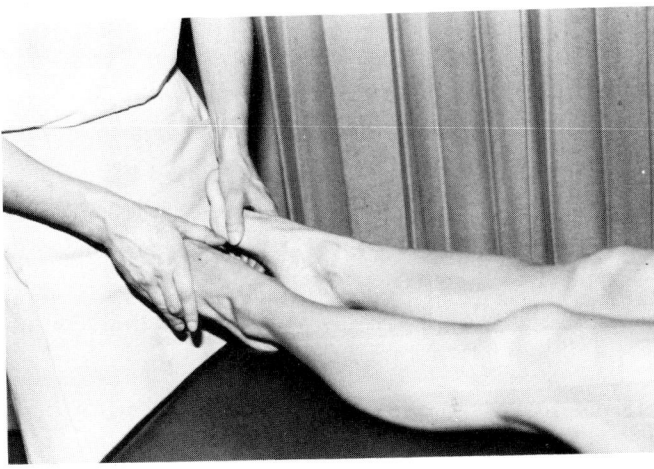

B

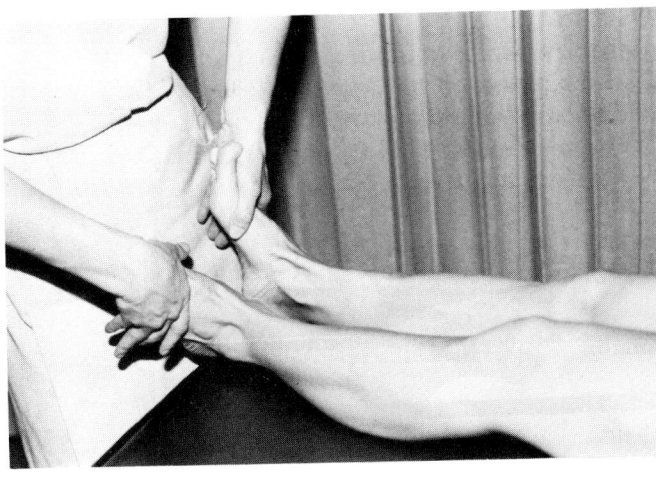

C

FIG. 1-143

Components of Motion

Free. In supine posture, head and shoulders may be elevated slightly so that eyes may follow foot and ankle movements. Hands may grip table edges for stability and reinforcement. Alternative postures: supine or sitting, knees flexed over table edge.

Resisted. Feet and ankles dorsiflex and inversion of right and eversion of left.

A. Lengthened Range

Commands. *Preparatory.* "You are to pull your feet up and to the left as you turn your heels to the left." *Action.* "Lift your toes! Pull your feet up and to the left!"

Suggested Techniques. Traction, stretch and resistance; slow reversals.

B. Middle Range

Commands. "Hold! Now lift your feet up and to the left! Again! More! Again! And again!"

Suggested Techniques. Repeated contractions.

C. Shortened Range

Commands. "Lift your toes up and to the left! Push, down and to the right! Lift up! Push down! And lift up! Hold! And relax."

Suggested Techniques. Quick reversals of this and its antagonistic pattern, ending with an isometric hold to emphasize foot and ankle dorsiflexion.

Antagonistic Pattern

(BA): D2 ex, left, and D1 ex, right (Fig. 1-144).

Related Unilateral Patterns

Lower extremity D1 fl with knee straight (Fig. 1-64); D2 fl with knee straight (Fig. 1-70).

Lower trunk flexion and extension: D1 fl of right foot and ankle, and D2 fl of left foot and ankle (Figs. 1-38, 1-39, and 1-40).

Related Total Patterns (Mat Activities)

Rising to plantigrade (Fig. 1-175, *C*).

Standing balance, compensatory movements (Fig. 1-187). Bilateral asymmetrical flexion to left of foot and ankle can be challenged by pushing the patient slightly off balance, backward and to the right; left, D2 fl, right, D1 fl).

Lower Extremity

Emphasis on Foot and Ankle: Asymmetrical (BA) Extension, Right

EXTENSION – ABDUCTION – INTERNAL ROTATION (D1 ex), RIGHT; EXTENSION – ADDUCTION – EXTERNAL ROTATION (D2 ex), LEFT

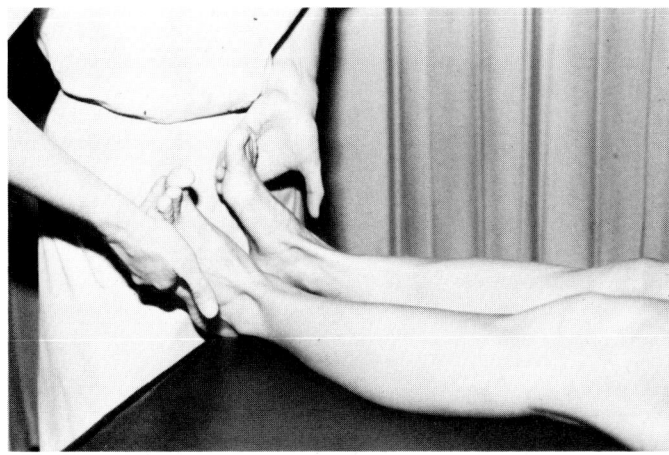

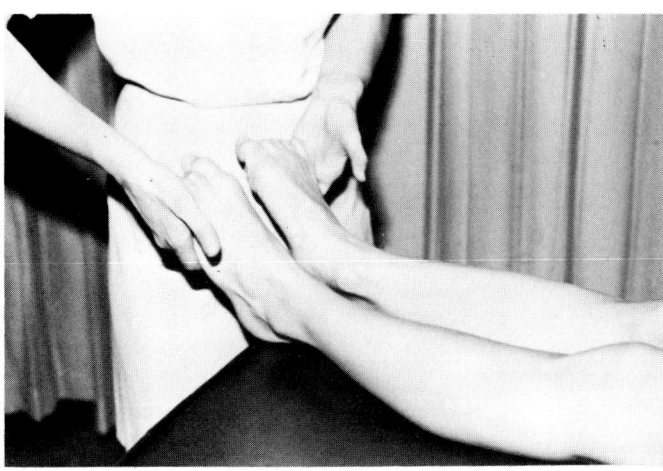

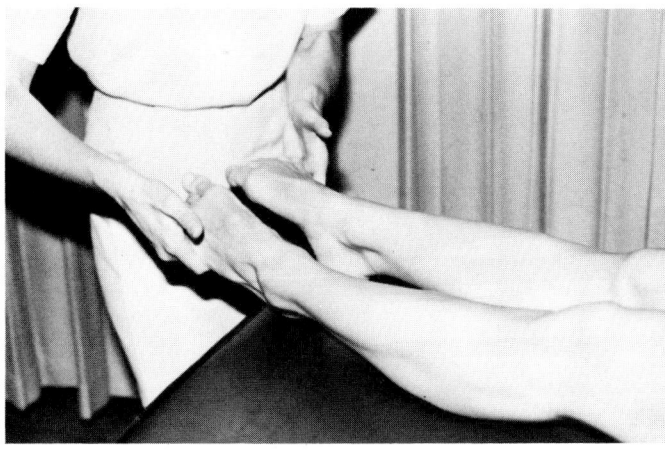

C

FIG. 1-144

Components of Motion

Free. In supine posture, head and shoulders may be elevated slightly so that eyes may follow foot and ankle movements. Hands may grip table edges for stability and reinforcement. Alternative postures: supine or sitting, knees flexed over table edge.

Resisted. Feet and ankles plantar flex with eversion of right and inversion of left.

A. Lengthened Range

Commands. Preparatory. "You are to push your feet down and to the right, turning your heels to the right." *Action.* "Bend your toes! Push your feet down to me!"

Suggested Techniques. Stretch and resistance.

B. Middle Range

Commands. "Hold it! And hold, and hold, and hold it! Now, change! Lift your toes up and to the left!" At lengthened range: "Hold again! And hold! And relax."

Suggested Techniques. Rhythmic stabilization followed by a reversal to lengthened range and completed with rhythmic stabilization in the lengthened range.

C. Shortened Range

Commands. "Now hold! Hold both feet still, and hold, and hold! And relax."

Suggested Techniques. Rhythmic stabilization, which can effectively be followed by repeated contractions progressing to slow reversals through this and its antagonistic pattern.

Antagonistic Pattern

(BA): D1 fl, right, and D2 fl, left (Fig. 1-143).

Related Unilateral Patterns

Lower extremity D1 ex with knee straight (Fig. 1-67); D2 ex with knee straight (Fig. 1-73).

Lower trunk flexion and extension: D1 ex of the right foot and ankle; D2 ex of the left foot and ankle (Figs. 1-41, 1-42, and 1-43).

Related Total Patterns (Mat Activities)

Pelvic elevation toward left with left foot in D2 ex and right foot D1 ex (Fig. 1-163). Elevating toward the right puts right foot in D2 ex and the left in D1 ex.

Rising to plantigrade (Fig. 1-175, *C*).

Standing balance, compensatory movements (Fig. 1-187). Bilateral asymmetrical extension to the right: foot and ankle can be challenged by pulling the patient slightly off balance forward and to the left; right ankle: D1 ex; left ankle: D2 ex.

Emphasis on Foot and Ankle: Reciprocal (BR, SD)

EXTENSION – ABDUCTION – INTERNAL ROTATION
(D1 ex), LEFT; FLEXION – ADDUCTION – EXTERNAL
ROTATION (D1 fl), RIGHT

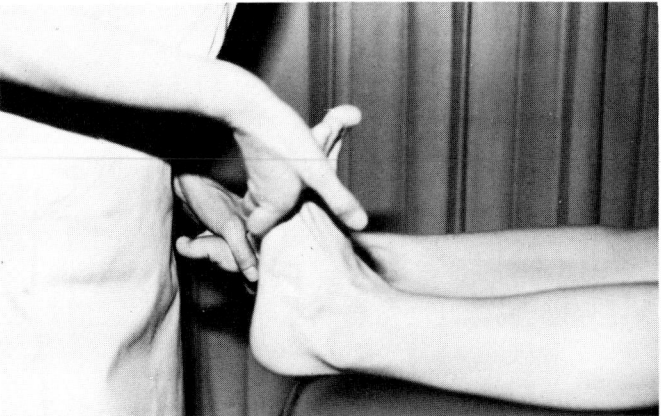

A

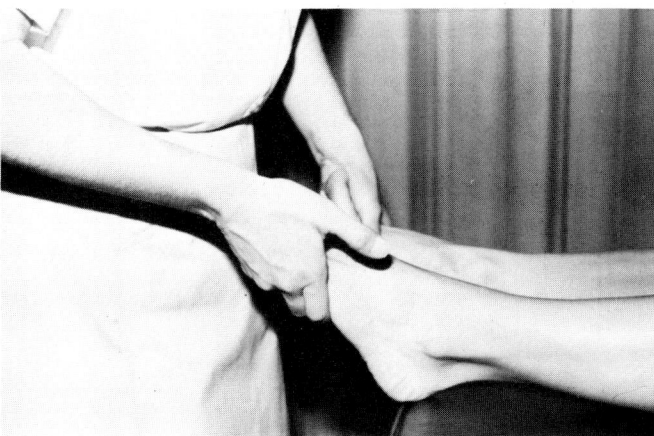

B

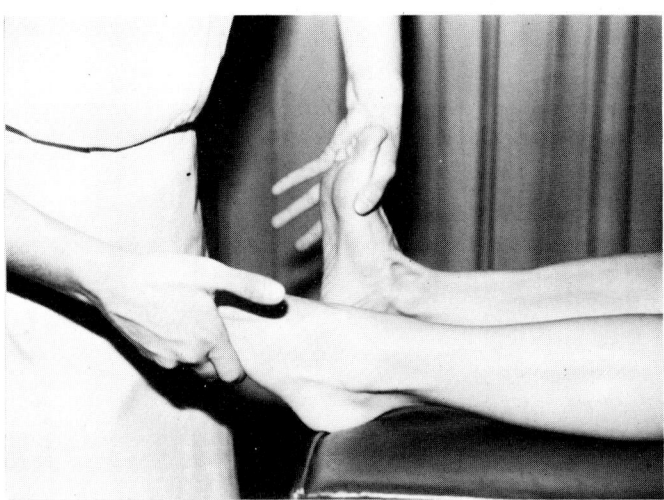

C

FIG. 1-145

Components of Motion

Free. In supine posture, head and shoulders may be elevated slightly so that eyes may follow foot and ankle movements. Hands may grip table edges for stability and reinforcement. Alternative postures: supine or sitting, knees flexed over table edge.

Resisted. Left foot and ankle plantar flex and evert with extremity internal rotation as right foot and ankle dorsiflex and invert with extremity external rotation.

A. Lengthened Range

Commands. *Preparatory.* "You are to push your left foot down and out [D1 ex], and pull your right foot in and up [D1 fl]." *Action.* "Push down and out with your left! Pull in and up with the right!"

Suggested Techniques. Stretch and resistance; slow reversal.

B. Middle Range

Commands. "Hold with your right! Push the left down and out! More! Again! And again! And relax."

Suggested Techniques. Maximal resistance for "hold" on right; repeated contractions on left; rhythmic stabilization followed by repeated contractions on left. Reverse and repeat sequence at various points in the range, *A* through *C*.

C. Shortened Range

Commands. "Hold everything! And hold, and hold, and hold it! Now change! Push down and out on the right; pull in and up on the left!" At middle range: "Hold again, and hold! And relax."

Suggested Techniques. Rhythmic stabilization followed by reversal to midrange, followed by stabilization.

Antagonistic Pattern

(BR, SD): D1 fl, left, and D1 ex, right (Fig. 1-146).

Related Unilateral Patterns

Lower extremity D1 fl with knee straight (Fig. 1-64); D1 ex with knee straight (Fig. 1-67).

Lower trunk flexion and extension: D1 fl of right foot and ankle (Figs. 1-38, 1-39, and 1-40); D1 ex of right foot and ankle (Figs. 1-41, 1-42, and 1-43).

Emphasis on Foot and Ankle: Reciprocal (BR, SD)

FLEXION – ADDUCTION – EXTERNAL ROTATION (D1 fl),
LEFT; EXTENSION – ABDUCTION – INTERNAL
ROTATION (D1 ex), RIGHT

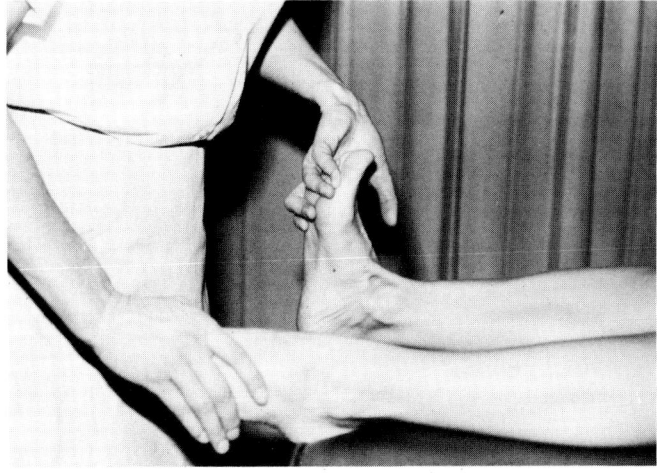

A

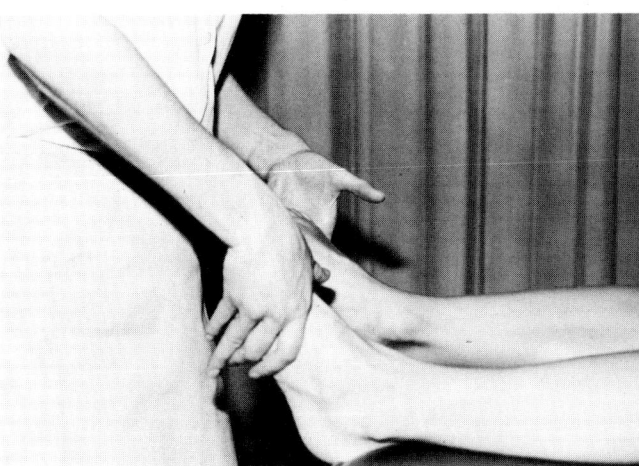

B

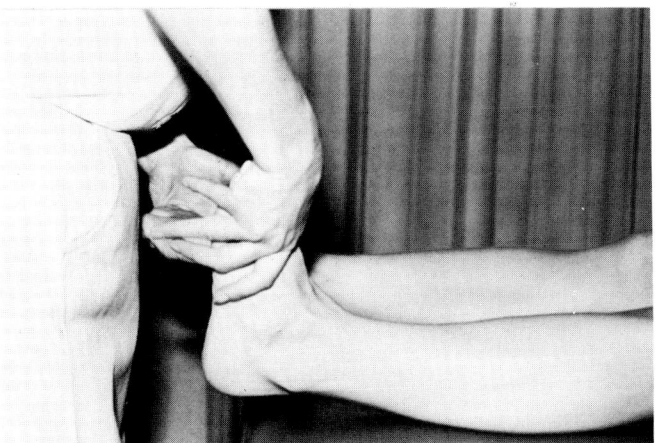

C

FIG. 1-146

Components of Motion

Free. In supine posture, head and shoulders may be elevated slightly so that eyes may follow foot and ankle movements. Hands may grip table edges for stability and reinforcement. Alternative postures: supine or sitting, knees flexed over table edge.

Resisted. Left foot and ankle dorsiflex and invert with extremity external rotation as right foot and ankle plantar flex and evert with extremity internal rotation.

A. Lengthened Range

Commands. Preparatory. "You are to pull your left foot in and up [D1 fl], and push your right foot down and out [D1 ex]." *Action.* "Pull in and up with your left! Push down and out with your right!"

Suggested Techniques. Stretch and resistance; slow reversal.

B. Middle Range

Commands. "Hold everything! Now keep the hold on the right! Pull in and up on the left! More! Again! And again! And relax."

Suggested Techniques. Maximal resistance for "hold" on right to facilitate repeated contractions of the left from middle range to shortened. Rhythmic stabilization may be effectively added.

C. Shortened Range

Commands. "Hold it! Now change; pull the right in and up and push the left down and out! Hold it! Now change; right down and out, left in and up. Hold it! Now change! Hold! And change! Hold! Now hold the right and pull the left in and up! Again! And again! And again! Hold it! And hold! And hold! And hold! And relax."

Suggested Techniques. Slow reversal – hold, *A* through *C*, followed by repeated contractions on left, ending with rhythmic stabilization.

Antagonistic Pattern

(BR, SD): D1 ex, left, and D1 fl, right (Fig. 1-145).

Related Unilateral Patterns

Lower extremity D1 fl with knee straight (Fig. 1-64); D1 ex with knee straight (Fig. 1-67).

Lower trunk flexion and extension: D1 fl of right foot and ankle (Figs. 1-38, 1-39, and 1-40); D1 ex of right foot and ankle (Figs. 1-41, 1-42, and 1-43).

Emphasis on Foot and Ankle: Reciprocal (BR, SD)

FLEXION – ABDUCTION – INTERNAL ROTATION (D2 fl),
LEFT; EXTENSION – ADDUCTION – EXTERNAL ROTATION
(D2 ex), RIGHT

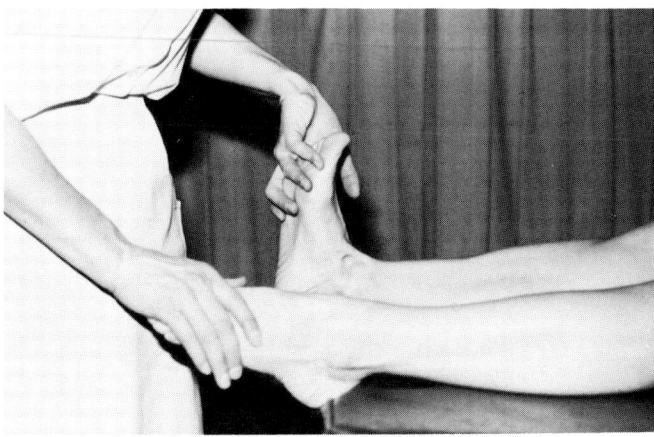

A

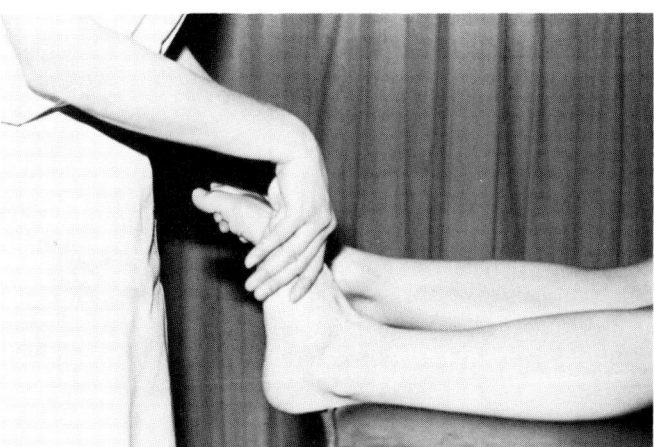

B

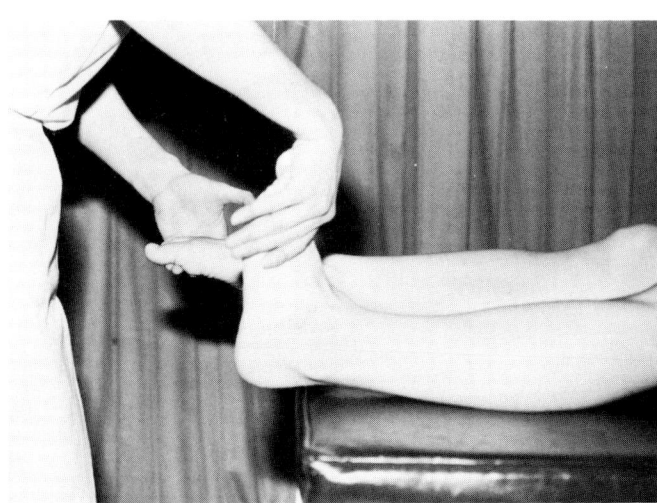

C

FIG. 1-147

Components of Motion

Free. In supine posture, head and shoulders may be elevated slightly so that eyes may follow foot and ankle movements. Hands may grip table edges for stability and reinforcement. Alternative postures: supine or sitting, knees flexed over table edge.

Resisted. Left foot and ankle dorsiflex and evert with extremity internal rotation as right foot and ankle plantar flex and invert with extremity external rotation.

A. Lengthened Range

Commands. *Preparatory.* "You are to pull your left foot up and out (D2 fl), and push your right foot down and in (D2 ex)." *Action.* "Lift your toes, pull your left foot up and out! Bend your toes and push your right foot down and in!"

Suggested Techniques. Stretch and resistance; slow reversal.

B. Middle Range

Commands. "Now hold! And hold, and hold, and hold! Now hold with the right and pull up and out with left again. And again, and relax."

Suggested Techniques. Rhythmic stabilization, repeated contractions.

C. Shortened Range

Commands. Reverse manual contacts: "Pull your right foot up and out, your left down and in." Place hands as in *A*: "Pull up with the left, push down with the right! Hold it! Now push with the right. Keep on holding with the left! And push with the right. Keep on holding with the left! And push with the right! And again! Once more. And relax."

Suggested Techniques. Stretch, resistance; repeated contractions of right with reinforcement by holding of left.

Antagonistic Pattern

(BR, SD): D2 ex, left, and D2 fl, right (Fig. 1-148).

Related Unilateral Patterns

Lower extremity D2 fl with knee straight (Fig. 1-70); D2 ex with knee straight (Fig. 1-73).

Related Total Patterns (Mat Activities)

Crawling forward on elbows (Fig. 1-164).

Crawling backward on elbows (Fig. 1-165). Reciprocal movements of lower extremities: flexed extremity producing D2 fl, extended extremity D2 ex.

Lower Extremity

EXTENSION – ADDUCTION – EXTERNAL ROTATION
(D2 ex), LEFT; FLEXION – ABDUCTION – INTERNAL
ROTATION (D2 fl), RIGHT

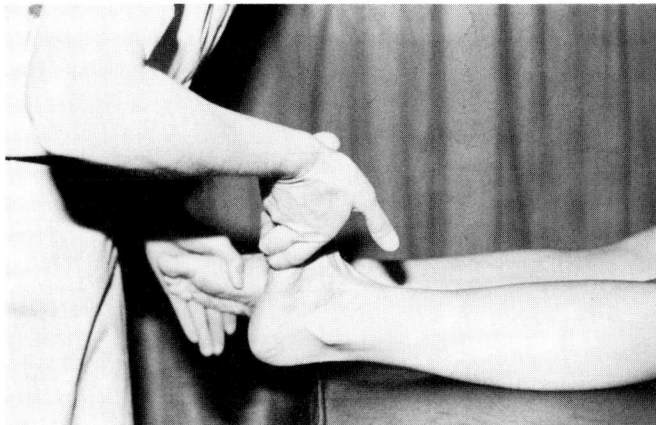

A

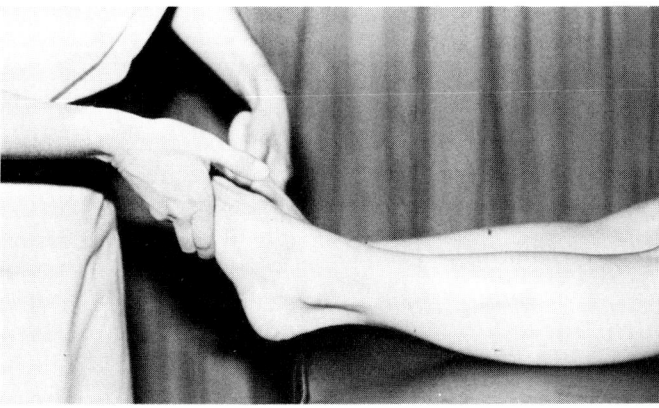

B

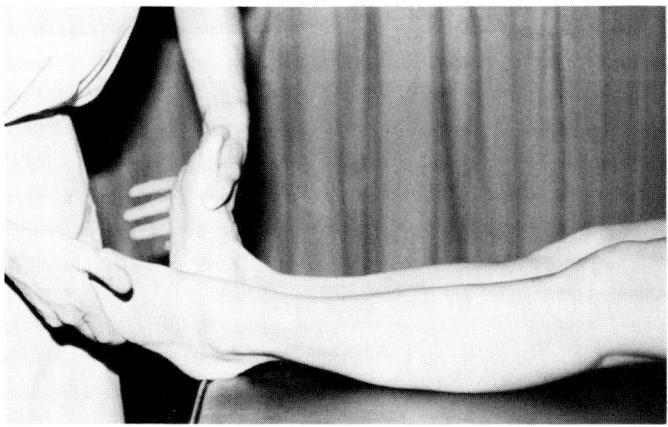

C

FIG. 1-148

Components of Motion

Free. In supine posture, head and shoulders may be elevated slightly so that eyes may follow foot and ankle movements. Hands may grip table edges for stability and reinforcement. Alternative postures: supine or sitting, knees flexed over table edge.

Resisted. Left foot and ankle plantar flex and invert with extremity external rotation as right foot and ankle dorsiflex and evert with extremity internal rotation.

A. Lengthened Range

Commands. *Preparatory.* "You are to push your left foot down and in [D2 ex], and pull your right foot up and out [D2 fl]." *Action.* "Bend your toes, push your left foot down and in! Lift your toes, pull your right foot up and out!"

Suggested Techniques. Stretch and resistance; slow reversal.

B. Middle Range

Commands. "Hold! Now pull up and out with the left and push down and in with the right. Hold! And change! Hold! Change! Hold! Change! Hold! And relax."

Suggested Techniques. Slow reversal – hold to various points in middle range.

C. Shortened Range

Commands. "Now hold the left foot! Don't let me move it! Pull the right foot up and out! Pull it up! Again! And again! Now hold it! Push the left foot down and in! Push it down! Again! And again! Hold everything! Now pull the left up and out and the right down and in. Hold! Change! Hold! and relax."

Suggested Techniques. Repeated contractions on right with hold on left, followed by repeated contractions on left with hold on right, ending the sequence with slow reversal – hold.

Antagonistic Pattern

(BR, SD): D2 fl, left, and D2 ex, right (Fig. 1-147).

Related Unilateral Patterns

Lower extremity D2 fl with knee straight (Fig. 1-70); D2 ex with knee straight (Fig. 1-73).

Related Total Patterns (Mat Activities)

Crawling forward on elbows (Fig. 1-164).

Crawling backward on elbows (Fig. 1-165). Reciprocal movements of lower extremities: flexed extremity producing D2 fl; extended extremity D2 ex.

Lower Extremity

Emphasis on Foot and Ankle: Reciprocal, in Crossed Diagonals (BR, CD)

FLEXION – ABDUCTION – INTERNAL ROTATION (D2 fl),
LEFT; EXTENSION – ABDUCTION – INTERNAL
ROTATION (D1 ex), RIGHT

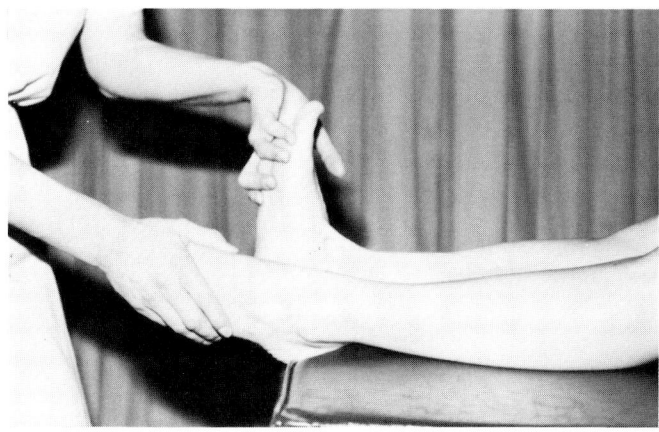

A

B

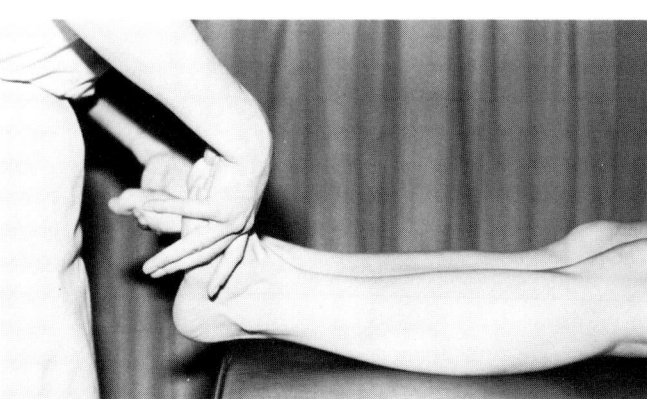

C

FIG. 1-149

Components of Motion

Free. In supine posture, head and shoulders may be elevated slightly so that eyes may follow foot and ankle movements. Hands may grip table edges for stability and reinforcement. Alternative postures: supine or sitting, knees flexed over table edge.

Resisted. Left foot and ankle dorsiflex and evert with extremity internal rotation as right foot and ankle plantar flex and evert with extremity internal rotation.

A. Lengthened Range

Commands. *Preparatory.* "You are to pull your left foot up and out [D2 fl] as you push your right foot down and out [D1 ex]." *Action.* "Lift your toes! Pull your left up and out. Bend your toes! Push the right down and out!"

Suggested Techniques. Stretch and resistance; slow reversal.

B. Middle Range

Commands. "Hold with your right! And pull your left up and out! More! Again! And again! And relax."

Suggested Techniques. Maximal resistance for "hold" on right; repeated contractions on left. Repeated contractions may be preceded or followed by rhythmic stabilization. Slow reversals may follow with this sequence of techniques performed at various points in the range.

C. Shortened Range

Commands. "Hold it! And hold! And hold! Now keep the hold on the left and don't let me move your right foot! Come on, hold it! Relax the right! Now push it down and out! Again! And again! And relax."

Suggested Techniques. Rhythmic stabilization followed by hold – relax for increased right plantar flexion followed by repeated contractions of right plantar flexion.

Antagonistic Pattern

(BR, CD): D2 ex, left, and D1 fl, right (Fig. 1-150).

Related Unilateral Patterns

Lower extremity D1 ex with knee straight (Fig. 1-67); D2 fl with knee straight (Fig. 1-70).

Lower trunk flexion and extension: D1 ex of right foot and ankle (Figs. 1-41, 1-42, and 1-43); D2 ex of left foot and ankle (Fig. 1-38, 1-39, and 1-40).

Related Total Patterns (Mat Activities)

Creeping forward to left (Fig. 1-171, 1-172, and 1-173).* Reciprocal movements of lower extremities: left leg uses foot and ankle D2 fl in swing and D2 ex in stance, while right leg uses foot and ankle D1 ex in stance and D1 fl in swing.

* Patterns of the lower extremities can be changed by changing the direction of the diagonal progression. Flexion and extension dominance can be reversed by reversing the forward or backward movement.

Lower Extremity

Emphasis on Foot and Ankle: Reciprocal, in Crossed Diagonals (BR, CD)

EXTENSION – ADDUCTION – EXTERNAL ROTATION (D2 ex), LEFT; FLEXION – ADDUCTION – EXTERNAL ROTATION (D1 fl), RIGHT

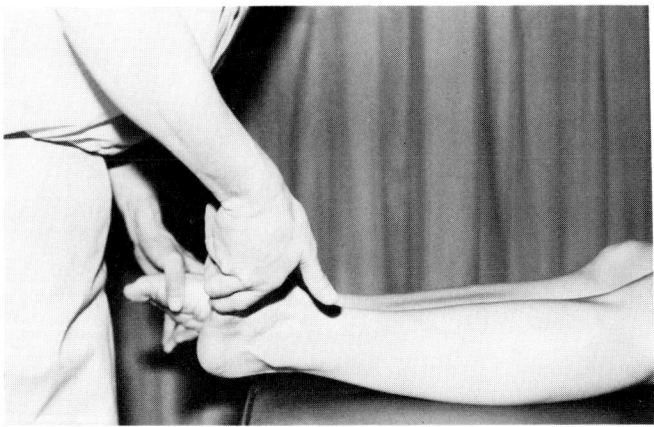

A

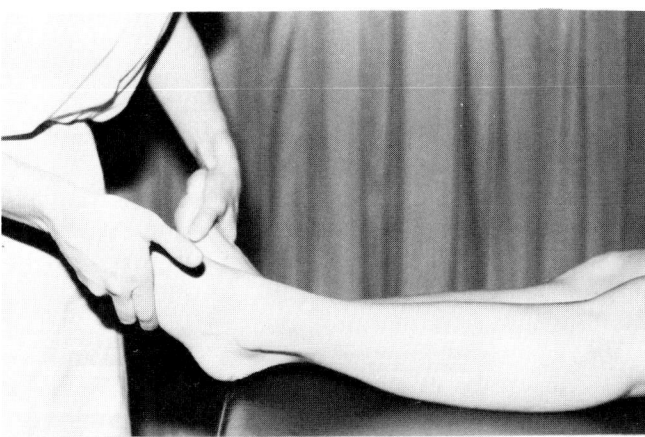

B

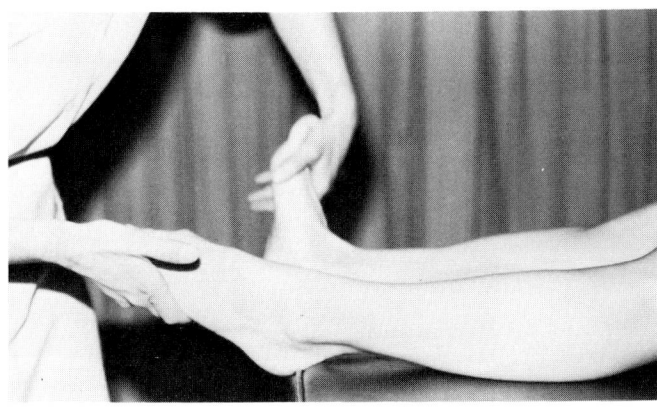

C

FIG. 1-150

Components of Motion

Free. In supine posture, head and shoulders may be elevated slightly so that eyes may follow foot and ankle movements. Hands may grip table edges for stability and reinforcement. Alternative postures: supine or sitting, knees flexed over table edge.

Resisted. Left foot and ankle plantar flex and invert with extremity external rotation as right foot and ankle dorsiflex and invert with extremity external rotation.

A. Lengthened Range

Commands. *Preparatory.* "You are to push your left foot down and in [D2 ex] as you pull your right in and up [D1 fl]. Heels turn toward each other." *Action.* "Bend your toes! Push your left foot down and in! Lift your toes! Pull your right up and in!"

Suggested Techniques. Stretch and resistance; slow reversal.

B. Middle Range

Commands. "Hold! Now keep the hold on the right and push down and in with the left! Again! And push! And hold on the left! Now pull in and up on the right! And again! Hold on left! In and up on the right! And rest!"

Suggested Techniques. Repeated contractions on left as right holds. Emphasize left, then hold with left and emphasize right.

C. Shortened Range

Commands. "Now hold! Hold both feet, and hold, and hold! And relax."

Suggested Techniques. Rhythmic stabilization. This may be followed by repeated contractions for emphasis, or slow reversal, slow reversal – hold.

Antagonistic Pattern

(BR, CD): D2 fl, left, and D1 ex, right (Fig. 1-149).

Related Unilateral Patterns

Lower extremity D1 fl with knee straight (Fig. 1-64); D2 ex with knee straight (Fig. 1-73).

Lower trunk flexion and extension: D1 fl of right foot and ankle (Figs. 1-38, 1-39, and 1-40); D2 ex of left foot and ankle (Figs. 1-41, 1-42, and 1-43).

Related Total Patterns (Mat Activities)

Bipedal walking forward to right (Fig. 1-188).* Reciprocal movements of lower extremities: right leg uses foot and ankle D2 fl in swing and D2 ex in stance, while left leg uses foot and ankle D1 ex in stance and D1 fl in swing.

* Patterns of the lower extremities can be changed by changing the direction of the diagonal progression. Flexion and extension dominance can be reversed by reversing the forward or backward movement.

RELATED ASPECTS OF MOTOR BEHAVIOR

The development of motor behavior is expressed in pattern movement. An ordered sequence of motor acts emerges in the normal process of growth. The overt manifestations of growth and development bear analysis. Hooker observed early fetal activity, and Humphrey identified the corresponding anatomical patterns.[23,24] Gesell and his coworkers, and McGraw recorded their observations of the ever-changing and interweaving of activities as motor behavior grows and matures after birth.[11,35] The observations of these workers are, in a sense, "clinical" observations. That which can be seen has been noted. The "total structure in action" can be seen; developing patterns of movement can be observed. The component patterns of total movement patterns can be analyzed.

Motor Development

TOTAL TO INDIVIDUATED

Motor development has certain elements and characteristics that have been identified. Hooker, in his studies of early fetal activity, found that a response occurs first to sensory stimulation around the mouth, and that the response is a total one; all segments that are functioning participate in a mass movement.[23] The head and neck flex lateralward. This is followed by lateral flexion of the trunk with extension of the arms. Later in the developmental process, an individual segment may be stimulated and will respond specifically without a total, mass response. Fetal movements are reflex in nature and may be termed primitive for the human species. However, they are the forerunners of purposeful movement.

PROXIMAL–DISTAL TO DISTAL–PROXIMAL

The development of motor function in the fetus has direction.[23] The direction is from head to foot (cephalocaudad) or from superior to inferior regions of the body. The direction is also from proximal to distal, that is, movements of the neck and shoulders occur before movements of the hand are evident. Gesell has simply stated, "The organization of behavior begins long before birth, and the general direction of this organization is from head to foot, from proximal to distal segments. Lips and tongue lead, eye muscles follow, then neck, shoulder, arms, hands, fingers, trunk, legs, feet."[11] Sensory development, too, is cephalocaudal, but when sensation has arrived in the feet and hands, stimulation of a segment produces a sequence of movement in a distal to proximal direction, for exam-ple, when the palm is stimulated, the fingers flex and the wrist flexes.[23] Such is the beginning of timed, coordinated movement.

REFLEXIVE TO DELIBERATE

After birth, while the developmental process continues in a cephalocaudad and proximal–distal direction, the first movements and postural attitudes as observed by McGraw and by Gesell and his co-workers are reflex in character.[11,35] The response to a startling stimulus (Moro reflex) is a total response of bodily movement. The asymmetric tonic neck reflex induces a postural attitude of the total structure. These reflexes have components used later in rolling from supine to prone. In the newborn, the turning of the head, the roving movements of the eyes, grasping of the fingers, rapid flexion and extension of the lower extremities, and stepping movements are reflex responses ready for transition to functional movements. As the growth process continues and the repertoire of activities enlarges, movements take on an automatic quality; the child appears to practice a newly acquired movement as, for example, while rolling from supine to prone.[35] He repeats rolling well in advance of using the movement to assume a sitting posture. As he progresses, his rolling movements become more deliberate and he incorporates them in functional activities. He uses rolling from supine as he arises to a sitting position. He rolls from supine to prone as preparation for progression in the prone position. In the entire course of development of motor behavior, primitive responses give way to controlled movements and postures that may be achieved automatically or deliberately as the occasion requires.[35] See Table 1-5, Equilibrium Reactions (Compensatory Movements).

MOTILE TO STABILE

Another characteristic of developing motor behavior is that movement precedes sustained posture. When the fetus is stimulated, resultant movement fades and terminates. After birth, motility is a striking feature of a newborn's behavior.[35] The newborn infant moves his extremities rapidly, but unless he cries these movements are rarely seen as a sustained effort. The postural and righting reflexes are invoked by movement, by alterations of the position of the head in space and in relation to the trunk and extremities, or the trunk and extremities in relation to the head.[40] As with other aspects of developing motor behavior, the righting response is composed of reflexes that have developed in a cephalocaudad direction.[35] From quiescent positions, such as supine, lateral (sidelying), or prone,

Table 1-5. Equilibrium Reactions (Compensatory Movements)

Stimuli		Rate of Stimulus	Response
Experimental*	**Natural**		
Tilt of supporting surface	"Follow the leader": walking a board laid across a stream; standing on a bus: sudden jerk or stopping, or sway while turning corner	Fast or quick disturbance	Fast or quick response through stimulation of labyrinths
Tilt of body in space	Being jostled in a crowd. Playing football (contact sport).	Slow or gradual disturbance	Slow or gradual response through stimulation of proprioceptors

* After Weisz S: Studies in equilibrium reaction. J Nerv Ment Dis 88:150, 1938 (Cites Magnus, Rademaker, Schaltenbrand, Hoff and Schilder, and others)

movement is necessary to alter position. In this respect, movement may be considered more primitive than sustained posture. Yet, as motor behavior matures, the stability of sustained posture is necessary for purposeful movement.

OVERLAPPING TO INTEGRATIVE

Motor abilities develop in sequence, and those that appear early in the sequence overlap with or contribute to those that emerge later. This characteristic of development may be observed in the normal child. There is an interweaving of component movement patterns and component postures. One activity prepares the way for another. For example, rolling is a component of the human righting response, the achievement of an erect posture.[35] Thus, the ability to roll leads to the ability to assume and sustain a sitting posture. The ability to assume and sustain a sitting posture leads to the ability to assume and sustain a standing posture. The ability to roll from supine to prone and from prone to supine prepares for the ability to creep. The ability to roll and the ability to creep lead to the ability to walk. The entire process is in continuum. Within the sequence of interrelated activities, motor behavior becomes integrated and movement becomes coordinated, functional, selective, and versatile.

GROSS TO SELECTIVE

While the development of component movement patterns interweaves and overlaps, the participation of bodily segments in relation to the neck and trunk becomes more controlled, more varied in degree and range of movement, and, therefore, more complex. At first, movement tends toward full ranges: complete range of flexion, then complete range of extension. There is an oscillation between extremes.[35] Then later, as integration occurs, with controlled posture and movement interacting as necessary, direction and range of movement are subservient to the total activity

or pattern of movement. See Table 1-6, Counterparts of Direction.

A total pattern of purposeful movement, such as walking, has direction that may be continued, discontinued, or reversed at will. Reversal of movement occurs within a total pattern, that is, the reciprocation of extremities during walking. Although the total pattern of walking has a forward movement, the forward direction is achieved through reversing movements. That is, there is an alternation of activity between opposite component patterns of movement as in dorsiflexion, then plantar flexion of the foot and ankle. Thus, alternation of activity, reversal of movement, occurs between component patterns of movement and within component patterns, and the total pattern may be reversed.

By the time motor ability has matured, innumerable combinations of movement of head and neck, trunk, and upper and lower extremities may be performed. There is selectivity and combining of movement patterns. See Table 1-7, Interaction of Segments.

The extremities contribute component patterns

Table 1-6. Counterparts of Direction

Direction	Total Patterns	Anatomical Planes
Vertical	Forward/backward (up/down)	Flexion/extension
Horizontal	Sideward, L/R	Abduction/adduction
Circular	Clockwise/counter-clockwise	External/internal rotation
Oblique/diagonal	Forward to L/R; backward to R/L	Diagonal flexion, L/R; diagonal extension, R/L

Gesell observed and reported that the sequence of development of direction is from vertical to horizontal to circular to oblique.[10] The counterparts of direction above are expressed in terms of a total pattern of movement or of posture.

Table 1-7. Interaction of Segments

Combined Movements of Paired Extremities

Symmetrical: perform like movements at the same time

Asymmetrical: perform movements toward one side at the same time

Reciprocal: perform movements in opposite direction at the same time

Combined Movements of Upper and Lower Extremities

Ipsilateral: extremities of same side move in same direction at same time

Contralateral: extremities of opposite sides move in same direction at same time

Diagonal reciprocal: contralateral extremities move in same direction at same time while opposite contralateral extremities move in opposite direction

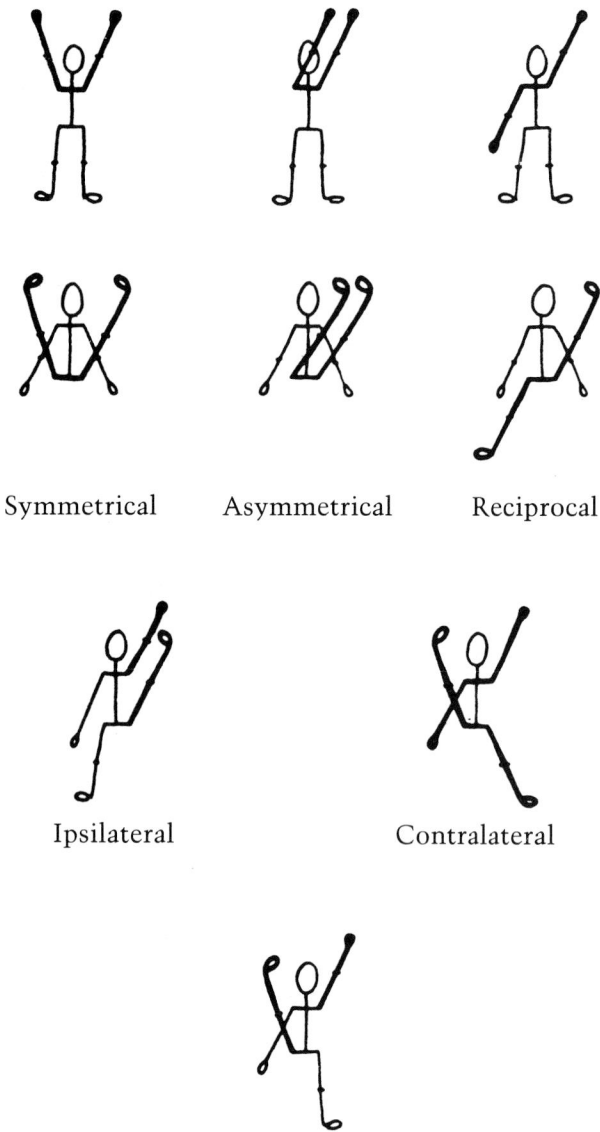

Symmetrical   Asymmetrical   Reciprocal

Ipsilateral   Contralateral

Diagonal reciprocal

to a total pattern in various ways. At first, in the supine position, movements of the upper and lower extremities tend to be symmetric (like movements of upper or lower extremities at the same time), although asymmetric (movement of upper or lower extremities to one side at the same time) and alternating movements do occur.[11] As the child learns to roll, ipsilateral movements (arm and leg of same side) participate. In the prone position, ipsilateral or symmetric movements occur as well as alternating movements of arms and legs.[35] As prone progression is achieved, simultaneous movements of an upper extremity and the contralateral (of the opposite side) lower extremity contribute reciprocally to crawling and creeping.

In fetal activity and in newborn behavior, flexion truly dominates extension.[35] Although flexion and extension continue to be the major components of motion, combinations of these with the components of adduction and abduction, external rotation and internal rotation become increasingly apparent as the child's repertoire of movements enlarges. He is not limited to one direction of movement. He uses combined components as he moves forward, backward, turns in a circle, and moves sideward and diagonally in all directions (see Table 1-6). All component patterns of motion within the activity, the total movement pattern, serve his purposes in varying degrees at various times as he needs them. In the sitting posture, the child is free to move his upper extremities bilaterally in symmetric and asymmetric movements or in unilateral movements (one arm, or one leg, at a time), or in a reciprocal fashion (opposite movements of opposite extremities at the same time). In walking, he uses reciprocal motions of upper and lower extremities. He jumps with bilateral movements. Hopping is a unilateral activity for one lower extremity. Skipping and leaping require reciprocation of the extremities.

INCOORDINATE TO COORDINATE

During the time that the infant is developing his neuromotor ability, maturation of his special senses, too, is progressing.[35] Developing vision serves movement and movement serves vision. Hand–eye coordination in reaching and prehension are sensorimotor activities, certain foundations for which were laid down in the tonic neck reflex pattern.[11] The developing child looks or gazes at the object for which he reaches and grasps. Movements of the hand and arm (and of the head, neck, trunk, and other segments as the occasion demands) may follow the visual phase of moving the eyes and looking, and, in turn, the visual act may follow movement of the hand. When an object is within reach, the child may regard it either before or after he grasps it. Locomotor activities and prone postures where the hands and arms reach or support weight must contribute to the development of prehension and manipulative skills. When the infant is prone, his fingers extend as he supports his weight on his palms with elbows extended. When he releases support on his arms, he reaches an arm forward and may flex his fingers and pull on the surface.[35] This type of finger extension and flexion precedes and promotes functional grasp and release of objects. The development of auditory responses, too, plays an important role in the development of motor behavior. As the infant begins to locate the sources of sounds, he turns his head appropriately.[11] Sound becomes a stimulus for movement. As he interprets sound and language, he begins to move in response to sounds and words.

Coordinated Movement

The striking feature of *mature* movement is that it is coordinated. Other features such as strength, endurance, and rate of movement that support coordination are evident well in advance of purposeful and functional movement. The infant exhibits strength as he grasps, and strength of the total musculature during crying. He exhibits endurance for repeating movement. He moves his extremities rhythmically and rapidly or slowly, although in random fashion. However, except for movements that have to do with vital activities, such as breathing, sucking, swallowing, peristalsis, micturition, and defecation, the newborn's movements lack a purposeful quality. As he grows, as motor behavior becomes organized from head to foot, the coordination of his movements, too, proceeds from head to foot. The upper extremities reveal coordinated movement, as in precise prehension, before the lower extremities are fully developed for independent walking.[11]

TIMED INTERACTION

In order for a movement to be coordinated it must have a sequence of action and interaction within and between segments. The sequence and timing of a movement permits ease of movement with economy of effort. There is a neat balance and counteraction between antagonistic components. For example, in rolling from supine to prone toward the left, the head turns toward the left and the neck proceeds into extension. As the head and neck move and the spine extends, the right upper extremity is prepared to lead, while the foot of the right lower extremity may push against the surface to elevate the pelvis; then the right upper and lower extremities lift across toward the chin side (to the left). Ordinarily the upper extremity leads the rolling movement, but variations on this sequence may occur. Later, the lower extremity may be lifted first and then the upper extremity may follow.[35] Nevertheless, the act is coordinated and exhibits a timed sequence of component patterns of movement of the extremities in relation to the head, neck, and trunk. As the timed sequence is established, the movement is

reproducible on demand.

In coordinated, mature movement the sequence within the extremities is from distal to proximal. Again, in the act of rolling, the leading hand and arm move before the shoulder girdle is completely elevated. If the shoulder were to move first, the movement of the hand and arm would appear to be an "afterthought." If the pelvis were to be completely elevated and rotated before the foot pushed against the surface or proceeded to lift across, the lower extremity would deter rolling rather than enhance it.

SEQUENTIAL ACTION OF MUSCLES

Coordinate movement with body parts interacting in sequence includes a sequential action of muscles. Those muscles necessary to the accomplishment of a movement will respond in the necessary sequence, and in a distal to proximal direction, although the development of the musculature has been from proximal to distal.[12] As in rolling to prone, when the foot pushes on the surface, plantar flexion with eversion serves through action of the toe flexors, the peroneus longus, and the gastrocnemius. Having pushed, the foot then serves the lifting of the extremity by dorsiflexing with inversion through action of the toe extensors and the anterior tibial, since the lifting phase is toward the midline of the body. However, if the lower extremity is lifted without push-off, it is lifted with the foot dorsiflexing, and there is no need for plantar flexion with eversion of the foot. Plantar flexion without push-off would deter the forward movement of the lower extremity by introducing an antagonistic movement; it would disturb the sequence of the total pattern of muscle action, and thus the coordination of the movement.

Summary

In summary, the development of motor behavior is expressed in an orderly sequence of patterned movements. Growth of sensorimotor activity has a cephalocaudad and proximal–distal direction, but coordinated movement has a distal to proximal sequence. Movements that are primitive and reflex in nature are altered by growth so that movement becomes automatic and then deliberate or purposeful. Upon maturity, coordinated, functional movement may have both automatic and deliberate aspects. Movement precedes postural control; movement is necessary to alter position or posture; posture is necessary to purposeful movement. In the sequence of developmental activities, the component patterns of movement and posture that make up one activity contribute to or overlap with the components of other activities in the sequence. Sensory development and motor development progress together and are inseparable. The end result of the process is a vast repertoire of coordinated movements and combinations of movements.

RATIONALE

The fundamental motor activities of the developmental sequence are interrelated and universal. Every human being who is capable of normal movement and balanced postures has learned to roll from supine to prone and from prone to supine, to progress or move in the prone position, to assume a sitting position, to arise to an erect posture, and to walk, run, jump, hop, skip, and leap. Individual variations occur in mode of performance and sometimes in sequence, for according to McGraw, the impulse to progress is "somewhat specific and may be 'grafted onto' any postural form predominant at the time the urge to progress is manifest."[35]

By the time the child has matured in his motor activities, he can perform in a coordinate fashion all activities in the sequence. Primitive patterns of movement have been altered by growth; mature movements of a willed or voluntary nature have become dominant, but they retain automatic and reflex aspects. The normal adult may revert to more primitive responses in stress situations. If when lying on the beach a person senses impending danger (approaching flames from a fire, a snake passing by, a man with a dull instrument raised overhead), he may automatically roll away from the hazard. The act of rolling serves his immediate need best. He may then from a prone position, or by rolling to sitting, scramble to his feet and walk or run away as the situation demands. He has used automatically a sequence of developmental activities that had their origin before birth, that matured within the first few years of life, and that may not have been used in sequence for a number of years, but that were immediately available on demand.

The ingredients from which normal movement is made, the emergence of specific patterns of movement from total patterns of response, the primitive and reflex aspects that underlie controlled posture and movement, the direction of development from head to foot, the distal – to – proximal direction of coordinate movement, the refinement of movement from full range to partial and specific ranges — are all characteristics of the developmental process that provide a basis for development or restoration of motor function in persons who lack normal ability to move or to sustain posture.[25] For these persons, a recapitulation of the developmental sequence is a means to the end: the ability to care for one's body, to walk, and to engage in productive work.

PRINCIPLES

Certain principles guide the use of developmental activities when patterns and techniques of proprioceptive neuromuscular facilitation are superimposed.

Develomental activities are useful as a basis for treatment of patients of all ages. The chronological age and the level of development must be considered. Aging is a normal process of human development in which alterations occur in postural form and configuration of movement.[7]

The reflex mechanisms underlying normal movement are recognized as potent forces for influencing movement and postures.[21] The sequence of developmental activities, by virtue of the normal process of growth and development, provides for activation of postural and righting reflexes. The coordination of visual – motor mechanisms and of auditory – motor mechanisms are taught and are used in training.

Development or restoration of motor abilities, including self-care and the ability to walk, are concomitants of motor learning. Patterns and techniques of proprioceptive neuromuscular facilitation are used to hasten motor learning by providing appropriate "sensory cues." The selection of sensory cues is the task of the physical therapist or teacher.[16]

Repetition of coordinate movement is used to increase strength and endurance and to adjust the rate of movement.[18] Resistance is applied during repetitions but is graded according to the needs and abilities of the patient.

In the developmental process, the development of movement is from proximal to distal, and total patterns of movement become individuated.[23] In using the developmental sequence with emphasis first on training of head and neck and trunk patterns, the proximal – to – distal relationship and the progression from total patterns of movement to individual component patterns are heeded.

That coordinate movement proceeds in a distal – to – proximal direction is recognized as essential to development or improvement of motor abilities.[23] In applying patterns and techniques of proprioceptive neuromuscular facilitation, a timed sequence of movement from distal to proximal is used.

Developmental activities are total patterns of movement and posture to which patterns and techniques of proprioceptive neuromuscular facilitation are applied precisely. The component patterns of a total pattern are readily converted to spiral and diagonal patterns of facilitation for maximum selectivity of response. Techniques based on isotonic contraction of muscle encourage movement; those based on isometric contraction encourage stability and sustenance of posture.

For optimum development of motor function, the patient must be helped to recapitulate the developmental sequence insofar as he possibly can. Each phase of the sequence has significance in that one activity lays the foundation for a more advanced activity. If a phase is omitted, function may be altered unfavorably and certain deficiencies may be retained unnecessarily. The acts of assumption of positions are necessary to maintaining balance in the positions.

The stronger component patterns of a total pattern and the stronger pivots of action within a component pattern are used for augmentation of weaker components. By using the patient's abilities to lessen his inabilities, an activity within the developmental sequence may be learned more readily.

The progress of the patient is enhanced by adequate performance of an activity within the sequence rather than by inadequate performance of a variety of activities. Performance of more primitive activities, insofar as is possible, should be instructed before attempting more complex activities that are completely beyond the ability of the patient.

The physical therapist becomes a part of the total movement or effort of the patient. The therapist must approach the patient in a mutually advantageous way. When patterns of movement have a diagonal direction, the therapist assumes and moves in a diagonal direction as the patient moves. This principle applies wherever activities are performed: on a gymnasium mat, a bed, a treatment table, or in an open area during gait training.

The program of activities is selected in accordance with the patient's needs and potentials. Long-term and short-term goals must be determined. All activities must be integrated and directed toward suitable goals.

Thus, the total approach of proprioceptive neuromuscular facilitation has denominations of total patterns of movement, specific patterns of facilitation combined for training of total patterns, and techniques for hastening motor learning.

USE OF THE DEVELOPMENTAL SEQUENCE

The developmental sequence is limited to those activities most typical of *human* development. McGraw's reminder that the human species has a long history of evolution serves as a guide to selection of primitive activities.[35] Every person concerned with development or restoration of motor ability in others can readily learn and apply the sequence.

As selected and adapted from McGraw and Gesell, the developmental sequence provides for a progression from primitive movements and postures to more complex and advanced movements and postures.[11,35] Briefly, the sequence of total patterns of movement with their related or ultimate positions and postures proceeds as follows: rolling from supine to prone, and from prone to supine; prone progression, as in pivoting, crawling, creeping, and plantigrade walking; rising to sitting; rising to kneeling, and knee walking; rising to standing, and bipedal walking; ascending and descending stairs and ramps; running; jumping;

hopping; and skipping. Table 1-8, Progression of Activities, portrays the progression of the elementary activities in the sequence. Within the sequence, movement is used to alter position and posture. Movement is enhanced by use of the hands following the eyes, or the eyes following the hand movements. Movement and posture, including eye–hand coordination, become interwoven. The sequence provides for total patterns wherein the head and neck, the trunk, and the four extremities participate in various relationships such as ipsilateral, bilateral symmetrical, bilateral asymmetrical, and reciprocal movements. Within a total pattern, certain segments may move while other segments adjust to the movement.

In the sequence, as position is altered by movement, balance and posture are developed and maintained in the altered position before movement leads to another position. That is, when the hand and knee (creeping) position is achieved, balance in this position precedes the creeping movement. Balance in a position is not limited to neutral positions of the extremities; positioning of the extremities in various ranges of motion and for reciprocation is used.

Provision is made for flexor dominance of a movement and for extensor dominance. As an illustration, the sitting position is assumed by initial rolling from supine toward prone (flexor dominance), and then by pushing up from the prone position (extensor dominance). Also, when balance is to be maintained in a certain position, the flexor components are required to alternate with extensor components. This alternation occurs when balance is disturbed in an anterior-to-posterior direction and then in a posterior-to-anterior direction. For instance, when a patient attempts to maintain himself in a lateral (sidelying) position, flexors dominate if balance is disturbed toward the supine position, and extensors dominate if balance is disturbed toward the prone position. In prone progression, such as in creeping, dominance is altered by changing direction from forward (flexor dominance) to backward (extensor dominance). As identified in Table 1-8, dominance is influenced by direction and by performance against resistance.

The developmental sequence promotes the ability to perform with isotonic contractions of related muscle groups during movement and with isometric contractions during performance of balancing activities. Transition from isometric contraction to isotonic contraction also occurs. Sherrington pointed out that, "Naturally, the distinction between reflexes of attitude (posture) and reflexes of movement is not in all cases sharp and abrupt. Between a short-lasting attitude and a slowly progressing movement, the difference is hardly more than one of degree. Moreover, each posture is introduced by a movement of assumption, and after each departure from the posture, if it is resumed, it is reverted to by a movement of compensation. Hence the taxis of attitude must involve not only static reactions of tonic maintenance of contraction, but innervations that execute reinforcing movements and compensatory movements."[44] If balance is disturbed so that the position must be recovered, recovery is achieved through isotonic contraction. During movement, stability of supporting segments must be maintained through isometric contractions as one segment advances with isotonic contractions of the responsible muscle groups. However, transitions between and intermingling of types of muscle contraction are not sharply distinct.

Ultimately, the use of developmental activities contributes to independence in self-care and gait activities. As an example, rolling movements are closely related to turning in bed, to rising and sitting on the edge of the bed, to dressing while supine, and when the component movements of the upper extremity are considered, to feeding and other activities requiring hand-to-face movements. Locomotion in the prone position and rising to standing prepare one for bipedal walking. A patient's potential for performance may be limited by pathology, but insofar as is possible the performance of the developmental sequence should promote optimum recovery of purposeful movement.

Mat Activities

Practical application of the principles for use of developmental activities requires proper physical facilities. A gymnasium mat should be firm, smooth, and pliant enough to be comfortable and to protect the patient from abrasions and undue stress should he fail to maintain his balance. An uninterrupted surface, without seams or tufts, which can be easily cleansed, seems best.

A mat's surface should be large enough to accommodate the patient and the therapist for creeping and walking activities with several repetitions of movement before direction is changed. For an adult, a useful size is 6 feet by 8 feet; for a child, 4 feet by 6 feet. Elevation on a platform the height of the seat of a standard wheel chair is desirable so that transferring from chair to mat may be incorporated as a related self-care activity. If a mat is used on the floor, a small ramp with hand rails allows some patients to descend from chair to mat and then return to the chair with minimal guidance and protection. For working with an individual patient, one mat of suitable size is sufficient. However, a series of mats covering an area of at least 24 feet by 24 feet will permit a number of patients to be supervised in those activities they can perform independently.

Motor activity on a gymnasium mat has certain advantages. There is an element of security for patients who are fearful of falling. Total patterns of movement may be performed without limitation such as exists when the patient is treated on a table. Postural and righting reflexes may be induced more effectively because a variety of positions and postures may be used, and because balance may be disturbed without the hazard of falling from a height. In-bed activities may be simulated and practiced safely as a means of teaching self-care, inasmuch as the sequence provides for a close relationship with self-care activities. Furthermore, when mat activities are done in an open area where patients can observe each other, there are indirect influences, such as learning from others, motivation through competition, and socialization, all of which may enhance performance.

Precise use of patterns of facilitation and application of techniques must be in keeping with the abilities and needs of the individual patient. Whereas the progression of activities is outlined in terms of total patterns of movement and related positions of balanced posture, precise use demands further analysis of a total movement or posture. The component patterns within the total movement or posture must be identified throughout the neck, trunk, and extremities. By so doing, the components of motion within a component pattern can be used for augmentation and reinforcement of the patient's effort to perform the total pattern, since all movement proceeds in the same direction.

A total pattern of movement and each component pattern have a point of initiation, a range of movement, and a point of completion. The point of initiation is termed the lengthened range (Le-R); midway within the range of movement is the middle range (Mid-R); and the point of completion is the shortened range (Sh-R). A total movement, or one of its component patterns, may be initiated in the lengthened range with isotonic contraction of responsible muscle groups. Movement may be initiated in the shortened range or the middle range with isometric contraction followed by repeated isotonic contractions. If movement is initiated in the lengthened range the direction proceeds toward the middle or, if possible, the shortened range. If movement is initiated in the middle or shortened ranges, the direction is still toward the shortened range, the point of completion. In this instance, however, repetitions of effort are controlled in retrograde in order to increase the range through which a movement is performed. This becomes necessary to the development of the complete range of a movement; the technique of repeated contractions is used (see Table 1-8).

A total movement may take several directions, such as forward, backward, sideward, or turning in a circle. As direction is changed, the component patterns and components of motion change accordingly. Flexor dominance of a movement may be altered to extensor dominance by changing direction from for-

Table 1-8.   Progression of Activities

Total Pattern of Movement	*Position for Balance*
Rolling from supine to prone: flexor dominance (FD)	Lateral (sidelying)
Rolling from prone to supine: extensor dominance (ED)	Lateral (sidelying)
Prone pivoting: alternate FD and ED	Prone on elbows and pelvis
Rising to elbows and knees from prone: ED	Prone on elbows and knees
Pulling to sitting from supine: FD	Sitting with hands reaching forward
Rising to sitting from hyperflexion: ED	Sitting with hands supporting forward
Crawling on elbows and knees: forward, FD; backward, ED	Prone with elbows and knees in various positions
Rising to hands and knees from prone: ED	Prone with hands and knees in various positions
Rocking on hands and knees: forward, ED; backward, FD	Prone on hands and knees while rocked forward, and backward
Creeping on hands and knees: forward, FD; backward, ED	Prone on hands, one knee and one foot
Rising to sitting from prone: ED	Sitting with and without hands supporting backward
Rising to sitting from supine: FD	Sitting with and without hands supporting forward
Rising to plantigrade position from prone: ED	Plantigrade, hands and feet in alternate ipsilateral
Plantigrade walking: forward, FD; backward, ED	Plantigrade with diagonal reciprocation, and with one extremity free of support
Pulling to upright from hands and knees (stall bars): FD	Upright for climbing with hands grasping and with support on one knee and one foot
Climbing and descending (stall bars): ascent, FD; descent, ED	Climbing with reciprocation
Rising to kneeling from sitting (buttocks on heels): FD	Kneeling on both knees
Rising to kneeling from prone: ED	Half-kneeling, one knee and one foot
Walking on knees: forward, FD; backward, ED	Kneeling with diagonal reciprocation
Pulling to standing from squat or sitting: FD	Standing with hands and feet parallel positions
Rocking on feet with hands supported: forward, ED; backward, FD	Standing in ipsilateral position with and without hands supported

(Continued)

Table 1-8. (*Continued*)

Total Pattern of Movement	Position for Balance
Lowering to squat or to sitting: FD	Near-squat and near-sitting with and without support of hands
Rising to standing from prone: ED	Standing with reciprocation with and without hands supported
Rising to standing from supine: FD	Standing with reciprocation with hands supported and with one foot free
Foot lifting and stamping: alternate FD, ED	Standing with reciprocation with one hand free and one foot free
Bipedal walking: forward, FD; backward, ED	Standing with reciprocation with both hands and one foot free, and on tiptoe
Ascending and descending ramp on hands and feet: forward ascent, FD; backward descent, ED	Plantigrade with reciprocation, and with one extremity free
Ascending and descending ramp in upright: forward ascent, FD; forward descent, FD; backward ascent, ED; backward descent, ED	Standing with both hands supported, one hand free, one hand and foot free, hands free and one foot free
Climbing and descending stairs on hands and feet: forward ascent, FD; backward descent, ED	Plantigrade with bilateral position and reciprocation
Ascending stairs in upright (advancing one foot; advancing alternately): forward ascent, FD; backward descent, ED	Standing with both hands and feet supported, one hand free, and hands free
Descending stairs in upright (advancing one foot; advancing alternately): forward descent, FD; backward ascent, ED	Standing with both hands and feet supported, one hand free, one hand and foot free, hands free
Running, jumping, hopping, and skipping	

Note: Chronology of the sequence has been omitted. The sequence is used in accordance with a patient's needs; chronological age is one factor of evaluation and treatment.

Solid lines indicate progression from assumption of a position to balance or posture related to the position, and from balance in one position to a more advanced form of movement or locomotion. Interrupted lines show relationships within prone postures and locomotion.

Dominance is influenced by direction and by superimposing manual resistance.

ward to backward. Lateralward (abduction) movements in a sideward direction may be altered to medialward (adduction) movements by changing direction to the opposite side. Turning in a circle and changing direction provides for lateralward and medialward movements of contralateral upper and lower extremities. Diagonal movements combine the flexion or extension components with abduction and adduction components. Diagonal movements permit greater selectivity than is possible with straight forward or straight backward movement.

The physical therapist approaches the patient in such a way as to be in line with the movement of the patient. Techniques of proprioceptive neuromuscular facilitation may be applied to each total pattern of movement. Through maximal resistance, stronger component patterns will augment the response of weaker component patterns. When the goal is to *move*, movement must be permitted; but the stronger patterns must be resisted strongly. To reinforce a weaker component pattern by a stronger component pattern, the technique of timing for emphasis is used. The patient is instructed to move; as he moves he is asked to sustain his effort ("hold" with isometric contraction) at the strongest phase, and then repeated isotonic contractions of the weaker pattern are demanded and commanded.

When the goal is to *maintain balance* in a certain position or posture, a stronger segment, or pattern within a segment, is again used to augment the ability of a weaker segment to sustain posture. The patient is instructed to maintain the position, and as he does so, the technique of rhythmic stabilization is used along with approximation applied to the weight-bearing segments. First, resistance is applied to the isometric contractions (holding) of stronger patterns or segment, and then an isometric contraction is gradually developed in the weaker patterns or segment. Counterpressure with anterior and posterior manual contacts applied simultaneously promotes maximum stability and security. If balance is to be disturbed sufficiently to promote compensatory movements, both manual contacts may be anterior or posterior as necessary. Compensatory movements are resisted. Balance may be disturbed abruptly by brief and suddenly applied and withdrawn pressure. Manual contacts must be selected so that the desired patterns will be evoked. When balance is disturbed in this fashion, the response is quick, and resistance is not used.

While the various techniques may be applied, the use of timing, reinforcement, maximal resistance, traction and approximation, stretch, reversal of antagonists including rhythmic stabilization, or repeated contractions seems most useful. When the ability to move is deficient, techniques that require isotonic contractions of muscles should be selected. When stability is deficient, isometric contractions should be used. As always, due regard must be given the prevention and correction of imbalances between antagonistic reflexes, patterns of facilitation, muscle groups, and components of motion. See Table 1-9, Support by Postural and Righting Reflexes.

Illustrations (Figs. 1-151 to 1-202)

The illustrations portray the use of selected activities from the developmental sequence. However, the sequence of the illustrations is not developmental. Rather, closely related activities appear in series; rolling activities are grouped together (Figs. 1-151 to 1-161), as are the activities related to prone progression (Figs. 1-164 to 1-176). Table 1-8 should be used as a guideline for appropriate overlapping between activities in various postures. Descriptions of standing balance and walking (see Figs. 1-189 to 1-195) are presented in the section on gait activities and should be read in conjunction with the related illustrations for mat activities.

To portray adequately all activities, all variations of posture, and all variations of the therapist's approach to the patient for performance to left and right

Table 1-9. Support by Postural and Righting Reflexes

Posture or Position	*Supportive Reflexes*
Supine: favorable for weak extensors	Tonic labyrinthine reflex (TLR): increased extensor tonus
Prone: favorable for weak flexors	TLR: decreased extensor tonus
Sidelying (uppermost limbs flexed, undermost extended): favorable for weak trunk flexors (toward prone) and extensors (toward supine)	TLR: asymmetric tonic neck reflex (ATNR); head turned to left or right, jaw limbs flex, skull limbs extend
Prone on elbows: favorable for stability of head and neck, and shoulder girdle	Labyrinthine righting acting on head; optical righting
Knee–chest and elbow–knees: favorable for stability of pelvic and shoulder girdles	Labyrinthine righting; optical righting
Hands and knees: favorable for rocking in all directions	
Head posture:	Symmetric tonic neck reflex (STNR)
Ventroflexed (down)	Head down: upper limbs flex, lower limbs extend
Dorsiflexed (up)	Head up: upper limbs extend, lower limbs flex
Rotated (left or right)	ATNR: skull limb flexes; jaw limb extends
Side-sitting: counter-rotation, shoulder girdle (upper trunk) and pelvic girdle (lower trunk), promotes stability	Body-on-body righting (asymmetric contact, body rights)
Long-sitting: favorable for weak extensors, lengthened range, and weak flexors, shortened range; demands lengthening of posterior structures	Labyrinthine righting acting on head; optical righting
Table-sitting, over edge: favorable for weak flexors, shortened range, and for weak extensors, lengthened range.	Labyrinthine righting acting on head; optical righting

Each basic posture has reflex support. Patients can be assisted in the assumption of a position, or passively positioned, more readily if regard is given to increasing or decreasing tonus through postural and righting reflexes. Also, these reflexes reinforce the voluntary attempt to maintain a certain position. The stretch reflex may help to initiate movement for recovery of balance.

See also Table 1-8, Progression of Activities. Note flexor dominance (FD) and extensor dominance (ED).

would require hundreds of illustrations. The series that follows is a sample. Some of the significant aspects of mat, gait, transfer, and self-care activities that are illustrated in Figures 1-151 to 1-202 are as follows:

Responses of the feet: The normal subject is shown with bare feet to reveal responses of the feet more clearly. (During mat activities neither patient nor therapist wears shoes. In gait and transfer activities shoes are worn.)

Movements of assumption of posture, the posture assumed, and the mode of progression related to the posture

The coordination, or combining, of component patterns of a total pattern wherein vision, head, and neck lead and give direction

The component patterns to which resistance or a technique is directed, and the component patterns of segments that may move free of manual contact, but not necessarily free of resistance, or that may adjust with a compensatory movement as balance is disturbed

Three phases of a total pattern of movement, or of a component pattern: lengthened, middle, and shortened ranges*; or three variations on a total pattern of posture during balancing activities

The therapist's approach to the subject (or patient) by taking a position that is on the diagonal if diagonal direction is expected, and by assuming a total posture that will permit movement to occur or posture to become stable, whichever is indicated

A variety of manual contacts, but not all-inclusive, that must be transposed for performance to the opposite side, which also requires that the therapist assume a transposed or adjusted posture

Commands that include some preparatory instructions as well as commands to perform, and in some instances commands that are in keeping with the suggested techniques (Commands for a specific technique should be gleaned from the text on the technique; inclusion here is only a guideline.)

Suggested techniques that may be superimposed (Many other techniques may be considered for use. Those suggested here should be treated as suggestions for learning.)

Antagonistic patterns, some of which are illustrated, some of which are not in order to permit portrayal of a variety of combinations of component patterns and of manual contacts (Performance of an antagonistic pattern requires adjustment of the therapist's position and manual contacts; where equipment is used, for example, a wheel chair, alteration of the position of the chair may be necessary.)

Augmentation: reinforcement of a total pattern of movement or posture by use of component patterns, or the use of a total pattern for augmentation of a component pattern (Reinforcement by postural and righting reflexes is evident in many of the illustrations.)

Notes that include comments on the therapist's and the subject's performance, additional suggestions for performance, and in some instances references to preparatory and related activities.

Within the sequence of activities as portrayed in Table 1-8, there is an overlapping between mat and gait activities. The most advanced activity illustrated as a mat activity is that of "Bipedal Walking" (Fig. 1-188). In general, prone progression, or locomotion, is best performed on a mat. Bipedal activities in the upright position that require a flat surface also may be performed on a mat. In fact, in walking barefoot on a mat, response of the feet is not hampered by close-fitting shoes, and action of the feet may be encouraged and observed more easily.

When the total structure is involved, the total patterns of developmental activities are used to hasten learning of total patterns of movement. When one segment is involved and the remainder of the total structure is intact, total patterns provide optimum reinforcements for the deficient segment. Any contraindications for weight bearing must be heeded. Given an intact skeletal system and integrity of joint structures, the use of total patterns promotes increasing ranges of motion and establishment of the proper interaction of antagonistic component patterns and interaction of segments.

* In some instances, the initial position is used, and in others, where the range is incomplete, indication as "approaching" middle or shortened range is used.

Rolling: Supine Toward Prone

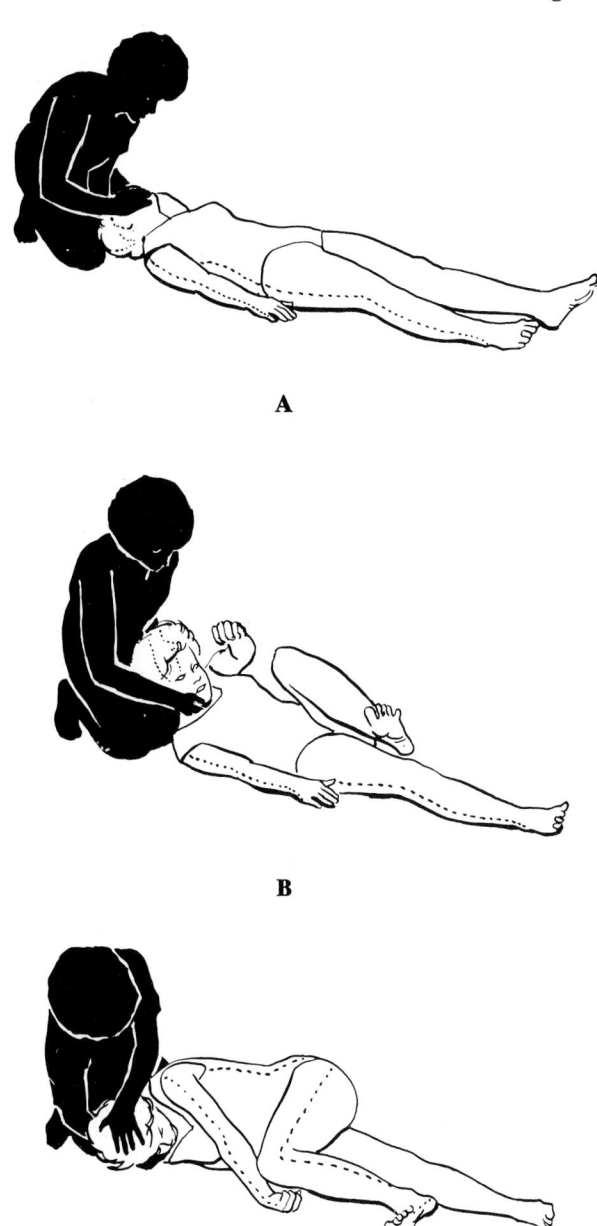

A

B

C

FIG. 1-151. Head and neck: flexion with rotation.

Component Patterns

Resisted. Head and neck, flexion with rotation to right.

Free. Left upper extremity, extension–adduction–internal rotation; left lower extremity, flexion–adduction–external rotation; right extremities adjust toward extension and adduction.

A. Lengthened Range

Commands. "Lift your head, look at your right hip, and roll! Pull your left arm down and across! Pull your left foot up and across! Roll!"

Suggested Techniques. Traction, stretch, and resistance.

B. Approaching Middle Range

Commands. "Pull your chin down some more! Roll on over!"

Suggested Techniques. Repeated contractions or, if patient cannot complete roll, slow reversal followed by repeated contractions.

C. Approaching Shortened Range

Commands. "Hold it! Don't let me pull you back!"

Suggested Techniques. Repeated contractions, rhythmic stabilization (see Fig. 1-157), slow reversal, slow reversal–hold.

Antagonistic Pattern

Rolling from prone toward supine: head and neck extension with rotation to left (Fig. 1-58). Left extremities move in antagonistic patterns (see Fig. 1-158, *Note*).

NOTE: Intermediate joints, elbow and knee, of moving extremities may flex, extend, or remain straight.

Mat Activity

Rolling: Supine Toward Prone

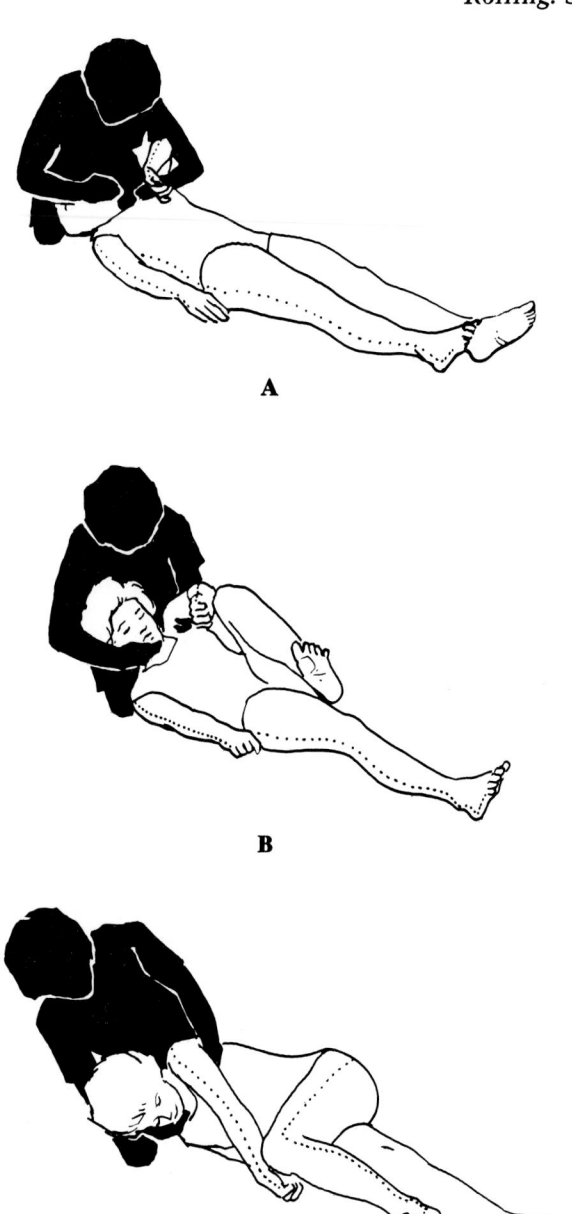

A

B

C

FIG. 1-152. Head and neck: flexion with rotation, contralateral scapula.

Component Patterns

Resisted. Head and neck, flexion with rotation to right; left upper extremity, extension – adduction – internal rotation, scapula depresses anteriorly.

Free. Left lower extremity, flexion – adduction – external rotation; right extremities adjust in extension and adduction.

A. Lengthened Range

Commands. "Pull your chin to your chest, pull your arm down and across, and roll over! Pull your left foot up and across! Roll!"

Suggested Techniques. Stretch and resistance.

B. Approaching Middle Range

Commands. "Reach for your right hip! All the way!"

Suggested Techniques. Repeated stretch, repeated contractions, or slow reversal followed by renewed effort to roll.

C. Approaching Shortened Range

Commands. "Hold it! Pull again!"

Suggested Techniques. Repeated contractions, rhythmic stabilization (see Fig. 1-157), slow reversal, slow reversal – hold.

Antagonistic Pattern

Rolling from prone toward supine: head and neck extension with rotation to left. Left upper extremity flexion – abduction – external rotation, scapula elevates posteriorly. Left lower extremity moves in antagonistic pattern.

NOTE: Intermediate joints, elbow and knee, of moving extremities may flex, extend, or remain straight.

Rolling: Supine Toward Prone

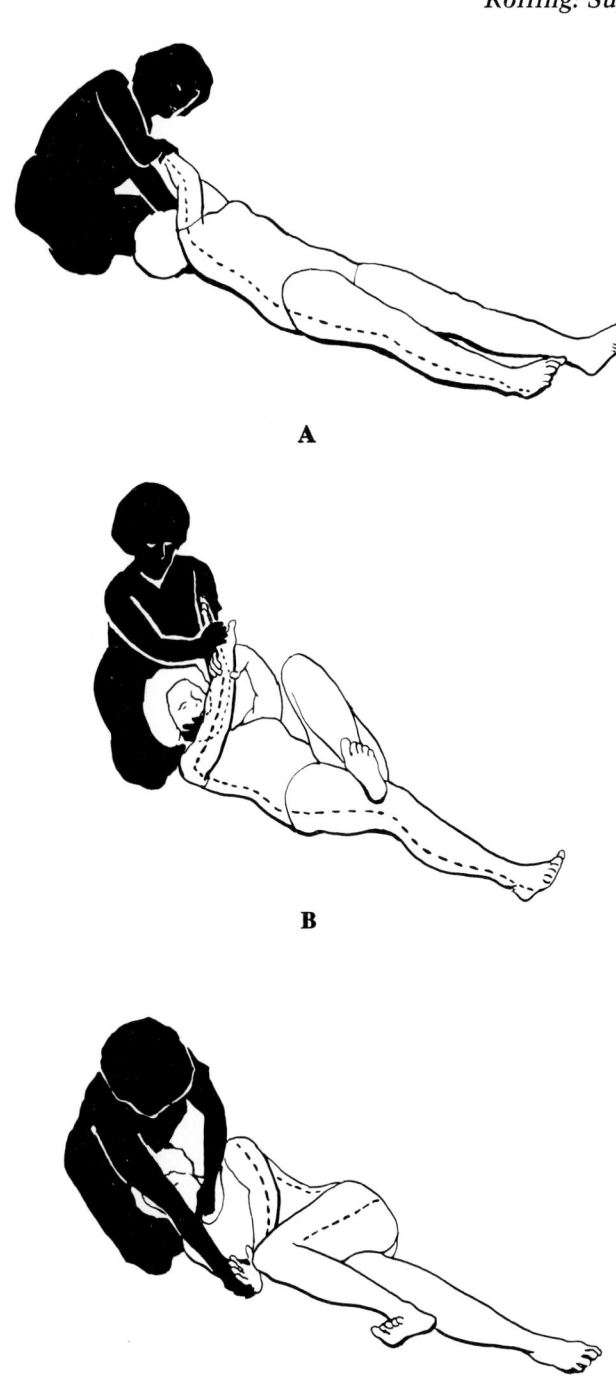

A

B

C

FIG. 1-153. Head and neck: flexion with rotation, bilateral asymmetrical upper extremities.

Component Patterns

Resisted. Head and neck, flexion with rotation to right; upper extremities, asymmetrical extension (chopping) to right.

Free. Left lower extremity, flexion–adduction–external rotation; right lower extremity adjusts in extension and adduction.

A. Lengthened Range

Commands. "Pull your arms down toward your right hip, lift your head, and roll over! Pull your left foot up and over! Roll!"

Suggested Techniques. Traction to upper extremities, stretch and resistance.

B. Approaching Middle Range

Commands. "Pull your arms down! Roll! Pull your knee on over! Roll!"

Suggested Techniques. Repeated stretch, repeated contractions.

C. Approaching Shortened Range

Commands. "Hold! Don't let me pull you back!"

Suggested Techniques. Slow reversal followed by repeated contractions, rhythmic stabilization.

Antagonistic Pattern

Rolling from prone toward supine: head and neck extension with rotation to left. Bilateral asymmetrical flexion of upper extremities (lifting) to left (Fig. 1-159). Left lower extremity moves in antagonistic pattern.

NOTE: Intermediate joints (elbows and knees) of moving extremities may flex, extend, or remain straight.

Rolling: Supine Toward Prone

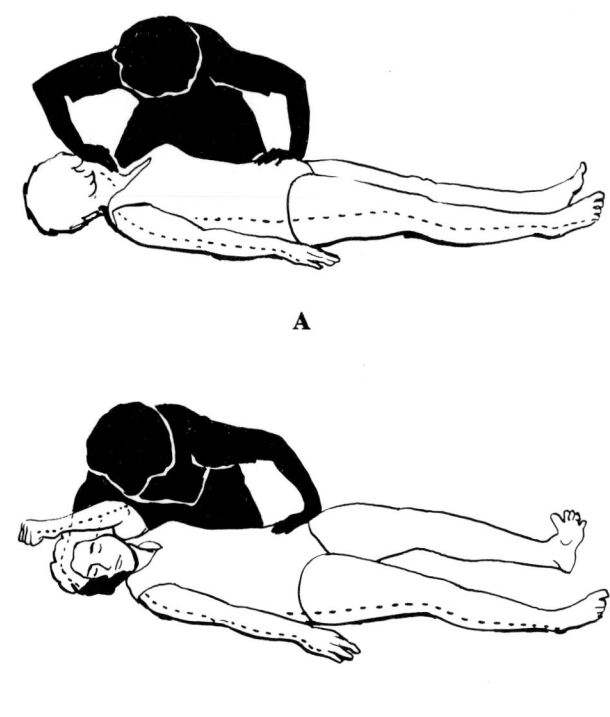

A

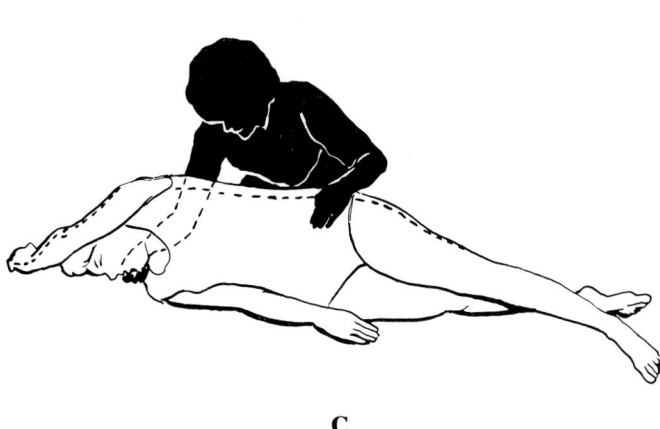

B

C

FIG. 1-154. Head and neck: rotation.

Component Patterns

Resisted. Head and neck, rotation to right; lower trunk, rotation to right.

Free. Left upper extremity, flexion–adduction–external rotation; left lower extremity, flexion–adduction–external rotation; right extremities adjust in extension and adduction.

A. Lengthened Range

Commands. "Turn your head toward your right shoulder, pull your hand across your face, and roll! Lift your left foot up and across! Roll over!"

Suggested Techniques. Stretch and resistance.

B. Approaching Middle Range

Commands. "Open your hand now and reach for the mat! Pull your left foot across! Roll!"

Suggested Techniques. Repeated stretch, repeated contractions.

C. Approaching Shortened Range

Commands. "Pull your left hip down to the mat! Hold it! Don't let me pull you back!"

Suggested Techniques. Repeated contractions, rhythmic stabilization (see Fig. 1-157).

Antagonistic Pattern

Rolling from prone toward supine: head and neck rotation to left, lower trunk rotation to left. Lower extremities move in antagonistic patterns (see Figs. 1-160 and 1-161).

NOTE: Head and neck rotation, as with all patterns of head and neck, activates the related trunk patterns. In this total pattern of rolling, upper and lower trunk rotate from lateralward extension on the left to lateralward extension on the right, as do head and neck.

Left upper extremity may thrust with opening of hand toward ulnar side and with elbow, initially positioned in flexion, extending. Knee may flex or extend.

Rolling: Supine Toward Prone

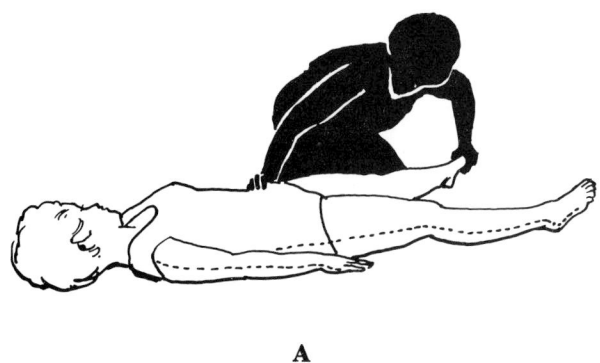

A

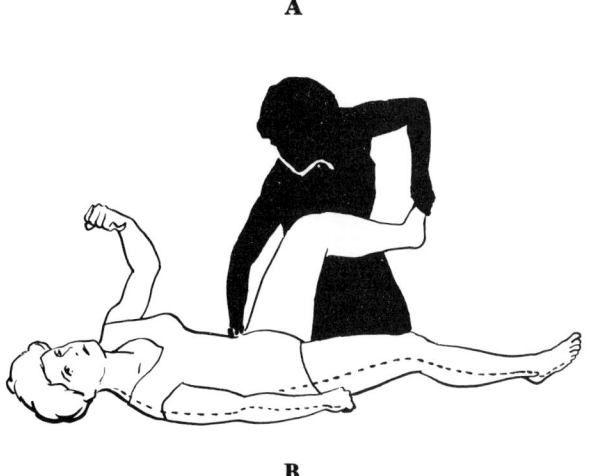

B

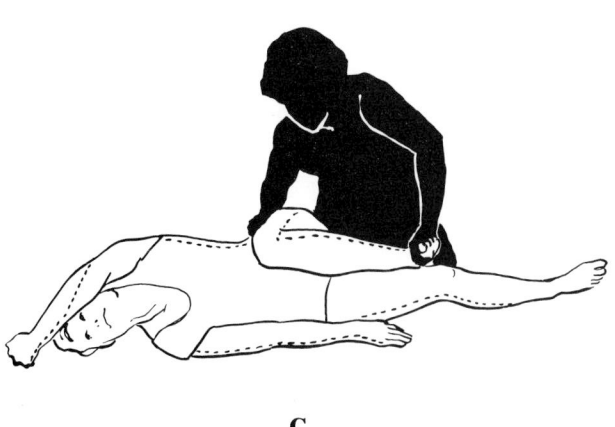

C

FIG. 1-155. Head and neck: extension with rotation, contralateral lower extremity flexion.

Component Patterns

Resisted. Left lower extremity, flexion–adduction–external rotation.

Free. Head and neck, extension with rotation to right; left upper extremity, flexion–adduction–external rotation; right extremities adjust in extension and adduction.

A. Lengthened Range

Commands. "Look up over your right shoulder, pull your foot up and bend your knee, and roll! Reach your hand up and across your face! Roll!"

Suggested Techniques. Traction, stretch and resistance.

B. Approaching Middle Range

Commands. "Bend your knee and pull it across! Reach for the mat, turn your head! Roll!"

Suggested Techniques. Slow reversal followed by renewed effort to roll.

C. Approaching Shortened Range

Commands. "Pull your knee down to the mat, and hold it!"

Suggested Techniques. Repeated contractions, slow reversal, slow reversal–hold.

Antagonistic Pattern

Rolling from prone toward supine: left lower extremity, extension–abduction–internal rotation; head and neck flexion with rotation to left. Left upper extremity moves in antagonistic pattern (see *Note*, Fig. 1-156).

NOTE: In *A*, subject may be asked to lift head and look at left foot before extending head and neck with rotation to right. Left upper extremity may thrust in flexion–adduction–external rotation (see *Note*, Fig. 1-154). Note that flexion–adduction–external rotation patterns of left extremities have been combined with head and neck extension with rotation, and with head and neck rotation patterns (see Fig. 1-154).

Rolling: Supine Toward Prone

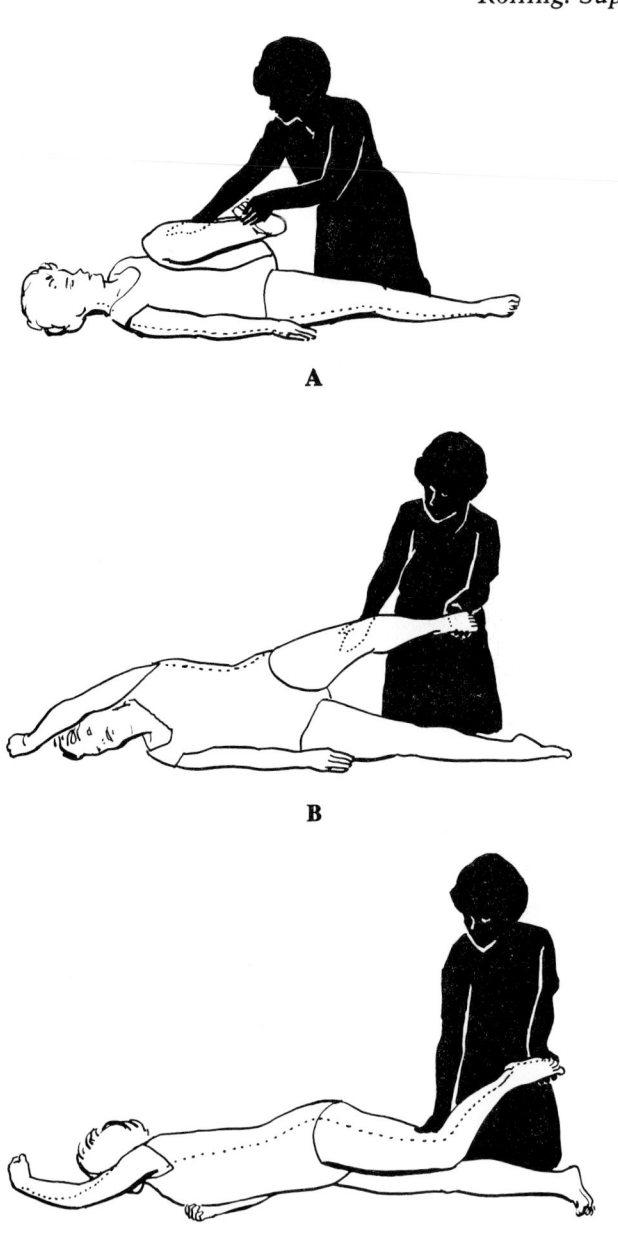

Component Patterns

Resisted. Left lower extremity, extension – abduction – internal rotation.

Free. Head and neck, extension with rotation to right; left upper extremity, flexion – adduction – external rotation; right extremities adjust in extension and adduction.

A. Lengthened Range

Commands. "Look up to your right, push your foot to me, and roll over! Turn your head, look up, and push!"

Suggested Techniques. Stretch and resistance.

B. Approaching Middle Range

Commands. "Push to me! Roll over!"
Suggested Techniques. Repeated stretch.

C. Approaching Shortened Range

Commands. "Straighten your knee!"
Suggested Techniques. See *Note.*

NOTE: An adversive movement, extension of the lower extremity in a thrusting pattern, has been used to initiate rolling toward prone. The normal child may initiate rolling by pushing against the surface. The subject, in this instance, pushes against the therapist's hand. The subject, as with the child, could push against the surface (mat) while the therapist resisted other component patterns.

The extension – abduction – internal rotation pattern may be used to initiate rolling from prone toward supine. This may be visualized by superimposing the position of the left lower extremity, as shown in *A*, on the position of head and trunk, as shown in *C*. In Figures 1-158 to 1-161, the extension – abduction – internal rotation pattern of the lower extremity is used consistently in rolling from prone to supine, while in Figures 1-151 to 1-155 the flexion – adduction – external rotation pattern of the lower extremity is used consistently in rolling from supine toward prone. The opposite diagonal of lower extremity patterns is not used to promote rolling.

FIG. 1-156. Head and neck: extension with rotation, contralateral lower extremity extension.

Rolling: Supine Toward Prone

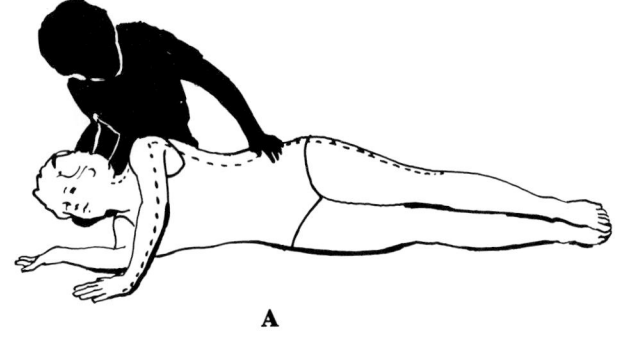

A

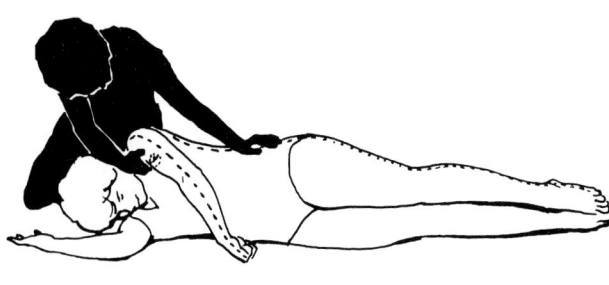

B

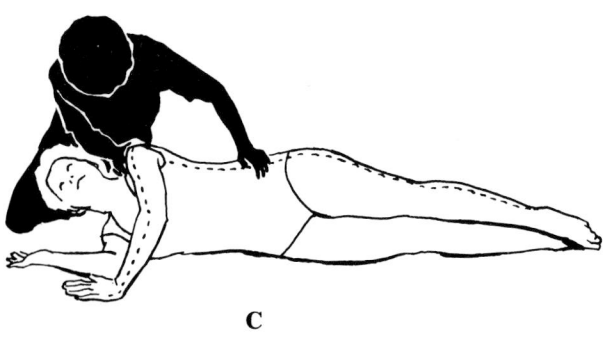

C

FIG. 1-157. Sidelying balance.

Component Patterns

A. Resisted. Head and neck, extension with rotation to right; lower trunk, rotation.

Free. Left upper extremity stabilizes in diagonal of flexion–adduction–external rotation and extension–abduction–internal rotation patterns. Right upper extremity stabilizes against surface as necessary. Lower extremities are in close approximation.

B. Resisted. Left upper extremity, extension–adduction–internal rotation, scapula depressed anteriorly; lower trunk, rotation.

Free. Head and neck, flexion with rotation to right; lower extremities in close approximation.

C. Resisted. Left upper extremity, flexion–adduction–external rotation, scapula elevated anteriorly; lower trunk, rotation.

Commands

A and *B* : "Hold, don't let me move you in any direction." *C*: "Hold. Don't let me pull you back!"

Suggested Techniques

A and *B*: rhythmic stabilization of flexion and extension components at the same time. *C*: Rhythmic stabilization of flexion, then extension components.

NOTE: Balancing, maintaining a position or posture, requires stability. Balancing against resistance promotes stability especially when antagonistic patterns are resisted at the same time, as in *A* and *B*. As performed in *C*, stability is threatened so that balance must be recovered by isotonic contraction in compensatory movements.

The sidelying or lateral position may be used to initiate rolling toward supine or toward prone where the patient cannot initiate against resistance from supine or prone positions. Because gravity will assist in either direction, weak patterns may be resisted.

Rolling: Prone Toward Supine

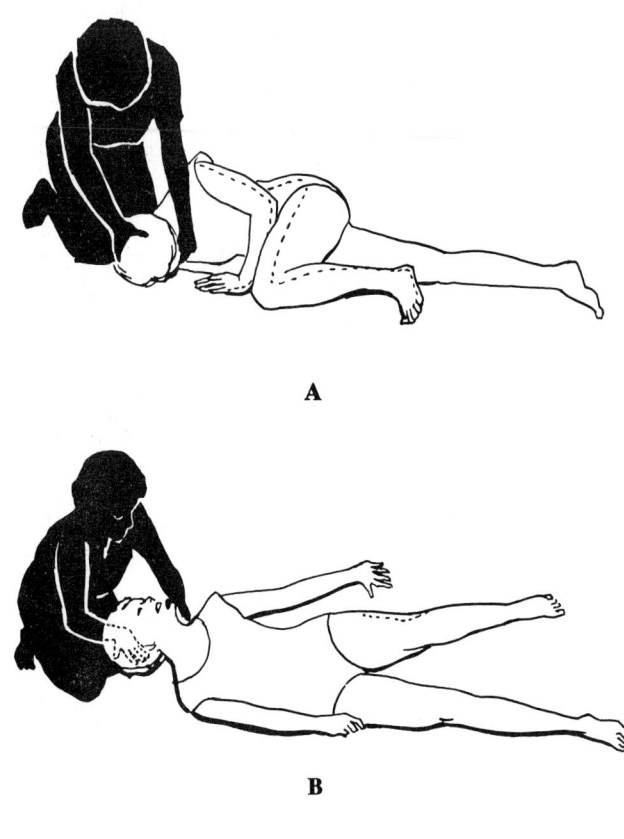

A

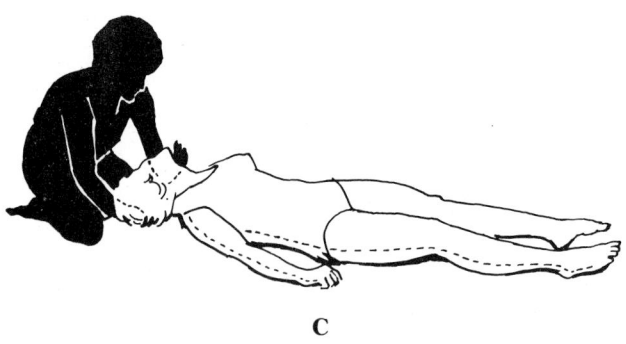

B

C

FIG. 1-158. Head and neck: extension with rotation.

Component Patterns

Resisted. Head and neck, extension with rotation to left.

Free. Left upper extremity, extension – abduction – internal rotation; left lower extremity, extension – abduction – internal rotation; right extremities adjust in extension and abduction.

A. Lengthened Range

Commands. "Look up at me, lift your head back to me, and roll! Push with your left hand! Lift your leg back! Roll!"

Suggested Techniques. Stretch and resistance.

B. Middle Range

Commands. "Push down to the mat! Look back here!"

Suggested Techniques. Slow reversal, repeated contractions.

C. Shortened Range

Commands. "Hold it! Don't let me lift you from the mat!"

Suggested Technique. Slow reversal.

Antagonistic Pattern

Rolling from supine toward prone: head and neck, flexion with rotation. Right upper extremity moves in extension – adduction – internal rotation pattern (Fig. 1-151). left lower extremity moves in antagonistic pattern.

NOTE: Intermediate joints, elbow and knee, of moving extremities extend or remain straight.

In this instance, because of the position of the therapist, the subject has used the left upper extremity in the extension – abduction – internal rotation pattern rather than the more closely related flexion – adduction – external rotation pattern as combined for "lifting," as in Figure 1-159. Therefore, the combinations used in Figures 1-151 and 1-158 are not directly antagonistic for the left upper extremity.

Rolling: Prone Toward Supine

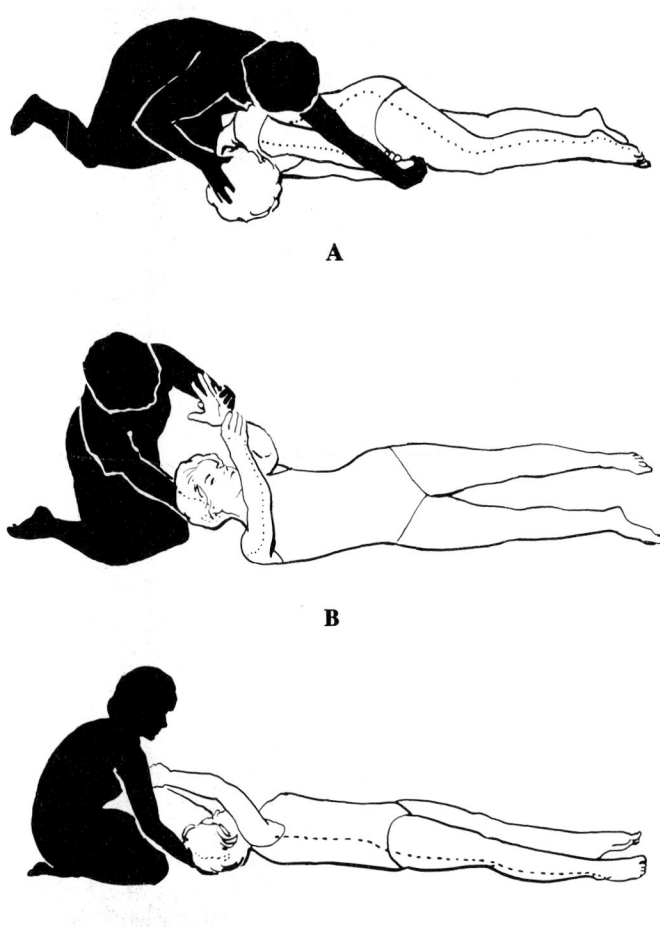

A. Lengthened Range

Commands. "Look at me, lift your head and hands to me, and roll! Lift your left leg back! Roll!"

Suggested Techniques. Traction to upper extremities, stretch and resistance.

B. Middle Range

Commands. "Look back at me! Lift your arms!"

Suggested Techniques. Rhythmic stabilization, repeated contractions, slow reversal, slow reversal–hold.

C. Shortened Range

Commands. "Hold! Don't let me lift you!"

Suggested Techniques. Approximation to upper extremities, repeated contractions.

Antagonistic Pattern

Rolling from supine toward prone: head and neck flexion with rotation to right; bilateral asymmetrical extension of upper extremities (chopping) to right (Fig. 1-153). Left lower extremity moves in antagonistic pattern.

NOTE: Intermediate joints of upper extremities may flex, extend, or remain straight. Approximation is used with extending or extended elbows.

If the position of head and upper extremities, as shown in *A*, is superimposed upon the supine body position in *C*, the use of this combination to initiate rolling from supine toward prone to the left can be visualized. Thus, extension with rotation of head and neck may be used to promote rolling toward supine, and rolling toward prone.

FIG. 1-159. Head and neck: extension with rotation, bilateral asymmetrical upper extremities.

Rolling: Prone Toward Supine

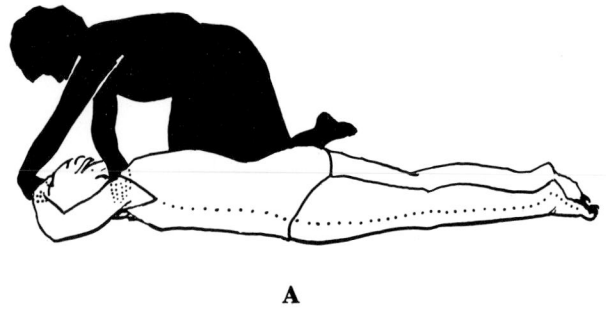

A

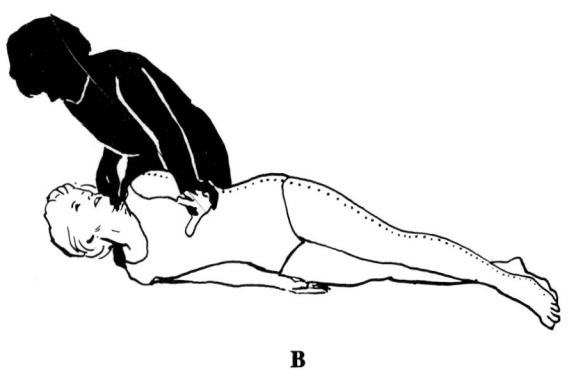

B

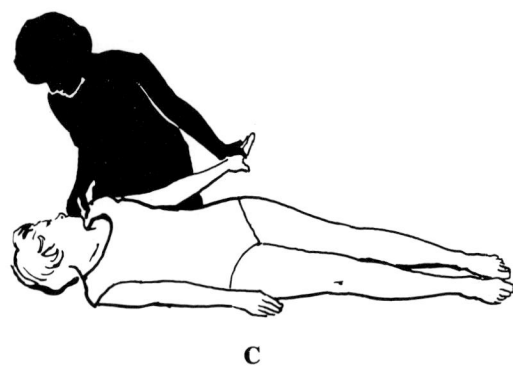

C

FIG. 1-160. Head and neck: rotation, ipsilateral upper extremity.

Component Patterns

Resisted. Head and neck, rotation to the left; left upper extremity, extension–abduction–internal rotation.

Free. Left lower extremity, extension–abduction–internal rotation. Right extremities adjust in extension and abduction.

A. Lengthened Range

Commands. "Open your hand, turn your head, and roll toward me! Lift your left leg back to the mat! Roll!"

Suggested Techniques. Stretch and resistance.

B. Approaching Middle Range

Commands. "Hold! Now, push on back here! Lift that foot back here!

Suggested Techniques. Repeated contractions, rhythmic stabilization (see Fig. 1-157).

C. Approaching Shortened Range

Commands. "Push some more! Hold it! Push again!"

Suggested Techniques. Approximation to left upper extremity followed by repeated contractions, slow reversal, slow reversal–hold.

Antagonistic Pattern

Rolling from supine toward prone: head and neck rotation to right. Left extremities move in antagonistic patterns (Fig. 1-154).

NOTE: Intermediate joints, elbow and knee, of moving extremities extend or remain straight. If, as the middle range is approached (B), the subject were to flex the left knee, the foot could contact the mat to thrust in the extension–abduction–internal rotation pattern as described in the *Note*, Figure 1-156.

Rolling: Prone Toward Supine

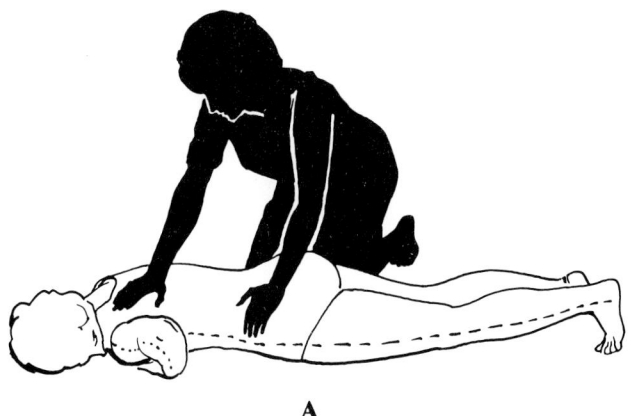

A

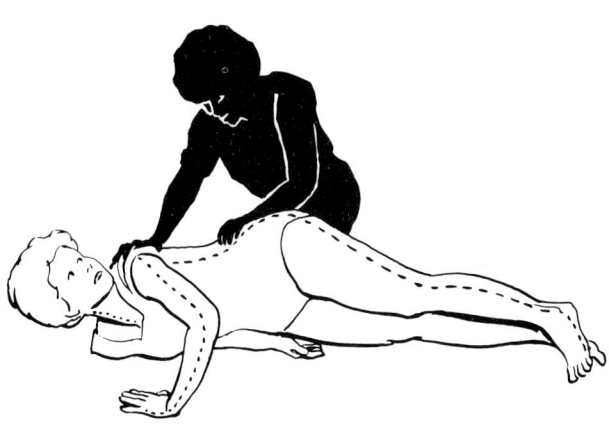

B

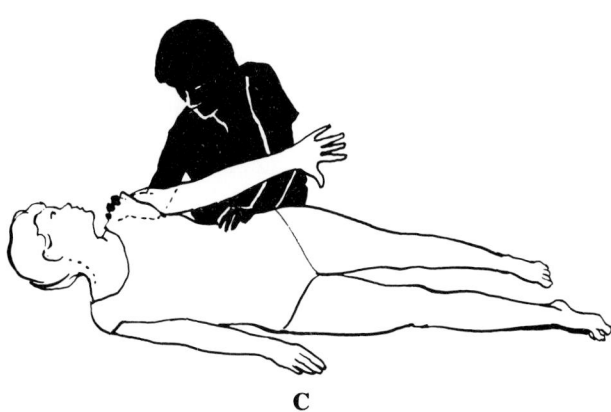

C

FIG. 1-161. Head and neck: rotation, ipsilateral scapula and pelvis.

Component Patterns

Resisted. Left upper extremity, extension – abduction – internal rotation, scapula depresses posteriorly; lower trunk rotation to left.

Free. Head and neck, rotation; left lower extremity, extension – abduction – internal rotation; right extremities adjust in extension and abduction.

A. Lengthened Range

Commands. "Turn your head to me, push with your left hand, and roll! Lift your left leg back toward me! Roll!"

Suggested Techniques. Stretch and resistance.

B. Approaching Middle Range

Commands. "Push! Roll back here!"

Suggested Techniques. Approximation to left upper extremity, repeated contractions, slow reversal – hold.

C. Approaching Shortened Range

Commands. "Come on back! Turn all the way!"

Suggested Techniques. Rhythmic stabilization (see Fig. 1-157), repeated contractions, slow reversal, slow reversal – hold.

Antagonistic Pattern

Rolling from supine toward prone: head and neck rotation to right; lower trunk rotation to right. Left extremities move in antagonistic patterns (Fig. 1-154).

NOTE: Intermediate joints, elbow and knee, of moving extremities extend, or remain straight.

In *A*, subject could have placed left hand near her forehead to more specifically activate the extension – abduction – internal rotation pattern of the left upper extremity.

Lower Trunk (Inferior Region)

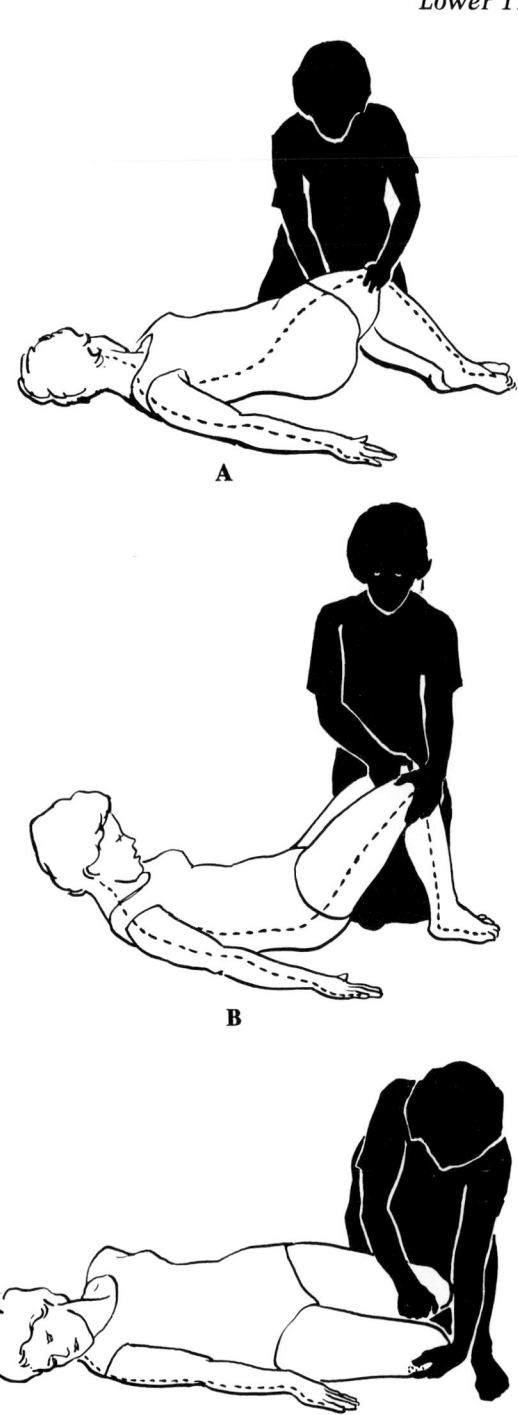

A

B

C

FIG. 1-162. Lower trunk: rotation, supine.

Component Patterns

Resisted. Lower trunk, rotation (with hips and knees flexed) to right.

Free. Head and neck, rotation; upper extremities adjust in extension and abduction.

A. Lengthened Range

Commands. "Turn your head and knees to the right! Pull away from me!"

Suggested Techniques. Stretch and resistance.

B. Middle Range

Commands. "Turn your head, and pull your knees on over!"

Suggested Techniques. Rhythmic stabilization followed by repeated contractions.

C. Shortened Range

Commands. "Hold! Don't let me pull you back!"

Suggested Techniques. Repeated contractions, slow reversal, slow reversal–hold.

Antagonistic Pattern

Lower trunk rotation to left.

NOTE: If necessary, lower trunk rotation with bilateral asymmetrical flexion of lower extremities may be used to initiate the ability to roll from supine toward prone. For completion of rolling, the left upper extremity should contribute with the flexion–adduction–external rotation pattern (see Fig. 1-154). If the head is rotated to the left while the lower trunk is rotated to the right, adversive movements produce stability of trunk.

As with head and neck rotation, lower trunk rotation proceeds from lateralward extension on the left, through flexion, to lateralward extension on the right. In *B*, subject has flexed head and neck as flexion phase is active in lower trunk. Usually, head and neck rotate without lifting from contact with surface.

Lower trunk rotation, supine, activates extensors. If performed in prone position (hips extended, knees flexed), flexors are activated.

Lower Trunk (Inferior Region)

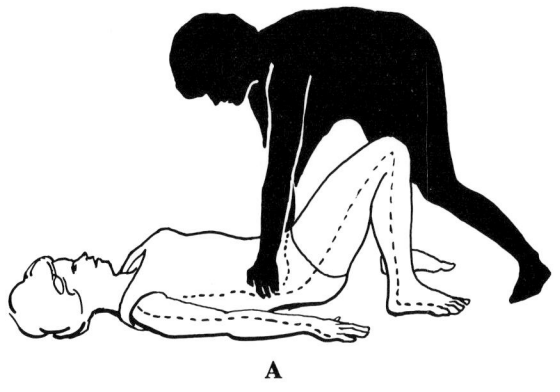

A

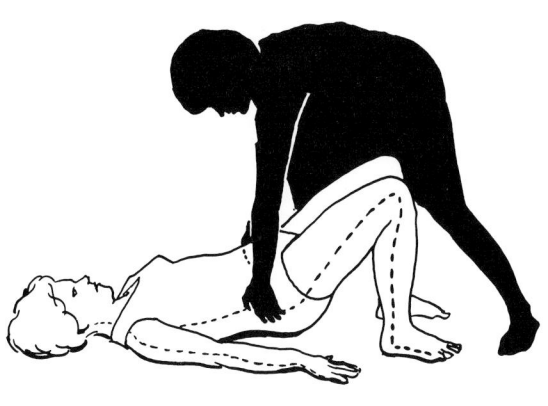

B

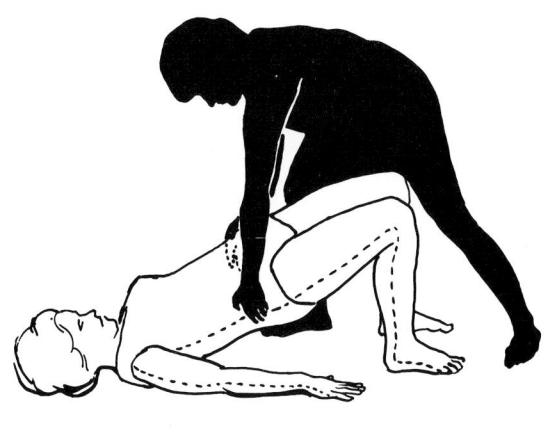

C

FIG. 1-163. Pelvic elevation, supine.

Component Patterns

Resisted. Pelvic elevation with extension of lower trunk (bridging).

Free. Head and neck adjust in mid-position; upper extremities adjust in extension and abduction.

A. Lengthened Range

Commands. "Push with your head and your feet, and lift your hips!"

Suggested Techniques. Stretch and resistance.

B. Middle Range

Commands. "Keep on pushing up! Hold it! Push again!"

Suggested Techniques. Repeated contractions, rhythmic stabilization, slow reversal.

C. Shortened Range

Commands. "Hold it! Don't let me push you down!"

Suggested Techniques. Rhythmic stabilization, slow reversal.

Antagonistic Pattern

Reversal to supine position with hips and knees flexed.

NOTE: This activity is resisted diagonally by commanding the subject to push toward one side while resistance is graded to promote range toward that side.

Pelvic elevation supine, if viewed by rotating illustration 90°, can be seen to be related to kneeling position (see Fig. 1-182). The total pattern would be that of rising from heel-sitting, feet plantar flexed, to kneeling.

Prone Progression: Crawling

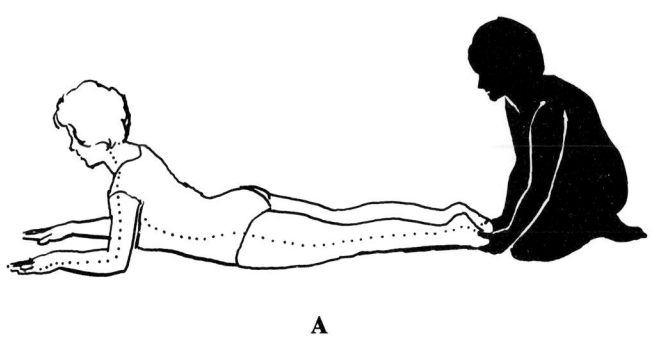

A

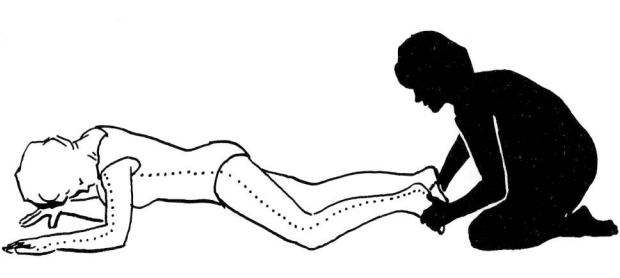

B

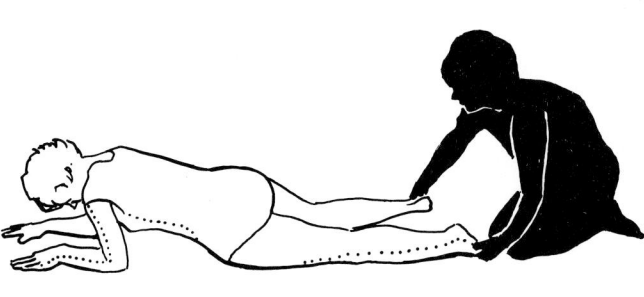

C

FIG. 1-164. Crawling forward on elbows.

Component Patterns

Resisted. Lower extremities, flexion–abduction–internal rotation, alternately.

Free. Head and neck, flexion with rotation toward left as left lower extremity flexes with abduction, toward right as right lower extremity advances. Upper extremities adjust alternately between flexion with abduction and extension with adduction. Lower extremity which has flexed then adjusts in extension–adduction–external rotation as opposite extremity flexes.

A. Lengthened Range, Left

Commands. "Pull your left foot and your knee up and out, and pull yourself forward!"

Suggested Techniques. Traction, stretch, and resistance.

B. Approaching Middle Range, Left

Commands. "Pull your knee forward!"
Suggested Techniques. Repeated contractions.

C. Approaching Shortened Range, Right

Commands. "Pull yourself forward! Use your hands!"

Suggested Techniques. Slow reversals of right and left extremities alternately.

Antagonistic Pattern

Crawling backward on elbows (Fig. 1-165).

NOTE: The amount of resistance used will influence movement of head and neck. With less resistance subject would be inclined to maintain head and neck in extension.

In the most primitive form, head and neck are not elevated so that rotation from one side to the other is used. Head turns to left when left upper and lower extremities advance in flexion with abduction, an ipsilateral combination. Other combining movements include alternating reciprocal of upper, then lower extremities; and diagonal reciprocal with contralateral upper and lower extremities advancing at the same time.

Mat Activity

Prone Progression: Crawling

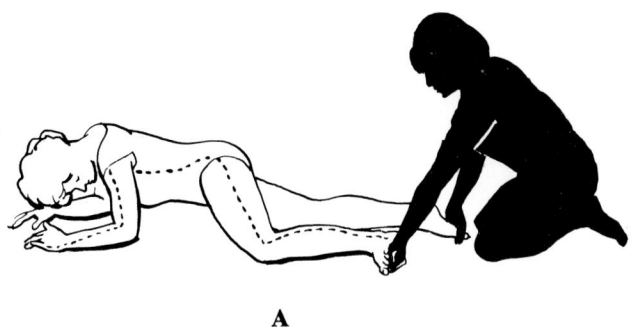

A

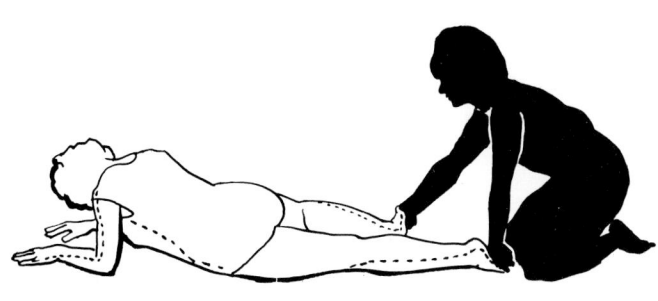

B

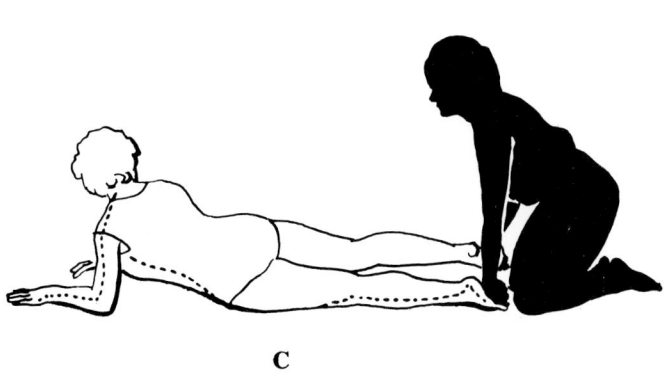

C

FIG. 1-165. Crawling backward on elbows.

Component Patterns

Resisted. Lower extremities, extension–adduction–external rotation, alternately.

Free. Head and neck, extension with rotation toward left as left lower extremity extends with adduction, toward right as right lower extremity extends with adduction. Upper extremities adjust alternately between extension with adduction and flexion with abduction. Lower extremity which has extended then adjusts in flexion after opposite extremity extends.

A. Middle Range, Left

Commands. "Push with your hands, and push your left foot back to me!"
Suggested Techniques. Stretch and resistance.

B. Lengthened Range, Right

Commands. "Now! Push your right foot back, and push with your hands!"
Suggested Techniques. Stretch and resistance.

C. Approaching Shortened Range, Right

Commands. "Push all the way!"
Suggested Techniques. Slow reversals of left and right extremities alternately.

Antagonistic Pattern

Crawling forward on elbows (Fig. 1-164).

NOTE: See *Note*, Figure 1-164.
Crawling forward and backward on elbows requires elevation of superior region, head and neck and thorax. Elevation of superior region is assumed, as shown in Figure 1-166, *A*. Rhythmic stabilization may be used to promote head control and stability of shoulder girdle.
When a diagonal direction is attempted, the total pattern resembles circular pivoting (prone). Circular pivoting should be performed first without elevation of superior region so that total body is in contact with surface.

Prone Progression: On Elbows and Knees

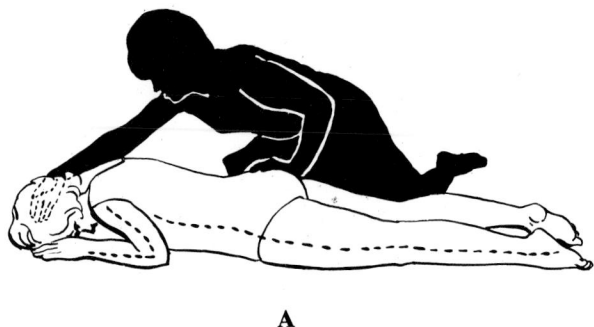

A

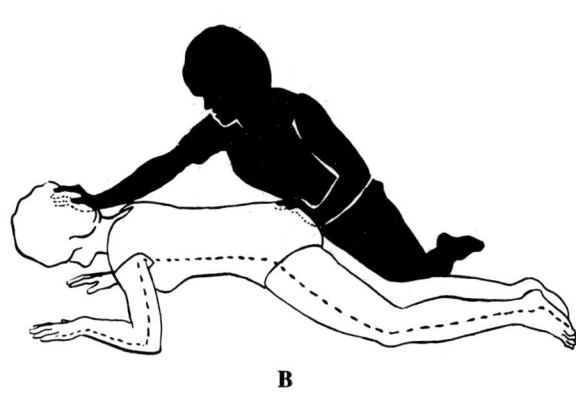

B

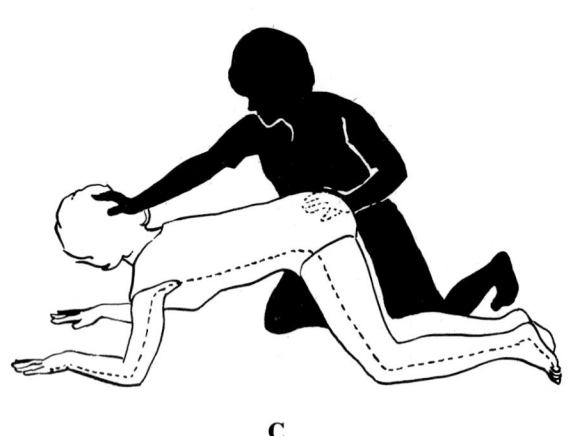

C

FIG. 1-166. Rising to elbows and knees.

Component Patterns

Resisted. Head and neck, extension with rotation to right; lower trunk, flexion with rotation toward right.

Free. Upper extremities adjust with bilateral asymmetrical flexion toward left. Lower extremities adjust with flexion toward right.

A. Lengthened Range

Commands. "Lift up to me! Get your head up! And your hips!"

Suggested Techniques. Stretch and resistance.

B. Middle Range

Commands. "Hold it! Now push some more!"

Suggested Techniques. Repeated contractions.

C. Approaching Shortened Range

Commands. "Move your left arm back a little. Now your right. Now, push your hips back!"

Suggested Techniques. Resistance.

Antagonistic Pattern

Reversal to prone position

NOTE: Diagonal direction promotes elbow extension on the left when total movement is backward to the right. Rocking forward and backward, and diagonally, develops ability to maintain balance with trunk free of contact with surface.

If necessary, as an intermediate activity, the superior region may remain in contact with surface while the inferior region, lower trunk, is resisted, or assisted to a chest and knees position. Rocking movements of the inferior region in all directions and rhythmic stabilization may be used to promote stability of inferior region.

Prone Progression: On Elbows and Knees

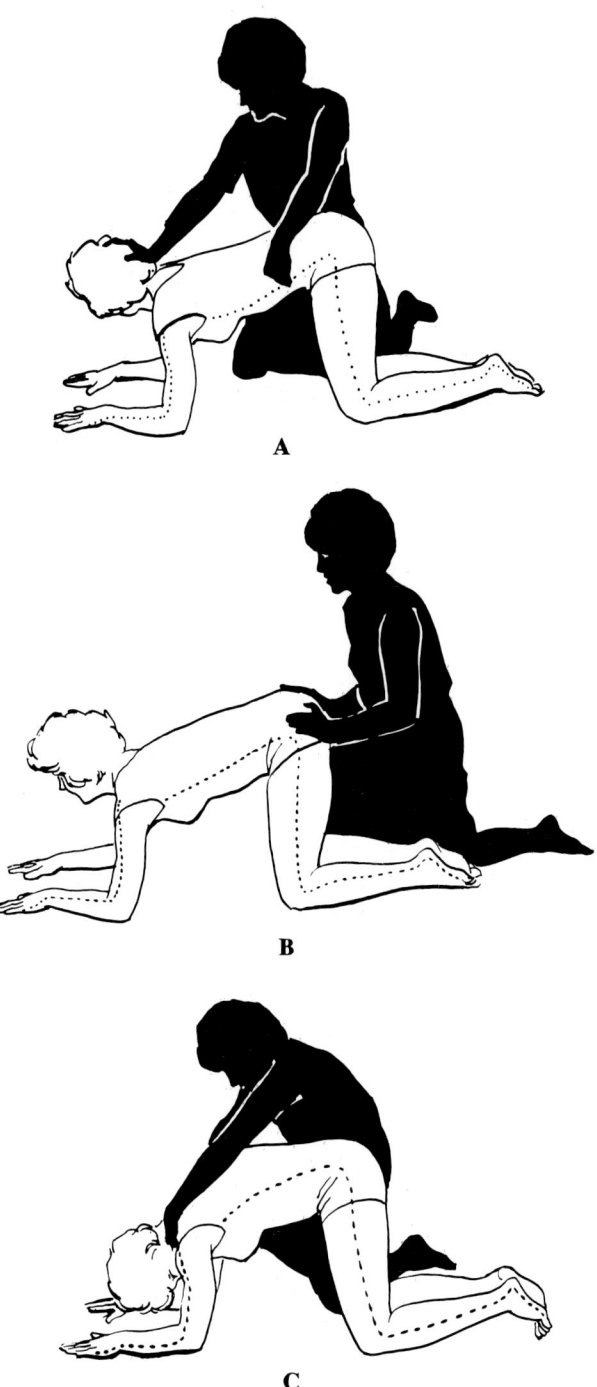

A

B

C

FIG. 1-167. Balance on elbows and knees.

Component Patterns

A. Resisted. Head and neck, extension with rotation to right; lower trunk, rotation to left.

Free. Upper extremities adjust with asymmetrical flexion toward left. Lower extremities adjust with asymmetrical flexion toward left.

B. Resisted. Lower trunk, flexion with rotation to right.

Free. Head and neck, extension with rotation to right. Upper extremities adjust with asymmetrical flexion toward left. Lower extremities adjust with asymmetrical flexion toward left.

C. Resisted. Lower trunk, extension with rotation toward left.

Free. Head and neck, flexion with rotation toward left. Upper extremities adjust with asymmetrical extension toward right. Lower extremities adjust with asymmetrical extension toward left.

Commands

A: "Hold! Don't let me push your head down! Don't let me pull your hips toward me! Stay there!"

B: "Don't let me push you forward! Hold still!"

C: "Don't let me pull you back! Hold!"

Suggested Techniques

A: Rhythmic stabilization of upper and lower trunk.

B: Rocking forward toward extension, and backward toward flexion, then rhythmic stabilization.

C: Holding alternately with hip extensors, then flexors.

NOTE: In *A*, rotation components combined with extension of upper trunk and with flexion of lower trunk are resisted at the same time so that stability is achieved. In *B*, flexion of trunk is necessary to maintain position. If pelvis is pulled toward heels by therapist, extension of lower trunk may be resisted. In *C*, extension of lower trunk is necessary to maintain position. If therapist pushes subject forward from scapular and axillary regions, subject will elevate head and will flex lower trunk. In *B* and *C*, stability is threatened alternately; disturbance of equilibrium promotes compensatory movements with isotonic contractions of muscle groups in order to recover position. See Figure 1-170 for other combinations of manual contacts.

Prone Progression: On Hands and Knees

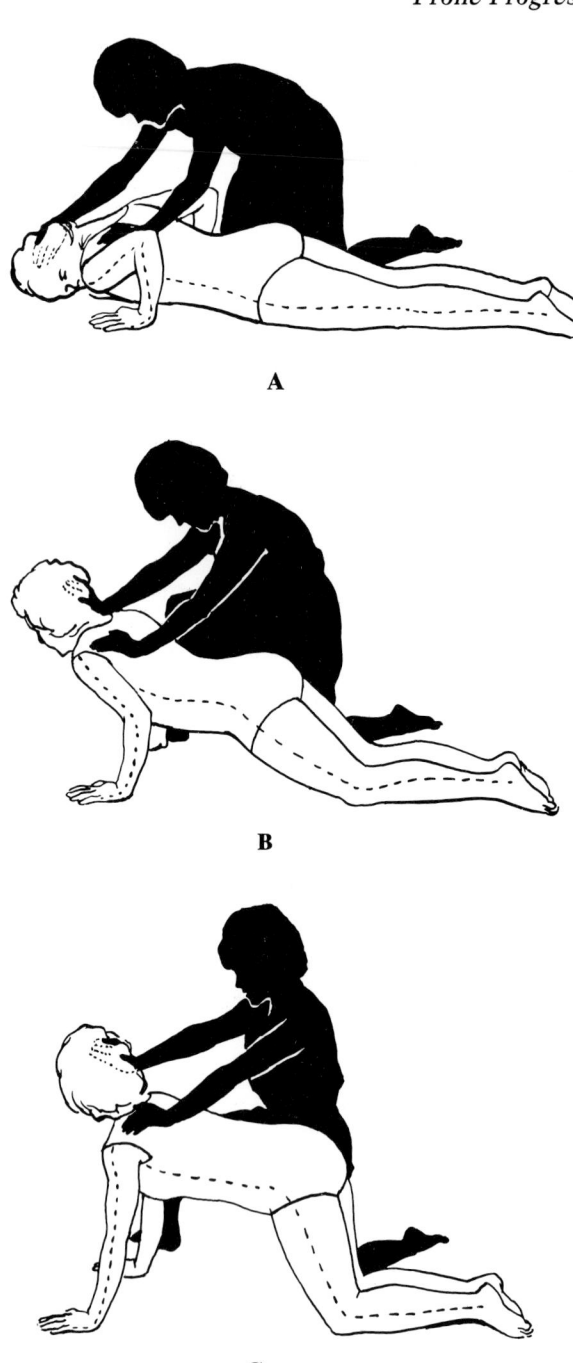

A

B

C

FIG. 1-168. Rising to hands and knees.

Component Patterns

Resisted. Head and neck extension with rotation to right; left upper extremity, flexion–abduction–external rotation.

Free. Right upper extremity, flexion–adduction–external rotation. Lower trunk, flexion with rotation to left. Lower extremities adjust with flexion toward left.

A. Lengthened Range

Commands. "Lift your head toward me, push with your hands, and push back to me!"
Suggested Techniques. Stretch and resistance.

B. Middle Range

Commands. "Come on up, on your hands and knees!"
Suggested Techniques. Repeated contractions, slow reversal.

C. Shortened Range

Commands. "Hold! Straighten your elbows!"
Suggested Techniques. Approximation to left upper extremity, rhythmic stabilization.

Antagonistic Pattern

Reversal to prone position.

NOTE: Emphasis is on extension of elbows. Subject could assume elbows and knees position first (see Fig. 1-166, *C*), and then rise to hands and knees by extending one elbow first, and then the other.

For complete verticality of thighs and upper extremities, subject must adjust upper extremities toward extension. Rocking toward one side and then the other permits the adjustment to be made. See Figures 1-167 through 1-170 for related balancing activities and a variety of manual contacts.

Prone Progression: On Hands and Knees

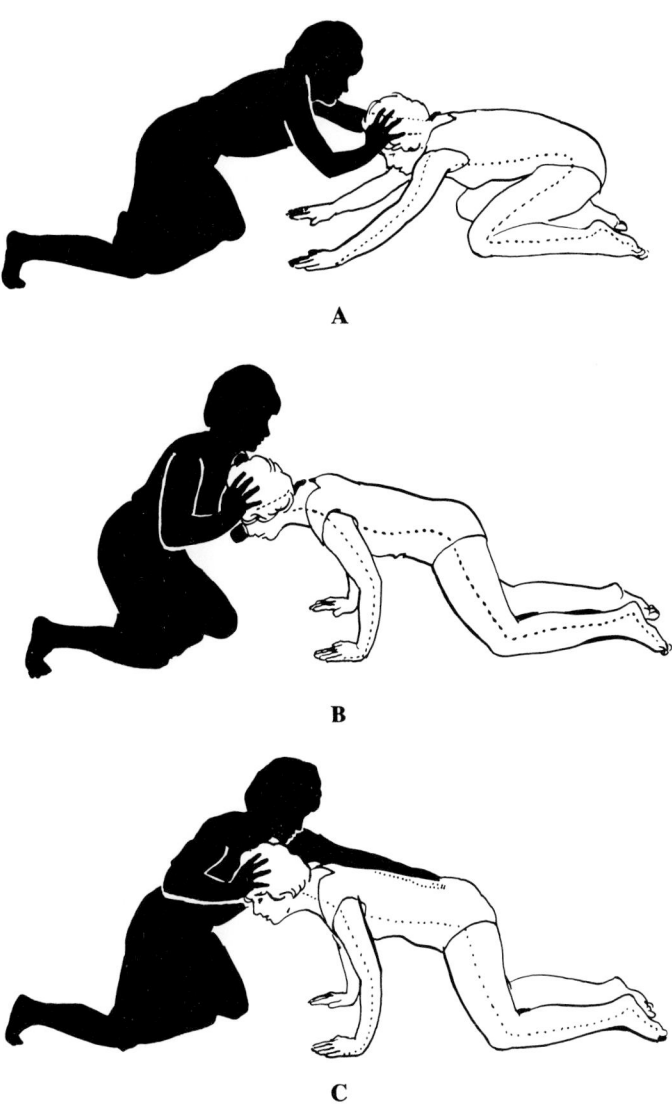

A

B

C

FIG. 1-169. Rocking on hands and knees.

Component Patterns

Resisted. Head and neck, extension with rotation toward left.

Free. Lower trunk, extension with rotation toward right. Upper extremities adjust with asymmetrical extension toward right. Lower extremities adjust with extension toward right.

A. Lengthened Range

Commands. "Push yourself forward toward me!"

Suggested Techniques. Approximation of trunk, stretch and resistance.

B. Approaching Shortened Range

Commands. "Hold! I'm going to push you back!"

Suggested Techniques. Slow reversal, slow reversal–hold.

C. Approaching Middle Range

Commands. "Straighten your elbows, and hold!"

Suggested Techniques. Rhythmic stablization, slow reversal (forward and backward).

Antagonistic Pattern

Rocking forward is antagonistic to rocking backward and the reverse.

NOTE: In *A*, head is positioned in middle range rather than in lengthened range of extension to use approximation and stretch of hip extensors.

Rocking may be performed through extreme ranges, from position in *A* forward and beyond position in *B*; or, rocking may be performed through brief excursions of range. Performance with decrements in range using slow reversal–hold technique promotes balance at middle range, the hands and knees position.

The position shown in *A* may be used for forward assumption of hands and knees position by extension of inferior region, while in Figure 1-168 position was assumed by flexion of inferior region and moving backward.

Acts of assumption, such as rolling into the sidelying position, rising to sitting, and rising to hands and knees, enhance the ability to maintain the assumed position. Rocking movements, performed in all possible directions, further enhance the ability to locate the point of balance and to recover equilibrium when it is disturbed deliberately or inadvertently.

Prone Progression: On Hands and Knees

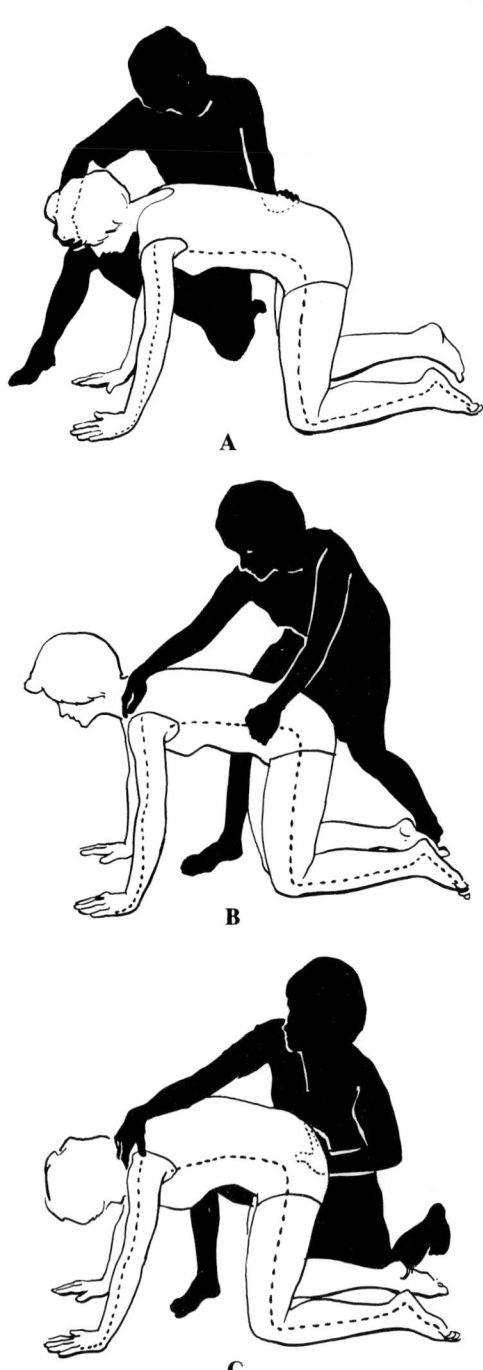

FIG. 1-170. Balance on hands and knees.

Component patterns

A. Resisted. Head and neck, flexion with rotation to left. Lower trunk, extension with rotation toward right.

Free. Upper extremities adust with assymetrical extension toward left.

B. Resisted. Left upper extremity, flexion–abduction–external rotation. Lower trunk, rotation to right.

Free. Head and neck adjust in extension toward left. Right upper extremity adjusts with flexion–adduction–external rotation. Lower extremities adjust with asymmetrical flexion toward right.

C. Resisted. Left upper extremity, flexion–abduction–external rotation. Lower trunk, flexion with rotation to right.

Free. Head and neck, flexion with rotation to left. Right upper extremity, flexion–adduction–external rotation. Lower extremities adjust with flexion toward right.

Commands

A: "Hold! Don't let me lift you up! Now, push your back!"

B: "Hold, and keep your left hand and knee on the mat."

C: "Don't let me push your hips to the left!"

Suggested Techniques

A: Rhythmic stabilization.

B: Stretch with disturbance to demand that subject reach for mat.

C: Approximation of trunk to promote elevation of head.

NOTE: In *A* and *B*, subject may be disturbed sufficiently to promote reaching for mat with open hand and with right knee, *A*, and left knee, *B*. For stability it is necessary to perceive weight bearing on the supporting segments. In *C*, superior region is disturbed from left to right while inferior region is disturbed from right to left. Because counterpressures and adversive directions are used, subject becomes stable. See Figures 1-167 and 1-169 for other appropriate manual contacts.

Prone Progression: On Hands and Knees

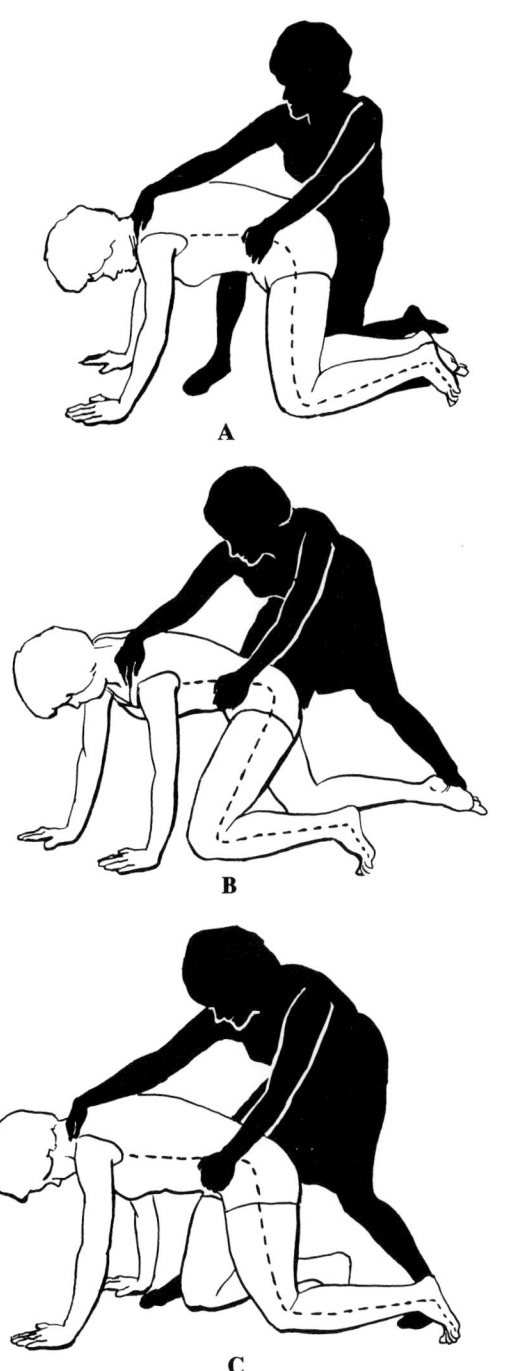

FIG. 1-171. Creeping forward to left, ipsilateral scapula and pelvis.

Component Patterns

Resisted. Left upper extremity, flexion–abduction–external rotation; left lower extremity, flexion–abduction–internal rotation.

Free. Right upper extremity, flexion–adduction–external rotation; right lower extremity, flexion–adduction–external rotation; head and neck adjust as necessary.

A. Initial Position

Commands. "Move your right arm forward to the left."

Suggested Techniques. Prepare to resist movement forward to left.

B. Shortened Range, Left Lower Extremity

Commands. "Pull your left foot and knee forward to the left! Now, move your left arm forward and sideward!"

Suggested Techniques. Resistance, rhythmic stabilization.

C. Shortened Range, Right Lower Extremity

Commands. "Pull your right knee toward your left shoulder!"

Suggested Techniques. Decrease resistance at pelvis so that subject bears more weight on left knee.

Antagonistic Pattern

Creeping backward to right (Fig. 1-174).

NOTE: Subject fails to elevate head to look in direction of movement because therapist is pulling diagonally backward yet is lifting the subject away from the surface so that trunk flexors are activated. Head and neck adjust accordingly. Manual contacts favor flexion–abduction patterns of left upper and lower extremities, which must advance if progression is to occur. At the same time, the subject is inclined to use extension of the right hip and knee.

Sequence is that of diagonal reciprocation: right upper, left lower, left upper, right lower extremities. Other less advanced combinations may be used: ipsilateral with left upper then left lower advancing, or with left extremities advancing together; bilateral asymmetrical placement of upper extremities followed by alternating reciprocal of lowers, left then right; or alternating reciprocal of upper extremities followed by alternating reciprocal of lower extremities.

Prone Progression: On Hands and Knees

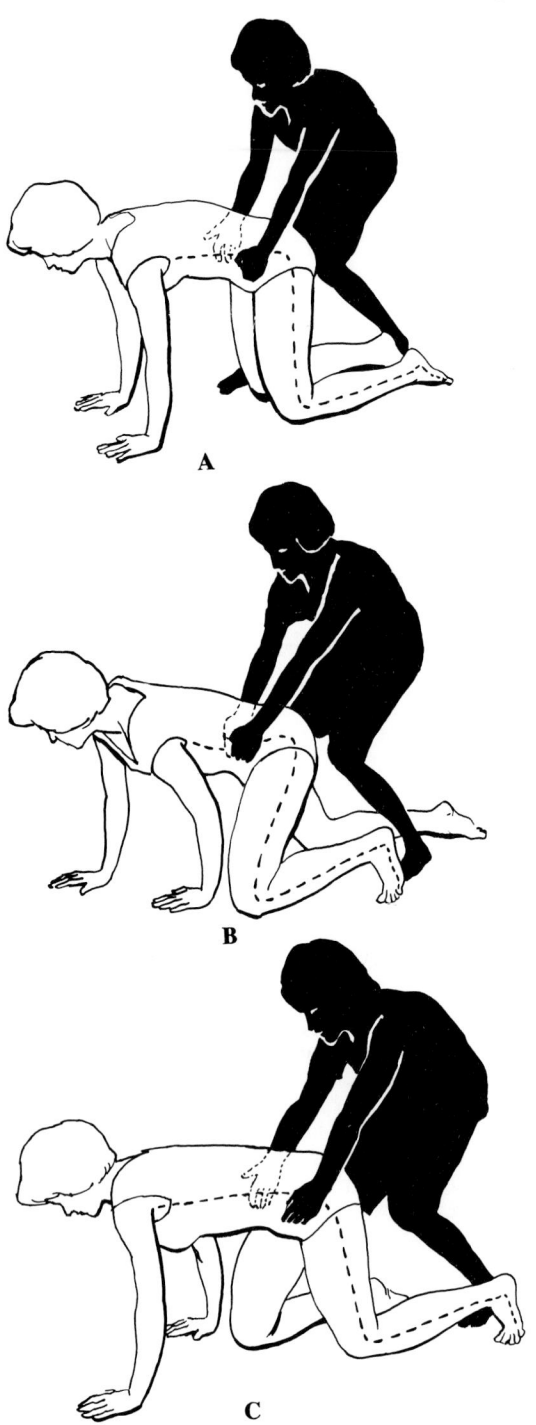

FIG. 1-172. Creeping forward to left, pelvis.

Component Patterns

Resisted. Left lower extremity, flexion–abduction–internal rotation; right lower extremity, flexion–adduction–external rotation.

Free. Head and neck adjust in extension; right upper extremity, flexion–adduction–external rotation; left upper extremity, flexion–abduction–external rotation.

A. Initial Position

Commands. "Hold! Now, move your right arm forward to the left."

Suggested Techniques. Rhythmic stabilization to rotation of pelvis.

B. Shortened Range, Left Lower Extremity

Commands. "Put your weight on your left knee, and move your right arm forward to the left."

Suggested Techniques. Resistance.

C. Shortened Range, Right Lower Extremity

Commands. "Pull your right knee toward your left shoulder!"

Suggested Techniques. Increase resistance on right, pulling upward and backward.

Antagonistic Pattern

Creeping backward to right (Fig. 1-174).

NOTE: Because, as compared with Figure 1-171, there is less activation of trunk flexors, head and neck adjust with extension.

Other combinations of extremity movements may be used as described in the *Note*, Fig. 1-171. Other appropriate manual contacts include resistance applied at head and neck with head and neck extension resisted during diagonal creeping forward and backward, and with head and neck flexion resisted during creeping backward. Appropriate contacts with head and mandible should be used. Manual contacts may be used at shoulders bilaterally, or at head and shoulder as in Figure 1-169, *A* and *B;* or at head and pelvis, as in *C.*

All manual contacts may be adjusted for creeping diagonally backward, or sideward, or in a circle: head, head and shoulder, shoulders, shoulder and pelvis, and pelvis.

Mat Activity

Prone Progression: On Hands and Knees

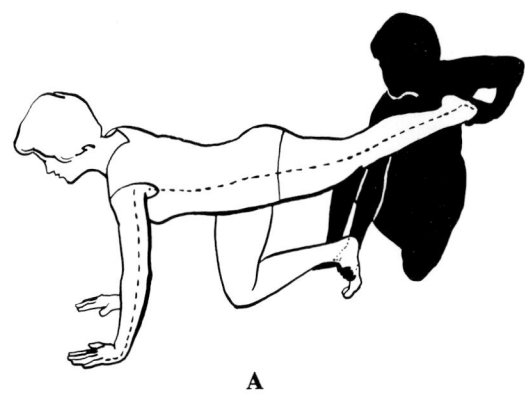

A

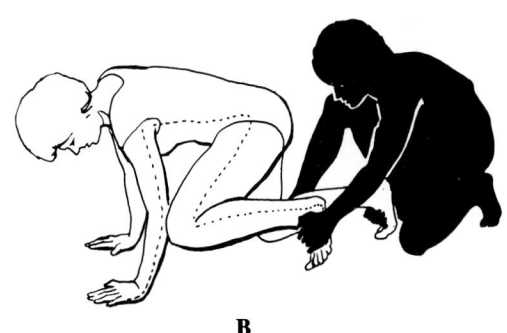

B

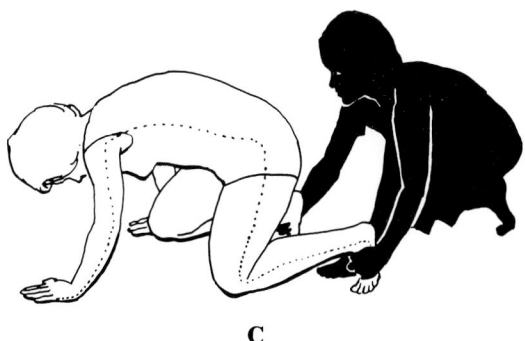

C

FIG. 1-173. Creeping forward to left, lower extremities.

Component Patterns

Resisted. Left lower extremity, flexion–abduction–internal rotation; right lower extremity, flexion–adduction–external rotation.

Free. Head and neck adjust from extension toward flexion. Upper extremities stabilize and adjust to movement of lower extremities.

A. Lengthened Range, Left Lower Extremity

Commands. "Pull your left foot and knee forward to your left! Pull! Bend your knee"

Suggested Techniques. Traction, stretch, and resistance.

B. Shortened Range, Left Lower Extremity

Commands. "Hold it! And let me have your right leg."

Suggested Techniques. Stretch and resistance to right lower extremity.

C. Shortened Range, Lower Extremities

Commands. "Hold with your right, and let me have your left leg."

Suggested Techniques. Repeat flexion patterns of lower extremities.

Antagonistic Pattern

Creeping backward to right (Fig. 1-174).

NOTE: Subject has contacted surface with feet only. Contacting surface with knees would be less difficult but would permit less range of flexion patterns.

In this position, lower extremity patterns as used in creeping may be emphasized, although subject does not actually progress forward. Extension patterns may be emphasized in a similar fashion by adjusting manual contacts. Reversal techniques may be used. Also, for greater control of an extremity, therapist may use both hands on one extremity while the other remains stable with knee in contact with surface. See Figure 1-174 for manual contacts for extension patterns.

Prone Progression: On Hands and Knees

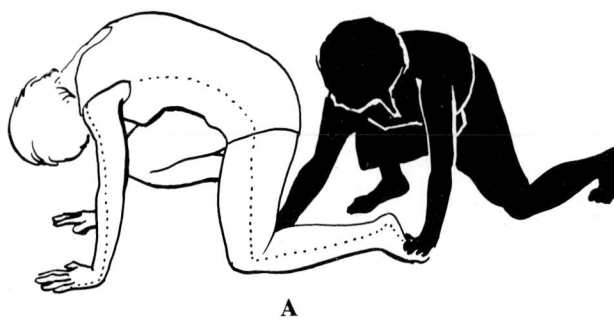

A

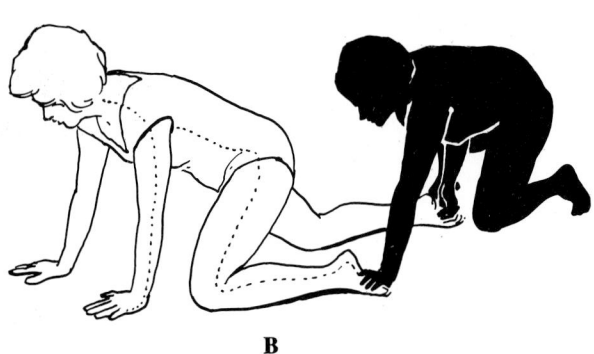

B

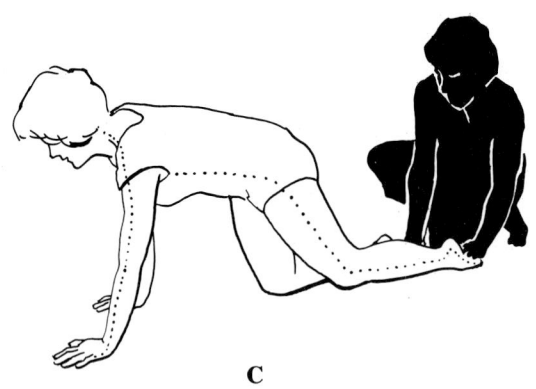

C

FIG. 1-174. Creeping backward to right.

Component Patterns

Resisted. Right lower extremity, extension–abduction–internal rotation; left lower extremity, extension–adduction–external rotation.

Free. Head and neck adjust from flexion toward extension; left upper extremity; extension–adduction–internal rotation; right upper extremity, extension–abduction–internal rotation.

A. Lengthened Range, Right Lower Extremity

Commands. "Push your right foot back to me! Move your left arm back!"

Suggested Techniques. Stretch and resistance.

B. Approaching Middle Range, Left Lower Extremity

Commands. "Now, push your left foot back, and then your right arm."

Suggested Techniques. Resistance.

C. Shortened Range, Left Lower Extremity

Commands. "Put more weight on your left knee. Move your left arm back to the right, and push your right foot back toward me."

Suggested Techniques. Prepare to resist right lower extremity.

Antagonistic Pattern

Creeping forward to left (Figs. 1-171 to 1-173).

NOTE: Sequence is that of diagonal reciprocation. Other combinations of extremity patterns may be used as described for Figure 1-171. Extension patterns may be emphasized as for flexion patterns, Figure 1-181.

For complete development of the total pattern, creeping should be performed in all directions, forward and backward diagonally toward left and right, sideward to left and right, and in a circle toward left and right. Creeping promotes mass flexion and extension of lower extremities. Plantigrade walking promotes more advanced patterns wherein hip flexion is combined with knee extension and hip extension with knee flexion, Figure 1-176.

Prone Progression: On Hands and Feet

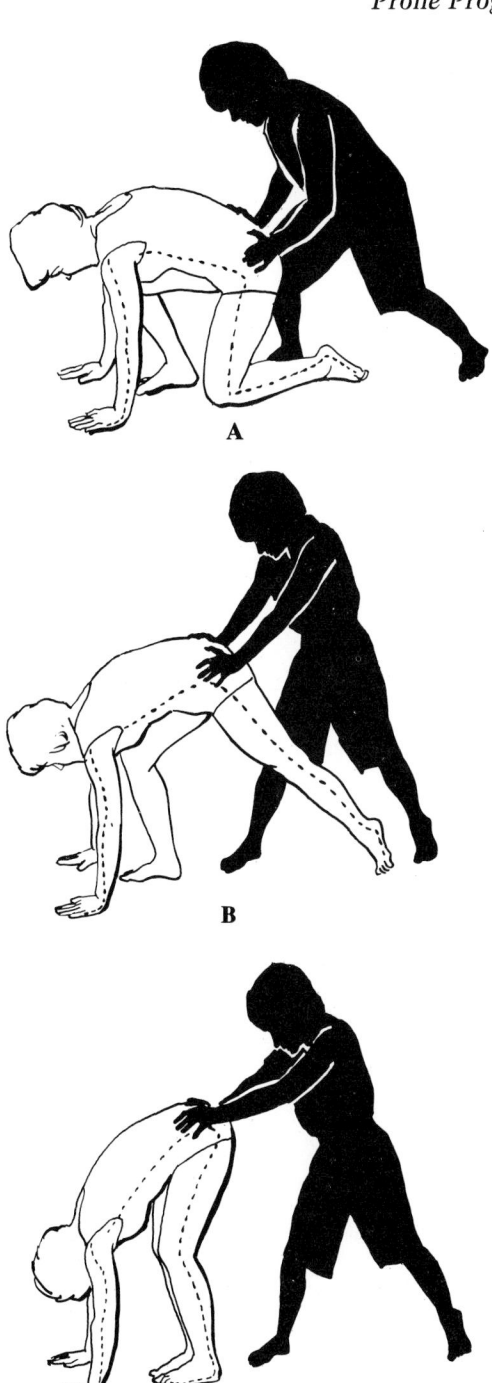

FIG. 1-175. Rising to plantigrade.

Component Patterns

Resisted. Elevation of pelvis; right lower extremity, extension–adduction–external rotation.

Free. Head and neck adjust in extension; upper extremities stabilize and adjust as necessary. Left lower extremity, flexion–adduction–external rotation.

A. Initial Position, Quadrupedal Half-Kneeling

Commands. "Push with your right foot, and straighten your knee!"

Suggested Techniques. Stretch and resistance.

B. Middle Range

Commands. "Push with your right foot, and pull your left leg forward!"

Suggested Techniques. Repeated contractions, slow reversal.

C. Shortened Range

Commands. "Hold it! Now, push some more! Straighten your knees!"

Suggested Techniques. Approximation, rhythmic stabilization to rotation of pelvis.

Antagonistic Pattern

Reversal to quadupedal half-kneeling.

NOTE: Subject has achieved almost complete extension of knees. Many normal subjects will not extend knees if hips are flexed as is right lower extremity in *B*. Or, if knees are extended, will not flex hips so that both lower extremities assume position of left lower extremity in *B*. In order for plantar surfaces to contact mat, subject should be permitted to flex hips and knees. Then, approximation may be used to encourage further extension of knees. See walking posture, Figure 1-176.

Plantigrade position may be assumed with bilateral extension of lower extremities by assuming creeping position, as shown in Figure 1-173, *C*.

Balancing and rocking activities should be carried out.

Squat-sitting and standing position may be assumed from plantigrade posture.

Prone Progression: On Hands and Feet

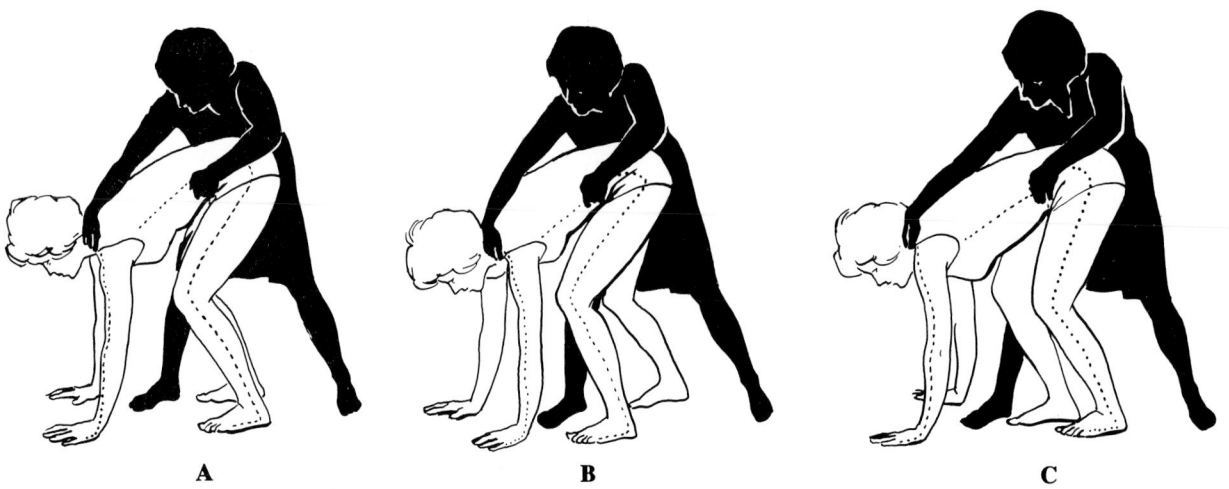

FIG. 1-176. Plantigrade walking forward to left.

Component Patterns

Resisted. Left upper extremity, flexion–abduction–external rotation; left lower extremity, flexion–abduction–internal rotation.

Free. Head and neck adjust in extension; right upper extremity, flexion–adduction–external rotation; right lower extremity, flexion–adduction–external rotation.

A. Initial Position

Commands. "Move your right arm forward to the left, and step with your left foot."
Suggested Techniques. Resistance.

B. Shortened Range, Left Lower Extremity

Commands. "Move your left arm forward and outward, push with your right foot, then pull it forward to the left."
Suggested Techniques. Decreased resistance at pelvis so that subject can bear weight on left.

C. Approaching Shortened Range, Right Lower Extremity

Commands. "Push with your left foot, and pull your right foot toward your left shoulder."
Suggested Techniques. Approximation to left lower extremity for increased extension.

Antagonistic Pattern

Plantigrade walking backward to right.

NOTE: While resistance is applied on the left, the advancement of left extremities is favored. In *B*, as therapist pulls pelvis backward to the right, weight is shifted to right foot so that left lower extremity can advance. Therapist may also use both hands at pelvis, or may move forward and resist superior region, as described in 1-172. *Note*, Figure 1-172. For combining movements of extremities, other than diagonal reciprocation, see 1-171. *Note*, Figure 1-171. See also *Note*, Figure 1-174.

Because in crawling and in creeping, plantar surfaces of feet do not necessarily contact surface, plantigrade walking is a highly desirable activity preparatory to bipedal walking. Knee extensors begin to cooperate with hip flexors as necessary to swing phase of normal walking.

Sitting

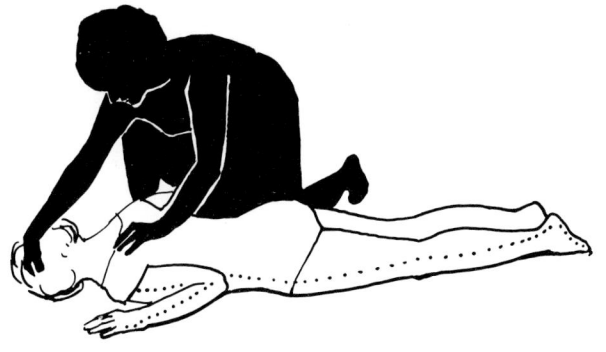

Component Patterns

Resisted. Head and neck, rotation to left; upper trunk rotation to left; upper extremities, asymmetrical thrusting to right.

Free. Lower trunk, flexion with rotation to right; lower extremities, asymmetrical flexion to right.

A. Lengthened Range

Commands. "Turn your head to the left, push with your arms, and sit up toward me! Push!"

Suggested Techniques. Stretch and resistance.

B. Middle Range

Commands. "Push some more! Shift your left hand back toward me! Turn! Hold it!"

Suggested Techniques. Repeated contractions, slow reversal, approximation to left upper extremity.

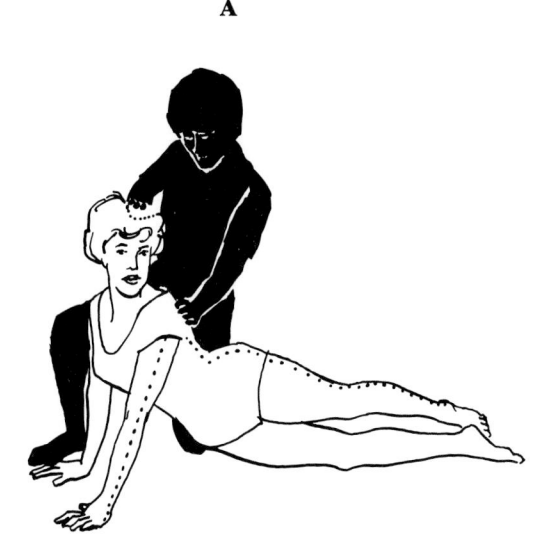

C. Approaching Shortened Range

Commands. "Turn all the way, and shift your right hand forward and closer to your hip!"

Suggested Techniques. Rhythmic stabilization (see Fig. 1-180, slow reversal).

Antagonistic Pattern

Reversal to prone position.

NOTE: Assumption of sitting from prone is an asymmetrical total pattern requiring adversive movements of upper and lower trunk. True asymmetry would be evident had subject flexed hips and knees toward the right. Had this occurred, adjustment of lower extremities toward symmetry would have followed symmetrical adjustment of upper extremities and upper trunk.

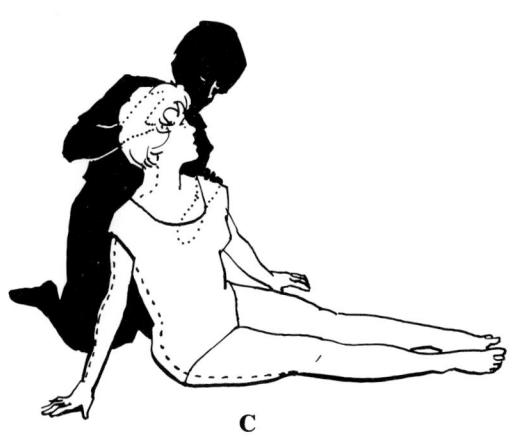

FIG. 1-177. Rising to sitting from prone.

Sitting

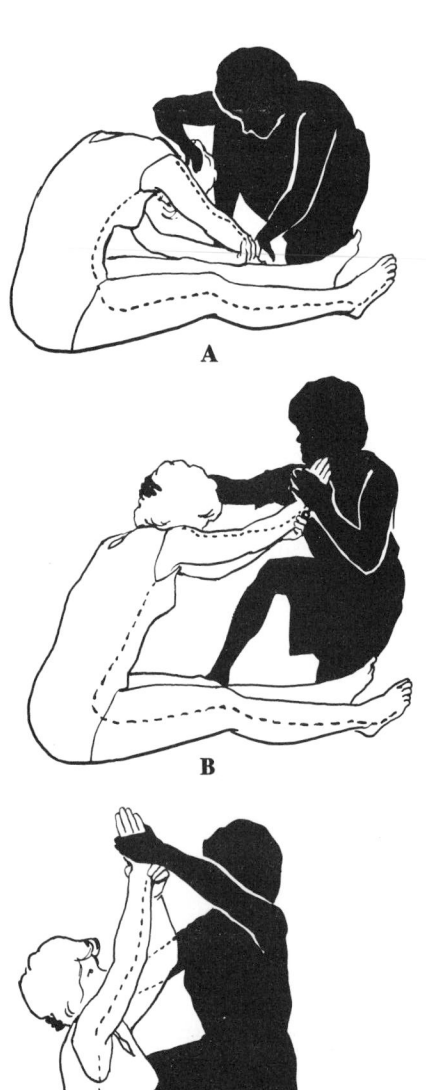

A

B

C

FIG. 1-178. Rising to sitting from hyperflexion.

Component Patterns

Resisted. Head and neck, extension with rotation to right; upper trunk, extension with rotation to right; upper extremities, asymmetrical flexion to right (lifting).

Free. Lower extremities adjust with bilateral asymmetrical extension of hips.

A. Lengthened Range

Commands. "Turn your head and lift up away from me! Lift your arms up and away! Sit up!"

Suggested Techniques. Stretch and resistance, traction to upper extremities.

B. Middle Range

Commands. "Hold it! Now lift up some more! All the way!"

Suggested Techniques. Repeated contractions, slow reversal.

C. Shortened Range

Commands. "Hold! Don't let me pull you down!"

Suggested Techniques. Approximation to upper extremities, rhythmic stabilization (see Fig. 1-180), slow reversal, slow reversal–hold.

Antagonistic Pattern

Reversal to hyperflexion.

NOTE: Lower trunk and lower extremities will adjust with asymmetry toward the left in proportion to the extent of rotation occurring in the upper trunk. The knees, which would be inclined toward more flexion in most subjects when trunk is hyperflexed, proceed from partial flexion in *A* to full extension in *C*. As the pattern is reversed from sitting to hyperflexion, the knees are again inclined to flex.

If total pattern were continued from *C*, the supine position would be assumed. To prevent further extension and to maintain sitting balance, head and neck and trunk flexor patterns must interact with extensor patterns.

Sitting

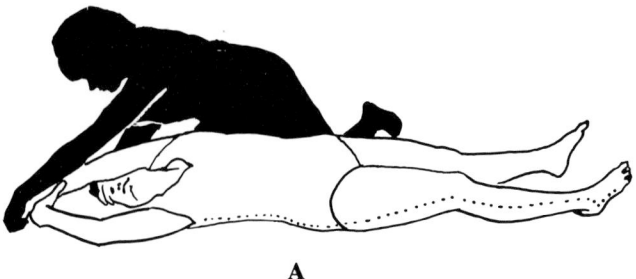

A

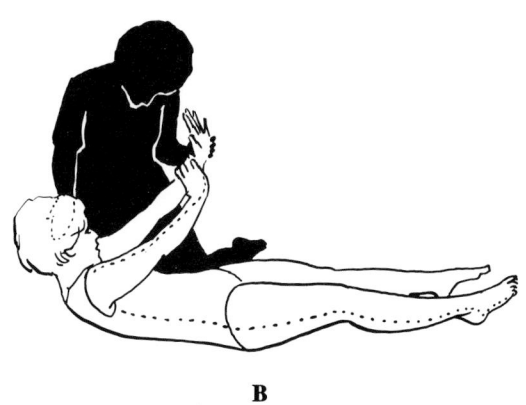

B

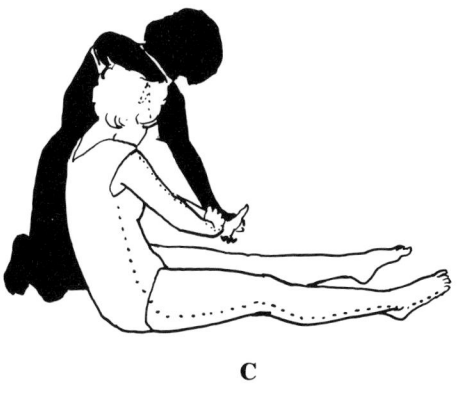

C

FIG. 1-179. Rising to sitting from supine.

Component Patterns

Resisted. Head and neck, flexion with rotation to left; upper trunk, flexion with rotation to left; upper extremities, asymmetrical extension to left (chopping).

Free. Lower extremities adjust with bilateral flexion of hips.

A. Lengthened Range

Commands. "Pull your arms down, lift your head toward me, and sit up!"

Suggested Techniques. Traction to upper extremities, stretch and resistance.

B. Approaching Middle Range

Commands. "Push your arms down! Hold it!"

Suggested Techniques. Repeated contractions, slow reversal.

C. Shortened Range

Commands. "Hold it! Don't let me push you back!"

Suggested Techniques. Approximation to upper extremities, rhythmic stabilization (see Fig. 1-180).

Antagonistic Pattern

Reversal to supine position.

NOTE: Lower trunk and lower extremities will adjust with asymmetry toward the right in proportion to the extend of rotation of the upper trunk to the left. The knees, extended in *A*, will incline toward flexion as shortened range of total pattern is approached, *C*.

If total pattern were continued, hyperflexion (Fig. 1-178, *A*) would be assumed. To achieve erect posture, and to maintain sitting balance, head and neck and upper trunk extensor patterns must interact with flexor patterns.

Configuration of head, neck, and trunk should be compared with configuration in Figure 1-178. Total movement from position *A*, Figure 1-178, to position *A*, this figure, and reversal to position *A*, Figure 1-178, are antagonistic movements of which erect sitting is approximately middle range.

Sitting

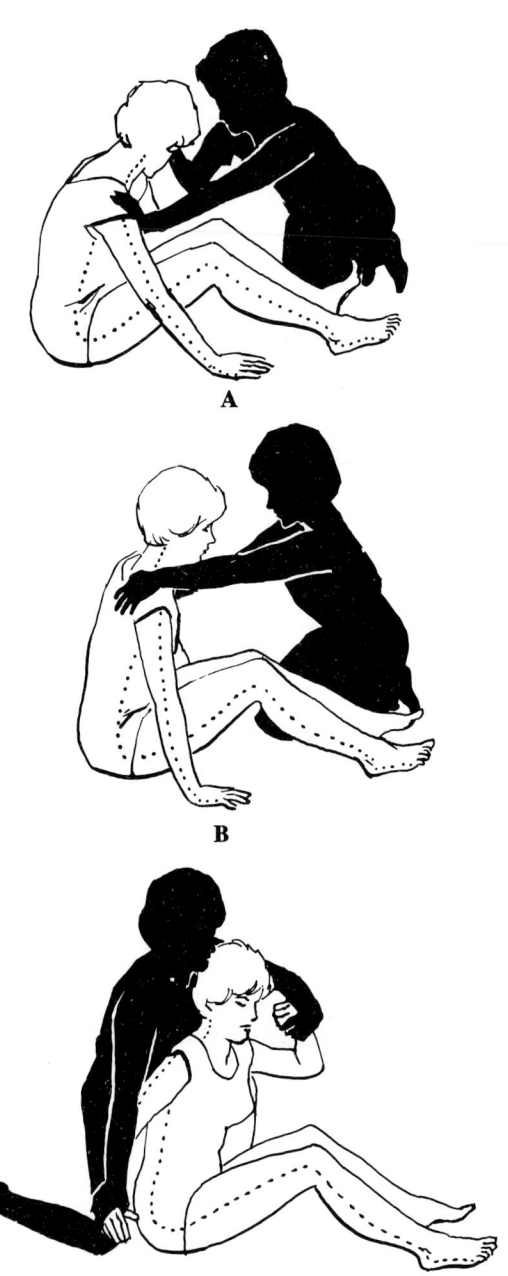

FIG. 1-180. Sitting balance.

Component Patterns

A. Resisted. Head and neck, flexion with rotation to left; right upper extremity, extension–adduction–internal rotation, scapula depressed anteriorly.

Free. Left upper extremity, extension–abduction–internal rotation; lower extremities adjust with asymmetrical flexion toward right.

B. Resisted. Upper trunk rotation toward right.

Free. Head and neck, mid-position with inclination toward rotation to left. Left upper extremity adjusts in extension with adduction, right in extension with abduction. Lower extremities adjust with asymmetrical flexion toward left.

C. Resisted. Upper extremities, reciprocal flexion–adduction–external rotation of left and extension–abduction–internal rotation of right.

Free. Head and neck, trunk and extremities adjust with symmetry.

Commands

A: "Hold! Don't let me push you back!"
B: "Hold! Don't let me turn you!"
C: "Hold! Don't let me move you!"

Suggested Techniques

A: Rhythmic stabilization of flexion, then extension components.
B: Rhythmic stabilization.
C: Rhythmic stabilization.

NOTE: To promote sitting balance, antagonistic patterns are resisted alternately, with manual contacts shifted from anterior, *A*, to posterior; or at the same time, *B* and *C*, with anterior and posterior manual contacts. Whenever possible, approximation is applied at head, or shoulders, and is followed immediately by rhythmic stabilization. Equilibrium may be disturbed slowly without defeating ability to maintain position, or abruptly so that equilibrium must be recovered. Rocking movements against resistance should also be performed.

Other forms of sitting, side-sitting, long-sitting, sitting in a chair or on a table with feet free of support, and squat-sitting should be used. Resistance and rhythmic stabilization may be applied.

Sitting

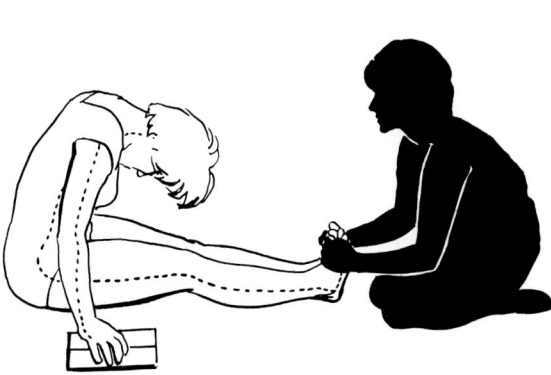

A

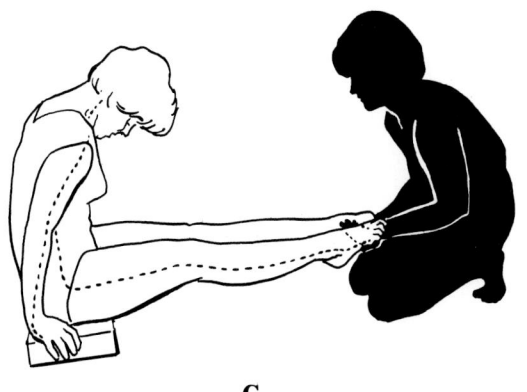

B

C

FIG. 1-181. Sitting: lower trunk rocking.

Component Patterns

A. Approaching Middle Range, Rocking Backward. Resisted: Lower trunk, pulling backward. Free: Upper extremities elevate and support trunk free of contact with surface; head and neck, flexion.

B. Shortened Range, Rocking Backward. Resisted: Lower trunk, pulling backward. Free: Upper extremities maintain trunk elevation free of contact with surface; head and neck, flexion.

C. Approaching Middle Range, Rocking Forward. Resisted: Lower trunk, thrusting forward. Free: Upper extremities support trunk elevation and assist thrusting of lower trunk; head and neck, flexion.

Commands

"Push on your hands and lift yourself from the mat."

A: "Hold it!"
B: "Now, pull your hips back and away from me!"
C: "Push your hips toward me!"

Suggested Techniques

Slow reversal, slow reversal – hold.

Antagonistic Pattern

Rocking forward is antagonistic to rocking backward, and the reverse.

NOTE: Rocking movements promote balance in various postures. Here rocking of lower trunk backward and forward while body is free of surface contact promotes ability to perform transfer activities, as shown in Fig. 1-200, *B*. Lower extremities may be resisted alternately or reciprocally, if ability permits.

Kneeling Progression

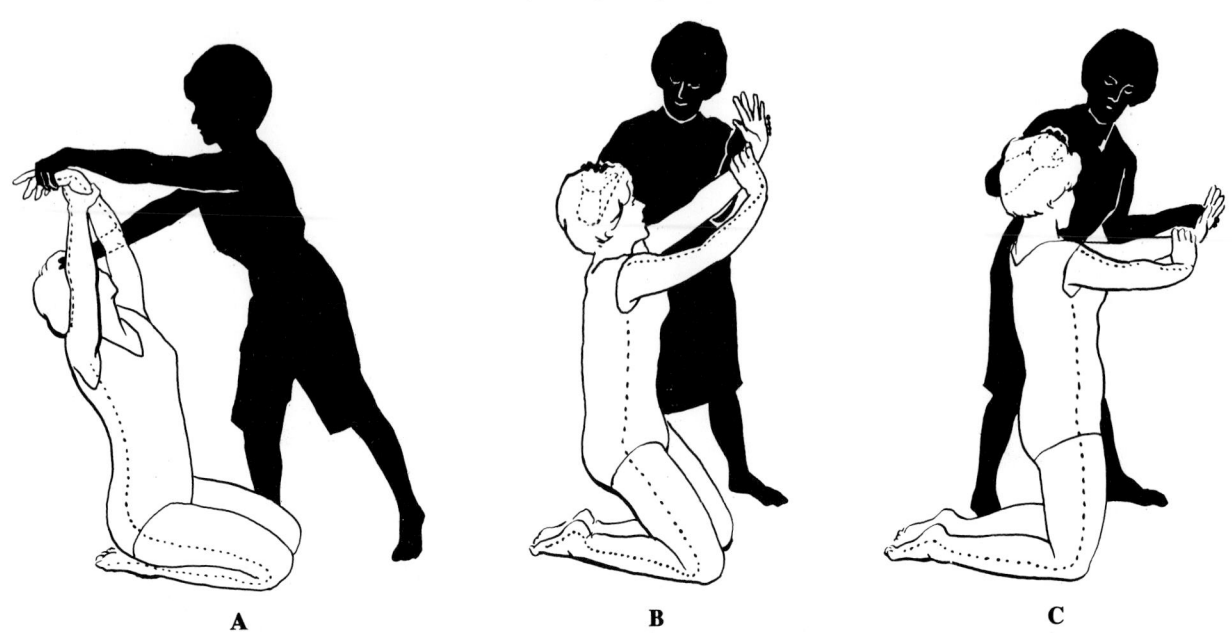

A   B   C

FIG. 1-182. Rising to kneeling toward left.

Component Patterns

Resisted. Head and neck, flexion with rotation to left; upper extremities, bilateral asymmetrical extension to left (chopping).

Free. Lower trunk adjusts in extension; lower extremities adjust with hips extending, knees flexed.

A. Initial Position: Heel-Sitting, Upper Trunk Extension to Right

Commands. "Pull your arms and your head down toward me, and get up on your knees!"

Suggested Techniques. Stretch and resistance.

B. Middle Range

Commands. "Up on your knees! Push with your head and arms!"

Suggested Techniques. Maintain head and neck at middle range so that subject can push up onto knees.

C. Shortened Range

Commands. "Hold it! Stay here!"

Suggested Techniques. Rhythmic stabilization, slow reversal

Antagonistic Pattern

Reversal to initial position with lifting.

NOTE: This total pattern uses flexor patterns of upper trunk performed from lengthened range. In *B*, subject could flex elbows and pull to kneeling. For completely erect posture, upper trunk must shift toward extension.

Kneeling may be assumed from a position of total flexion, head on knees, with resistance applied at head, or at head and with upper extremities lifting; or, from heel sitting with trunk erect and resistance given at pelvis, or shoulders; or, subject may pull up on a stationary object (see Fig. 1-185). Rising with total extension is a more difficult and more advanced activity than is rising with flexion as shown in this figure.

Kneeling Progression

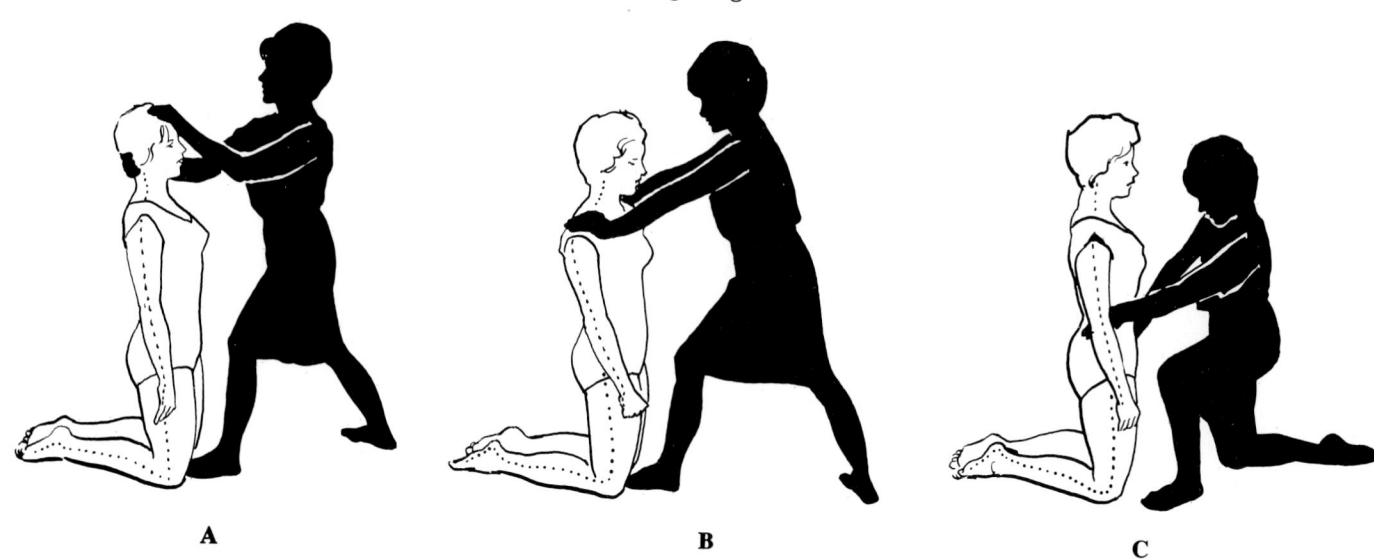

FIG. 1-183. Kneeling balance.

Component Patterns

A. Resisted. Head and neck, flexion and extension with rotation.

Free. Trunk and lower extremities adjust with flexion and extension patterns. Upper extremities adjust with compensatory movements if balance is disturbed.

B. Resisted. Upper trunk, rotation to left.

Free. Head and neck shift toward rotation to right. Upper trunk adjusts with flexion and extension toward left. Lower trunk adjusts in midposition or toward right. Upper extremities adjust with compensatory movements, left in adduction, right in abduction.

C. Resisted. Lower trunk rotation to right.

Free. Head and neck and upper trunk shift toward rotation to left. Upper extremities adjust with compensatory movements as necessary. Lower extremities adjust toward right, extension and abduction of right, flexion and adduction of left.

Commands

A: "Hold everything! Don't let me move you!"
B: "Hold! Now turn to the left, and hold!"
C: "Hold! Don't let me turn you!"

Suggested Techniques

A: Rhythmic stabilization.
B: Slow reversal–hold, rhythmic stabilization.
C: Approximation to right hip, rhythmic stabilization.

NOTE: Other appropriate manual contacts include head and shoulder, shoulder and pelvis on opposite sides. All manual contacts are combined for stability: one is anterior, the other posterior. Rocking movements against resistance should be used as well as abrupt but guarded disturbance of equilibrium.

Kneeling balance demands that knee flexors cooperate with hip extensors and that knee extensors interact with hip flexors. Thus, more advanced patterns of lower extremities are activated (see *Note,* Fig. 1-176).

Kneeling Progression

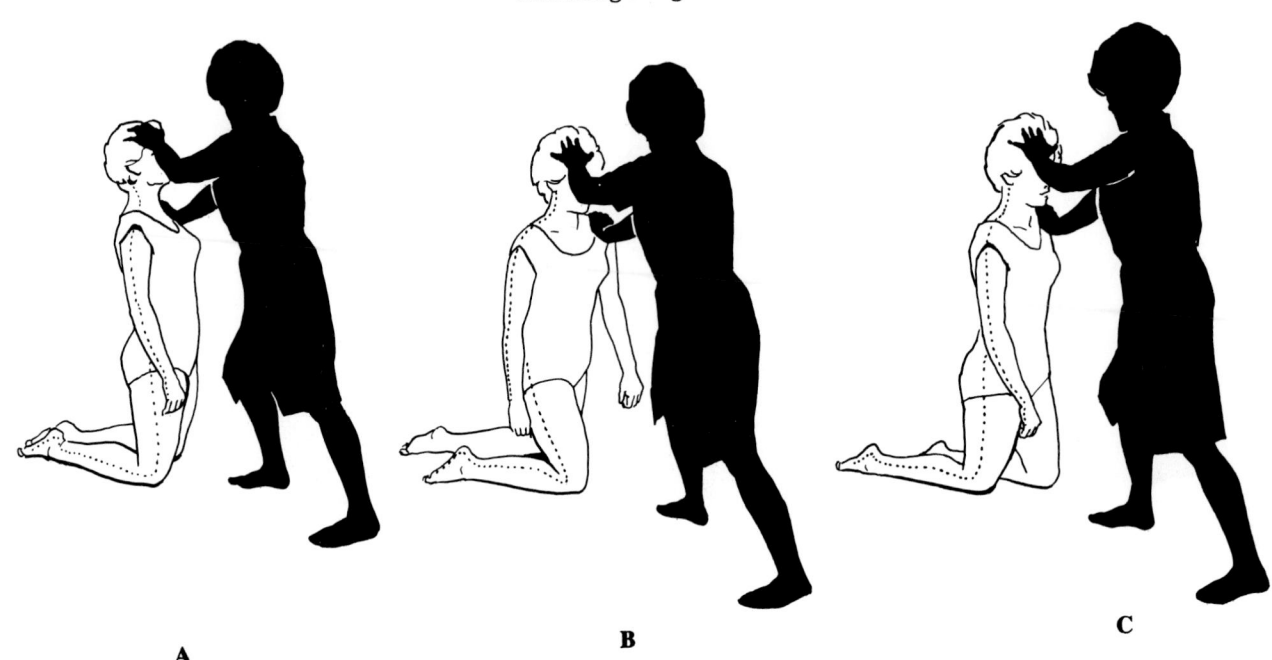

A   **B**   **C**

FIG. 1-184. Knee-walking forward to right.

Component Patterns

Resisted. Head and neck, flexion with rotation to right; upper trunk, flexion with rotation to right.

Free. Upper extremities adjust alternately between adduction and abduction. Right lower extremity, flexion – abduction – internal rotation. Left lower extremity, flexion – adduction – external rotation.

A. Initial Position

Commands. "Pull your head and left shoulder toward me, and hold! Now move your right knee forward toward me!"

Suggested Technique. Resistance.

B. Shortened Range, Right Lower Extremity

Commands. "Put your weight on your right knee!"

Suggested Techniques. Maintained resistance at head and shoulder.

C. Approaching Shortened Range: Left Lower Extremity

Commands. "Pull your left knee toward the right and put your weight on it."

Suggested Techniques. Maintained resistance at head and shoulder.

Antagonistic Pattern

Knee-walking backward to left.

NOTE: Other appropriate manual contacts include head alone, shoulders, shoulder and pelvis on opposite sides, and pelvis with therapist kneeling or half-kneeling (see Fig. 1-183).

Developmentally, the child does not walk on his knees before performing various patterns of bipedal walking. Nevertheless, normal children and adults use knee-walking when it is the most convenient mode of progression. Knee-walking may be used to promote stability for bipedal walking.

Bipedal Progression

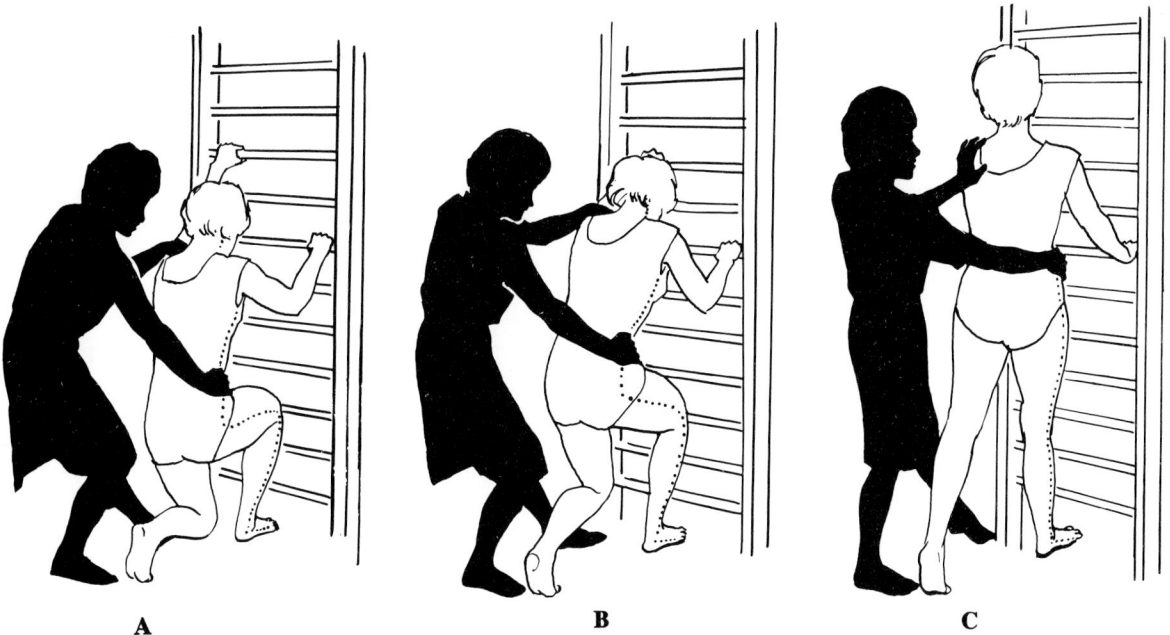

FIG. 1-185. Pulling to standing, stall bars.

Component Patterns

Resisted. Upper trunk, flexion with rotation to right, extension with rotation to left. Right lower extremity, extension–abduction–internal rotation.

Free. Head and neck adjust from flexion toward left to extension toward right. Left upper extremity extends toward adduction with elbow flexing, then extending. Left lower extremity, extension–adduction–external rotation.

A. Initial Position, Half-Kneeling

Commands. "Pull yourself forward, and push with your right foot!"
Suggested Techniques. Stretch and resistance.

B. Middle Range

Commands. "Now push with both feet! Lift your head to the left! Stand up!"
Suggested Techniques. Approximation at shoulder and hip, resistance.

C. Shortened Range

Commands. "Hold! Now pull your left foot forward and step on it."
Suggested Techniques. Rhythmic stabilization, slow reversal.

Antagonistic Pattern

Reversal to half-kneeling.

NOTE: Assumption of erect posture from half-kneeling, squat-sitting, or sitting in a chair requires that the total pattern be initiated with flexion followed by extension to upright. Head and neck lead the movements. Pulling to standing from sitting is shown in Figure 1-197.

Other activities to be performed at stall bars include rising to kneeling (see Fig. 1-182) and climbing activities. Climbing may be considered upright quadrupedal locomotion. Lower extremity patterns may be emphasized while subject maintains position with upper and the opposite lower extremities (see Fig. 1-173).

Bipedal Progression

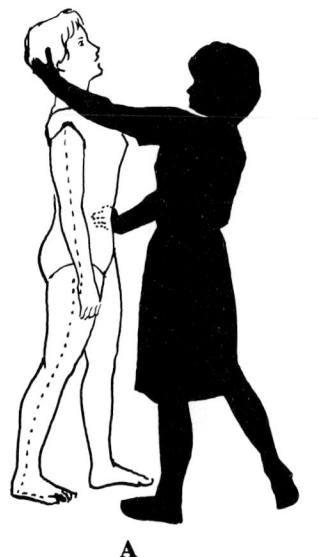 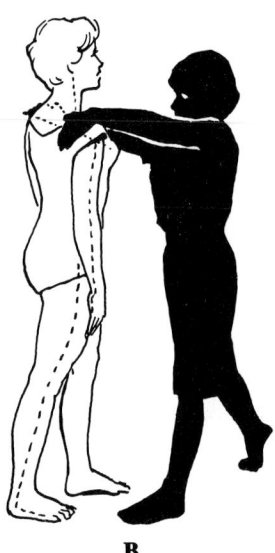 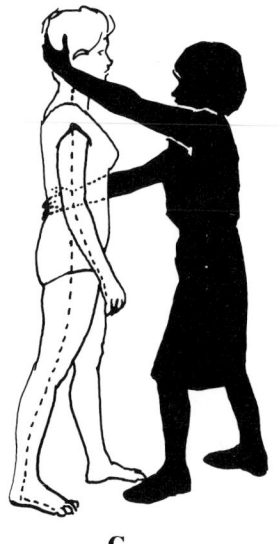

A	B	C

FIG. 1-186. Standing balance, stability.

Component Patterns

A. Resisted. Head and neck, extension with rotation to right; lower trunk, rotation to right.

Free. Right lower extremity adjusts with weight-bearing. Left lower extremity adjusts toward flexion and swing phase. Upper extremities adjust with compensatory movements.

B. Resisted. Upper trunk, rotation to right.

Free. Head and neck shift toward rotation to left. Upper extremities adjust with compensatory movements. Right lower extremity adjusts in extension–abduction–internal rotation. Left lower extremity adjusts in flexion–adduction–external rotation.

C. Resisted. Head and neck, extension with rotation to right. Lower trunk, rotation toward left.

Free. Upper extremities adjust with compensatory movements. Right lower extremity, extension–abduction–internal rotation. Left lower extremity, extension–adduction–external rotation.

Commands

A: "Hold! Don't let me pull your head forward! Don't let me push your hip back!"

B: "Hold! Don't let me turn you to the left!"

C: "Hold! Don't let me pull you forward!"

Suggested Techniques

A: Maintain resistance at head, increase pressure at hip.

B: Rhythmic stabilization, slow reversal–hold.

C: Rhythmic stabilization, approximation on right.

NOTE: In *A* and *B*, balance is stable because one manual contact is anterior, the other is posterior. In *C*, both contacts are posterior. As subject is pulled forward to disturb balance, response of extension patterns of lower extremities is demanded.

Other appropriate manual contacts include head alone, shoulder and pelvis at opposite sides, and pelvis on both sides. See also Figure 1-187.

Standing may be assumed from half-kneeling, squat-sitting, sitting in a chair, and plantigrade. Except for the plantigrade position where trunk is flexed, all assumptions of standing have an initial phase of flexion of head and neck, and of upper trunk, followed by the extension phase. See Figure 1-197, for rising to standing from sitting in wheel chair.

Bipedal Progression

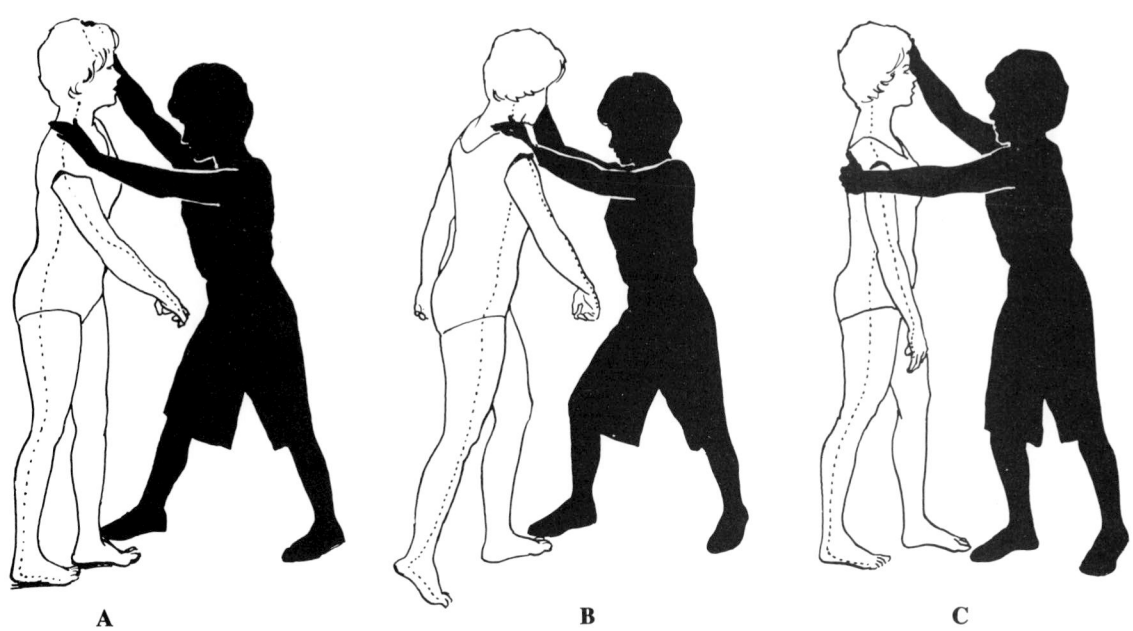

FIG. 1-187. Standing balance, compensatory movements.

Component Patterns

A. Resisted. Head and neck, flexion with rotation to left; upper trunk, flexion with rotation to left.

Free. Upper extremities adjust with compensatory movements; right, extension–adduction–internal rotation; left, extension–abduction–internal rotation. Left lower extremity, flexion–abduction–internal rotation. Right lower extremity, flexion–adduction–external rotation.

B. Resisted. As in *A*.

Free. Upper extremities, as in *A*. Left lower extremity, extension–adduction–external rotation. Right lower extremity, extension–abduction–internal rotation.

C. Resisted. Head and neck, flexion with rotation to left; upper trunk, rotation to right.

Free. Upper extremities adjust with compensatory movements. Lower extremities adjust alternately between flexion patterns, *A*, and extension patterns, *B*.

Commands

A: "Hold! Don't let me push you back!"
B: "Come back to me!"
C: "Now stand tall, and hold!"

Suggested Techniques

A: Pressure and stretch.
B: Resistance.
C: Rhythmic stabilization, alternate increase of pressure at head, then at shoulder.

NOTE: Whereas in Figure 1-186, subject was encouraged to remain stable, in this instance balance has been disturbed to elicit compensatory movements through range, *A* and *B*. In *C*, subject is again stabilized; one manual contact is anterior, the other, posterior.

Rocking movements should be performed against resistance. Abrupt disturbance of equilibrium may be done using a variety of manual contacts. For completeness, positions of feet should be reversed; symmetrical positions should be used as well.

Bipedal Progression

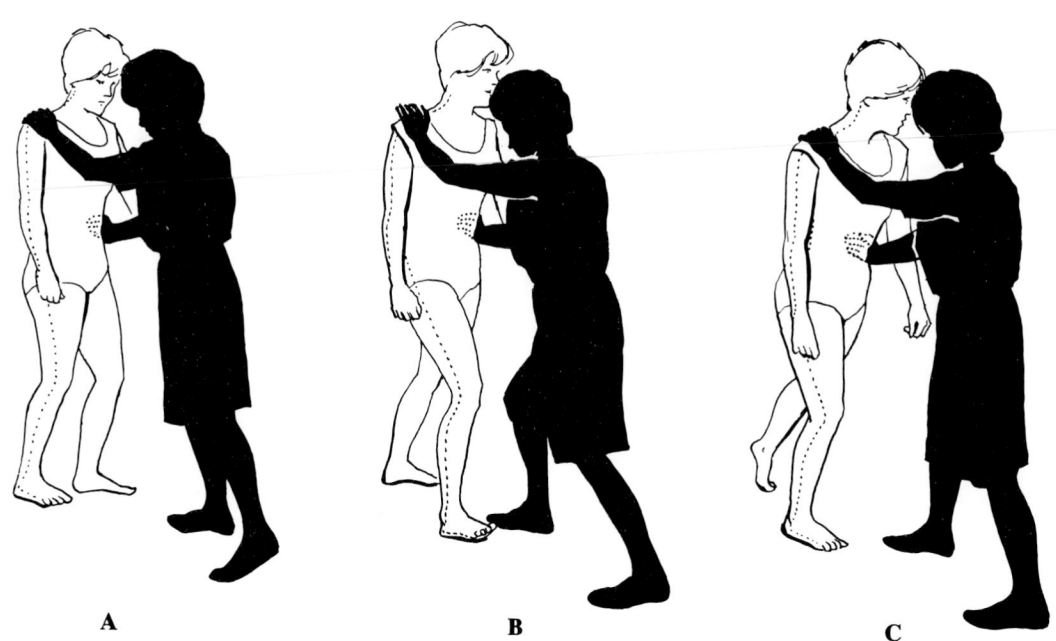

A   **B**   **C**

FIG. 1-188.   Bipedal walking forward to right.

Component Patterns (see Note)

Resisted.   Upper trunk, rotation to left; lower trunk, rotation to right.

Free.   Upper extremities adjust with compensatory movements. Right lower extremity alternates between flexion–abduction–internal rotation and extension–adduction–external rotation. Left lower extremity alternates between extension–abduction–internal rotation and flexion–adduction–external rotation.

A. Initial Position

Commands.   "Lift your right foot forward to the right."

Suggested Techniques.   Approximation on left, resistance on left.

B. Heel Strike, Right Lower Extremity; Stance Phase on Left

Commands.   "Step on your right foot, and push with your left."

Suggested Techniques.   Resistance.

C. Stance Phase, Right Lower Extremity; Preparatory for Swing Phase of Left

Commands.   "Pull your left foot forward!"

Suggested Techniques.   Approximation to right, resistance on left.

Antagonistic Pattern

Bipedal walking backward to left.

NOTE: Positions of therapist and subject have been adjusted for purposes of illustration. Therapist should be positioned toward right. Because therapist is not in the diagonal position, subject has not moved in a diagonal direction. Although instructed to walk toward the right, subject proceeds to move toward therapist. This figure illustrates the importance of the therapist's assuming a position on the diagonal if a diagonal direction or movement is expected. Other distortions include *B*, failure of subject's right upper extremity to extend toward abduction although left upper extremity has flexed toward adduction, and incomplete eversion of left foot; *C*, excessive leaning of subject toward therapist with failure of head to shift toward right lower extremity in approaching stance phase.

Manual contacts for alternating resistance to swing phase with approximation on stance phase should be shifted to level of pelvis bilaterally, as for therapist's right hand.

Gait Activities

The ability to walk erect materializes from the performance of less advanced activities. When methods of facilitation are used to hasten motor learning, the ability to walk may be enhanced by intensive performance of less advanced preparatory activities. Thus, the training of gait patterns begins with rolling and proceeds with prone locomotion on a flat surface provided by a gymnasium mat. Assuming sitting, quadrupedal, kneeling, and standing postures, too, are preliminaries for walking in the upright position. The ability to roll, creep, and stand does not ensure the ability to walk, but the quality of a gait pattern may be improved and the patient's potentials may be more fully developed by intensive performance of less advanced activities.

Assuming an erect posture and walking are goals for the majority of patients. Walking may be an unattainable goal for severely disabled patients. Some patients may achieve quadrupedal upright walking (two crutches or two canes) or tripedal walking (one crutch or one cane). Others may only acquire the ability to cruise in a walker. Those with gross deficiencies may be limited to manual locomotion in a wheel chair. Nevertheless, the urge to walk is basic to the human species. Maximal effort should be made to achieve the highest level of ability that has functional significance for the patient.

The developmental activities related to locomotion in the upright position are shown in Table 1-8. The overlapping between mat activities and gait activities is evident. The least advanced form of assuming erect posture is that of "pulling to standing from sitting." Using parallel bars for pulling to standing is portrayed as a wheelchair activity. Patterns and techniques of proprioceptive neuromuscular facilitation are used in gait activities with all type of patients and with various kinds of support, such as parallel bars, braces, crutches, and canes.

Standing Balance

Once the patient has assumed an erect position, standing balance is necessary to maintenance of posture. Maintenance of erect posture and postural adjustments during bipedal activity are dependent upon postural and righting reflexes and a neat interaction between antagonistic pairs of muscle groups.

When the normal subject attempts to maintain himself in an erect position with feet firmly planted, and when, for example, his balance is disturbed by pushing against his forehead, the dorsiflexors contract in an effort to maintain the position of the feet and ankles. As resistance is increased, the antagonistic muscles, the plantar flexors, contract in cooperation with the dorsiflexors. The effort to maintain position is expressed in isometric contraction of the responsi-

ble muscle groups and a co-contraction of antagonists may result. If balance is disturbed sufficiently, the plantar flexors, by isotonic contraction, contribute to recovery of the position through movement. Furthermore, a whole complex of muscle groups reinforces the effort. Related muscles of the neck, trunk, and the extremities respond. Those responses which entail dorsiflexion of the foot and ankle prepare for the swing phase of walking; responses of plantar flexion prepare for the stance phase and propulsion.

To stimulate postural responses and to facilitate response of specific groups of muscles, patterns and techniques of proprioceptive neuromuscular facilitation are used in the training of standing balance, as shown in mat activities. Pressure and resistance, maximal for the occasion, are applied through specific manual contacts. Other techniques, including rhythmic stabilization, repeated contractions, reversal of antagonists, and approximation, may be superimposed. Selectivity of response is achieved by disturbing balance in a diagonal direction.

Just as the specific patterns of facilitation are composed of two diagonals of movement which, in turn, consist of two pairs of antagonistic patterns, so are there two diagonals and two pairs of antagonistic patterns within the total pattern of erect posture. Balance may be disturbed by applying pressure at the head, shoulder girdle, or pelvis in a direction from left anterior to right posterior, or in the reverse direction, from right posterior to left anterior. In this way, one pair of antagonistic patterns or the patterns of one diagonal may be stimulated. If pressure is applied in a direction from right anterior to left posterior, or in the reverse direction from left posterior to right anterior, the second pair of antagonistic patterns of the second diagonal responds.

Rotation components within the neck and trunk and the extremities may be used to promote security and balance in the erect posture. Various combinations of extremity positions may be used as in a symmetric posture or reciprocation. To facilitate the response of rotation components, pressure is applied in an anterior–posterior direction on one side of the body and, at the same time, in a posterior–anterior direction on the opposite side of the body.

Gait Patterns: Combining Movements

A person who has suffered illness or injury may need to alter his normal gait pattern to adjust to the deficiencies that are present. He may require support of various kinds for various reasons. The combinations of movements that he uses are influenced by the pathological condition that has produced the deficiencies, and by the type of support that is necessary. In general, the goal is to assist the patient to develop or to restore a gait pattern that is as nearly normal as possible.

Table 1-10. Examples of Combining Movements in Crutch Gait Patterns (Primitive to Advanced)

Combining Movement	Type of Patient	Name of Gait	Level of Stability
Bilateral symmetrical	Paraplegic	Swing-through*†	Poor, as stable as jumping with feet held together
Alternating ipsilateral	Arthritic with ankylosed hips	Two-point amputation*	Fair, more stable than turning a corner on one foot
Alternating reciprocal (combined with bilateral symmetrical of upper extremities	Postoperative knee; fractured hip	Three point*	Good; base may be broadened as necessary
Diagonal reciprocal	Quadriparetic, paraparetic, arthritic	Four point*†	Most stable; base may be broadened as necessary

* Deaver GG, Brown ME: The Challenge of Crutches. Arch Phys Med July – Nov 1945
† Buchwald E: Physical Rehabilitation for Daily Living. New York, Blakiston Division, McGraw-Hill, 1952

As with any form of therapeutic exercise, gradation of demand is possible. Demand may be increased or decreased by altering the type and degree of support, the rate of walking, and the relationship with gravity, as, for example, use of a level, smooth surface as compared with ascending and descending ramps or stairs. An acceptable gait pattern must be safe for the patient's use in the environment in which he will have to use it. The pattern and the devices used to support the pattern must protect the segments to be protected, or must lessen the deficiency, and, hopefully, will permit the patient to improve his gait pattern through use. Altered gait patterns include combining movements of upper and lower extremities in ways that are more primitive than is diagonal reciprocation as follows:

Combining Movements: Primitive to Advanced
Bilateral symmetrical: upper extremities advance, then lower extremities follow

Alternating ipsilateral: upper extremity and lower extremity of the same side advance, then the extremities of the opposite side follow in a like manner

Alternating reciprocal: one upper extremity advances, then the other upper extremity follows in a like manner; then the lower extremities advance in a like sequence

Diagonal reciprocal: one upper extremity advances as the opposite lower extremity advances; the other upper extremity and its opposite lower extremity then advance in a like manner or sequence

Other Combinations Used for Altered Gait Patterns
Bilateral symmetrical combined with alternating reciprocal: one pair of extremities, upper or lower, advances with symmetrical movements; the other pair, upper or lower, advances with alternating reciprocal movements

These are the basic combinations of movement used in gait training. Some patients may use diagonal reciprocation, the most advanced form, from the beginning. Other patients may never be able to perform diagonal reciprocation with its neat interaction of extremities. The selection of an appropriate pattern is the task of the physician and the physical therapist. Elderly patients usually will perform better if they are allowed to select, or reveal, within the limits of safety, those combinations that are easiest for them. Examples are given in Table 1-10.

Gait training may begin by use of parallel bars. The patient may progress from the use of the bars to the use of a walker, to crutches, to canes, to freedom from support by devices. Or, selected patients may begin by using crutches or canes, or may never need these devices but may require training under supervision. The various patterns of walking in parallel bars, or using crutches, or using canes may be analyzed in terms of the combining movements used. Crutches or canes may be considered extensions of the upper extremities. The total pattern may be considered upright quadrupedal walking since, when two crutches or two canes are used, all four extremities are supported, or contact the surface.

Gait Activity

Parallel Bars

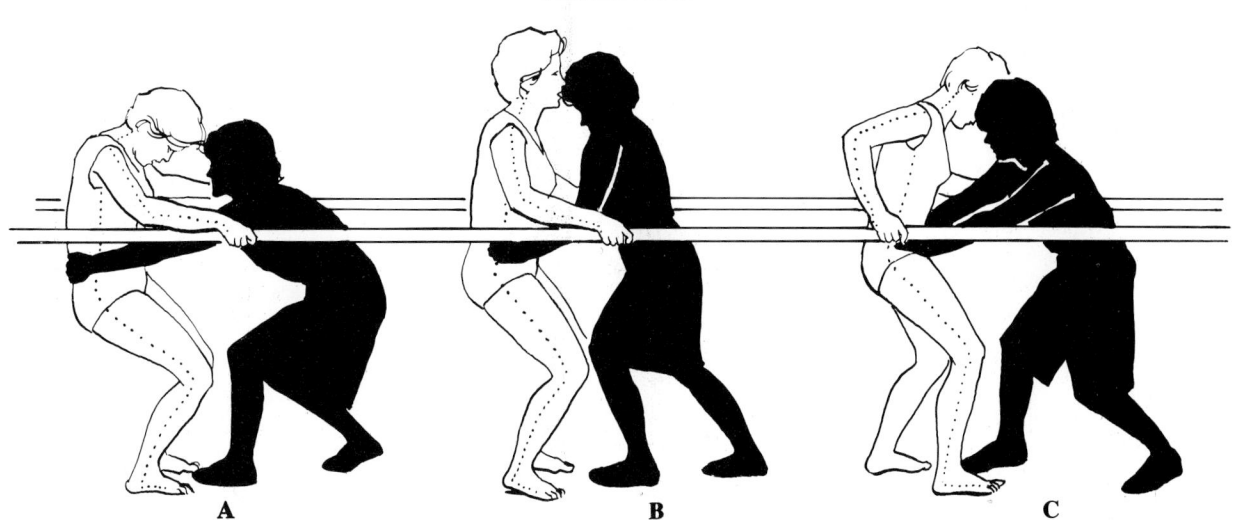

FIG. 1-189.   Sitting to standing balance.

Component Patterns

A. Resisted. Approaching symmetrical total flexion as in lowering from standing to sitting in a chair.

Free. Head and neck, trunk, and lower extremities adjust in flexion; upper extremities prevent lowering to squat-sitting.

B. Resisted. Approaching symmetrical total extension as in rising from sitting to standing.

Free. Head and neck, trunk, and lower extremities adjust toward extension; upper extremities prevent lowering toward sitting.

C. Resisted. Approaching total extension with extremities in diagonal reciprocation.

Free. Head and neck and trunk adjust in flexion in effort to align superior region with support on feet; left upper extremity pulls as right pushes to assist alignment of superior region.

Commands

A: "Hold! Don't let me pull you forward!"

B: "Hold! Don't let me push you back! Now pull with your arms, and come on up toward me!"

C: "Hold! Now push up to me, and lift your head up!"

Suggested Techniques

A and *B*: Slow reversal – hold with rocking backward and forward, rhythmic stabilization.

C: Rhythmic stabilization.

NOTE: Subject has not approached the shortened range of extension of lower extremities. Therefore, approximation at hips cannot be used to stimulate extensor reflexes. In *C*, manual contact for head and neck extension would promote total extension.

The ability to maintain a semi-flexed posture is useful in the initial phase of rising to standing from sitting, and in lowering to sitting in a chair. Resistance applied at various ranges of a total pattern hastens the ability to move through increased range. If assistance to upright is given, rocking movements should be used to promote control and the ability to rise independently. Pulling to standing in parallel bars is shown in Figure 1-197.

Balancing activities in an erect posture are shown in Figure 1-190. Figures 1-186 and 1-187 portray training of standing balance in an open area.

Parallel Bars

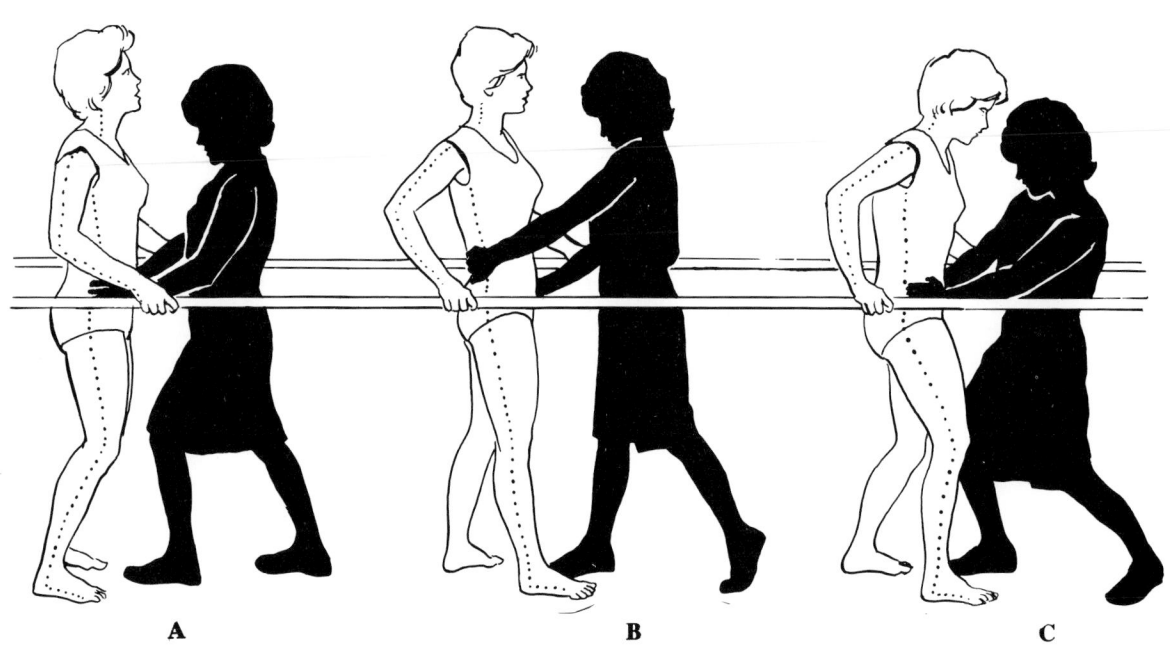

A   **B**   **C**

FIG. 1-190. Standing and walking.

Component Patterns

A. Resisted. Lower trunk, rotation to left.

Free. Head and neck shift toward left as extension of left lower extremity is activated. Right lower extremity has flexed prior to extending. Upper extremities adjust with stabilization.

B. Resisted. Lower trunk, rotation to right.

Free. Head and neck adjust toward left, away from advanced right lower extremity. Extremities, positioned in diagonal reciprocation, adjust with stabilization.

C. Resisted. Right lower extremity, approaching stance phase; left lower extremity, approaching swing phase.

Free. Head and neck adjust toward left. Upper trunk adjusts toward right. Lower trunk adjusts toward left. Left upper extremity pulls to assist swing of right lower extremity; right upper pushes to assist propulsion of left lower.

Commands

A and *B:* "Hold! Don't let me turn you!"

C: "Step on your right foot, and move your right hand forward. Now pull your left foot forward."

Suggested Techniques. A and *B:* Rhythmic stabilization, approximation.

C: Approximation on right, resistance on left.

NOTE: In *A* and *C,* approximation is needed to promote extension of weight-bearing lower extremities. For other appropriate manual contacts, see Figures 1-186 to 1-188.

Diagonal patterns of the lower extremity may be elicited as the patient moves sideways between parallel bars. This activity is termed *braiding.* The patient faces one bar and grips the bar with both hands. In moving to the right the following sequence occurs: step forward R foot, D2 fl; step backward L foot, D2 ex; step backward R foot, D1 ex; step forward L foot, D1 fl. To activate the same patterns in the opposite limbs, move from right to left. Braiding may be performed while ascending or descending stairs with both hands on rail. See also Fig. 1-195 and footnote, p. 344.

Crutches

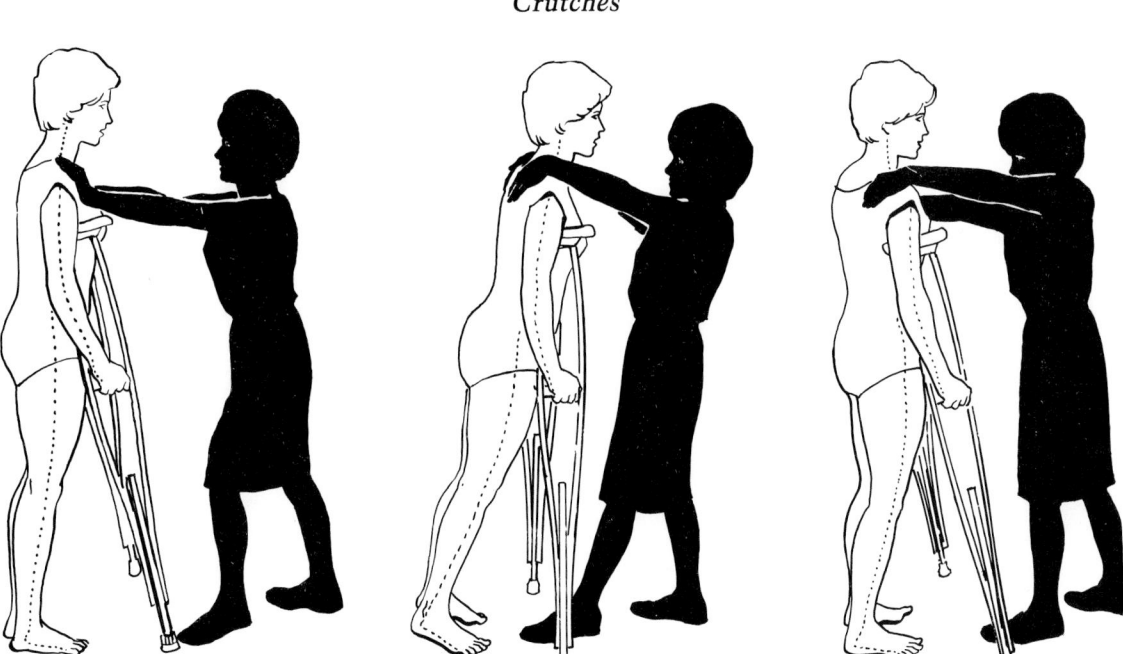

FIG. 1-191. Superior region balance.

Component Patterns

A. Resisted. Upper trunk, flexion.
Free. Head and neck adjust with flexion. Upper extremities thrust downward and backward. Lower trunk adjusts with flexion. Lower extremities adjust with activation of dorsiflexors.
B. Resisted. Upper trunk, extension.
Free. Head and neck adjust with extension. Upper extremities thrust downward and forward. Lower trunk adjusts with extension. Lower extremities adjust with activation of plantar flexors.
C. Resisted. Upper trunk, rotation toward right.
Free. Head and neck adjust toward right. Lower trunk adjusts with rotation toward left. Upper and lower extremities adjust with stabilization.

Commands

A: "Hold! Don't let me push you back!"

B: "Hold! Don't let me pull you forward!"
C: "Hold! Don't let me turn you to the left!"

Suggested Techniques

A and B: Pressure and resistance.
C: Approximation to right shoulder, rhythmic stabilization.

NOTE: In A and B, stability is threatened so that compensatory movements may be necessary to recover equilibrium. In C, stability is encouraged through resistance applied simultaneously to flexion and extension of trunk. Other appropriate manual contacts include head, and head and shoulder on opposite sides.
Resistance may be given at subject's wrist as a crutch is shifted in position, and as the crutch is maintained in position. Subject may be instructed to hold one crutch free of contact with surface as resistance is applied in various combinations. Various combinations of foot and crutch positions should be used. Rocking movements may be done with crutches lifted as subject rocks backward, with crutches replaced in contact as subject rocks forward.

Gait Activity

Crutches

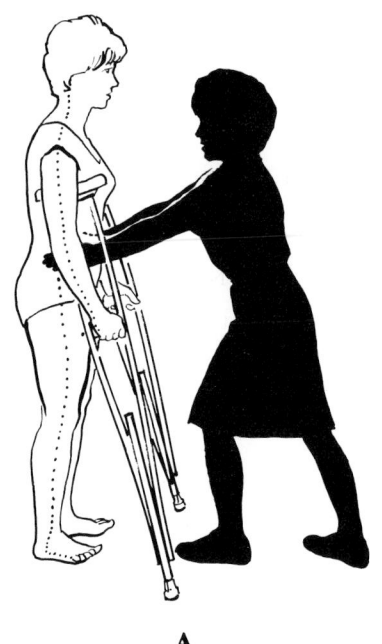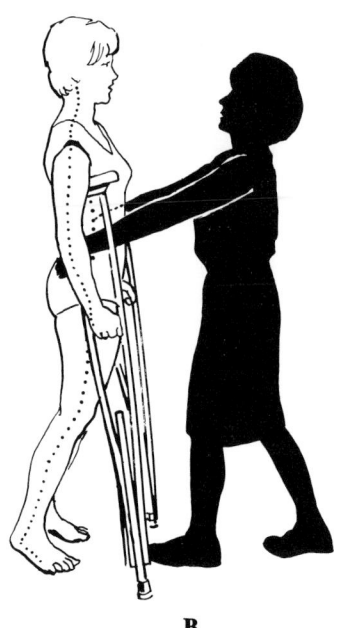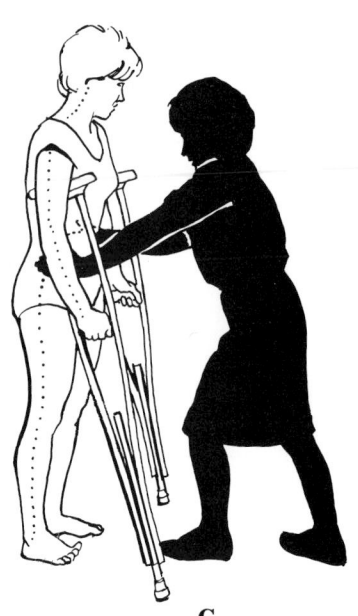

A **B** **C**

FIG. 1-192.   Inferior region balance.

Component Patterns

A. Resisted.   Lower trunk, flexion.

Free.   Head and neck and upper trunk adjust with flexion. Upper extremities thrust downward and backward. Lower extremities adjust with activation of dorsiflexors.

B. Resisted.   Lower trunk, extension.

Free.   Head and neck and upper trunk adjust with extension. Upper extremities thrust downward and forward. Lower extremities adjust with activation of plantar flexors.

C. Resisted.   Lower trunk, rotation toward left.

Free.   Head and neck adjust toward left. Upper trunk adjusts with rotation toward right. Upper and lower extremities adjust with stabilization.

Commands

A: "Hold! Don't let me push you back!"
B: "Hold! Don't let me pull you forward!"
C: "Hold! Don't let me turn you to the right!"

Suggested Techniques

A and *B:* Pressure and resistance.
C: Approximation at left hip, rhythmic stabilization.

NOTE: In *A* and *B*, as in Figure 1-191, stability is threatened. In *C*, stability is encouraged. Various combinations of foot and crutch positions, one crutch free of contact, and one foot free of contact with surface, may be used.

During balancing activities in the erect posture, whenever extension of hips and knees is incomplete at the appropriate time, approximation should be used to promote response of postural reflexes, except where skeletal structures are not intact.

Balance in any position may be disturbed abruptly with appropriate guarding for safety. Balancing in side-lying, on elbows and knees, on hands and knees, on hands and feet, and in various forms of sitting contribute to the development of standing balance. Assumption of various postures also contribute to assumption of standing and to maintenance of upright posture.

Walking

Normal gait involves smooth, rhythmical, and continuous transition among component patterns of the total movement. Even though walking proceeds from a swing phase (flexion) through a stance phase (extension), and the movement of one lower extremity is timed with alternating phases of the other lower extremity, all components of motion within the neck and trunk and extremities are used as necessary.

Walking against resistance in a diagonal direction may be regarded in much the same way as is standing balance when disturbed and recovered in a diagonal direction. In walking there is a transition from balance or sustained posture to movement. Whereas in balancing activities effort and movement are directed centrally toward a point of balance, bipedal progression requires continuous effort in the direction of the total movement. The first phase of response that occurs when balance is disturbed in an anterior–posterior direction is related to the swing phase of walking forward; the phase of recovery of balance is related to the stance and propulsive phase. Thus, patterns of movement necessary to walking are developed during standing balance activities.

During standing balance activities the emphasis is on stability of segments promoted by isometric contractions and co-contraction of antagonistic muscle groups, but movement with isotonic contraction of muscle group supports the effort to recover balance. In walking against resistance, the emphasis is on movement of the segments promoted by isotonic contractions of muscle groups, but balance and posture with isometric contractions of related muscle groups support the effort to move. When in standing balance a co-contraction of antagonists is promoted by maximal resistance there is no movement; the segments of the body unite to form a stable pillar. When the effort to walk is resisted, the segments of the body interact in unison and depart toward a goal.

A normal person walking into a gale of 50 miles per hour leans forward as he walks. The flexion component dominates the movement. If he turns and walks backward into the wind, he extends his neck and trunk so that the extension component dominates the movement. When manual resistance is used the result is much the same. In walking forward, the tendency is to lean into the resisting force. When walking backward, the tendency is the same: to lean into the resisting force. By so doing, the propulsive effort becomes more effective. To encourage the maintenance of an upright posture and to discourage the patient's dependence on the therapist for support, resistance must be adjusted for control of the head and neck and trunk. If, for example, related component patterns of the head and neck and shoulder are resisted, the patient is resisted strongly and then is required to "hold" or maintain the position of his head and shoulder as he moves his extremities. In this way he learns to control his entire body as he moves.

The direction of the diagonals, the pairs of antagonistic patterns, the direction of pressure and resistance, and the manual contacts used are the same for resisted walking as for standing balance. The therapist's approach is the same; the therapist must accommodate the patient's effort and movement.

ILLUSTRATIONS

Specific comments on illustrations and text that follow the discussion on mat activities apply to those that portray walking and the use of stairs.

Bipedal walking without support has been portrayed as a mat activity, Figure 1-188. Walking while using support of parallel bars has been shown in Figure 1-190, *C*. Use of crutches is portrayed in Figure 1-193; and ascent and descent of stairs are shown in Figures 1-194 and 1-195.

As a patient walks, his gait pattern may deteriorate because of fatigue, imbalances between antagonistic patterns or muscle groups, or pain. The intermittent use of balancing activities with rhythmic stabilization applied to the segment of concern may help to restore proper interaction of segments and antagonistic muscle groups. A change in direction may alleviate fatigue.

To firmly establish a proper gait pattern, use of the pattern is necessary. If additional support in the form of braces or crutches permits a patient to use a desirable pattern for longer periods of time, support should be used. Gripping parallel bars or crutches during resisted balance and walking provides additional reinforcement. Supportive devices should be viewed as tools that permit the patient to put forth greater effort for longer periods in good form. Although some patients may need supportive devices permanently, other patients may abandon support sooner by intensive use against resistance. Although braces limit movement and although they provide security, the proximal-to-distal effect of resisted balancing and walking activities permits response of related patterns and muscle groups insofar as the potential for response is present. The influence of postural and righting responses dominates.

Resistance should be applied to give security or to challenge the patient according to his needs. The task of the physical therapist is to provide the patient with an opportunity to improve and to progress. Wisely, challenge should be interspersed with security to help the patient toward independence.

Crutches

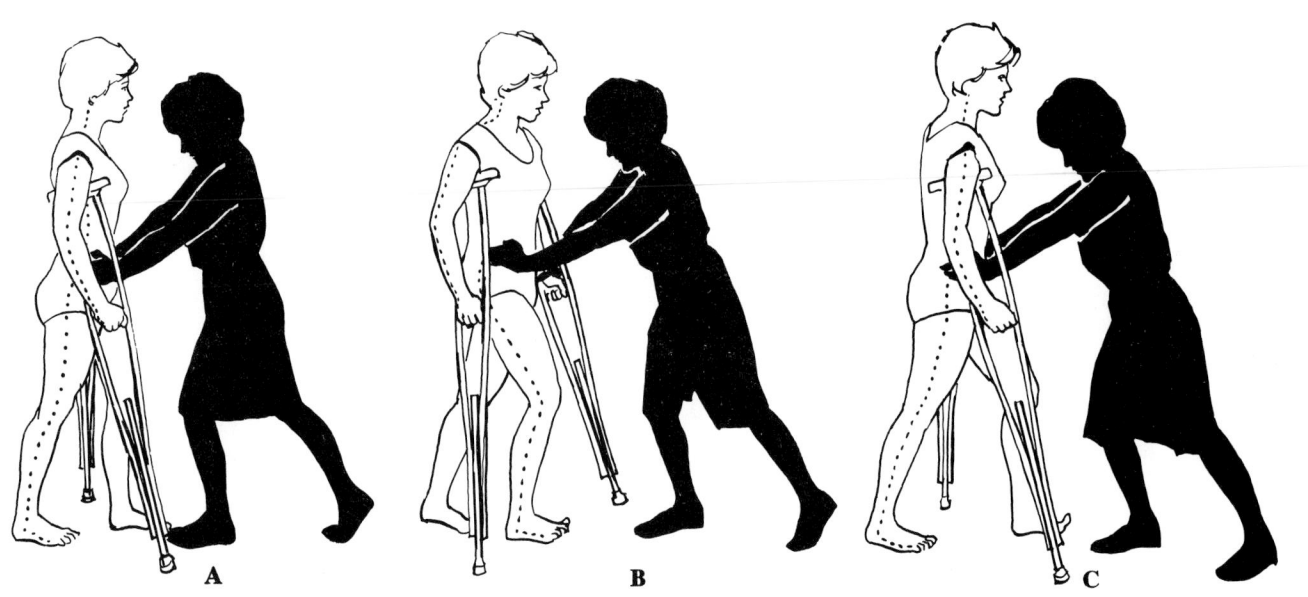

FIG. 1-193. Walking forward.

Component Patterns

Resisted. Lower extremities, alternating swing and stance phases.

Free. Head and neck adjust toward extremity in stance phase. Upper trunk adjusts toward extremity in swing phase. Lower trunk adjusts toward extremity in stance phase. Upper extremities reciprocate with lower extremities.

A. Initial Position

Commands. "Move your left crutch, then your right foot forward."

Suggested Techniques. Approximation on left, resistance on right.

B. Approaching Stance Phase on Right, Propulsion and Swing on Left

Commands. "Step on your right foot; move your right crutch and your left foot forward."

Suggested Techniques. Resistance on left, approximation on right.

C. Approaching Heel Strike on Left, Propulsion on Right

Commands. "Step on your left foot, and move your left crutch forward."

Suggested Techniques. Approximation on right, resistance on left.

Antagonistic Pattern

Walking backward.

NOTE: Subject is walking with diagonal reciprocation using a four-point gait. Other crutch-gait patterns may be trained with appropriate adjustments of the therapist's position, manual contacts, and commands. Walking forward and backward emphasizes flexion and extension components. Side-stepping, turning or pivoting, and walking diagonally forward and backward toward left and right should be used.

The use of crutches ascending and descending ramps and stairs, rising to standing, and lowering to sitting in a chair may be trained in a similar fashion. Safety is always of primary concern. Training by use of preparatory activities of the developmental sequence lessens the hazards of locomotion in the upright posture.

The use of other types of crutches, of a cane, or of canes may be taught with proper adaptations according to the type of support.

Stairs

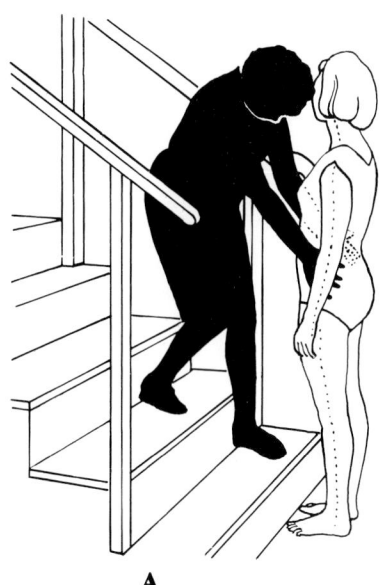 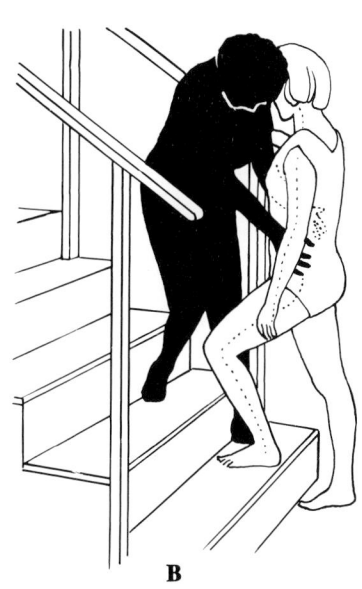 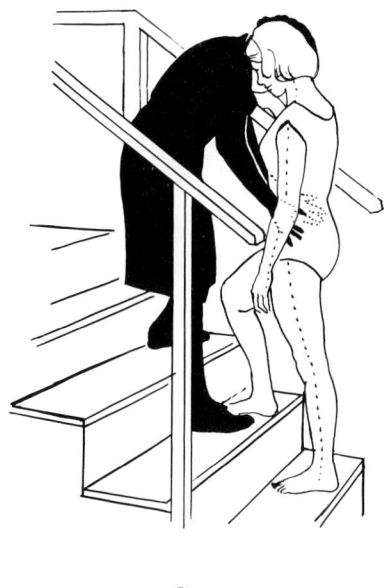

A   B   C

FIG. 1-194.   Ascending forward.

Component Patterns

Resisted.   Lower extremities, alternating flexion and extension.

Free.   Head and neck adjust toward extending lower extremity. Right upper extremity pulls on hand rail to assist left lower extremity. Left upper extremity reciprocates with right lower extremity. Upper trunk adjusts toward flexing lower extremity. Lower trunk adjusts toward extending lower extremity.

A. Initial Position

Commands.   "Hold! Now step up with your left foot."

Suggested Techniques.   Approximation at pelvis, resistance on left.

B. Approaching Extension on Left, Flexion on Right

Commands.   "Push with your left foot, and step up with your right."

Suggested Techniques.   Approximation on left, resistance on right.

C. Approaching Flexion on Left, Extension on Right

Commands.   "Push with your right foot, and step up with your left."

Suggested Techniques.   Approximation on right, resistance on left.

Antagonistic Pattern

Descending backward.

NOTE: Balancing activities with rhythmic stabilization may be used. Manual contacts for head and pelvis, shoulder and pelvis may be used. By taking a position behind subject, therapist may resist flexion patterns of lower extremity as shown for creeping forward, Figure 1-173; if possible, both hand rails may be grasped, or both hands may grasp one hand rail. When necessary, one lower extremity may lead the total pattern repeatedly while the other is brought to the level of the first rather than advancing to the next step.

Ascending forward and descending backward may be done as a plantigrade activity. Ascending backward and descending forward may be done while sitting. Other activities include balancing while using crutches or canes, and ascending and descending while using supportive devices. Ascending and descending a ramp may be considered as preparatory to ascending and descending stairs.

Stairs

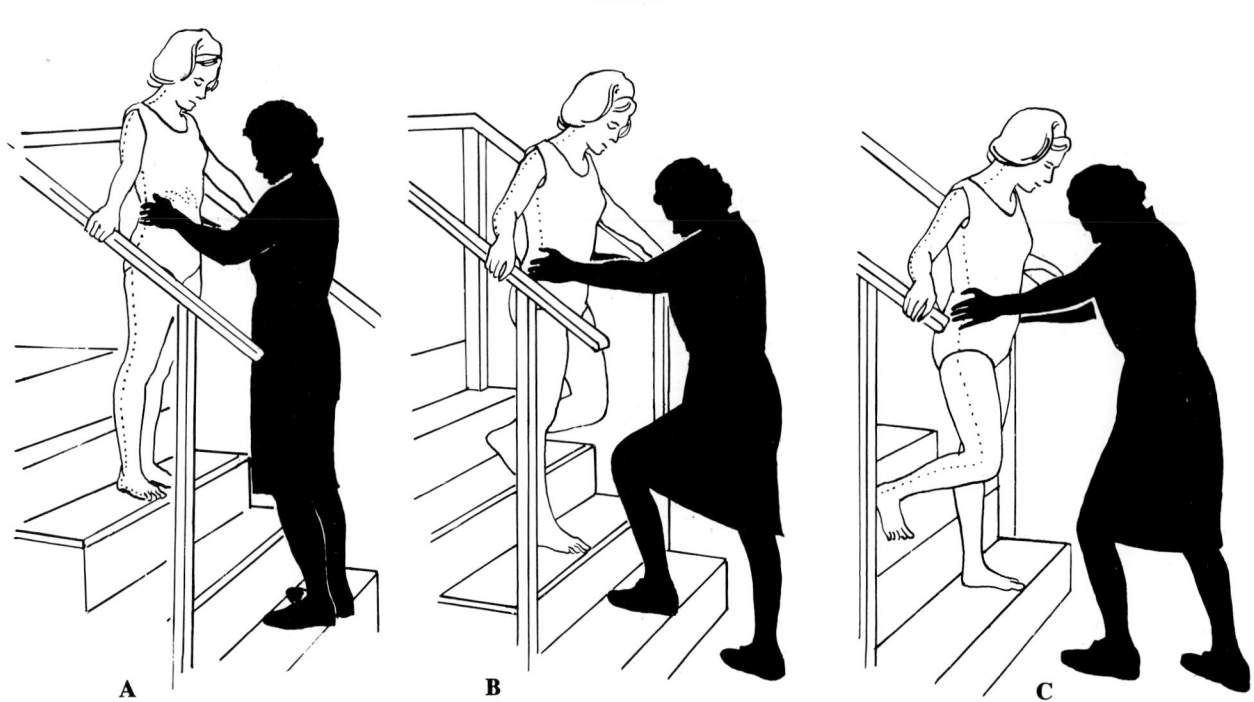

FIG. 1-195. Descending forward.

Component Patterns

Resisted. Lower extremities, alternating flexion and release of extension.

Free. Head and neck adjust toward extended lower extremity. Upper extremities support releasing lower extremity. Upper trunk adjusts toward extension and releasing lower extremity. Lower trunk adjusts toward extension and extended lower extremity.

A. Initial Position

Commands. "Hold! Now reach down with your right foot."

Suggested Techniques. Approximation, left and right, followed by resistance on right.

B. Approaching Flexion on Left, Release of Extension on Right

Commands. "Reach with your left foot, and bend your right knee slowly!"

Suggested Techniques. Approximation on right, resistance on left.

C. Approaching Flexion on Right, Release of Extension on Left

Commands. "Now hold back with your left knee, and reach down with your right foot."

Suggested Techniques. Approximation on left, resistance on right.

Antagonistic Pattern

Ascending backward.

NOTE: In *B*, left lower extremity is about to advance forward and downward with flexion of hip and extension of knee as right lower extremity enters phase of releasing extension of hip and knee, as shown in *C*. The patient may face and grasp the handrail so that his stronger side leads, permitting braiding or stepping sideward in sequence. As an example, the left (stronger) side leads. Sequence for ascent: D2 fl, L; D2 ex, R; D1 ex, L; D1 fl, R. Sequence for descent: D1 ex, R; D1 fl, L; D2 fl, R; D2 ex, L. Therapist maintains manual contacts at patient's pelvis. If right hand is weak, a mitt may be used to maintain contact near left wrist, as for lifting on ascent, and reversal of lift on descent.

Wheelchair and Transfer Activities

As the normal child grows, he is often provided with toys that promote, to a degree, his motor development. The child who moves a toy with foot pedals or by cooperative effort of upper and lower extremities is developing movement patterns necessary to balanced posture and walking. Unless the child is handicapped by physical disability, he does not normally use a wheelchair. However, the proper use of a wheelchair by a patient as a means of locomotion may further his recovery.

In the adapted developmental sequence, certain activities are closely related to wheelchair activities. Assuming and maintaining a sitting position, rising to standing from sitting, lowering to a squat position and sitting, and foot lifting and stamping prepare the patient to use a wheelchair. Bilateral movements of the upper extremities usually provide the force necessary to wheel a chair. However, ipsilateral use of one upper and one lower extremity may be the best means of propulsion for some patients. Again, the performance of related mat activities prepares for more complex functional activities.

Wheeling a chair demands coordination of body segments in balance and in movement. The ability to sustain and to recover a sitting posture is necessary to the patient's safety. The ability to move extremities while sitting permits the patient to propel the chair and to use it efficiently. Manipulation of brakes, foot plates, and wheels are necessary to operation. Entering, sitting, and arising from the chair are goals for the majority of patients. Learning to use a wheelchair skillfully may be hastened by application of proprioceptive neuromuscular facilitation.

As with other activities, using a wheelchair may be regarded as a total pattern of movement made up of component patterns. Resistance may be applied to the total pattern by restricting movement of the chair itself. In this way, some patients may improve their strength and increase their speed of performance.

In promoting the ability to transfer from chair to bed or table, or to and from an automobile, the individual patient's potentials and needs determine the method to be used and the selection of component patterns to be trained. Techniques of facilitation, including maximal resistance, approximation, reversal of antagonists, repeated contractions, rhythmic stabilization, and relaxation, may be used in training. Techniques are superimposed upon patterns of facilitation insofar as specific patterns contribute to training and upon functional movements, such as reaching for and lifting foot plates, placement of a transfer board, or removal of an arm of a chair.

Illustrations

An example of training of a specific component pattern necessary to the management of a wheelchair is shown in Figure 1-196. Pulling to standing at parallel bars, and transfer to bed and automobile are shown in Figures 1-197 to 1-200; transfer to toilet is shown as a self-care activity, Figure 1-201.

The guidelines that accompany the illustrations and text for mat activities apply to all subsequent illustrations and text.

Training in the use of a wheelchair is viewed as a phase of the patient's total treatment program. Just as related mat activities prepare the patient to use a wheelchair, properly performed wheelchair activities prepare the patient for more advanced activities, such as household tasks. There should be an overlapping of various phases of treatment, with emphasis on those activities that will hasten the achievement of goals.

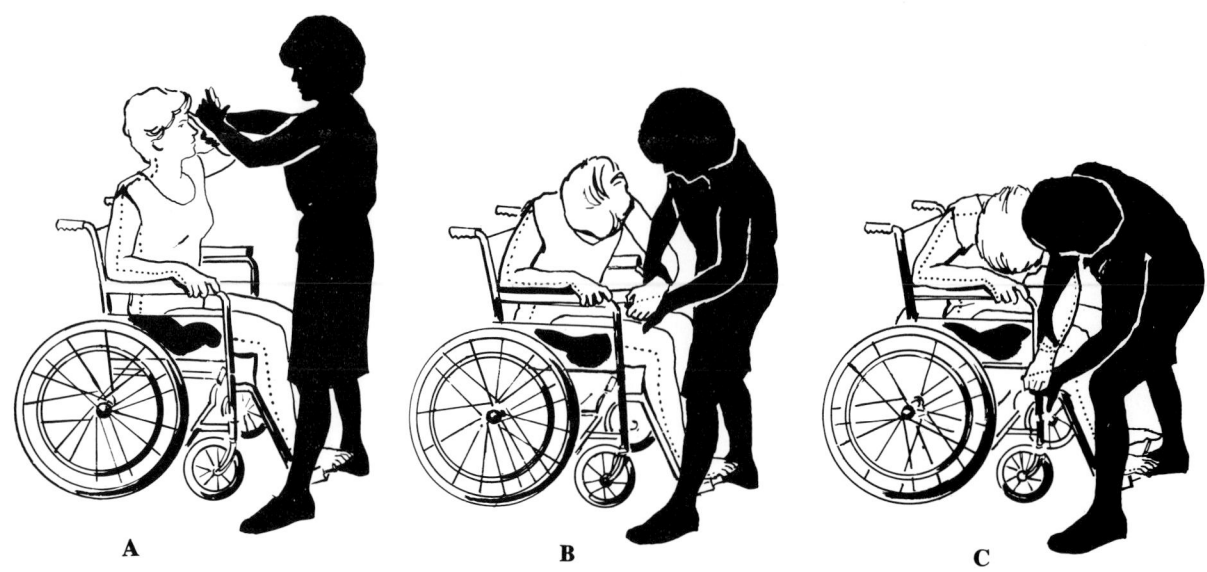

FIG. 1-196. Use of hand brake.

Component Patterns

Resisted. Left upper extremity, extension–adduction–internal rotation.

Free. Head and neck and upper trunk, flexion with rotation to right. Right upper extremity grasps arm of chair for security and to reinforce left upper extremity. Lower trunk and lower extremities adjust for stability.

A. Lengthened Range

Commands. "Squeeze my hand, and reach down and across to the brake."

Suggested Techniques. Stretch and resistance.

B. Middle Range

Commands. "Hold it! Now reach again!"

Suggested Techniques. Repeated contractions, slow reversal.

C. Shortened Range

Commands. "Now open your hand and grasp the brake. Don't let me pull you away from it."

Suggested Techniques. Resistance, repeated contractions.

Antagonistic Pattern

Rising to sitting toward left.

NOTE: Radial extensor thrust may be used with hand opening rather than closing. As shown, the goal is to train the ability to flex the upper trunk with rotation. If thrusting is used, inclination to extend trunk may occur.

In *C*, opening and closing of the hand may be performed against resistance. The effort to unlock and lock the brake may be resisted. The entire pattern of movement from *C* to *A* may be resisted with reversal of antagonist techniques. Other appropriate manual contacts include head and left upper extremity at wrist.

The same pattern with reversal may be used in training the ability to reach for the right knee and, if necessary, to assist the lifting of the right lower extremity away from and placement on foot plate. The manipulation of foot plates may be trained in a similar way.

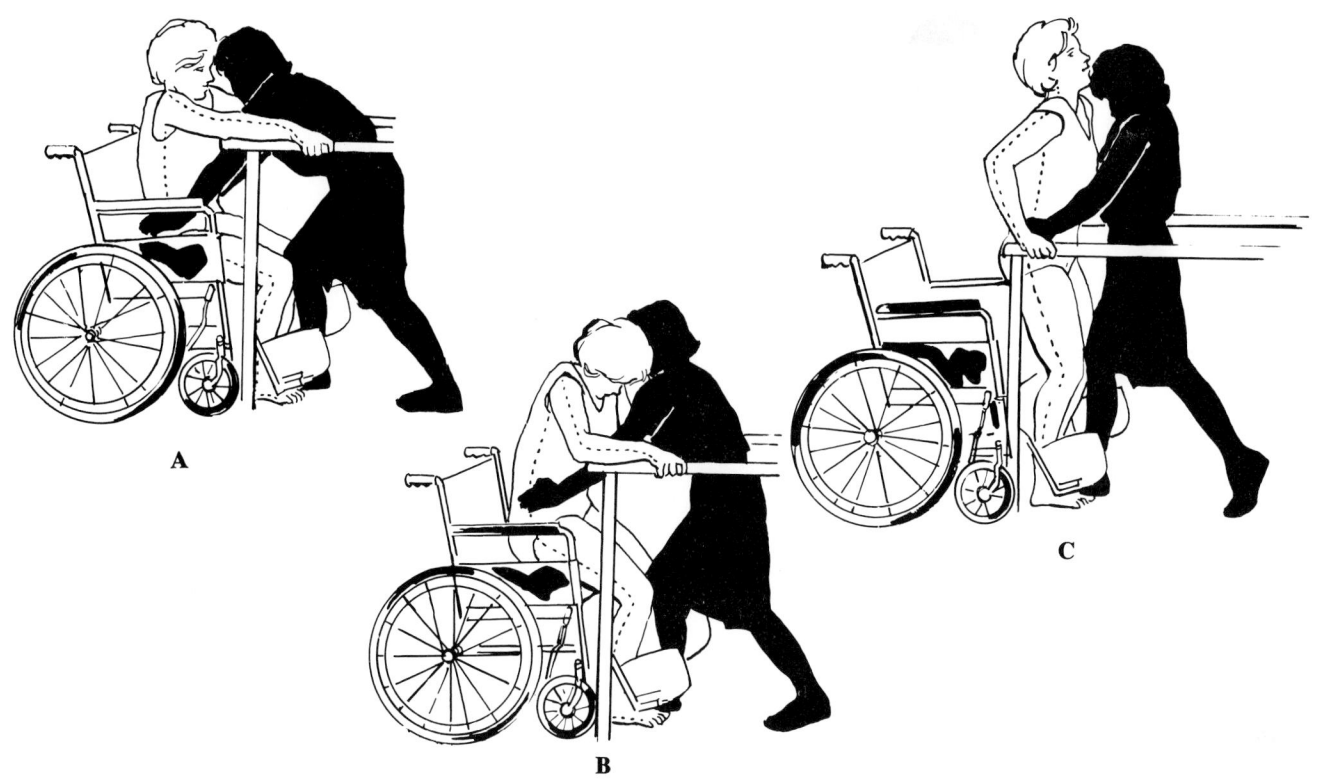

FIG. 1-197. Pulling to standing.

Component Patterns

Resisted. Lower trunk and lower extremities, extension.

Free. Head and neck and upper trunk adjust in flexion, then extension. Upper extremities grasp and pull on bars with elbows flexing, then extending.

A. Initial Position

Commands. "Pull on the bars, pull toward me!"
Suggested Techniques. Approximation, resistance.

B. Middle Range

Commands. "Lift your head, look up here, and push!"
Suggested Techniques. Resistance, repeated contractions, slow reversal.

C. Approaching Shortened Range

Commands. "Hold it! Now push up all the way!"

Suggested Techniques. Approximation, rhythmic stabilization.

Antagonistic Pattern

Reversal to sitting.

NOTE: Pulling to standing is the least advanced form of rising to standing. Therapist places right knee against subject's right knee (as for patient's less involved side) to promote stability.

Pushing to standing with subject's hands on arms of chair may be done by having subject extend head and neck and upper trunk from a hyperflexed position with head near left or right knee. Extension then proceeds toward the opposite side, right or left. Manual contacts with head and pelvis on opposite sides may be used.

Subject may also use one hand on bar, the other on arm of chair. Manual contacts may be made at shoulder on side of hand on chair arm, and at pelvis on side of hand on bar.

Component patterns that may be resisted include placement of feet with knees flexed, shifting forward in seat of chair by rocking from side to side, and reaching for parallel bars.

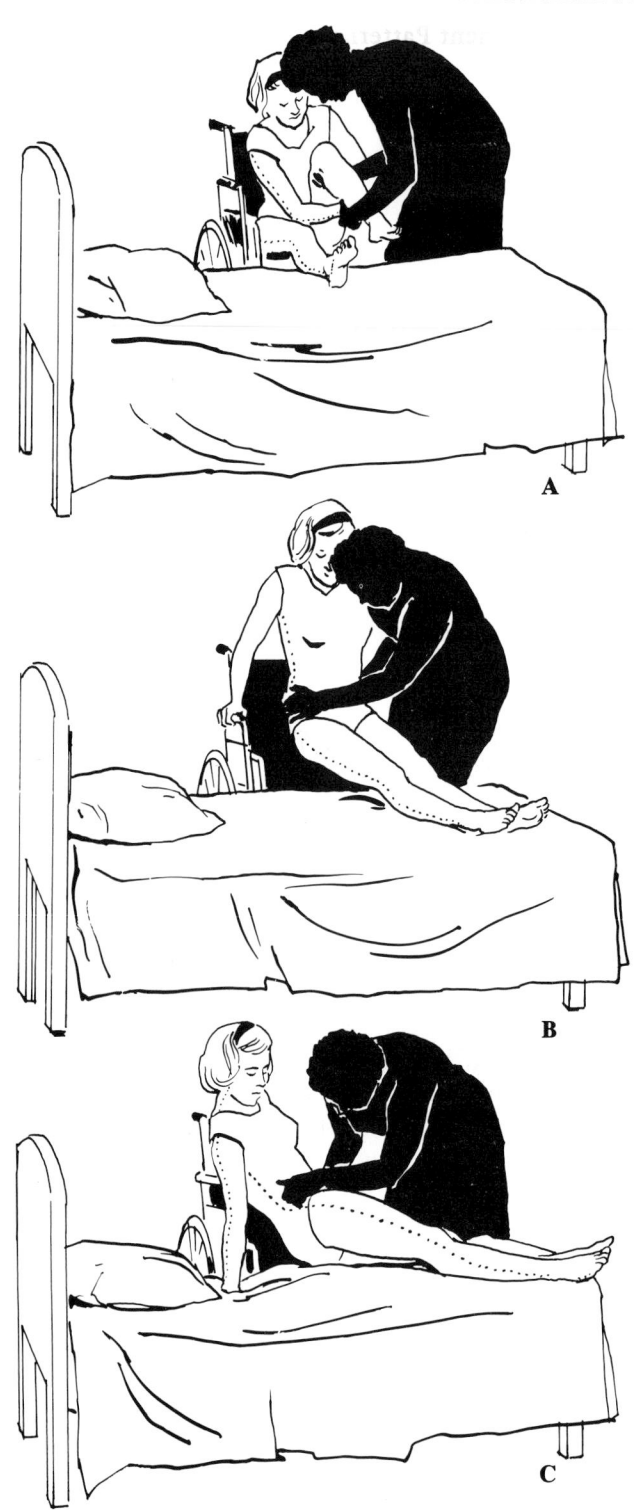

FIG. 1-198.   From chair to bed.

Component Patterns

Resisted. Upper extremities, placement of lower extremities on bed. Lower trunk, elevation and rotation toward left.

Free. Head and neck adjust with flexion, then flexion with rotation toward right. Upper trunk adjusts with flexion, then rotation toward right, and releases toward extension and supine position. Upper extremities flex to assist lower extremities, then thrust in extension for elevation of lower trunk.

A. Initial Position

Commands. "Pull your knee away from me and toward your chest. Now push it forward to the bed."

Suggested Technique. Resistance.

B. Elevation of Lower Trunk

Commands. "Push with your hands and lift up!"

Suggested Techniques. Approximation for initiation, resistance, rhythmic stabilization, slow reversal.

C. Rotation of Lower Trunk

Commands. "Put your right hand on the bed, and turn your hips toward me. Shift your hand to the right, again!"

Suggested Techniques. Guidance and resistance to lower trunk rotation.

Antagonistic Pattern

Rising from bed to chair.

NOTE: In *A*, therapist grasps subject's hands and left lower extremity and thereby resists subject's effort to elevate and place lower extremity. At the same time, guidance, resistance, or protection may be given to the lower extremity. In *B* and *C*, therapist guides, resists, and protects as necessary.

Preparatory mat activities include rising to sitting from supine (Fig. 1-179), sitting balance (Fig. 1-180), and lower trunk rocking (Fig. 1-181). Related activities include transfer from chair to bed, sideward approach with arm of chair removed; transfer from chair to mat platform; and transfer from chair to table using side approach with chair arms in place.

Wheelchair and Transfer Activity

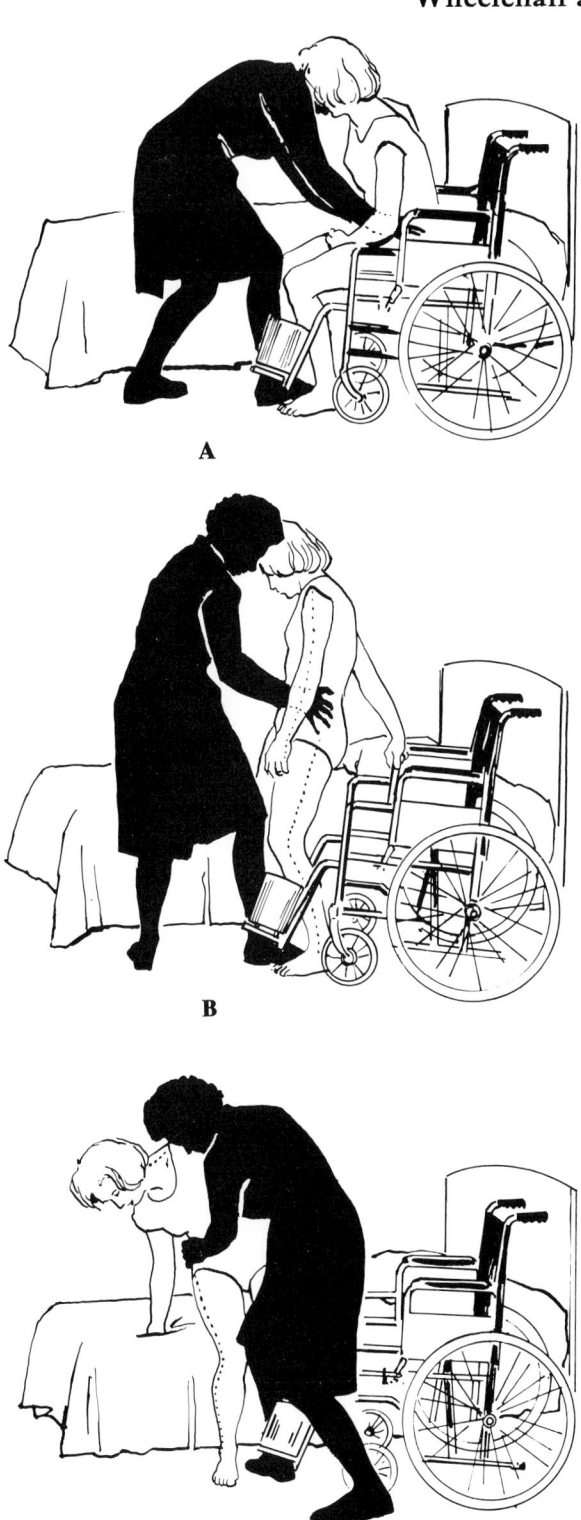

A

B

C

FIG. 1-199. From chair to standing to bed.

Component Patterns

Resisted. Lower trunk and lower extremities, extension with rotation toward left, then release to flexion toward left.

Free. Head and neck and upper trunk adjust toward flexion with rotation toward right. Right upper extremity thrusts in extension. Left upper extremity does not contribute to total pattern.

A. Initial Position

Commands. "Lean toward me, push with your right arm, and stand up! Straighten your knees!"

Suggested Techniques. Approximation and resistance.

B. Approaching Shortened Range, Standing

Commands. "Hold it! Now reach your right hand to the bed!"

Suggested Techniques. Approximation at pelvis.

C. Approaching Shortened Range, Sitting

Commands. "Now sit down slowly!"

Suggested Techniques. Guidance and resistance to lower trunk.

Antagonistic Pattern

Rising from sitting to standing to chair (wheelchair placed at angle at foot of bed).

NOTE: Subject is using extremities of right side to achieve transfer. Therapist has placed right knee against subject's right knee to ensure one pillar of support. Approximation and rotation of lower trunk toward left promotes stability of left lower extremity, *B.* Also in *B*, subject has achieved the maximum of extension which is limited by right upper extremity's contact with arm of chair. With approximation, freeing of right hand, and extension of head and neck, subject may achieve complete extension before turning and reaching for bed. Note that in transfers from chair to bed, also Figure 1-198, as in any total pattern, head and neck lead and subject looks toward goal.

Preparatory mat activities include adversive rotation of upper trunk to right and lower trunk to left while lying on right side, balance sidelying (Fig. 1-157), sitting balance (Fig. 1-180), and standing balance (Figs. 1-180, 1-186, and 1-187).

Wheelchair and Transfer Activity

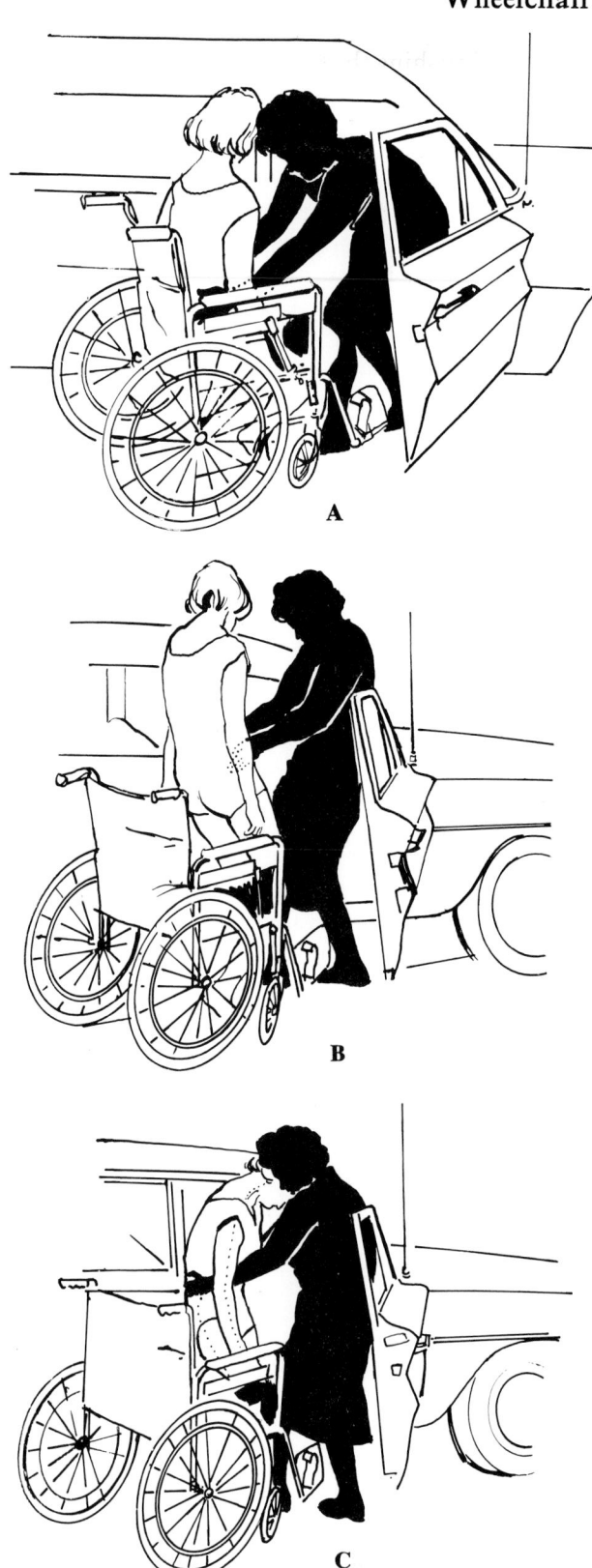

Component Patterns

Resisted. Lower trunk and lower extremities, extension with rotation toward right, then release to flexion toward right.

Free. Head and neck and upper trunk adjust toward flexion with rotation toward left. Left upper extremity thrusts in extension. Right upper extremity does not contribute to total pattern.

A. Initial Position

Commands. "Lean forward, push with your left arm, and stand up!"

Suggested Techniques. Approximation and resistance.

B. Approaching Shortened Range, Standing

Commands. "Hold it! Straighten your knees!"

Suggested Technique. Approximation.

C. Approaching Middle Range, Sitting

Commands. "Reach your left hand to the seat, and sit down slowly."

Suggested Techniques. Guidance and resistance to lower trunk.

Antagonistic Pattern

Rising from sitting to standing to chair.

NOTE: Subject is using extremities of left side to achieve transfer. Therapist has placed left knee against subject's left knee for stability of left lower extremity, which is primarily responsible for control of inferior region.

Preparatory mat activities are as for transfer shown in Figure 1-199 with appropriate adjustments made for developing use and emphasis of right side of body.

FIG. 1-200. From chair to standing to automobile.

Self-Care Activities

By common definition, self-care activities are related to personal care, including feeding, using the toilet, bathing, and dressing. The normal child acquires these abilities through development and training. For the normal adult of sedentary occupation, bathing and dressing may constitute the most varied exercise of his daily life. The handicapped child needs to develop self-care abilities. The handicapped adult needs to relearn self-care. Because of their personal nature, self-care activities are of utmost importance to the patient's morale and motivation. In the total treatment of the patient, activities directed toward goals of self-care are given primary emphasis.

Training for self-care begins when the patient attempts to roll on a mat. The individuated patterns as used, for example, in feeding may have their origin in rolling from supine to prone and from prone to supine. Because the human being is capable of innumerable combinations of movement, each alteration of position places a different demand on the neuromuscular mechanism. To fully develop a self-care activity, analysis of related component patterns in a variety of positions may be necessary to adequate performance of the activity. An example is given in Table 1-11.

With a good basis for function developed through mat activities and specific facilitation, a transition from gross to refined movement can be made. If, for example, a patient has achieved sitting balance and at the same time can move his upper extremities without disturbing his balance, it is obvious that he can more easily feed himself than if he were completely dependent upon a chair for support. If a patient can roll with ease and is able to use his extremities to accomplish the act, he can more readily learn to bathe and dress himself in bed.

Table 1-11. Activity for Analysis: Primitive* Washing of Face and Neck

Hand(s)	Side(s) of Face	Diagonal and Sequence†	Combined Diagonals
R	L, then R	D1, then D2	
L and R	Both sides	D1, then D2	BS
L contacts, R wrist	L, then R	L, D2, then D1 R, D1, then D2	BA, chop and lift
R contacts, L wrist	R, then L	L, D1, then D2 R, D2, then D1	BA, chop and lift

BS: Both hands use *bilateral symmetry*, same diagonal

BA: One hand uses the first diagonal (D1) as the other uses the second (D2). Hands are placed in contact as for "chopping and lifting"; this permits one hand to guide or "track" the other. This *bilateral asymmetrical* combination of diagonal patterns may be useful with hemiplegic patients, among others.

* Primitive: using hands and running water; without washcloth

† Diagonals change and interact as hand crosses midline of face, nose, or mouth.

The transition from gross to refined movements, such as those required for feeding, shaving, dressing the hair, and brushing the teeth, may be encouraged by superimposing techniques of facilitation on the functional movement or self-care activity itself. The left hand is superior to the right in locating hidden or out-of-sight objects.[30] Thus, the patient who lacks use of his dominant right hand may find that if he must button his shirt or coat with his left hand alone, the task may be easier if he lets his hand find buttonhole and button as he looks elsewhere. Performance in a position of functional use is desirable because it is conducive to eye–hand coordination. As coordination is acquired, the patient is free to attend other matters, and his movements serve the matter which he is attending.

Resistance graded to encourage isotonic contraction of related muscle groups in the desired range of movement and repetition of a movement are adjuncts to training in self-care. Refinement of postural control for intricate movements is encouraged by performance of isometric contractions at specific ranges within a movement. Functional activities require reversing movements so that performance of reversal of antagonists techniques may hasten the learning of an activity. Other techniques, including relaxation techniques, may be used as necessary.

Illustrations

Figure 1-201, transfer from chair to toilet, and Figure 1-202, dressing in bed, are two examples of self-care activities. Although all activities are related to self-care and independence, certain related in-bed activities (most of which are obvious) may be considered. The components of functional activities can be recognized more specifically if various combinations of elbow motions, and reversal of direction of total patterns and of component patterns are visualized:

Turning, bathing, dressing	Rolling (Figs. 1-151 to 1-161)
Adjusting clothing at hips	Lower trunk activities (Figs. 1-162 and 1-163)
Use of bedpan	Elevation of pelvis (Fig. 1-163)
Moving headward and footward	Crawling (Figs. 1-164 and 1-165)
Reaching for feet	Sitting (Figs. 1-178 to 1-180)

Self-care is a goal of treatment. If the potential exists for performance of an activity in a coordinate manner, training in the position of functional use may be hastened by use of resistance and other techniques of facilitation. However, if imbalances exist, if coordination is lacking, or if there is need to alter the rate of movement, these factors are not favorable to adequate self-care. The manifestation of bizarre and inadequate attempts to perform is evidence that the patient has been asked to perform beyond his level of ability and that he has need for additional work in more primitive patterns and in specific patterns of facilitation. Meeting this need may ultimately result in improved performance of self-care activities. The infant does not lace his shoes; he develops this ability through performance of a variety of less skilled activities.

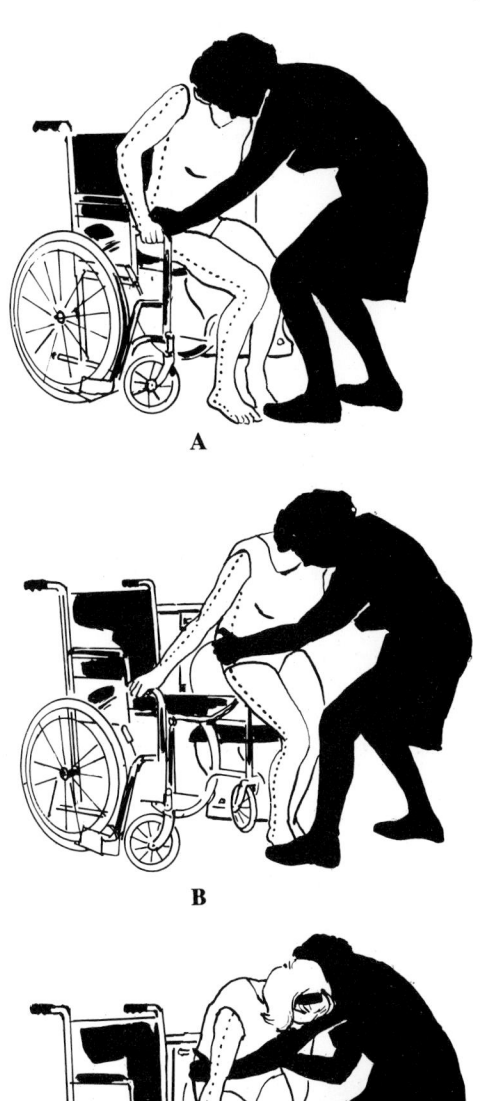

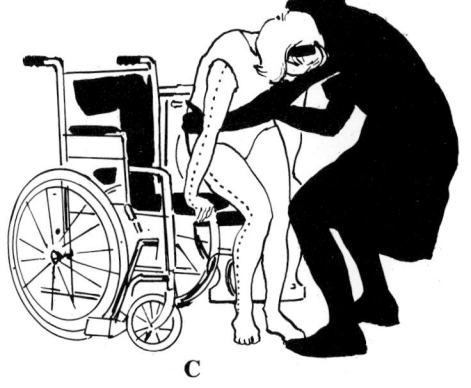

FIG. 1-201. From chair to toilet.

Component Patterns

Resisted. Lower trunk, elevation.

Free. Head and neck and upper trunk adjust with flexion toward left. Upper extremities thrust downward, then alternately support and shift for progression toward left, then release with elbows flexing. Lower extremities do not contribute to total pattern.

A. Initial Position: Arm of Chair Removed

Commands. "Reach your left hand to the toilet seat; now push with your hands, and lift up."

Suggested Techniques. Guidance and resistance for lower trunk.

B. Middle Range

Commands. "Hold! Now put your right hand on the seat of your chair."

Suggested Techniques. Guidance and resistance, rhythmic stabilization.

C. Approaching Shortened Range

Commands. "Swing your hips to the left, and sit down slowly."

Suggested Techniques. Guidance and resistance at pelvis.

Antagonistic Pattern

From toilet to chair.

NOTE: Component patterns that may be trained with subject sitting in chair include elevation of lower trunk, sideward rocking of pelvis while elevation is maintained, and reaching for seat of toilet. Where hand grips or rails are conveniently placed, training includes their use.

Transfer from chair to edge of bathtub or seat in shower stall may be carried out in a similar fashion including the use of hand rails. If a bench is to be used in a bathtub, transfers to benches of varying heights may be done as a preparatory mat activity.

As shown for transfer from chair to bed, Figure 1-199, subject may be trained for transfer to toilet. For transfer from toilet to chair, position of chair and of therapist must be adjusted.

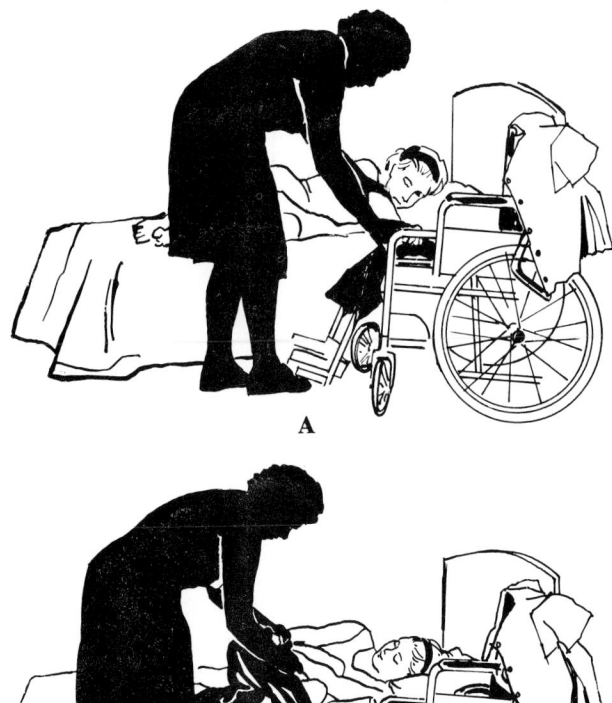

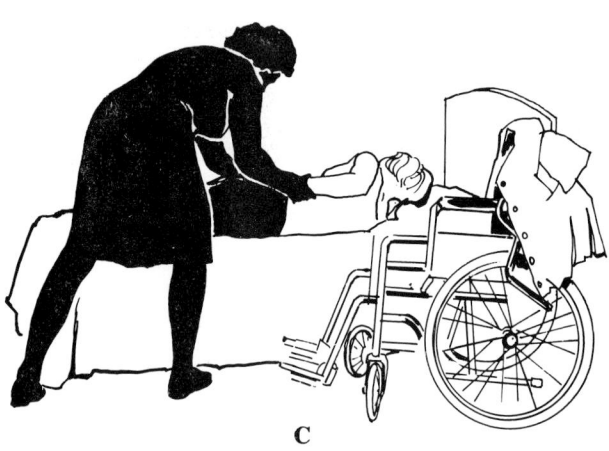

C

FIG. 1-202. Dressing in bed, inferior region.

Component Patterns

Resisted. Reaching to wheelchair for slacks. Asymmetrical extension of upper extremities toward right lower extremity; left hand grasps ankle, right grasps slacks. Pulling slacks up to waist.

Free. Rolling to left with asymmetrical flexion of lower extremities. Flexion of head and neck and upper trunk right. Extension of right lower extremity into leg of slacks. Rolling to right with head and neck rotation.

A. Reaching to Chair

Commands. "Reach, take hold of your slacks, and pull them to you."

Suggested Techniques. Resistance, slow reversal.

B. Placing Right Lower Extremity

Commands. "Take hold of your right ankle with your left hand, and your slacks with your right. Pull your right foot toward you some more. Don't let me pull your right hand off your slacks. Now push your right leg down with your left hand, and pull your slacks up with your right."

Suggested Techniques. Resistance during various phases.

C. Adjusting Slacks at Waist

Commands. "Pull with your left hand. Now roll toward me, then pull with your right."

Suggested Techniques. Resistance during various phases.

Antagonistic Pattern

Undressing inferior region.

NOTE: Component patterns to be trained include asymmetrical flexion of lower extremities with rolling to left, thrusting of right upper extremity from shoulder extension with elbow flexion, *A;* "chopping" to right with elbow extension, *B;* rolling to right and to left, and, if possible, lower trunk activities, elevation of pelvis and lower trunk rotation, Figures 1-162 and 1-163.

Manipulation of zippers, buttons, and Velcro fastenings may be resisted. Also, of course, putting on and removal of socks and shoes, and braces, may be trained by use of resistance. Sitting over edge of bed or in chair may be assumed for dressing of superior region.

Supplementary Activities

In the process of development and in motor learning, the child practices and uses the total and component patterns he has mastered. He may try and fail but he repeats his efforts until he succeeds. Once he has learned an activity, it is a part of him. He can use it automatically or deliberately, as the occasion demands. The handicapped child or adult needs opportunity to practice the activities he is learning and to use those he has mastered. In this way he advances his own progress.

Supervised classes provide an opportunity for continued motor learning, for establishing more firmly those patterns of movement which have been learned, and for developing strength, endurance, and stability of posture. Individual patients have individual needs. The activities they perform in a class are selected to meet their needs and to fulfill specific goals. Several patients may have the same needs so that they may work together or compete with each other, but the concept of class work is supervision of individual programs of activity rather than group work of selected activities. Patients perform in different ways and at different speeds.

Class work carried out on gymnasium mats may include free activity and mechanically resisted activity. Free activity is based on the developmental activities. When possible, gymnasium equipment, including dumbbells, medicine balls, beach balls, and pulley weights, is used for increasing demands and challenging balance or stability of posture.[46] The patient is limited to those activities he can do in good form in accordance with normal timing; he is limited to coordinate movements or those movements that will improve his coordination. The supervisor is a teacher, a taskmaster, and sometimes an arbitrator. Patients are people. they play together, they compete, they win, they lose, they challenge each other, they help each other.[22] They learn again to be members of a group, to overcome self-centered attitudes. The wise supervisor enlists those patients who can help others. The hemiplegic adult may practice hand–knee balance while talking to and stimulating a brain-injured child. An active child competes with adults and challenges them. They may play together and may be taught to resist each other in useful movements. In a sense, a mat class is not a class but a community of activity.

Use of Wall Pulleys

Wall pulleys and weights are among the more versatile pieces of equipment because movements can be performed with them in diagonal directions as well as in vertical or horizontal directions. Horizontal direction represents movement in anatomical planes, while diagonal direction represents movement in combined planes.

The use of wall pulleys demands the attention of the patient and has built-in motivational factors. Because reversal of direction is used, movement tends to become rhythmical, and repetition is encouraged. The latter promotes retention of motor learning.

In keeping with developmental bases of PNF, a pulley program is directed toward strengthening movements of head and neck and trunk before emphasizing movements of distal parts, such as opening and closing of the hand. While a wrist strap to which the pulley is attached will permit opening and closing, usually the hand must grip the handle. This factor is offset by the vast need of most patients to strengthen muscles of trunk, shoulder, and pelvic girdles. To this end diagonal direction is used to demand interaction of the two sides of the body with segments crossing the midline. This kind of activity must yield a dividend in the training of proprioception and thus of perception.

Kabat determined clinically that *resistance to the antagonist* facilitated the agonist, the desired movement. Thus, happily, the *gravity-assisted motions may be resisted* with resultant facilitation of the agonist. During performance of upper trunk patterns while sitting in a chair, gravity-assisted flexion is resisted by pulley weights. When direction is reversed, *gravity-resisted extension is assisted* by pulley weights. This combination of factors should promote a balanced interaction between antagonistic movements.

Upper trunk patterns are activated by head and neck patterns and are reinforced by bilateral asymmetrical upper extremity patterns combined for "chopping" and "lifting." One hand grips the pulley handle as the other grips the opposite wrist. These movements cross the midline for reinforcement from the stronger side, which occurs through related head and neck, trunk, and upper extremity patterns.

According to Kimura, body touching, or self-touching, has bilateral representation in the brain.[30] This more primitive function may be used in training the patient. Chopping and reversal of the chop are used with contact between the extremities for strengthening upper trunk and shoulders. Self-touching, or body contact, is used as well in exercises for lower trunk with lower extremities in contact.

Pulley exercises for the *superior region*, upper trunk and upper extremities, can be performed while the patient is seated in a wooden armchair or in a wheelchair, or a mat may be useful. Exercises for the *inferior region*, lower trunk and lower extremities, are done as the patient lies or sits on a treatment table or a mat, or sits on a bench.

The chair and table are positioned *diagonally* when *asymmetrical movements* of the extremities are used. During *reciprocal and symmetrical combinations* the position of the chair and the table is *symmetrical.* On the mat the patient is positioned accordingly as total patterns are performed.

A limited number and choice of diagonal patterns are presented to demonstrate the use of wall pulleys at two levels: overhead (OL) and floor (FL). The selection is not designed as a program of treatment, although the examples given are frequently helpful to many patients. Each sequence includes Lengthened Range (Le-R), Middle Range (Mid-R), and Shortened Range (Sh-R).

In all sequences, wrist and ankle straps permit full range of appropriate movement of hand and foot. In this way the patterns of facilitation are complete. The use of wall pulley handles may encourage strength of grasp and stronger response in the more proximal muscles.

While the use of pulleys requires a reversal of antagonists and of diagonal direction, the aim is to develop a balanced antagonism. To achieve balance, a level of pulley (OL or FL) and the load of weights must be determined by assessing the patient's weakness and ability to control the load and to reverse direction smoothly. For example, in Figure 1-203 (FL), upper trunk extension with lifting (to the left) requires shortening–concentric–isotonic contraction of extensor muscles. Upon reversal, lengthening–eccentric–isotonic contraction of the extensors is de-manded for control. Anterior trunk flexors lengthen and shorten as necessary. The floor level pulley is used: concentric contractions lift the load; eccentric contractions lower the load. While isotonic contraction produces movement from Le-R to Sh-R, static–isometric–holding contraction is used to promote stability as in Mid-R. Holding can be used at selected points throughout the range.

In Figure 1-205 (OL), upper trunk flexion with reversal of lifting (to the right) requires shortening of flexors and lengthening of trunk extensors. The overhead pulley is used. Concentric contraction of trunk flexors lift the load. Eccentric contraction of flexors lower the load when lifting (to the right) is repeated. At the same time, concentric contraction of trunk extensors may be assisted by the lowering of the load.

The use of wall pulleys offers a vast repertoire from which a patient's program may be developed. Review Patterns as Active Motion and select appropriate Total Patterns such as Figures 1-159, 1-179, and 1-173; Bilateral Combinations, Figures 1-127 and 1-133; and Unilateral Patterns as necessary. Facilitation Techniques to be considered are SR, SRH, and RC. When two pulleys are used, RC is the technique of choice; hold with one, repeat with the other. (See Table 1-3, Acronyms.)

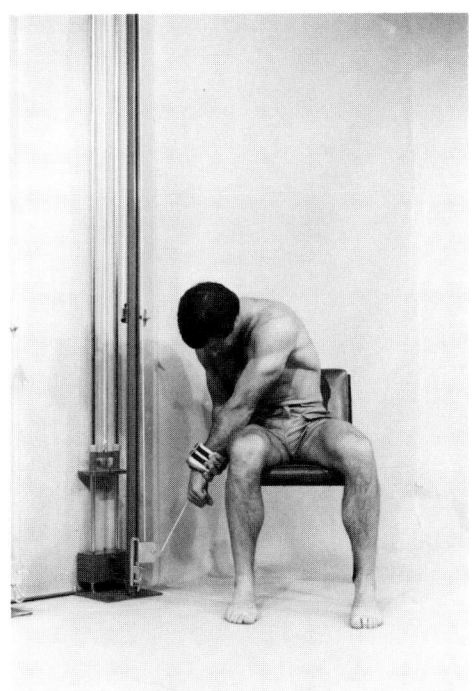

A   Le-R

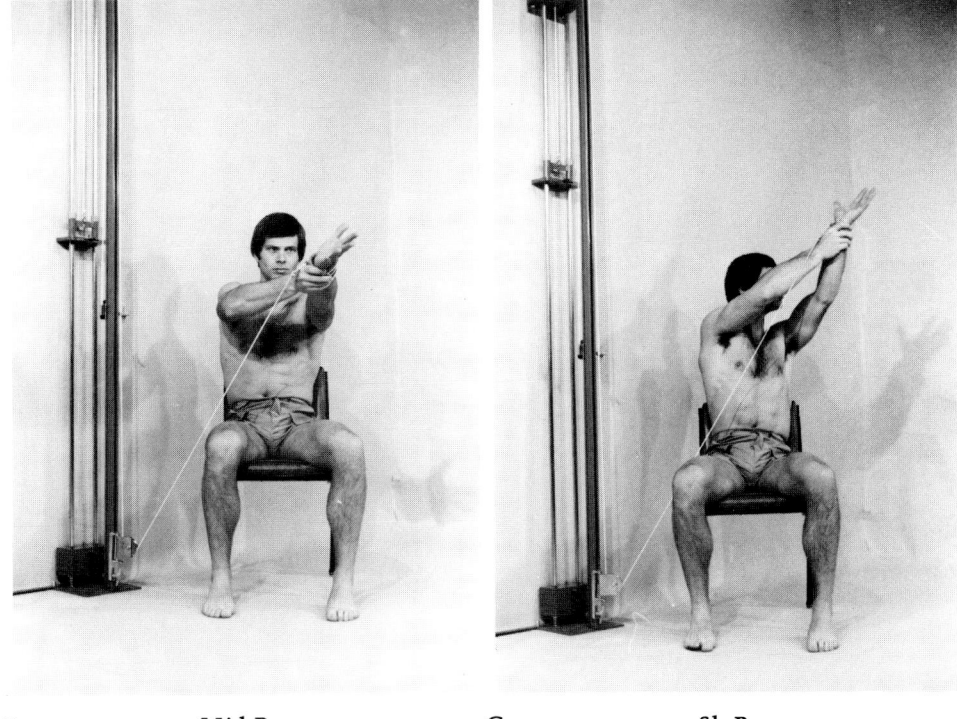

B   Mid-R   C   Sh-R

FIG. 1-203. Upper trunk extension with lifting (BA) to left (FL)

A. Lifting load: gravity resists; load resists
B. Holding load
C. *Reversal,* lowering load: gravity assists; eccentric control, extensors
Alternate postures: standing, kneeling, sidelying (rolling)

NOTE: Transpose direction for extension with lifting to right followed by reversal to left.

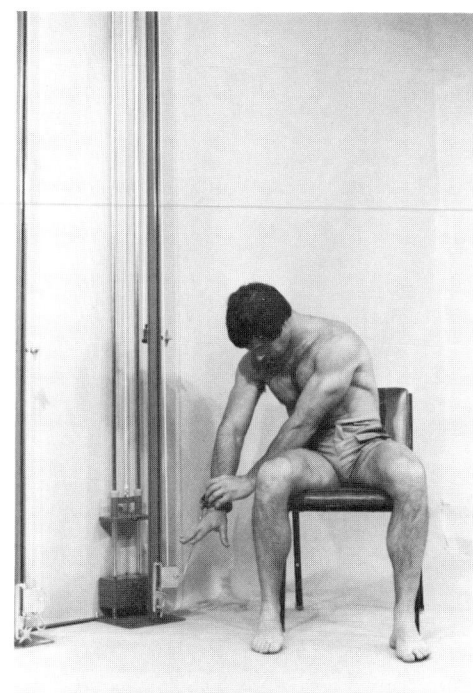

A   Le-R

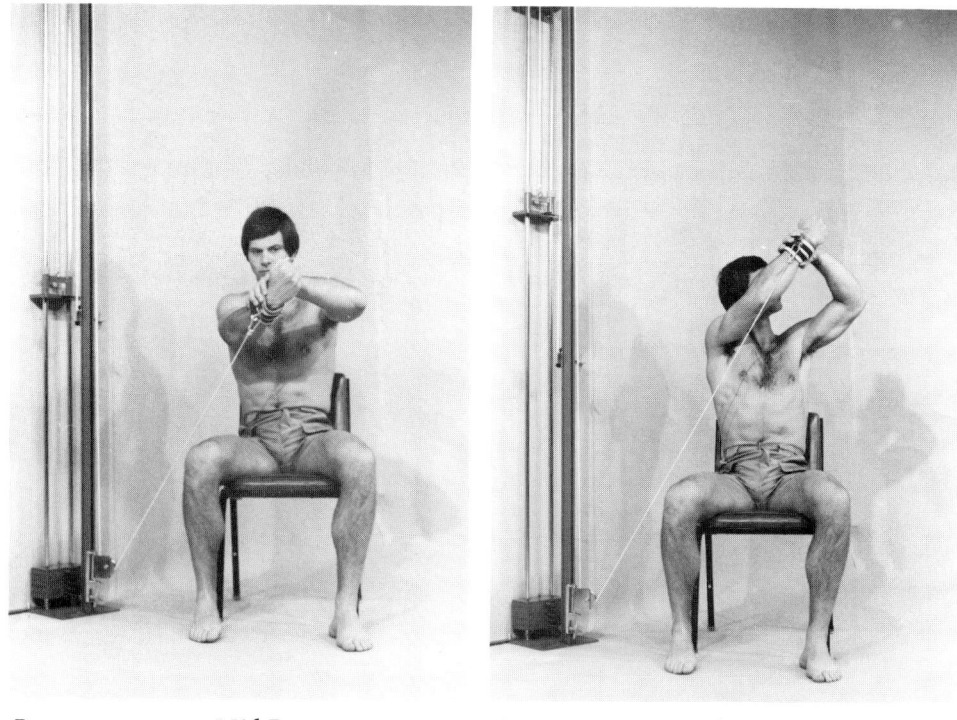

B Mid-R   C   Sh-R

FIG. 1-204. Upper trunk extension with reversal of chopping (BA) to right (FL)

A. Lifting load: gravity resists; load resists
B. Holding load
C. *Reversal,* lowering load: gravity assists; eccentric control, extensors
Alternate postures: standing, kneeling, sidelying (rolling)

NOTE: Transpose direction for extension with reversal of chopping to left.

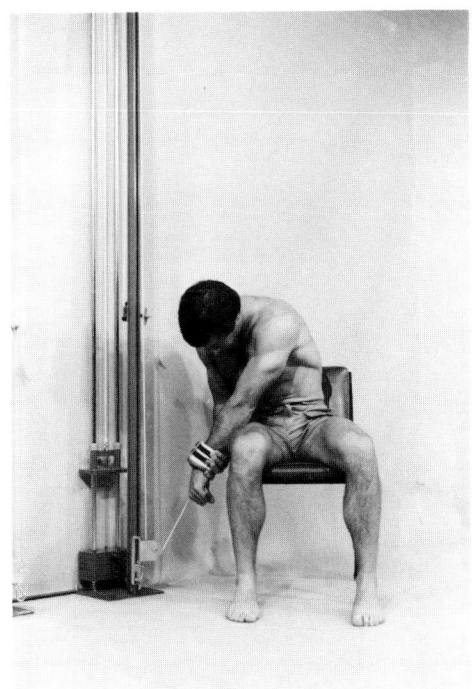

A   Le-R

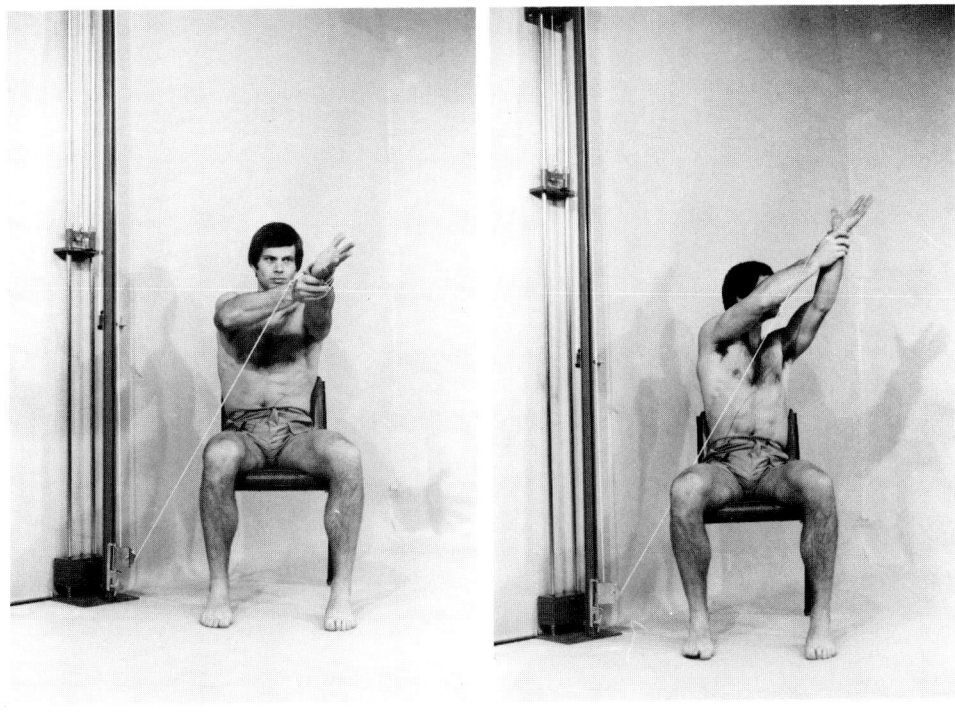

B   Mid-R   C   Sh-R

FIG. 1-203. Upper trunk extension with lifting (BA) to left (FL)

A. Lifting load: gravity resists; load resists
B. Holding load
C. *Reversal*, lowering load: gravity assists; eccentric control, extensors
Alternate postures: standing, kneeling, sidelying (rolling)

NOTE: Transpose direction for extension with lifting to right followed by reversal to left.

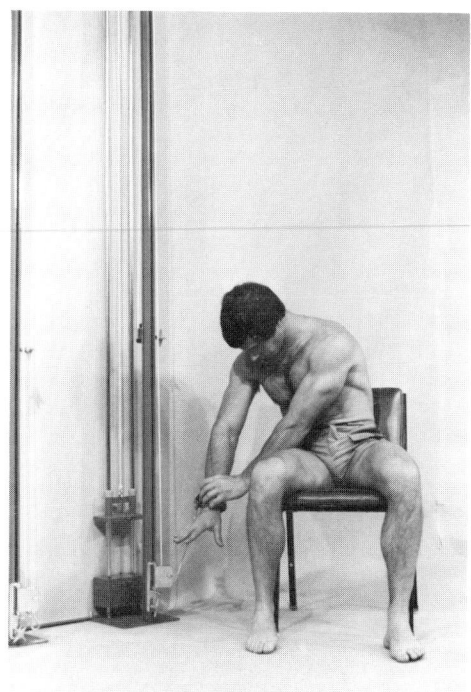

A   Le-R

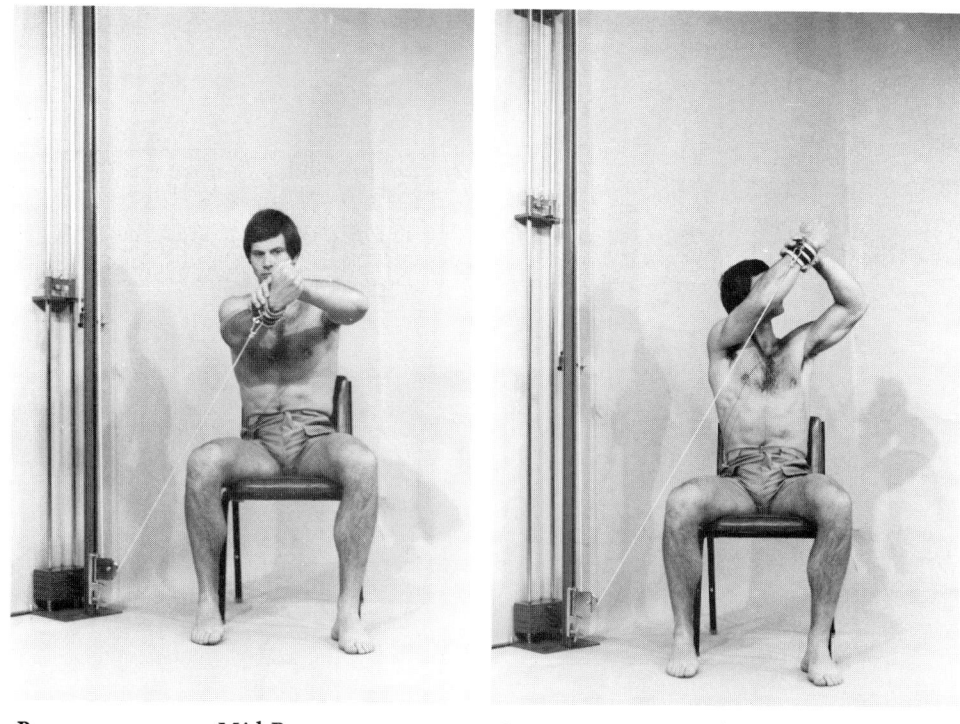

B   Mid-R   C   Sh-R

FIG. 1-204.   Upper trunk extension with reversal of chopping (BA) to right (FL)

A. Lifting load: gravity resists; load resists
B. Holding load
C. *Reversal*, lowering load: gravity assists; eccentric control, extensors
Alternate postures: standing, kneeling, sidelying (rolling)

NOTE: Transpose direction for extension with reversal of chopping to left.

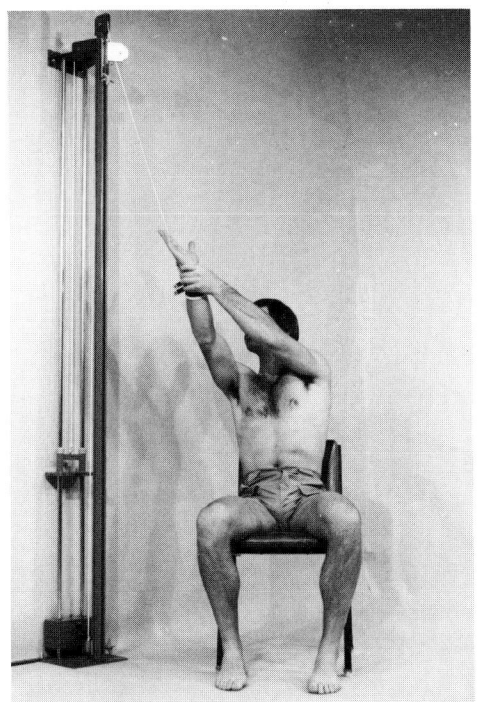

A   Le-R

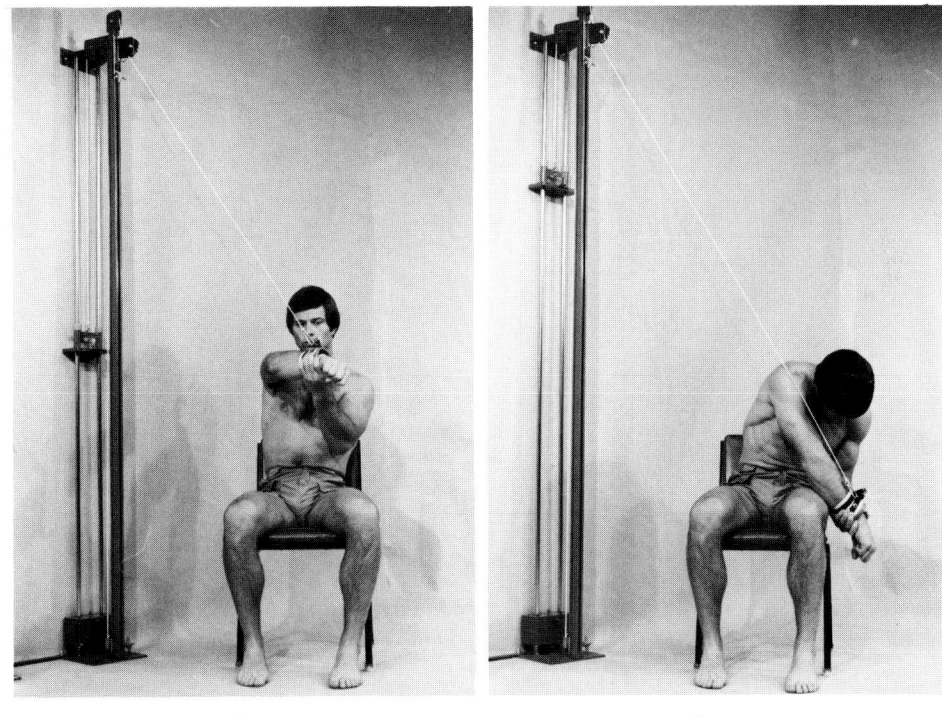

B   Mid-R   C   Sh-R

FIG. 1-205.   Upper trunk flexion with reversal of lifting (BA) to right (OL)

A. Lifting load: gravity assists; load resists
B. Holding load
C. *Reversal*, lowering load: gravity resists; load assists; eccentric control, flexors
Alternate postures: standing, kneeling, sidelying (rolling)

NOTE: Transpose direction for flexion with reversal of lifting to left.

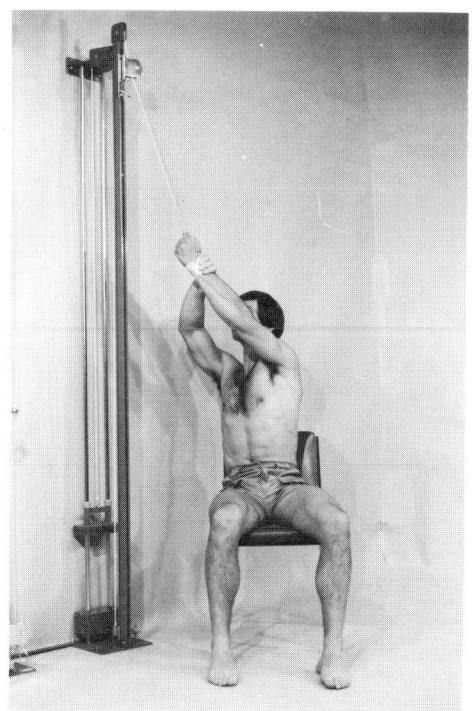

A   Le-R

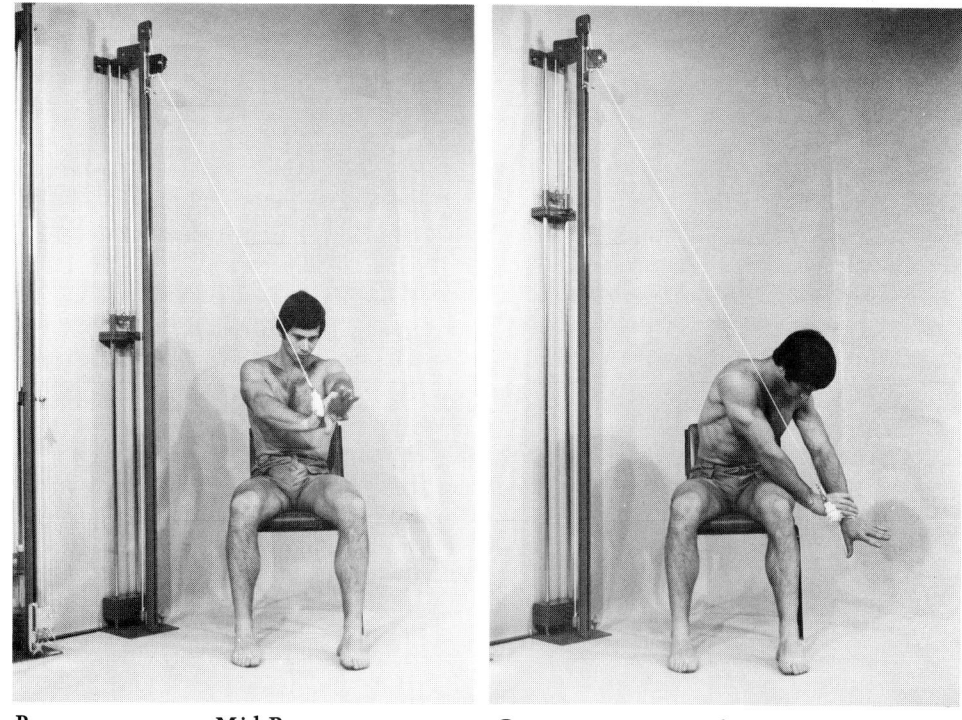

B   Mid-R   C   Sh-R

FIG. 1-206. Upper trunk flexion with chopping (BA) to left (OL)

A. Lifting load: gravity assists; load resists
B. Holding load
C. *Reversal,* lowering load: gravity resists; load assists; eccentric control, flexors
Alternate postures: standing, kneeling, sidelying (rolling)

NOTE: Transpose direction for flexion with chopping to right.

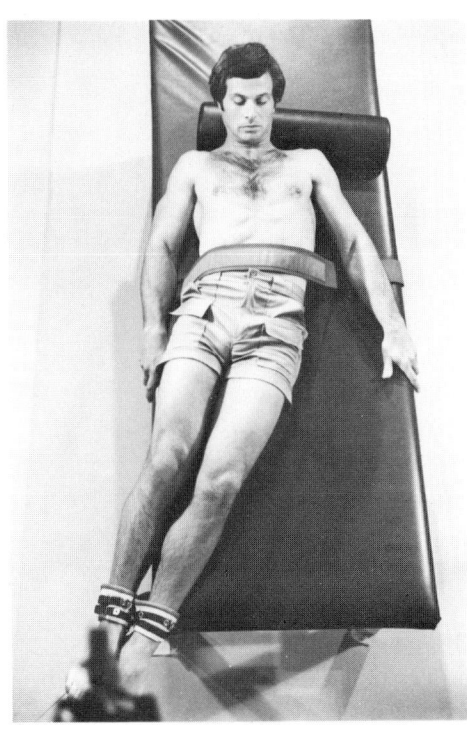

A   Le-R

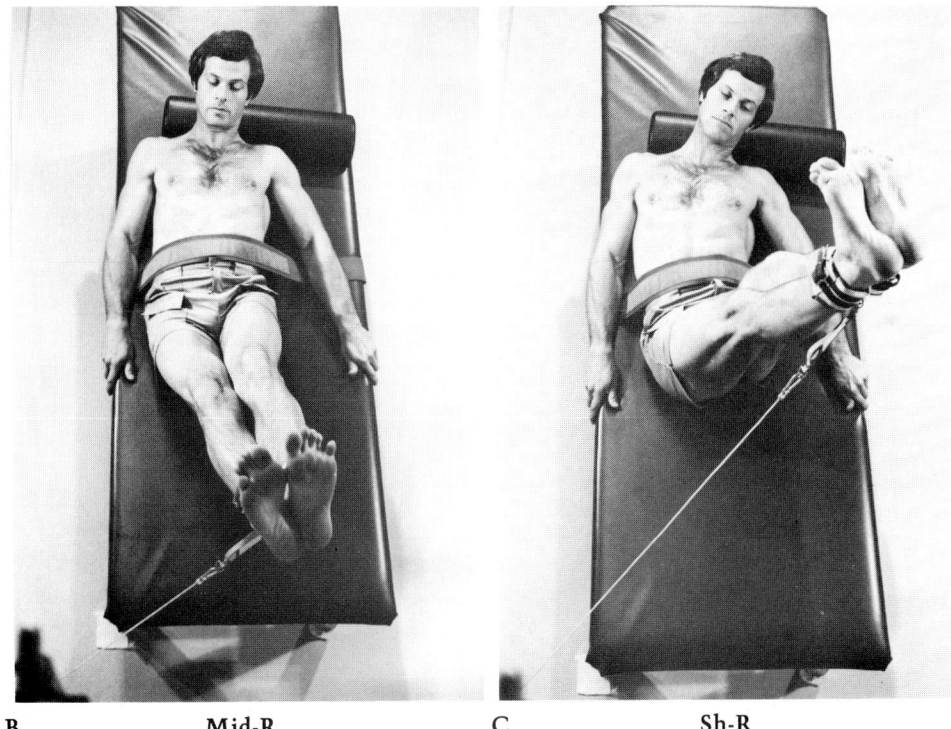

B   Mid-R   C   Sh-R

FIG. 1-207.   Lower trunk flexion with lower extremities (BA) to left (FL)

A. Lifting load: gravity resists; load resists
B. Holding load
C. *Reversal*, lowering load: gravity assists; eccentric control, flexors
Alternate posture: prone, lower trunk over table edge; gravity assists; load
  resists (OL)

NOTE: Transpose direction for flexion to right followed by reversal to left.

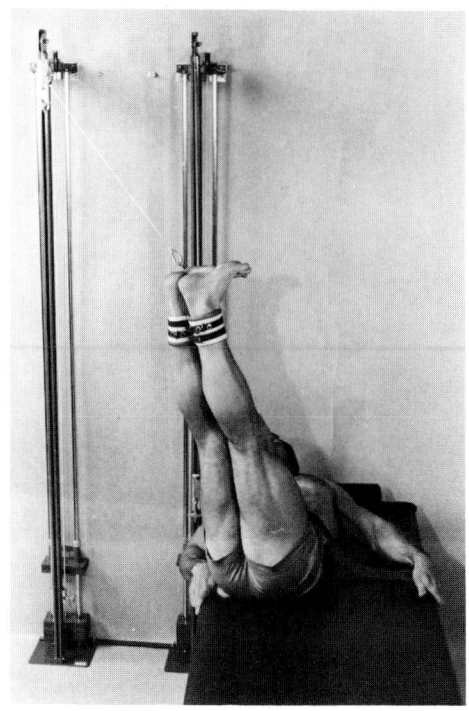

A　　　　Le-R

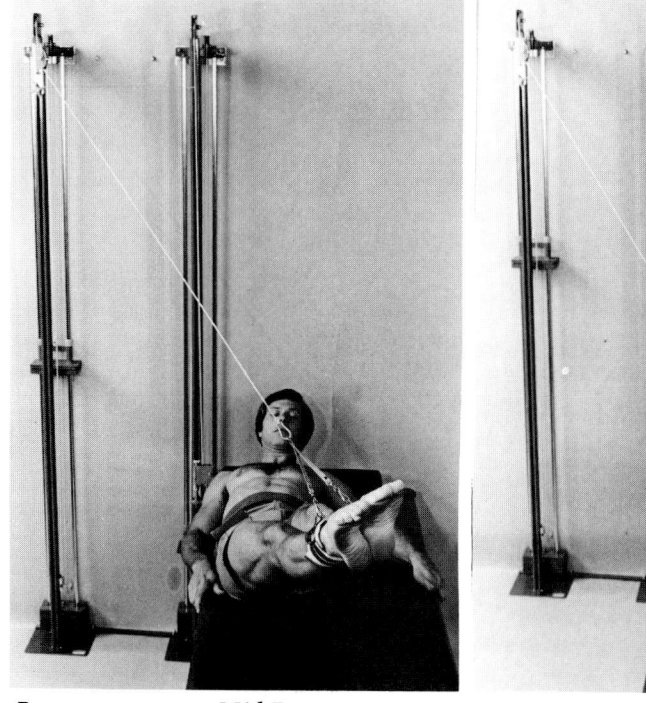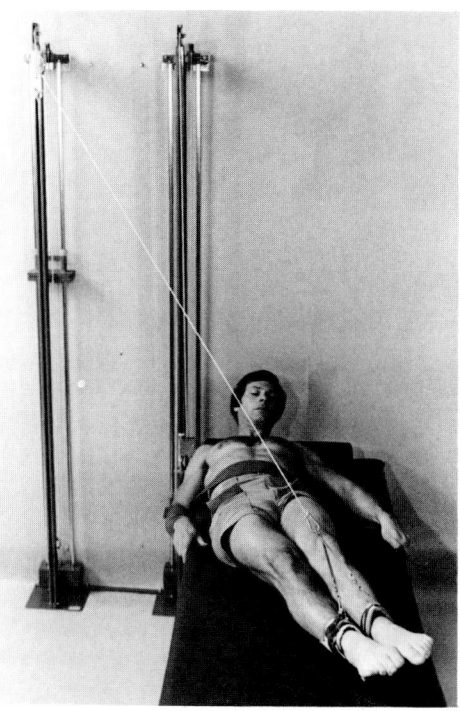

B　　　Mid-R　　　C　　　Sh-R

FIG. 1-208. Lower trunk extension with lower extremities (BA) to left (OL)

A. Lifting load: gravity assists; load resists
B. Holding load
C. *Reversal,* lowering load: gravity resists; eccentric control, extensors
Alternate posture: prone, lower trunk over table edge; gravity resists; load assists

NOTE: Transpose direction for extension to right followed by reversal to left.

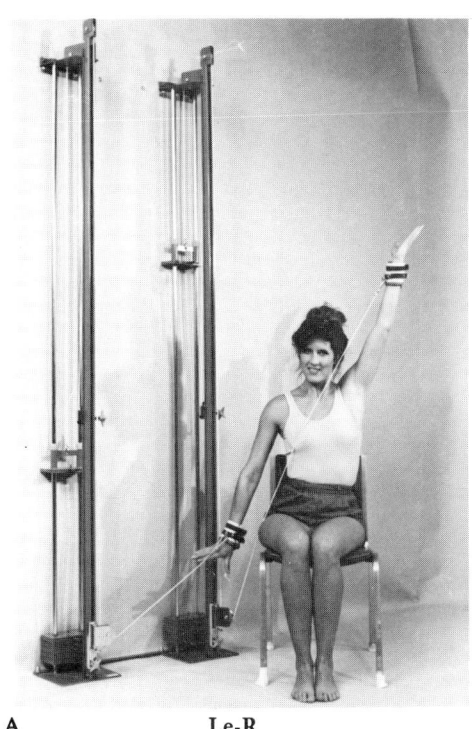

A   Le-R

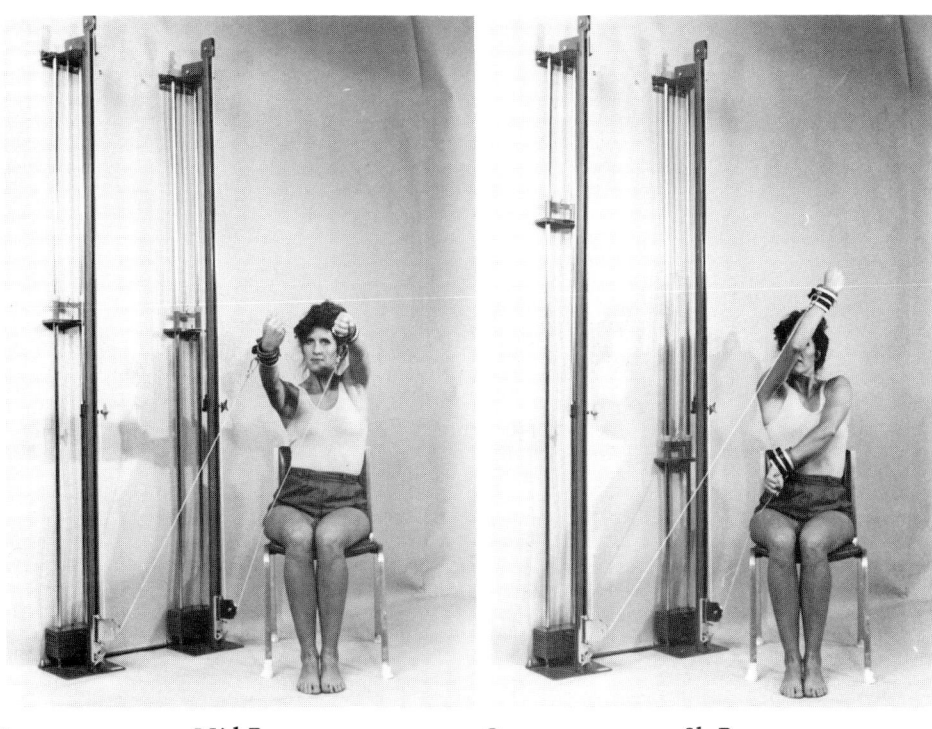

B   Mid-R   C   Sh-R

FIG. 1-209. Upper extremities, bilateral reciprocal (BR, CD) (FL)

A. Lifting load: R, D1, gravity resists; load resists. Lowering load: L, D2, gravity assists; eccentric control, extensors

B. Holding load

C. *Reversal:* lowering load, R; lifting load, L

Alternate postures: standing, kneeling

NOTE: Transpose diagonals: L, D1; R, D2.

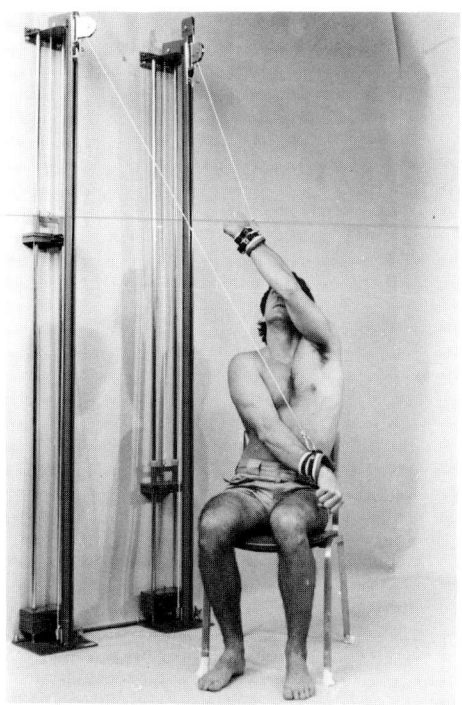

A   Le-R

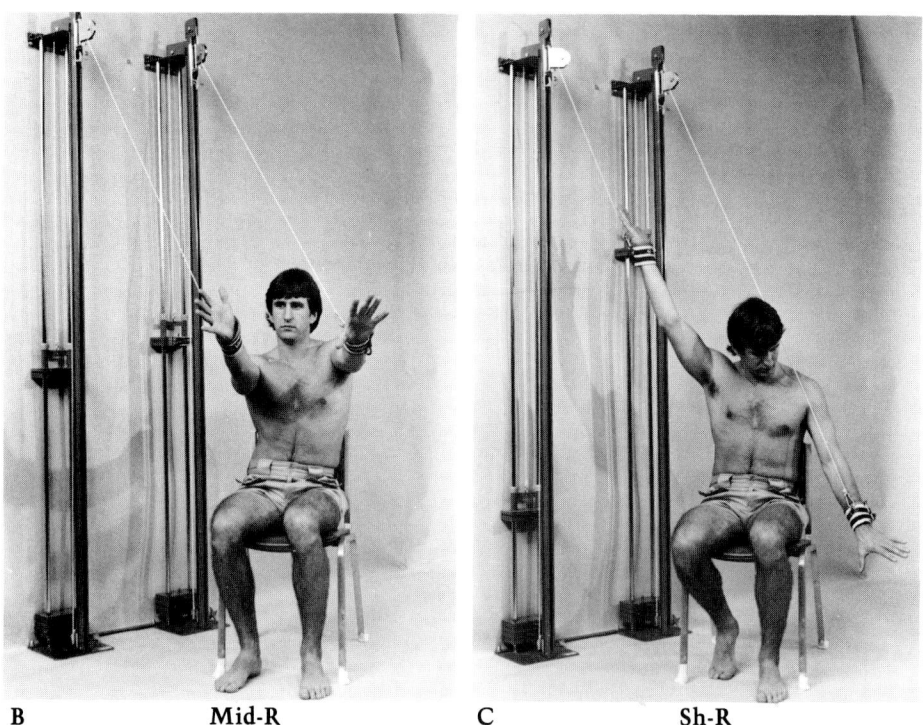

B   Mid-R   C   Sh-R

FIG. 1-210. Upper extremities, bilateral reciprocal (BR, CD) (OL)

A. Lifting load: L, D1, gravity assists; load resists. Lowering load: R, D2, gravity resists; load assists

B. Holding load

C. *Reversal:* lowering load, L; lifting load, R

Alternate postures: standing, kneeling

NOTE: Transpose diagonals: L, D2; R, D1.

TECHNIQUES FOR FACILITATION

2

Within the repertoire of techniques that are superimposed upon movement and posture, there are certain procedures that are considered basic to the approach. These basic procedures become a part of the treatment of every patient insofar as his medical condition permits their use. In the broadest sense, the basic procedures may be used with or without the patient's complete cooperation; if the patient moves, the physical therapist's maneuvers guide and influence the patient's response. The procedures have to do with how the therapist approaches the patient, how manual contacts are made effective, how the therapist communicates with the patient, how the therapist opposes the patient's effort and at the same time becomes a part of his effort, how coordination is brought about through timing, and how reinforcement is used to increase response and to circumvent fatigue.

Beyond the basic procedures there is a battery of specific techniques which are, for the most part, dependent upon the patient's cooperation and his voluntary effort. Whenever and wherever possible the patient's voluntary effort is used to promote volitional control of movement and posture. The coupling of the patient's voluntary effort with resistance, graded appropriately by the physical therapist, permits the use of specific techniques for stimulation or facilitation and for relaxation or inhibition. Facilitation and inhibition are inseparable: A technique that promotes response or facilitation of the agonist simultaneously promotes relaxation or inhibition of the antagonist.

The specific techniques may be analyzed as to whether they are directed primarily to the agonist; whether the antagonist is used primarily to facilitate the agonist; or whether the antagonist is used primarily for relaxation or inhibition of the antagonist itself. Again, because facilitation and inhibition are inseparable, there is an overlapping of effect. Techniques may be classified by their contributions to mobility and stability (Table 2-1).

The specific techniques are rarely used singly; they are usually combined in a sequence that promotes the desired effect. The use of techniques that employ the antagonist (reversal and relaxation techniques) is, more often than not, followed by the use of repeated contractions in order to emphasize movement in the desired direction. An arbitrary guide to selection of techniques cannot be given. The diversity of patients' problems, the degree of involvement, and the presence of pain are factors that influence selection. The Summary of Techniques, Table 2-2, provides certain guidelines to indications and contraindications.

The battery of specific techniques permits choice of the way or ways in which the basic procedures may be supplemented and adapted to the patient's needs. The patient's needs will be fulfilled most readily by combining basic procedures and specific techniques, all of which become more effective when superimposed upon the spiral and diagonal patterns of facilitation, as individual patterns, as combining patterns, and as total patterns of movement and posture.

Table 2-1. Promotion of Mobility and Stability

Techniques	Mobility	Stability
Manual contacts	Pressure over agonist, flexors or extensors	Pressure over agonists and antagonists, flexors *and* extensors
Commands	Strong and exclamatory: "Move!"	Moderate and soothing: "Hold"
Stretch	Quick repetitive to agonist; timed with "Move!"	Slow stretch of "hold" contraction without defeating hold
Traction	Distraction of joint surfaces for ease of movement	
Approximation	May promote ability to move after posture is stable	Compression of joint surfaces for postural response
Maximal resistance, reinforcement	Stimulation of isotonic contractions	Stimulation of isometric contractions
Directed to Agonist		
Repeated contractions	Increase range, endurance	
Rhythmic initiation	Assisted initiation of movement	
Hold–relax active motion	Isometric hold, shortened range, followed by isotonic contraction, lengthened range	
Reversal of Antagonists		
Slow reversal	Isotonic contraction of antagonists alternately	
Slow reversal–hold	As in slow reversal, followed by isometric hold	Isometric hold phase
Rhythmic stabilization	May promote ability to move after posture is stable	Simultaneous isometric contraction of antagonists: co-contraction
Quick reversal	Repetitive stretch of antagonists alternately	
Relaxation		
Contract–relax	In lieu of "passive stretching"	
Hold–relax	In lieu of "passive stretching"	
Rhythmic rotation	In lieu of "passive stretching"	
Slow reversal–hold–relax	Isotonic contraction of agonist following relaxation	

See Table 2-2, Summary of Techniques.

MANUAL CONTACT (MC)

Treatment of the patient frequently involves manual contact (MC) with the patient by the physical therapist. Manual contacts use pressure as a facilitating mechanism.[13] This may be demonstrated very simply in the normal subject. When elbow flexion is resisted with pressure over the biceps brachii, the subject will be able to pull with effectiveness and strength, and will be able to hold adequately in the shortened range of the motion. If a comparable degree of pressure is applied to the triceps as the subject flexes the elbow against resistance, he will be felt to contract the biceps less effectively and to hold less well against resistance in the shortened range of elbow flexion. This test will be most convincing when the amount of resistance given allows the range of motion to occur slowly with maximum effort by the subject.

Tactile stimulation by scratching the skin overlying an antagonistic muscle inhibits the agonist as it is tested for strength of an eccentric contraction.[38] That is, when shoulder abductors were tested at 90° before and after tactile stimulation of skin overlying shoulder adductors, a 19% decrease of strength of abductors was documented. While "scratching" would seem a noxious, attention-demanding stimulus as compared with pressure of manual contacts, the effects are similar. Pressure or scratching of skin overlying the antagonist inhibits the agonist. At the same time the antagonist may be facilitated. Thus, when enhancement of response of a specific muscle is desired, such as in the example of biceps and triceps, pressure of the therapist's hands or tactile stimulation must be applied specifically.

The specific manual contacts described for the patterns employ pressure to the skin overlying the groups of muscles, tendons, and joints responsible for the patterns and in line with the direction to which resistance is to be applied. Since the direction of the movement is diagonal, the therapist assumes a position in the diagonal. In this way, therapist and subject move together. If the therapist fails to move, or assumes a position away from the diagonal, the subject's efforts will be hindered and his movement may be distorted.

This interaction between therapist and patient is a form of social tracking. The therapist's response provides guidance by which the patient can direct his own movements.[45] The two hands of the therapist in contact with the patient can track two movements simultaneously. For example, bilateral reciprocal patterns of the upper extremities may be controlled precisely. If the therapist placed her hands an inch away from the patient's palms and moved in the desired directions, the patient would have great difficulty in visually tracking two hands moving in opposite directions. The role of the therapist is to track what the patient is doing and then to extend or refine the pattern of feedback control.[45]

Manual contacts may be varied somewhat with shifting pivots of emphasis and in special situations in order to make pressure more specific in relation to a given muscle or group of muscles, for example, in the axilla as a stimulus to the subscapularis when internal rotation is to be emphasized in the lengthened range of extension–adduction–internal rotation of the upper extremity. Manual contacts may be used to place a demand or they may be used to give the patient security. The latter applies when treating patients who have symptoms of pain. The contacts should then include pressure for both antagonistic and agonistic patterns in order to provide security.

Pressure may be used as a sensory cue to help the patient to understand the direction of the anticipated movement. For example, if a patient is to flex his neck with rotation toward the left, briskly tapping him on the chest above the left nipple will guide his movement.

Suggestions for Learning Manual Contacts

Practice placing hands for a specific pattern. Have the subject move actively through the available range of motion. The following questions will help you evaluate your performance:

> Did the position of your hands allow the full range of motion to occur, or did they impede the range of motion?
> Did you move as the subject moved?
> Was your body in line with the diagonal direction of the movement?
> Were your hands accurately placed so that the pressure was over the muscle groups, tendons, and joints participating in the movement?

COMMANDS AND COMMUNICATION

Communication with the patient depends upon sensory cues. Manually contacting the patient's skin, telling the patient what to do, and engaging vision to give movement direction are means of communication that demand the patient's attention. Skin can make both temporal and spatial discriminations, and vision is the great spatial sense, while audition is the great temporal sense.[13]

Verbal commands place a demand upon the subject. In order to provide an adequate stimulus, the developmental level of the subject and his ability to cooperate must be considered. Commands given to the lucid, normally innervated adult subject will obviously be very different from the type of motivation employed with a child of 6 months. Where the developmental or cooperative level is low, adequate stimulation may be more dependent upon physical demands and visual cues than upon verbal commands.

Tone of voice may influence considerably the quality of response.[2] Strong, sharp commands simulate a stress situation and are used when maximal stimulation of active motion is desired. Overuse of strong commands may result in adaptation by the subject; therefore, they should be reserved for demands for further effort. A moderate tone of voice should be used when the subject is responding with his best effort, and in giving preparatory commands. A soft tone of voice is desirable when security is needed by patients who have symptoms of pain.

Preparatory commands must be clear and concise. They may be made more meaningful by demonstration of the desired movement and by providing a visual cue. The therapist may point at an appropriate object on which the patient is to focus his attention. Using vision to lead movement encourages response. A child is frequently led to perform by enticing him to look at and pursue an object. In the adult, vision also reinforces movement and should be used with preparatory commands. Complete understanding of what is to be done is most important when pain is a factor. When understanding and confidence have been gained, when patterns have been learned and pain is relieved, preparatory commands play a lesser role.

Action commands must be short, accurate, and timed to the physical demands. "Push" or "pull" are commands for isotonic contractions. "Hold" is the command for isometric contraction. "Relax" or "let go" are the commands for voluntary relaxation. The timing of action commands is extremely important. A premature command results in poor initiation by the patient and loss of control of the motion by the physical therapist. Delayed commands result in a lessened response especially when a stretch is being used.

Rhythmic timing of verbal commands and auditory rhythmic beats of music may encourage rhythmic performance of motor activities. From creeping on the mat with manual resistance to repetitive use of wall pulleys and weights, and to the use of crutches in various gait patterns, all require a neat interaction of segments which builds endurance and establishes habit patterns. The technique of repeated contractions done rhythmically, as the therapist resists and guides the patient's movement, helps to condition reflexes through voluntary effort.

The effect of auditory rhythm on muscle (biceps and triceps) activity has been recorded by electromyograph (EMG). Even and uneven rhythms produced different changes in the variation of EMG activity. The even rhythm (1-2-3-4-5-6) produced significant decreased variation in the EMG pattern, whereas the uneven rhythm (1-2-3-4-5-6) caused significant increased variation. This increased variation appeared to be the result of uneven timing of the beat. As motor tasks performed to these rhythms (both in $^6/_8$ time) became new skills to be learned (metal peg hitting target board), increased EMG activity occurred in duration and co-contraction of antagonistic muscles. These changes are features of performance by untrained subjects as they seek control.[43]

Rhythms or beats of dance music may be useful or not, depending upon the motor skill to be learned. Two known beats, the waltz (da-da-da) and a so-called rock beat (da-da-da) have been studied. The selected rock beat when tested with normal males was found to have a "weakening effect" (the deltoid muscle was tested manually at 90° of shoulder abduction). The rock beat has a "stopped quality" at the end of each bar or measure unless the music is played at a rapid rate. The stopped quality, a weakening rhythm, is apparently counter to the normal physiological rhythm of the body. The waltz rhythm has the opposite quality and an even flow.[5]

The patient who is to use crutches with a four-point pattern should learn to walk with an even rhythm. Waltz music may help to set the pattern. The beat is da-da-da. In walking, arm swing precedes leg swing of the contralateral limb. In the four-point pattern crutch placement precedes foot placement. Verbal mediation (VM) may be used as the patient speaks aloud. The waltz beat may be spoken by therapist or patient, or music may be played.

Problem: Arthritis
Gait pattern: Four-point
Sequence: R crutch, L foot, L crutch, R foot
VM: *Reach* and step; *reach* and step
Waltz beat: *Da*, da, da; *da*, da, da

While the four-point gait pattern has a rhythmical, waltz-like quality, some gait patterns, such as the rock beat, have a stopped quality. The patient who has had a recent fracture of the right ankle is unable to bear weight on the right foot. As he places his crutches slightly in advance, he steps forward on his left foot. His left extremity must become stable with co-contraction of antagonistic muscles to permit simultaneous advancement of both crutches.

Problem: Fracture, R ankle
Gait pattern: Three-point

Sequence: Crutches, then L foot; crutches, then L foot

VM: Reach, step, and *stop*; reach, step, and *stop*

Rock beat: da, da, *da*; da, da, *da*

Thus, the rock beat is the reverse of the waltz rhythm, and the person who chants the rhythm, therapist or patient, must select and use an appropriate beat. Music to assist patients must be selected accordingly.

Self-direction through VM is useful in training patients in the performance of functional activities. Overt verbal mediation procedures lead the patient to express aloud the sequence and spatial relationships of a motor task. He directs his own performance. Children at ages 3 and 4 years speak aloud words that direct their action.[34] Thus, there is a developmental basis for encouraging patients to use self-direction.

For example, a patient who lacks control of eccentric contraction of extensors while lowering to sitting may be told to speak aloud, "I am going to sit down *slowly*, slowly, slowly, slow-ly." The therapist should demonstrate the task and the procedure when necessary.

Self-touching[30] is a normal reaction in the presence of pain, for pursuit of a fly near the eye, or for reinforcement by interaction of segments when control and power are needed. The baseball player at bat, except when bunting, places his hands in contact for control and power. In recent years some tennis players use two hands in contact for the same purpose. By so doing, the total body contributes to the motor act.

Self-touching or "hand-to-body discovery" begins soon after birth when the infant sucks his thumb or fisted hand. The developmental sequence proceeds from head to foot, and at about 6 months of age the foot has reached the mouth.[31]

In PNF, self-touching is used when one hand contacts the opposite forearm and wrist in "chopping and lifting." During these asymmetrical, diagonal movements, the head and neck and upper trunk patterns reinforce and, in turn, are reinforced by the upper limbs.

In treatment, a patient may touch his painful or weak limb. His touch or pressure may help to activate his muscles. The patient becomes the third hand of the physical therapist. Some patients can be trained to participate during rhythmic stabilization. For example, as the therapist stabilizes the hand (thumb and fingers), the patient may place his free hand on wrist and forearm. As the therapist resists extensors, the patient applies pressure and resistance to flexor muscles. The patient contributes to his own treatment.

Through self direction and self-touching, the patient learns to help himself and at the same time gains security and self-confidence.

Self-evaluation by the physical therapist may include the following questions:

Did my hands and my words help the subject to understand what was expected of him? Did I rely too much on too many words, rather than on careful use of my hands?

Did I command him to "push" or "pull" when I meant for him to hold?

Did he perform in accordance with normal timing?

Did my commands encourage normal timing?

Were my commands directed at the pivot of emphasis? Would the patient's response have been better if I had used a stronger tone of voice? If I had asked him to look in the direction of the movement, would he have performed more adequately?

STRETCH (STR)

Stimulus

That muscle responds with greater force after stretch has been superimposed is a fact of physiology.[17] Stretch, for this reason, may be used as a stimulus.

In order to achieve a stretch stimulus in any given pattern, the part must be placed in the extreme lengthened range of that pattern, which is the completely shortened range of the directly antagonistic pattern. This is the starting position of the pattern as portrayed by the black figure of the physical therapist in the illustrations of individual patterns. All components of the pattern must be considered to obtain a stretch stimulus. The component of rotation receives first and last consideration since it is the rotatory component that elongates the muscle fibers of the muscles in a given pattern. The part should be taken to the point where tension is felt on all muscle components of a given pattern.

Stretch Reflex

Once the position has been achieved with the stretch stimulus, a stretch reflex can be superimposed on the pattern. The reflex can be elicited manually by "quickly" taking the part past the point of tension, being certain that all components are stretched, especially proper rotation. At the exact same moment the reflex is elicited, the patient attempts the motion. To be certain that the stretch and the patient's efforts are synchronized, the command should be, "Now push," or "Now pull." This warns the patient to be prepared to attempt the motion.

Even in completely paralyzed muscles there may be a contraction over the reflex arc when a stretch reflex is elicited.[40] This contraction is followed by relaxation of the muscles stretched. Repetition of the stretch reflex with patient's efforts timed accurately is essential. The stretch reflex can be used to initiate voluntary motion as well as to increase strength and enhance a quicker response in weak motions. Use of stretch reflex aids the patient with intact innervation to learn and perform the patterns with greater ease. Pain should always be avoided in using the stretch reflex. It is contraindicated with patients who have the problem of pain or with patients whose skeletal, joint, or soft tissue structures should not be subjected to sudden movement.

When either stretch stimulus or stretch reflex is used, commands for voluntary motion are always used. By so doing, any potential for voluntary control will be tapped more readily. A proper balance of stretch reflexes is necessary to postural control. The stretch reflex may be used repeatedly, as in the technique of repeated contractions.

The use of the stretch reflex should be judicious, especially when stimulating flexion responses. Flexion reflexes may become dominant, creating an imbalance between flexion and extension.

Suggestions and Questions for Learning

Stretch stimulus
- Practice placement of a part in the lengthened range of a pattern to the point of tension
- Consider rotation at the proximal joint first, then all other components from proximal to distal.

Stretch reflex
- Practice taking the part to the point where tension is felt.
- "Quickly" move the part into and past the point of tension of components.
- Synchronize commands so that the physical therapist and the patient are working together.

Was rotation considered first and last?
Were the patient and physical therapist completely together?
Was pain avoided?

TRACTION AND APPROXIMATION (TR AND AP)

Traction (separating the joint surfaces) and approximation (compressing the joint surfaces) are directed toward the joint receptors. Joint receptors are responsive to alterations in joint position; the effect of joint receptor discharge upon motoneuron responses probably depends upon the position of the joint and upon the type of joint movement.[2] In treatment, the use of traction seems to promote movement, whereas approximation promotes stability or maintenance of posture.

Traction and approximation are used to stimulate the proprioceptive centers supplying the joint structures themselves. Either separating joint surfaces (traction) or compressing joint surfaces together (approximation) are helpful means of stimulation. Manual contacts make possible the use of traction or approximation. In general, traction is used where the motion is one of pulling, and approximation is used where the motion is one of pushing. This is in keeping with normal activities. For example, if one attempts to lift a weight, the joint surfaces are separated by the weight unless the muscles contract to perform the job of lifting. In pushing a heavy object, the joint surfaces are approximated because of contact with the object and contraction of the necessary muscle groups. When there is marked weakness, traction or approximation are maintained throughout the active range of motion. Traction and approximation may be contraindicated in patients having acute symptoms. However, in patients who have arthritis, traction often encourages range of motion.

Approximation may be used to stimulate postural reflexes. To encourage sitting balance, a suddenly applied pressure in a downward direction should be exerted on the shoulders. This maneuver will be most effective when the spinal column is in a nearly extended position. As the pressure is applied, the patient is commanded to "hold," at which time resistance is applied anteriorly at one shoulder and posteriorly at the other. The patient attempts to hold himself as rigidly as possible, thereby preventing rotation of his trunk. To encourage standing balance, approximation may be given at the pelvis. Again, the alignment of joint structures is important. The pelvis should be tilted by gripping the brim on either side while the extremities are in extension. Pressure is then applied suddenly downward through the pelvis and extremities with the command, "Hold." Resisting rotation at the pelvis as the patient sustains his position encourages stability.

During mat activities, postural responses in the upper extremities may be enhanced by superimposing pressure downward on the scapulae as the patient maintains himself in a creeping posture.

Approximation is always applied in resistive walking except where weight bearing is contraindicated. Approximation is most effective if it is applied alternately as the patient puts weight on his lower extremities during the stance phases. This can be done by downward pressure applied through the shoulders or the pelvis.

Suggestions and Questions for Learning Use of Traction (Tr) and Approximation (Ap)

Practice applying traction and approximation using specific manual contacts.

Did the subject perform with greater ease and strength?

Were traction and approximation applied without producing pain?

MAXIMAL RESISTANCE (MR)

Movement performed against resistance of sufficient degree to demand maximal effort produces an increase in strength.[17] When maximal effort is demanded, the amount of resistance used may be termed maximal. Performance with maximal effort may be hazardous to some patients.[17] The hazard is perhaps greater when mechanical resistance is used than when manually applied resistance is appropriately graded to the patient's effort. The Valsalva phenomenon can best be avoided by allowing the patient to move when the command for movement is given rather than requiring a prolonged effort to overcome the opposition provided by the physical therapist. Where sustained effort by the patient warrants precaution, prolonged repetition of isometric contractions, holding, should be avoided or used guardedly.

Maximal resistance as applied in techniques of PNF may be defined as the greatest amount of resistance that can be applied to an isotonic or active contraction allowing full range of motion to occur. When applied to an isometric contraction, maximal resistance is the greatest amount that can be applied without defeating or breaking the patient's hold. It therefore becomes necessary for the physical therapist to feel and sense the ability of the patient and to grade resistance accordingly. If these amounts of resistance were measurable, there would be a wide range of variation. The skill with which a physical therapist applies the manual contacts, and superimposes pressure, stretch, traction, or approximation on the pattern will affect the amount of resistance a patient can overcome. Many mechanical factors involving the relationship of levers, the axis of motion, and the effect of gravity play a role in determining the amount of resistance given, but there is only one criterion for judging maximal resistance. This criterion is that the patient must put forth maximum effort but must be allowed to move the part slowly but smoothly throughout a range of motion. When isometric contraction is resisted, the patient must again put forth maximum effort, but the physical therapist must not break or defeat the hold. Rather, the patient's ability to hold is developed by gradually increasing, from minimal to maximal, the

amount of resistance in keeping with the patient's response.

Resistance may also be graded to encourage speed and repetition of a motion, conducive to the development of endurance. Grading resistance for this purpose demands skill and perception on the part of the physical therapist. Here the objective is to allow the patient to repeat the motion as many times as possible, whereas in developing power throughout the range of motion, resistance is given so strongly that the patient may only succeed in a few repetitions of the pattern. As always, the needs of the patient determine the method. Patients who have normal innervation but with acute symptoms require very careful grading of resistance in specific, limited ranges of motion. The resistance used may be very slight but may be maximal for the patient's needs.

In treating patients who have deficiency of innervation, maximal resistance is one of the most important techniques when superimposed upon patterns of facilitation. It is maximal resistance that provides the means for securing overflow or irradiation from more adequate to less adequate patterns of movement of the head and neck, the trunk, and the extremities. Stronger muscle groups within a pattern and stronger patterns must be used to augment the response of weaker muscle groups and of weaker patterns through a process of timing. The timing of application is coupled with appropriate gradation of maximal resistance.

Suggestions and Questions for Learning Maximal Resistance

Position the part in the lengthened range of a pattern with proper attention to all components of the pattern. Check manual contacts for accuracy, apply stretch, traction, or approximation, and command the subject to pull or push. Grade resistance so that the subject performs smoothly and slowly through the available range of the pattern.

Did the subject perform through the full range of the pattern?

Did rotation enter the motion first? Did the line of movement become diagonal following initiation of rotation? Was performance in the "groove" of the pattern?

Did the manual contacts allow the subject to move all component parts through their full range of of motion?

Did the distal parts move first?

Did pressure, stretch, traction, or approximation produce pain?

Were commands timed with manual demands and performance?

TIMING

Normal timing is the sequence of muscle contraction that occurs in any motor activity, resulting in a coordinated movement. The importance of timing is realized in life when the normal subject attempts to learn a sport skill that involves a high degree of coordination. Routine activities of life involve timing and are learned through trial and error.[16] Witness the baby learning to feed himself: he may open his mouth, lift the spoon, then close his mouth before emptying the spoon, or he may empty the spoon before closing his mouth. The baby is in the process of learning the timing that establishes coordinated movements related to feeding himself.

In the normal process of development, proximal control is evident before distal control. After coordinated, purposeful movements have been acquired, timing or sequential contraction of muscles occurs from distal to proximal. An example of this difference is that of the approach to rolling from supine to prone by the infant as compared with the coordinated person. The infant makes his initial attempts by using neck and trunk motions and then learns to use the extremities effectively. The older child or adult will automatically use the extremities by placement and as reinforcement to assist in the process of rolling.

Distal to proximal timing is in keeping with the fact that the distal parts, the hands and feet, receive most of the stimuli for motor activities. Motions of the trunk that are proximal follow motions of the neck and extremities. For example, an article is grasped and lifted with action occurring first in the hand and proceeding to the elbow, shoulder, neck, trunk, and other extremities in accordance with demand.

Normal timing in patterns of facilitation may be demonstrated simply by superimposing resistance in the lengthened range of a specific pattern. The normal, coordinated subject will initiate the pattern by rotating the part first and then accomplishing the other components of the pattern from distal to proximal. Rotation always enters the motion first, and the diagonal direction of the pattern is controlled by the physical therapist through control of the rotation component. If rotation is not allowed to occur, the other components of motion cannot occur. After rotation is allowed to enter the motion, the normal subject will proceed to move first the distal pivots, and action proceeds from there to the proximal pivots.

For example, if resistance is applied to the lengthened range of the flexion–adduction–external rotation pattern, the subject will grasp and rotate the entire extremity, the fingers will flex and adduct toward the radial side, the wrist will proceed to flex toward the radial side, the forearm will supinate, and the shoulder will externally rotate. After this initial rotation has taken place, the distal parts complete their range of motion by the time the elbow has flexed to the middle range; the shoulder proceeds to flex and adduct. The elbow completes its range of motion before the shoulder has completely flexed and adducted.

Normal timing may be prevented by excessive resistance to the rotation component and to the distal pivots. If the fingers and wrist are not allowed to move, action cannot occur at the proximal pivots.

If normal timing in patterns of facilitation has not been developed or is deficient, it becomes one of the goals of treatment. Proximal deficiencies are corrected first in line with the normal process of development. Distal deficiencies are corrected after proximal control has been established. If proximal control is adequate, distal control must receive emphasis in accordance with normal timing.

Timing for Emphasis (TE)

Timing for emphasis is based upon Beevor's axiom that the brain knows not of individual muscle action but knows only of motion. The urge of the subject to accomplish a motion brings into action the muscles necessary to the performance of that motion.[9]

In timing for emphasis, maximal resistance is superimposed upon patterns of facilitation with due regard for normal timing in order that overflow or irradiation may occur from stronger to weaker major muscle components. The stronger muscle components must augment the weaker components; a weaker component cannot augment the response of a stronger component. Timing for emphasis provides the means for increasing response and stimulating action at a specific pivot within a pattern, a specific component in relation to that pivot, and a specific part of the range of motion of that pivot.[27]

Timing may be accomplished by using either the stronger distal parts or the stronger proximal muscle groups. The process of timing produces irradiation from one group of muscles to the other. It may be done either by preventing the stronger component motions of a pattern from moving through any appreciable range through application of manual maximal resistance, or by allowing the part to move against maximal resistance to the strongest point in the range of motion, at which point a maximal isometric or "hold" contraction is done. After the "hold" is completed the patient is asked to "pull" or "push" strongly with no joint motion being allowed except in the joint needing emphasis.

If wrist extension toward the radial side is the weakest component of the pattern and needs emphasis, the physical therapist could promote irradiation by resisting strongly the pattern of flexion–abduction–

external rotation of the shoulder allowing motion to occur only at the wrist joint. The resistance to wrist extension toward the radial side could be minimal or guided resistance to give the patient the feeling of motion occurring.

If the wrist extension toward the radial side is the strongest motion of the flexion – abduction – external rotation pattern, the physical therapist can apply enough resistance to prevent motion of the wrist joint from occurring but allow range of motion to occur in the shoulder joint. Resistance must be given slowly to allow maximal "build-up" if irradiation is to occur.

Timing may also be done in the two ways described by using the patterns of the stronger extremity to produce irradiation to the opposite extremity or extremities, such as arm or leg patterns or a combination of both. When these are used, maximal resistance is always given to the strongest part first. The weaker extremity is then guided and resisted into the desired pattern. Any strong pattern can reinforce another on the opposite side. They do not have to be corresponding motions on the two sides. Strong extensor patterns can promote irradiation to flexors on the opposite side as well as to the extensor groups.

DIRECTED TO AGONIST

Repeated Contractions (RC)

Repeated excitation of a pathway in the central nervous system promotes ease of transmission of impulses through that pathway.[27] Repetition of activity is necessary to the learning process and to the development of strength and endurance. Repeated activity of the weaker components of a pattern is obtained through a technique of emphasis, repeated contractions. In order to emphasize the response of a weak component of a pattern, or a weak pattern, motion is repeated until fatigue is evident in the performance of that motion. Fatigue will be delayed, and response will be enhanced if the stretch reflex is coupled with the patient's voluntary effort to initiate movement.

The less advanced form of repeated contractions involves only isotonic contractions stimulated by use of the stretch reflex as the patient attempts the movement. The response to stretch must be resisted by the therapist to enhance voluntary response and motor learning. Repeated isotonic contractions induced by stretch reflex may be the only choice when a patient cannot move voluntarily, or if the patient is unable to perform a ''hold'' with isometric contraction. When the stretch reflex is used, care must be taken to avoid creation of imbalances between flexor and extensor reflexes. Therefore, the skill lies in the ability to resist the response from stretching the muscle groups in the pattern and to time the use of resistance with the patient's voluntary effort.

The verbal commands are combined with stretch. That is, as stretch is given, the command, ''Now,'' is synchronized with the maneuver, and the command, ''Pull!'' follows immediately if flexion is being stimulated. For extensor movements the command becomes, ''Now (stretch) push! Now (stretch) push!''

The more advanced form of repeated contractions uses both isotonic and isometric contractions. If a patient is only able to perform the simpler form, the advanced form becomes a goal of treatment, that is, the therapist must keep in mind the need to teach the patient to hold and must not be satisfied by use of only isotonic contractions. As the patient's strength and endurance improves, performance of a ''hold'' contraction may become possible. The more advanced form is executed as follows.

After the subject has performed initially against resistance with resultant overflow to a weaker pivot of action, he is instructed to hold, with an isometric contraction, at the point where active motion is felt to be lessening in power. The physical therapist then se-

cures the hold by resisting all components of the pattern in turn from distal to proximal. Resistance is maximal but the goal is to encourage the subject to hold rather than to defeat or break the hold. When the entire part has become secure or, as it were, a complete unit by the patient having sustained his effort, the physical therapist maintains resistance to all pivots of action equally and then resists more strongly at the weaker pivot of action. At the moment that resistance is increased at the weaker pivot, the physical therapist instructs the subject to pull again or push again, thereby shifting from an isometric to an isotonic contraction. Having asked the subject to push or pull, it is again necessary to grade the resistance so that active motion of the weaker pivot may occur.

By repeating isotonic contractions, the patient may be allowed to work toward the shortened range of the pattern. If the initial response was secured in the shortened range, the response may be channeled toward the lengthened range by gradually decreasing the range of motion through resistance.

Example of Technique: Isotonic and Isometric

PATTERN TO BE EMPHASIZED

Flexion–adduction–external rotation of right upper extremity (Fig. 1-45).

PIVOT OF EMPHASIS

Action to be emphasized; elbow flexion.

STARTING POSITION

Lengthened range of pattern (stretch range).

TIMING FOR EMPHASIS OF ELBOW FLEXION (BICEPS BRACHII)

Resist strongly the fingers and wrist flexion to the radial side, the supination of the forearm, and the external rotation of the shoulder. Allow beginning rotation to occur at the fingers, wrist, forearm, and shoulder, but do not allow full range of finger and wrist flexion toward the radial side and shoulder flexion and adduction to occur until the elbow begins to flex. As the elbow begins to flex, allow the distal components to complete their range of motion (normal timing) and then allow beginning range to occur at the shoulder.

COMMANDS TO THE SUBJECT

For initiation of active motion with isotonic contraction: ''Squeeze my hand, turn it and pull it up and across your face. Bend your elbow!'' Patient pulls while the physical therapist resists the motion as outlined above.

For securing isometric contraction in preparation for repeated isotonic contractions: "Hold it!" "Hold" command is given when patient has achieved maximum elbow flexion. All major muscle components are resisted without defeating the hold at any pivot of action. The part becomes secure. Derotation is avoided.

For repetitions of elbow flexion: "Now pull, and pull, and pull, and pull again! And rest." The physical therapist, having felt the subject hold throughout the pattern, resists slightly the sustained hold contraction at the elbow, and proceeds to give the commands for repetitions of elbow flexion. Repeated application of resistance immediately precedes the commands. Increased range of motion is allowed to occur.

Repeated contractions technique is indicated where weakness and incoordination are primary problems. It is contraindicated where sustained effort is contraindicated and in very acute situations.

Hold – Relax – Active Motion (HRA)

Hold – relax – active motion (HRA) is a technique of emphasis that provides repetition of isotonic contraction without sustained effort. The physical therapist first elicits an isometric contraction in the shortened range of a pattern. When the hold has been secured and resisted strongly, the physical therapist commands the patient to let go. As soon as the patient has relaxed his hold, the physical therapist immediately and quickly moves the part passively into the lengthened range of the pattern and instructs the patient to pull. This procedure may be repeated several times until a buildup in power is felt to occur, or it may be repeated until fatigue is evident.

Commands for hold – relax – active motion would be as follows:

"Hold"—isometric contraction, shortened range—agonist
"Let go"—relaxation occurs; physical therapist moves the part quickly to the lengthened range
"Pull"—isotonic contraction, lengthened range—agonist

Good cooperation of the patient and precise commands and performance by the physical therapist are necessary to successful application of this technique. The passive movement of the part by the physical therapist must be done smoothly and quickly.

Hold – relax – active motion is indicated if a patient presents marked weakness in the lengthened range of a pattern, marked lack of endurance, or marked imbalance in favor of the antagonistic pattern. Repeated contractions places a greater demand than hold – relax – active motion, and the former should be given preference as a technique whenever possible.

Hold – relax – active motion is contraindicated if full range of passive motion and resisted motion are to be avoided because of pain.

Correction of Imbalances

Repeated contractions with timing for emphasis is the technique of choice in the correction of imbalances. In patterns of facilitation imbalances may present themselves with relation to the major muscle components of a specific pivot. For example, a weak anterior deltoid may be overpowered by a strong clavicular portion of the pectoralis major. Both muscles are related in the flexion – adduction – external rotation pattern. When this pattern is performed, response in the anterior deltoid is dependent upon maximal resistance to the stronger clavicular portion of the pectoralis major and to the component of external rotation. Emphasizing external rotation will prevent excessive adduction of the shoulder and will stimulate the anterior deltoid.

Imbalances may also occur in relation to the major muscle components of related patterns with reference to a specific pivot. For example, the ulnar flexor of the wrist may be stronger than the radial flexor. When the flexion – adduction – external rotation pattern is performed for shoulder emphasis, the wrist may fail to proceed to radial flexion and this will distort the pattern with regard to the proximal components. For emphasis of the shoulder pivot in a situation of this kind, the wrist must be guided into radial flexion and supination. For correction of the imbalance at the wrist, radial flexion must be considered a pivot of emphasis, and external rotation of the shoulder and supination of the forearm must be resisted strongly to stimulate the radial flexor. Correction of proximal imbalances will enhance the correction of distal imbalances.

Imbalances may also exist between antagonistic patterns in relation to various pivots of action. For example, a patient who has strong rhomboid and teres major muscles, and a weak anterior deltoid and clavicular portion of the pectoralis major has an imbalance in favor of extension – abduction – internal rotation of the shoulder. The same patient may have a strong biceps and a weak triceps, resulting in imbalance in favor of the flexion – adduction – external rotation pattern with reference to the elbow. If he has a weak ulnar extensor of the wrist and a strong radial flexor, he again presents an imbalance in favor of the flexion – adduction – external rotation pattern with reference to the wrist. Such a picture presents imbalances not only between antagonistic patterns but also within the components of both patterns. When techniques of facilitation are used, the stronger posterior scapular and shoulder muscles of the extension – abduction – internal rotation pattern must be used to stimulate the weaker triceps and ulnar extensor of the wrist. The distal power in the radial flexor of the wrist and the stronger biceps must be used to stimulate the weaker anterior deltoid and clavicular portion of the pectoralis major. Correction of imbalance at the shoulder deserves the first emphasis, but the imbalance at the elbow and wrist must also receive due emphasis.

Hyperactive Reflexes

Just as imbalances may exist between antagonistic muscle groups, so may imbalances exist between antagonistic reflexes. For example, if extensor spasticity is so severe that it prevents a patient from voluntarily flexing his left lower extremity, repeated use of stretch reflex coupled with his voluntary effort may be helpful. Positioning the patient on his right side or in the hand–knee position will promote response because of the favorability of these positions for flexor response. In this way the patient may be able to produce more voluntary movement on which resistance can be superimposed. Increased voluntary response will help to reduce hyperactivity of the antagonistic reflex. See Table 1-9, Support by Postural and Righting Reflexes.

Pivots for Emphasis

Determination of imbalances and selection of pivots for emphasis are based upon careful evaluation of the patient's strengths and weaknesses. In techniques of facilitation, the development of power and the correction of imbalances proceeds from proximal to distal in line with the normal process of development. Proximal power and control is essential to stability and to the process of overflow or irradiation. Therefore, weakness and imbalance of neck and trunk musculature receive first emphasis. The proximal pivots of the extremities, the shoulder and hip, receive second emphasis, and the more distal pivots receive third emphasis. Where generalized weakness exists, proximal emphasis is necessary and precludes emphasis of a weak distal pivot. Weak distal pivots receive a certain amount of stimulation during proximal emphasis because all components of the pattern are considered. In techniques of facilitation it becomes futile to attempt to strengthen a nonfunctional anterior tibial, if the muscle groups related by pattern are equally deficient.

Rhythmic Initiation (RI)

Rhythmic initiation (RI), or rhythm technique, is used to improve the ability to initiate movement. This technique involves voluntary relaxation, passive movement, and repeated isotonic contractions of the major muscle components of the agonistic pattern. Using rhythmic initiation is helpful to those patients who lack the ability to initiate movement because of rigid-

ity (parkinsonian) or severe spasticity. The patient is helped, too, to become aware of the direction of the movement. Those who are lethargic and are slow in their movement, the elderly, and those who have diminished position sense may be stimulated and guided by this method. The technique does not involve forced movement. If only a limited range of movement is possible, this is the starting point. Movement should not produce pain; pain will only limit movement.

Example of Technique

The physical therapist asks the patient to relax and "Let me move you." The therapist then moves the part through the available range of the pattern, giving attention to all components of the pattern with special attention to the distal parts. During the movement of the part, emphasis is in the direction of the agonistic pattern, although the part is returned, of course, toward the shortened range of the antagonistic pattern. As relaxation is felt to occur and movement is more easily accomplished, the patient is commanded, "Now help me just a little." Again, the emphasis is in the direction of the agonistic pattern. After the patient has assisted for several repetitions, the physical therapist gradually superimposes resistance and increases the amount as the patient's response is felt to increase. He is commanded to pull or push as the occasion requires. After several repetitions against resistance, the patient is allowed to move actively by himself to sense the increased ease of movement.

REVERSAL OF ANTAGONISTS

Reversal of antagonists techniques are related to normal responses, and good performance is indicative of normalcy of function.

Goal-centered activity has direction based on pursuit or avoidance. Normal persons may move toward the goal or may withdraw from the goal. The normal person may change direction at will; he may reverse direction of a total pattern—for example, in dancing he may move forward, then backward. Reversal of direction is a feature of developmental activities and is a basis for several specific reversal of antagonist techniques where the antagonist is used to facilitate the agonist.

In normal physical activity the reversal of antagonists plays an important role. The examples of sawing wood, chopping wood, rowing a boat, walking, running, grasping and releasing objects are trite but true illustrations of this phenomenon in life's activities. When antagonists fail to reverse in accordance with the demand of the activity, function is immediately impaired in relation to power, skill, or coordination. The objective of neuromuscular education or reeducation and of therapeutic exercise may be said to be the development or redevelopment of a normal reversal of antagonists through a normal range of motion. This implies correction of imbalances and development of strength, coordination, and endurance.

The techniques are based upon Sherrington's principle of successive induction.[44] The patient who does not respond well to reversal techniques and in whom the desired response can be achieved only by resistance in pattern with repeated contractions has severe involvement; for example, the hemiplegic patient who presents a picture of disturbed patterns and who responds to reversal with an increase in spasticity also demonstrates a low level of functional participation. He is the patient who, when his antagonists should reverse in a functional movement, "bumps" into his spasticity, and his function is impaired thereby. For such a patient, patterns must be reestablished with first emphasis on the proximal pivots, and the technique of repeated contractions is indicated. The reversal of antagonists becomes a goal of treatment rather than a technique of treatment.

The stimulation of the agonist by resisting a contraction, either isotonic or isometric, of the antagonist is readily demonstrated in the normal subject by determining the amount of resistance that can be overcome in performing a motion such as elbow flexion. If the motion of elbow extension is then performed against maximal resistance, a succeeding motion of elbow flexion should be performed more strongly, overcoming greater resistance than was possible on the initial attempt.

Techniques using the reversal of antagonists are superimposed upon patterns of facilitation, with proper attention given to the manual contacts, maximal resistance, and timing of the pattern. The potentials of reversal techniques are several because of the variations possible. Either isotonic or isometric contractions may be used, or a combination of both types of muscle contraction may be used.

There are four reversal techniques that may be used primarily for the purpose of stimulation, as evidenced by a buildup in power or a gain in range of motion. Slow reversal involves an isotonic contraction of the antagonist, followed by an isotonic contraction of the agonist. Slow reversal-hold involves an isotonic contraction, followed by an isometric contraction of the antagonist, followed by the same sequence of contractions of the agonist. Rhythmic stabilization involves simultaneous isometric contractions of antagonists and results in co-contraction. The fourth reversal technique is quick reversal, which requires rapidly alternating isotonic contractions of antagonists. Detailed descriptions of reversal techniques follow.

Slow Reversal; Slow Reversal–Hold (SR; SRH)

A patient may present weakness of the flexion–adduction–external rotation pattern of the right lower extremity with reference to the hip, with good power in the antagonistic pattern of extension–abduction–internal rotation. If the antagonistic pattern is to be used as a a means of stimulation by using reversal, the physical therapist must be prepared to resist the antagonistic pattern, but will vary the manual contacts in order to be able to apply maximum proprioceptive stimulation to the weaker pattern. The procedure should be to require the patient to perform the agonistic motion of flexion–adduction–external rotation, the physical therapist applying optimum manual contacts with maximal resistance, in order to determine the response of the patient. The physical therapist then shifts his manual contacts to those described for the extension–abduction–internal rotation pattern and asks the patient to perform this motion against maximal resistance. The therapist then shifts again to the agonistic pattern of flexion–adduction–external rotation and determines if the patient performs with greater power or with increased range of motion. The grading of resistance is essential in order to demand a strong contraction of the antagonist and to allow range of motion to occur when the agonistic pattern is performed. The manual contacts must be varied to the extent that it is possible for the physical therapist to shift contacts and resistance smoothly, making it possible for the patient to shift smoothly and effectively from one pattern to the other. If the patient gains little range by reversing at the point where the agonistic pattern of flexion–adduction–external rotation had become ineffective, a reversal should be attempted from the lengthened range of extension–abduction–internal rotation, allowing the patient to work to the strongest part of the range of this pattern before requiring a succeeding contraction of the agonistic pattern. The reversal process may be repeated several times with the agonistic pattern being resisted last. When the agonistic pattern has been stimulated, the patient is instructed to hold immediately following the gain in flexion–adduction–external rotation, and repeated contractions may then be used as a technique of emphasis in order to gain further range and develop power or endurance in the agonistic pattern.

The series of commands for slow reversal, using extension–abduction–internal rotation to stimulate flexion–adduction–external rotation, could be as follows:

"Push your foot down and out toward me"—extension–abduction–internal rotation—isotonic—antagonist

"And pull your foot up and across your body"—flexion–adduction–external rotation—isotonic — agonist

"And push down and out" — extension – abduction – internal rotation — isotonic — antagonist

"And pull up and over" — flexion – adduction – external rotation — isotonic — agonist

"And hold" — flexion – adduction – external rotation — isometric — agonist

"And pull, and pull, and pull again" — flexion – adduction – external rotation — isotonic — repeated contractions for emphasis — agonist

Slow reversal – hold requiring an isotonic and then an isometric contraction may be performed in the same manner, with a "hold" command inserted after each active command.

If slow reversal techniques are performed against maximal resistance, an increase in range or buildup in power should be felt on each successive isotonic and isometric contraction. The physical therapist should remember that on a "hold" command the rotation is resisted strongly, but the hold is not defeated or broken.

Rhythmic Stabilization (RS)

Whereas slow reversal technique employs isotonic contractions, and slow reversal – hold employs isotonic and isometric contractions, a third technique of stimulation, based upon reversal of antagonists, is rhythmic stabilization. Rhythmic stabilization employs isometric contraction of antagonistic patterns, which results in co-contraction of antagonists if the isometric contraction is not broken by the physical therapist. Because only isometric contractions are employed, rhythmic stabilization has a by-product of increasing circulation. Rhythmic stabilization performed on the normal subject results in a buildup of holding power so great that the hold cannot be broken unless rotation of the part is defeated. If the normal subject is instructed to hold the arm completely still or to hold it stiffly, he will do so by performing isometric contractions of all groups about a given joint, and the co-contraction of antagonists may be felt. If the normal subject thinks of holding his arm "up" or holding it "down," he will be felt to contract first one group, then the opposite group, with relaxation occurring between the isometric contractions. This is not rhythmic stabilization, for as the subject performs, he will be felt to shift into alternating isotonic contractions rather than to develop a co-contraction of antagonists. Careful grading of resistance to the "hold" contractions, with special consideration given to the rotation components, makes it possible for the subject to stabilize. The patient must not be defeated with so much resistance that he finds it necessary to contract isotonically

in order to recover or maintain his position. This becomes especially important in treating patients who have normal innervation but problems of pain. The grading of resistance will be as accurate as the physical therapist's ability to feel the patient's response. In order to develop the patient's ability to stabilize, the physical therapist may move the part through a slight range of motion so as to better bring in the antagonistic patterns, but this must also be done by sensing the patient's response and without defeating the patient's hold in the rotation components.

Where there is inability to perform isometric contractions, as in ataxia, rhythmic stabilization may be impossible for the patient to perform. The patient must be taught to "hold." One approach is to have him perform slow reversal – hold through decreasing ranges of motion until no motion occurs. If ataxia is severe, use of slow reversal with adjustment of decrements of range at various points, and attempts to hold at these points, will be necessary. Kabat identified rhythmic stabilization as a test of clinical value in the presence of mild cerebellar disease.[26]

Examples of Technique

Rhythmic stabilization of the trunk by use of manual contacts on shoulder and pelvic girdles readily elicits responses of anterior and posterior muscles simultaneously. As the therapist and the normal subject stand facing each other, the therapist places her left hand on the subject's right shoulder, and her right hand on the crest of the pelvis, left side. Pressure and resistance are applied anteriorly at the right shoulder and posteriorly at the left pelvis as the therapist gives the command, "Hold!" The therapist feels an impasse; no movement occurs. The therapist slowly shifts pressure to the posterior of the right shoulder and to the anterior surface of the pelvis, left side. On the command, "Hold," the therapist feels stability and continues: "Hold. And hold. And relax." The procedure has provided pressure alternately twice, two "holds" anteriorly and two posteriorly.

The therapist contacts the subject's left shoulder and the right side of the pelvis, and performs the procedure as before. Manual contacts are maintained; the direction of pressure is shifted from front to back, and from back to front. The two diagonals of the upper trunk patterns have been considered, right shoulder to left hip and left shoulder to right hip.

Rhythmic stabilization may be applied at any point in the range of a pattern. To stabilize upper trunk rotation the therapist places both hands on the shoulder girdle, left hand at the back of the subject's right sholder and right hand at the front of the subject's left shoulder. With pressure and resistance the therapist commands, "Look to your right! Push your right shoulder back and pull your left forward. Move! And hold! Now look to your left. Push back with your left as you pull forward with the right. Turn! Look behind your left shoulder. And hold. And hold. And hold. And hold. And relax." The subject first rotated his head and upper trunk to the right, then reversed the direction with head and upper trunk rotated to the left. Stabilization was carried out in the shortened range of rotation to the left (see Chap. 1, Free Active Motion, Head and Neck and Upper Trunk).

When an extremity is to be stabilized, the manual contacts permit a pair of antagonistic patterns to receive pressure and resistance simultaneously. For example, the flexion – adduction – external rotation pattern of the upper extremity and its antagonist, the extension – abduction – internal rotation pattern, are subjected to alternating pressure and, at the same time, there is pressure applied simultaneously. The therapist places one hand at the wrist, the other above the elbow. As the "hold" command is given, pressure is applied to the flexor surface distally, as pressure is applied to the extensor surface above the elbow. Thus, the flexion pattern has been resisted at the wrist as the extension pattern was resisted at shoulder. As pressure and resistance are shifted, the distal contact engages the extensor surface at the wrist slightly before the proximal contact moves to the flexor surface. Control of rotation at the wrist is more effective as contact is readily altered, as compared with contact on the arm. The entire procedure may be performed at any point in the range of the pattern. The command, "Hold," is used as pressure alternates. Slight movement of the part during "holding" may elicit eccentric contraction, a factor of control.

Quick Reversal (QR)

Quick reversal of antagonists, like slow reversal, uses isotonic contractions.* To facilitate the agonist, the antagonistic pattern is performed slowly from lengthened range to shortened range against maximal resistance. As the shortened range is approached, the direction is suddenly reversed by isotonic contraction of the agonist, with assistance to the shortened range given as quickly as possible. Immediately thereafter an isometric contraction of the agonist against maximal resistance follows. Repeated contractions or hold – relax active motion may be used for emphasis, or the quick reversal sequence may be repeated.

Example of Technique

Given weakness of the flexion – adduction – external rotation pattern with marked imbalance favoring the

* The quick reversal technique was developed by Luba Brisker, KKI, physical therapist.

antagonistic extension – abduction – internal rotation pattern, quick reversal may be the technique of choice. The following sequence of commands could be used.

"Push your foot down and out toward me!" (extension – abduction – internal rotation — isotonic — antagonist — slowly with maximal resistance)

"Now pull your foot up and across." (flexion – adduction – external rotation — isotonic — agonist — quickly with assistance to shortened range)

"And hold it." (flexion – adduction – external rotation — isometric — agonist — preparatory to hold – relax active motion technique)

"Let go." (relaxation — agonist — move quickly to lengthened range — flexion – adduction – external rotation)

"Now pull." (flexion – adduction – external rotation — isotonic — agonist — with graded resistance)

As isotonic contraction of agonist fatigues, quickly assist to shortened range of agonist.

"Hold it." (isometric — agonist — preparation for repeated contractions technique emphasizing shortened range, or working in decrements of range toward lengthened range)

"Now pull, and pull, and pull, and relax."

The quick reversal technique may be repeated with the sequence of techniques: hold – relax active motion and repeated contractions.

In summary, success in application of reversal of antagonists techniques will be dependent upon maximal resistance to the antagonistic pattern, control of antagonistic and agonistic patterns so that the motion may be performed smoothly, and careful grading of resistance between the stronger antagonist and the weaker agonist. Reversals may be performed in any desired part of the range of motion that gives the desired response. They may be performed through a full range of motion or a minimal part of the range of the antagonistic pattern, if that is adequate for stimulation of the agonist.

RELAXATION

A technique that demands contraction of one pattern of facilitation demands a lengthening reaction, relaxation, or inhibition of the directly antagonistic pattern. Any technique that demands or makes possible a gain in range of motion in one pattern has achieved relaxation of its antagonistic pattern. This relaxation, or inhibition, of the antagonist during facilitation of the agonist relies upon reciprocal innervation, which was demonstrated by Sherrington.[44] In the normal subject, the techniques of repeated contractions, slow reversal, slow reversal – hold, and rhythmic stabilization, superimposed upon a pattern of motion, will stimulate the agonist and relax the antagonist. This may be simply demonstrated in normal subjects who have adaptive or postural shortening of the biceps femoris. If the subject is required to perform the flexion – adduction – external rotation pattern with emphasis at the hip and knee against maximal resistance, he may perform through greater range than when he does unresisted motion. If he is then required to perform repeated contractions, he may gain further range; if rhythmic stabilization is performed at the end point of the range, he may again achieve added range. If at this point he is allowed to reverse through the antagonistic pattern of extension – abduction – internal rotation with maximal resistance, his performance in the agonistic pattern may be still further enhanced both in power and range of motion. Thus, stimulation and relaxation are inseparable.

The specific relaxation techniques are substitutes for passive stretching. The patient who seemingly has very little strength available may be able to produce a contraction of a shortened muscle of sufficient strength to encourage relaxation, providing the contraction is skillfully resisted. Use of these techniques obviates painful reactions to stretch and is far less hazardous.

Although relaxation techniques afford means to relaxation, the use of positioning to influence tonus, and maximum stimulation of related patterns may achieve more relaxation than will the application of a relaxation technique directed to a specific muscle group. For example, resisting the patient's efforts in creeping may bring about more relaxation of the extensors of the lower trunk than will contract – relax done in the supine position. These techniques of relaxation use maximal contractions of the antagonist followed by voluntary relaxation, which, whenever possible, is followed by resisted contraction of the agonist.

Contract – Relax (CR)

In patients presenting marked limitation of range of motion with no active motion available in the agonistic pattern, some relaxation of the antagonistic pattern may be achieved by using contract – relax. This technique involves an isotonic contraction of the antagonist, allowing range of motion in rotation against maximal resistance but no range of the other components, followed by a period of relaxation.

The procedure is to move the part passively into the agonstic pattern to the point where limitation is felt; at this point, the patient is instructed to contract isotonically in the antagonistic pattern. The physical therapist resists the rotation as strongly as possible and then instructs the patient to "relax." It is necessary to lighten the pressure and to wait for relaxation to occur. Having felt the patient "let go," the physical therapist again moves the part passively, through as much range as possible, to the point where limitation is again felt to occur. The entire procedure is repeated several times, following which an attempt should be made to have the patient perform the agonistic pattern actively from the lengthened range. If the patient is not able to perform or initiate from the lengthened range, he may be asked to move actively in the direction of the agonistic pattern after each contract – relax procedure. However, as always, the goal is to initiate from the lengthened range and to perform throughout the range.

The commands for contract – relax in such a situation would be as follows:

"Pull your foot down and in." (extension – adduction – external rotation — isotonic — range of external rotation against maximal resistance — antagonist)
"Let go." (lighten pressure, support part, and wait for relaxation to occur, move the extremity into flexion – abduction – internal rotation — agonist)

Repeat procedure, then place the part in the lengthened range for flexion – abduction – internal rotation — agonist.

"Now pull up and out toward me." (flexion – abduction – internal rotation — isotonic — agonist)
"And hold." (preparation for repeated isotonic contractions)
"And pull, and pull, and pull, *etc.*" (repeated isotonic contractions of agonistic pattern)

Hold – Relax (HR)

Hold – relax is a relaxation technique based upon maximal resistance of an isometric contraction. The technique is performed in the same type of sequence as contract – relax. Since an isometric contraction is involved, the command must be "hold" instead of "push" or "pull." Also, since no joint motion is implied, this technique may be performed as a method of achieving relaxation where muscle spasm is accompanied by pain. The isometric contraction must not be broken or defeated. In any acute situation, the technique should be demonstrated to the patient on a pain-free part. Exercise of the pain-free part has secondary benefits of general relaxation with reduction of pain, and, if resistance is maximal, irradiation to the painful area may occur without pain.

Example of Technique

The fracture patient who has just had a cast removed may be helped to relax the part or to gain range with this simple technique. For example, a patient who has a united fracture of the head of the radius and is to perform active motion to encourage elbow extension has already established a mechanism of inhibition for elbow extension. By performing hold – relax to the biceps, with slowly increasing amounts of resistance applied to the isometric contraction, relaxation of the biceps may be achieved with resultant stimulation of the triceps. The part, of course, should be supported by the physical therapist, and after hold – relax is performed, the patient is instructed to extend the elbow without resistance. The commands in such a situation would be as follows:

> "Just *hold* your elbow bent and don't let me move it." (Apply resistance gently and slowly to supination using the distal contact of the flexion – adduction – external rotation pattern. Resistance is greater at the radially flexed wrist than it is at the elbow.)
> "Let go." (Maintain gentle support of the extremity and wait for relaxation of the biceps to occur.)
> "Open your hand and push it down and away." (Use extension – abduction – internal rotation with elbow extension — isotonic without resistance.)

Success of the technique will depend upon gently increasing resistance, encouraging the isometric contraction without defeating it, supporting the part while relaxation occurs, and having the patient move the part actively in the desired motion. The procedure may be repeated and followed with repeated unresisted active contractions of the agonist. Unresisted reversing movements, emphasizing the rotation, may also be used as a follow-up procedure.

Slow Reversal – Hold – Relax (SRHR)

Slow reversal – hold – relax is a technique involving an isotonic contraction of the range-limiting pattern (the antagonistic pattern) followed by an isometric contraction of the antagonistic pattern, followed by a brief period of voluntary relaxation, followed by an isotonic contraction of the agonistic pattern. Relaxation must be achieved first at the exact point in the range where limitation presents itself. Maximal relaxation is dependent upon maximal resistance applied to the rotation component without allowing range of motion to occur in the other components of the antagonistic pattern.

Example of Technique

If a patient presents limitation of active motion at 15° of flexion – abduction – internal rotation of the lower extremity with reference to the hip, that is the part of the range where relaxation of the extension – adduction – external rotation pattern must begin in order to stimulate the agonist and develop inhibition of the antagonist. The point at which the relaxation technique is to be performed is best determined by having the patient perform actively as much range of the agonistic pattern as possible, and then proceed with slow reversal – hold – relax of the antagonistic pattern. Using the manual contacts that are optimal for the antagonistic pattern, the patient is resisted so strongly as he attempts an isotonic contraction of the extension – adduction – external rotation pattern that no motion occurs, except in the component of rotation. The physical therapist instructs the patient to hold, and resists the hold contraction with all the resistance applied to the rotation component. Having resisted the isometric contraction, the physical therapist instructs the patient to relax, and at once releases her pressure, just supporting the part without moving it. As soon as relaxation is felt to occur, the physical therapist demands an isotonic contraction of the agonistic pattern, applying manual contacts for that pattern, but allowing the patient to flex, abduct, and internally rotate through as much range as possible. At this point, the slow reversal – hold – relax technique may be repeated, or, if a definite gain in range has been achieved, the physical therapist may emphasize the recently gained portion of the range of motion by performing repeated contractions. Success in application of the technique will be dependent upon maximal resistance to the antagonistic pattern, allowing only range of rotation to occur, decrease in pressure by manual contacts when the patient is instructed to relax, and active motion against resistance following relaxation.

The commands for the technique as set forth in this example could be as follows:

> "Pull your foot up and out toward me as far as you can." (flexion – abduction – internal rotation — isotonic — agonist)
> "Now pull your foot down and in, and hold." (extension – adduction – external rotation —

isotonic — range of external rotation allowed and resisted as strongly as possible — isometric — antagonist)

"Relax." (lighten contact and shift manual contacts for optimal stimulation of agonist — flexion-abduction-internal rotation)

"Now pull up and out." (flexion-abduction-internal rotation — isotonic — agonist)

"And hold." (preparation for repeated contractions — isometric — agonist)

"And pull, and pull, and pull." (agonist — repeated isotonic contractions)

Rhythmic Rotation (RRo)

In rhythmic rotation the patient's voluntary effort is enlisted. When voluntary control is present, the patient may perform actively. When voluntary control is absent, the therapist performs rhythmic rotation passively. Whether done actively (self-directed) or passively (therapist directed), the components and sequence are the same. The by-product is relaxation.

Example of Self-Directed Technique

A normal person with intact innervation may demonstrate limited range of straight-leg raising (SLR), a traditional test of range of motion. With the subject supine, goniometric measurements are done before and after the subject performs as follows.

The person lies supine, hands at sides of body, and lower extremities in a comfortable position, usually with external rotation of hips and with toes pointed outward. The limbs may be rotated bilaterally, singly, or alternately. The commands are as follows:

"Roll your legs outward, toes away! Now turn your knees and feet inward. And roll outward again. And inward again.

"Now with toes pointed toward ceiling, spread your legs apart, as far as you can. Now roll out, all the way. And in again. And, relax. Spread your legs again. And roll out, and in, and relax."

SLR is remeasured singly and recorded as before. To further enhance a gain in SLR, the subject may perform reciprocal combinations in the same and opposite, or crossed diagonal, directions. Results may be recorded.

Example of Techniques in Sequence

The quadriparetic patient with flexor reflexes domi-

nant in the lower extremities may benefit from passive rhythmic rotation followed by repetitive rhythmical mass extension. Again, SLR may be used as a test with results recorded before and after the procedures.

These procedures are preceded by resisted breathing with the therapist's manual contact on sternum as lateral chest walls are compressed by therapist's other hand and forearm (see Chap. 3, Stimulation of Vital and Related Functions). Several series of repeated contractions may further encourage relaxation.

Rhythmic rotation is carried out by the therapist gripping the patient's heel with one hand as the other controls and rotates the limb by manual contact at the knee. As the limb is rotated deliberately and rhythmically, the muscles about the hip are tense. This tension decreases as the muscles relax. The command "Relax," or "Let go," may be helpful to the patient's voluntary effort and to the timing of the procedure. The limb may then be slowly and gently abducted. As the new point of tension is felt, the rotation procedure is repeated. After two or three repetitions, the SLR test may be done. Where one limb is more spastic than the other, rotation of the less spastic limb first may increase the ease of rotating the more spastic limb.

Rhythmic rotation is preparatory to the use of repetitive mass extension of hip and knee, thrusting of the lower extremity. The aim is to promote balance between flexor and extensor reflexes. Again, the less spastic limb should be approached first. The extremity may be rotated gently as the therapist moves it to the lengthened range of the extension-abduction-internal rotation pattern. Hip and knee are in maximum flexion. Stretch and mild resistance may be an adequate stimulus to produce complete extension after three or four repetitions. The extension-adduction-external rotation pattern may be facilitated in the same manner. After a brief period of relaxation, the limb may be moved to a greater range of abduction. When the mass extension has been done with both limbs, the therapist may contact both heels and gently spread the limbs apart. If increased range of SLR is obvious, other phases of treatment such as work with upper extremities may be done. At the end of the period, mass extension in the abduction pattern may be desirable.

Emphasis on extensor activity is a safeguard. Flexor reflexes are protective, and withdrawal responses are readily activated. A patient who is able to stand with extensor activity may be deprived of this ability if flexor reflexes are allowed to become and to remain dominant.

(Text continues page 312)

Learn the patterns as free active motion in accordance with normal timing. Begin with head and neck and upper trunk patterns with chopping and lifting. Practice with eyes leading the movement, and with eyes following the hands as the chop leads trunk flexion and the lift leads trunk extension. Proceed to upper extremity and then to lower extremity patterns. Perform the patterns in as many positions as possible including positions and postures of the developmental sequence. Analyze total patterns of movement and functional activities, and identify their component patterns.

Learn to apply manual contacts accurately.

Practice giving commands with a normal subject performing active range of motion in accordance with normal timing.

Learn techniques of facilitation in the following order:

Maximal resistance through full range of pattern in accordance with normal timing (isotonic)
Maximal resistance to "holding" in shortened range of pattern and various points in range (isometric)
Repeated contractions (emphasis of proximal pivot). Observe buildup in power or gain in range.
Timing for emphasis (proximal, intermediate and distal pivots). Follow with repeated contractions.
Slow reversal, slow reversal–hold, rhythmic stabilization: Work in various parts of the range of ago-
nistic and antagonistic patterns. Observe buildup in power or gains in range of motion.
Slow reversal–hold–relax, contract–relax, hold–relax: Observe relaxation and gains in active range and passive range.
Reinforcement of one pattern by a related pattern: Practice performance of related patterns for various parts of the range and various pivots of action. See Reference Tables 1 through 7 in the back of the text.

Practice all techniques with normal subjects and selected patients.

Learn application of techniques to vital related functions: breathing, tongue motions, facial motions, opening and closing of mouth, stimulation of soft palate.

Evaluate a normal subject to determine any variation in range of motion, coordination, and power.

Outline a treatment program directed toward correction of variations or deficiencies.

Evaluate patients and plan treatment programs including areas of emphasis, pivots of emphasis, selection of techniques, and reinforcement for patients who present flaccid paralysis, spasticity, incoordination, and orthopedic problems including postural deficiencies.

See Table 2-2 for a summary of the techniques described in the section.

Table 2-2. Summary of Techniques

Procedures and Techniques	Type of Muscle Contraction	Purposes and By-Products	Indications	Contra-indications
Manual Contacts: Deep pressure but not painful, applied to parts and muscle groups where response is desired. Manual contacts of the antagonistic pattern may be used when the agonistic pattern is performed passively for determining limitations in range of motion.	Isotonic or isometric	To stimulate proprioceptors in muscles, tendons, and joints. May be used with or without resistance.	Used whenever contact with patient by the physical therapist is necessary in an exercise procedure.	Manual contacts may provide demand or security depending upon patient's needs. Manual contacts are not contraindicated except where postoperative site or open wound does not permit contact as suggested.
Traction: Separation of joint surfaces by manual contact of physical therapist.	Superimposed upon isotonic or isometric contractions.	To stimulate proprioceptors related to stretch. To separate joint surfaces in order to make joint motion less painful.	Conditions where separation of joint surfaces is desirable. When maximal facilitation is used, superimposed upon patterns the motion of which is that of pulling.	Recent fractures where there is danger of separating fragments. Recent postoperative conditions if traction is generally contraindicated.

(Continued)

Table 2-2. *(Continued)*

Procedures and Techniques	Type of Muscle Contraction	Purposes and By-Products	Indications	Contra-indications
Approximation: Joint compression by manual contact of physical therapist.	Superimposed upon isotonic or isometric contractions.	To stimulate joint proprioceptors related to compression.	When maximal facilitation is used, superimposed upon patterns the motion of which is that of pushing.	Same as for Traction.
Stretch: Maximal stretch of major muscle components in lengthened range of pattern.	Superimposed upon isotonic contractions.	To demand increased response where response is inadequate to initiate active motion in lengthened range of pattern. To achieve increased response throughout the major muscle components.	Conditions where innervation is inadequate to produce active motion.	Acute orthopaedic conditions, recent fractures, recent post-operative conditions, pain.
Timing for Emphasis: Sequence of contraction of major muscle components from distal to proximal.	Superimposed upon isotonic or isometric contractions.	To develop coordinate movements. To make possible overflow and reinforcement when resistance is superimposed.	Conditions that permit active motion or motion against resistance.	Contraindicated only where any form of exercise is contraindicated.
Maximal Resistance: Graded according to patient's abilities and needs. May be a slight amount for weak components and a great amount for stronger components. Patient must be allowed to move if command is for active motion. Must not be so excessive that it prevents the patient from holding when the command is to hold.	Superimposed upon isotonic or isometric contractions.	To stimulate active motion. To obtain overflow from stronger components to weaker components and to reinforce weaker patterns with stronger related patterns. To develop power, endurance, coordination. To correct imbalances. To demand relaxation. To reverse adaptive shortening.	Conditions where weakness is a primary problem. Conditions that demand correction of imbalances and improvement of coordination. Conditions where relaxation is a prime need. Superimposed upon isometric contractions in recent fractures and acute orthopedic conditions.	May not be superimposed upon isotonic contraction in acute orthopaedic conditions. May not be superimposed upon a pattern favored by an imbalance unless that pattern provides stimulation of the weaker pattern, in reversal techniques. Must be used guardedly where sustained or prolonged effort may be harmful.
Reinforcement: Accomplished by resisted motion in strongest part of range of reinforcing components of pattern. Patterns selected as reinforcement must be related and stronger than the pattern to be reinforced.	Superimposed upon isotonic or isometric contraction.	To stimulate weaker components or weaker patterns. To establish coordination between combinations of patterns.	Conditions where weakness is a primary factor. Conditions that permit active motion against resistance.	Where pattern cannot be controlled in a coordinate manner unless two hands are used on the part. Acute conditions that do not permit active motion against resistance.

(Continued)

Table 2-2. *(Continued)*

Procedures and Techniques	Type of Muscle Contraction	Purposes and By-Products	Indications	Contra-indications
Repeated Contractions: Technique of emphasis. Sustained and repeated effort in one direction. May be performed at any desired point of range of motion.	Isotonic following initial isometric contraction.	To stimulate gains in range of active motion of agonistic pattern. To demand relaxation or lengthening reaction of antagonistic pattern. To improve endurance, coordination, and strength in a given pattern or a specific part of the range of motion of a specific pattern.	Conditions where weakness, lack of endurance, and imbalance exist as primary problems.	Conditions that do not permit sustained effort against resistance, such as acute orthopaedic and recent postoperative conditions, cerebrovascular accidents.
Hold–relax–active motion: Technique of emphasis. Repeated effort without sustained effort. Performed from shortened range to lengthened range.	Isometric, followed by voluntary relaxation, followed by isotonic contraction.	To stimulate response in lengthened range of pattern. To demand relaxation or lengthened reaction of antagonistic pattern. To improve endurance, strength, and coordination of the agonistic pattern.	Conditions where lack of endurance is a primary problem. Conditions where extreme weakness prevails in the lengthened range of a pattern. Conditions where sustained effort by the patient is not permissible. Conditions where marked imbalance exists in favor of the antagonistic pattern.	Conditions that do not permit full range of passive or resisted motion. Should be discarded in favor of more stimulating techniques as soon as possible.
Rhythmic Initiation–Rhythm Technique: Repeated movement without sustained effort. Performed from lengthened range to shortened range.	Voluntary relaxation, followed by assisted isotonic contraction, followed by resisted isotonic contraction.	To promote ability to initiate movement, and to increase rate of movement.	Conditions where rigidity (Parkinsonian) or spasticity prevents initiation of movement or results in less than desirable rate.	Conditions where passive movement is contraindicated.
Slow Reversal: May be performed through available range or partial range according to patient's response.	Simultaneous isometric contraction of antagonistic patterns.	To stimulate active motion of agonistic pattern. To redevelop normal reversal of antagonists. To develop coordination of two antagonistic patterns. To develop strength in two antagonistic patterns. To achieve relaxation as a result of stimulation of the agonistic pattern.	Conditions where weakness is a primary factor and where reversal provides stimulation of the agonistic pattern. Conditions that have passed the acute phase and in which normal reversal of antagonists is desired.	Conditions where reversal does not stimulate the agonistic pattern. Acute orthopaedic conditions.
Slow Reversal–Hold: May be performed through available range of motion or partial range according to patient's response.	Isotonic, then isometric of antagonistic pattern followed by isotonic, then isometric of agonistic pattern. Sequence repeated if necessary to increase response.	Same as Slow Reversal. To develop stability and ability to perform isometric contractions in specific patterns or specific parts of range of a pattern.	Same as Slow Reversal. Conditions where ability to perform isometric contractions is deficient.	Same as Slow Reversal.

(Continued)

Table 2-2. *(Continued)*

Procedures and Techniques	Type of Muscle Contraction	Purposes and By-Products	Indications	Contra-indications
Rhythmic Stabilization: May be performed at any point of available range of motion.	Isometric of agonistic pattern followed by isometric of antagonistic pattern.	To stimulate active motion of agonistic pattern. To develop stability of the part in specific ranges of motion. To achieve relaxation of antagonistic pattern as a result of stimulation of agonistic pattern. To stimulate circulation through isometric contraction.	Conditions where weakness is a primary factor and where stabilization provides stimulation of the agonistic pattern. Conditions where active motion is not permitted or impossible because of pain. Conditions where isometric contraction is deficient as in ataxia. Stability is a goal of treatment.	Conditions where stabilization does not stimulate agonistic pattern.
Quick Reversal: May be used to facilitate agonist by resistance to antagonist through full range followed by sudden reversal with isotonic contraction of agonist and with assistance to shortened range.	Isotonic, then isometric contraction of agonist.	To correct imbalance at shortened range of agonist by assisting agonistic pattern to shortened range.	Marked imbalance of antagonists with sufficient strength in shortened range of agonist to facilitate response through full range.	Any condition for which sudden movement may be hazardous.
Contract–Relax: May be performed at succeeding points of range of motion beginning with the point where limitation by antagonistic pattern presents itself.	Isotonic contraction of antagonistic pattern—no range of motion allowed—followed by passive motion of agonistic pattern. Procedure followed by attempted performance of agonistic pattern from stretch stimulus or from isometric contraction in shortened range.	To achieve relaxation of antagonistic pattern where active motion cannot be initiated from stretch range of agonistic pattern.	Conditions where spasticity is primary factor and no active motion is available from a stretch stimulus.	Conditions where active motion of the agonist is present. Acute orthopaedic conditions.
Hold–Relax: May be performed at any point of range where limitation presents itself as the result of pain and muscle spasm.	Isometric of antagonist followed by free active motion of agonist. Isometric contraction of agonist may follow initial contraction of antagonist.	To achieve relaxation of antagonist. To encourage active motion of agonist.	Conditions where pain prevents active motion. Acute orthopedic conditions.	Conditions where ability to perform isometric contraction is grossly deficient.

Table 2-2. *(Continued)*

Procedures and Techniques	Type of Muscle Contraction	Purposes and By-Products	Indications	Contra-indications
Slow Reversal–Hold–Relax: Performed at exact point of range of motion where limitation by antagonistic pattern presents itself.	Isotonic, then isometric of antagonistic pattern—no range of motion allowed —followed by voluntary relaxation, then by isotonic of agonistic pattern. Sequence repeated in order to promote further relaxation.	To achieve relaxation of antagonistic pattern. To stimulate agonist following relaxation of antagonist.	Conditions where limitation of range of motion is present and where motion against resistance is permitted. Conditions where limitation of motion is a primary factor.	Conditions where Slow Reversal–Hold–Relax does not achieve relaxation of antagonistic pattern. Conditions where active motion against resistance is not permitted.
Rhythmic Rotation: Repeated rotation of a segment at the point in the range where limitation is noted.	Voluntary relaxation when possible. When technique is self-directed, isotonic contraction of range-limiting muscles occurs.	To achieve relaxation of range-limiting muscles and stimulation of rotation components.	Conditions where imbalance of reflexes exists due to trauma of spinal cord. Orthopaedic conditions with lack of flexibility of soft tissue structures.	Acute orthopaedic conditions, recent postoperative conditions; circulatory conditions.

Certain physical agents specifically applied may enhance the patient's ability to perform, and at the same time may conserve the physical therapist's energy.[20] The agents are not new, but the method of application is different. As with other techniques of facilitation, application is superimposed upon patterns of facilitation, that is, the superficial structures related to the specific patterns. The antagonistic relationship of diagonally opposite patterns and structures is considered.

If movement, active or passive, is limited by adaptive shortening, spasm, or spasticity, or by localized pain, the factor of limitation usually lies within the antagonistic pattern of facilitation. The relaxation or alleviation of the limiting factor may be approached through direct relaxation of the antagonistic pattern, or through the direct stimulation of the agonistic pattern with subsequent relaxation of the antagonistic pattern.

Two physical agents, cold and electrical stimulation, have been used to good advantage with the majority of patients. The use of cold has a broader application and is discussed first. A third agent, mechanical vibration, came into use more recently.[14] See Table 2-3.

Table 2-3. Applications of Adjunctive Procedures

Agent and Method	Agonist	Antagonist	Antagonists
Cold			
Immersion (PNF)			R/I
Ice (Rood)	S/F (brief)		
Ice massage (Hayden)		R/I	R/I
Compress (PNF)	S/F (brief)	R/I	R/I
Electrical Stimulation			
Faradic-like (PNF)	S/F		
Vibration (PNF/Voss)			
One vibrator	S/F		
Two vibrators			
One pattern	S/F		
Two patterns (antagonists)			R/I stability

S/F = Stimulation/Facilitation
R/I = Relaxation/Inhibition
(After Hayden C: Cryokinetics in an early treatment program. J Am Phys Ther Assoc 44:990, 1964; Stockmeyer SA: An interpretation of the approach of Rood to the treatment of neuromuscular dysfunction. Am J Phys Med 46:900, 1967; and Voss DE: Proprioceptive Neuromuscular Facilitation. Am J Phys Med 46:838, 1967.)

COLD

Cold may be applied in several ways. One method may be selected or several methods may be combined. For direct relaxation of an antagonistic pattern that is limiting movement, turkish towels wrung from ice water are applied to the skin overlying the muscle groups of the antagonistic pattern, or, in the case of painful joints, the towels may be wrapped around the entire segment. For example, if the range of the flexion–abduction–external rotation pattern of the shoulder is limited, the cold compress is placed over the axillary and pectoral regions. The compress is used for about 3 minutes and within this time is replaced by another cold towel at least once. With the cold compress in place, the agonistic pattern is facilitated. Relaxation techniques may be directed to the antagonistic pattern at the point in the range where limitation is evident, thereby facilitating the agonistic pattern. Isometric contraction by use of rhythmic stabilization or hold–relax technique is indicated in the presence of pain. If possible, the patient should perform with isotonic contraction through the available range of motion so that a more lasting effect is obtained. If working with an extremity while the cold compress is in place seems cumbersome, related patterns of other segments may be performed while the cold is having its effect. Where pain is a dominant factor, this may be the procedure of choice.

Where a localized area of pain or limitation of movement exists, direct and specific application may be made by use of a ball of ice, formed by hand until smooth, or by use of an icicle formed on a wooden applicator.[42]* The ice is rubbed vigorously over the painful area, as, for example, a postsurgical scar that limits movement and produces pain. Application is continued until the patient no longer "feels" the cold, usually less than 1 minute. Hypersensitive responses to ice massage for 5 and 10 minutes to dorsolumbar areas has been reported, with the suggestion that a test application be carried out before beginning massage with ice.[4] Positioning and maintaining the part so that tension is present in the limiting muscle groups or soft structures is conducive to maximum relaxation provided that pain is not produced. If tension produces pain, the degree of tension should be reduced. In this way, the movement–pain–limitation cycle may be interrupted. The point of pain may have been altered. That is, movement may continue to produce pain, but the range of pain-free movement has been increased. When resistance is superimposed, it is applied most

* Margaret Rood used plastic trays commercially made for home use in preparing Popsicles for children. She has also extended the use of cold for discrete sensory stimulation and inhibition.

strongly to the pain-free components of a pattern; if movement of the proximal joint is painful, maximal resistance may be applied to distal muscle groups during performance of isometric and isotonic contractions. Again, the use of cold is coupled with exercise to use any relaxation that has been gained.

Selective stimulation or facilitation of a specific muscle or muscle group may be gained by discrete application of cold.[42] Using an ice ball or an icicle, a quick stroking of the skin overlying the muscles of the agonistic pattern may promote response of these muscles. If, for example, flexion–abduction–external rotation of the shoulder is painful, quickly and briefly stroking the areas of the trapezius muscle and the middle portion of the deltoid muscle may increase the pain-free range.

Immersion of a segment in ice water may be useful for relaxation of the distal musculature. The hand and forearm or the foot and leg may be immersed for a minute or less, and the time may be increased as tolerated. If tolerance for immersion is low, dipping the part briefly and repeating the process several times may be desirable at first. The distal part of the segment well be relaxed. Should limitation persist at the proximal joints, cold compresses may be used proximally. Upon completing the procedure, exercises and facilitation of the desired movements should be carried out.

Immersion of the lower region of the body and extremities in a cold bath, about 50°F, for 1 to 4 minutes may help to reduce marked spasticity in patients having generalized involvement. The procedure should be adapted to the patient's tolerance. Mead is of the opinion that contraindications for the use of cold are rare.[36] However, the individual patient must be assessed by his physician, and any possible contraindications must be heeded. Patients are not to be subjected to sudden application of cold without preparatory discussion. Physical therapists and physicians should undergo the treatment procedure in order to understand better their patients' reactions. In general, patients like cold, although in the beginning some are not completely receptive to the idea of its use.

Cold is used as preparation for exercise and movement, and for relief of pain experienced during movement. Thus, cold is used locally on a treatment table, on a gymnasium mat, or in a gait area. If necessary, mat and gait activities are carried out in the privacy of a treatment room so that the part to be treated may be exposed.

ELECTRICAL STIMULATION

The use of faradic or tetanizing current for relaxation of spasticity or of adaptive shortening is a useful preliminary to performance of patterns of facilitation.[32,33] As a procedure, electrical stimulation is more time consuming than is the use of cold. However, in selected patients, and where the use of cold is medically contraindicated, electrical stimulation may be preferred. Proper application requires that two physical therapists work together; one person controls the stimulation, the second moves the segment of the patient's body passively through the available range of motion as relaxation occurs.

For electrical stimulation, the usual preparations are carried out. The thoroughly moistened inactive electrode (about 3 inches by 4 inches) is placed at a distance from the part to be stimulated. That is, if the lower extremity is to be stimulated, the inactive electrode is placed near the midthoracic region so that contact will be maintained as the extremity is moved. The active electrode (about 1 inch in diameter) attached to a long-handled applicator is used for ease of control and application. The active electrode is applied to the skin with firm pressure. After the electrode is in place, the current is increased sufficiently to produce a tentanized contraction. The current is decreased before the electrode is withdrawn. In this way, the patient having intact sensation experiences less discomfort.

The therapist who is responsible for moving the segment determines the areas of limitation by passively moving the part through the available range of motion. The movement is carried out by moving the distal parts first, then progressing to the more proximal joints. If the patient is able to move the part actively or to assist, he is instructed to do so. The areas of limitation or points at which limitation becomes evident have been determined, the stimulation is done in a proximal-to-distal direction. The proximal muscles of a pattern are stimulated first; strict adherence to classical motor points is not essential. Application of the active electrode to skin overlying those muscles that are diagonally opposite the limiting pattern is important. For example, if the biceps femoris muscle is limiting complete extension of the knee, the vastus medialis muscle is stimulated. The therapist who is supporting and moving the segment waits for relaxation to occur. As tension lessens, the part is moved through additional range. A degree of relaxation having been achieved, the active electrode is moved to a somewhat more distal point over the same muscle or over a related muscle of the same pattern. The entire procedure is repeated and the distal muscles of the pattern are stimulated successively. The person who is moving the part is able to direct the person who is controlling the current because of his awareness of exact points of limitation. Because overlapping exists between the patterns of one diagonal and those of the second diagonal, it may be necessary to relax the antagonists of the second diagonal as well. This is not done in a haphazard fashion. Again, all components of the second diagonal are considered, and the procedure is conducted from proximal to distal.

After stimulation has been completed, the passive and active range of motion may be tested to determine the degree of success. In any case, the agonistic pattern should be facilitated as soon as possible by use of maximal resistance. Repeated contractions should be performed so as to promote a more lasting effect. If possible, the patient should perform actively the movement or activity in whose interest the procedure was done. It follows that the greater the potential for performance actively and against resistance, the greater the lasting effect.

MECHANICAL VIBRATION

In coupling vibration with PNF, the voluntary effort of the patient is enlisted; the use of vibration is not a passive procedure. The tonic vibration reflex (TVR) is stronger under isometric than under isotonic conditions, and the reflex response induced is sustained contraction of the vibrated muscle with simultaneous relaxation of the prime antagonist.[14]

The three-dimensional PNF patterns of motion are based on the topographical alignment of muscles. Stretch is used to activate the pattern in its lengthened range. Isotonic–concentric contraction occurs upon the command, "Pull!" If, for example, the biceps brachii muscle is weak with limited flexion of the elbow, an active vibrator placed over the muscle belly will serve as a further stretch stimulus with increased strength of response and further flexion of the elbow.

If, during use of RS technique, isometric contractions of antagonistic patterns are produced, two identical vibrators applied and activated simultaneously will elicit greater response and stability through co-contraction of antagonistic muscles. For example, the vastus medialis and the biceps femoris would contribute stability during weight bearing. If the knee joint failed to extend as it should during the swing phase of walking, one active vibrator applied over the vastus medialis during the swing phase could yield improved extension. Because the response of the vastus medialis was used functionally, the effectiveness of the vibration may be longer lasting than if the vibrator were used with "quadriceps setting." See Observations on Effects of Vibration, below.

OBSERVATIONS ON EFFECTS OF VIBRATION

Standing

Extension of relaxed wrist in response to vibration: Vibrate extensor surface at wrist. Observe response.

Hand opening: Test resistance through range, hold at end of range. Vibrate extensor surface at wrist. Evaluate initiation and strength of hold.

Hold 0.5 pounds in D1 fl with index finger to nose. Test strength of hold. Vibrate flexor–adductor surface at shoulder. Evaluate strength of hold.

Rise on tiptoe of one foot; both hands give support by contact with table. Observe rate and range for sign of fatigue. Vibrate hip extensor–abductor surface when fatigue is apparent. Evaluate increase in rate, range, or ease of movement, reversal of fatigue.

On Hands and Knees

Elbow extension on hands and knees at end of table. Test hold in elbow extension: (1) head toward, (2) head away, and (3) head away plus vibration. Vibrate triceps near elbow. Evaluate strength of hold. Compare (1) with (2); (1) with (3); (2) with (3).

D1 ex, lower extremity, hands–knees position. Test (1) hold in shortened range; (2) hold as in (1) plus vibration on hip extensor surface; (3) hold as in (1) plus vibration on hip flexor surface. Evaluate (1) > (2); (2) > (1); (2) > (3); (3) > (2).

STIMULATION OF VITAL AND RELATED FUNCTIONS

3

Vital and related proximal functions may be defined as those functions of the body which are primarily under reflex control but which may be inhibited at will. They include motions of respiration, facial motions, eye motions, opening and closing of the mouth, tongue motions, swallowing, micturition, and defecation. Performance of patterns of facilitation against maximal resistance stimulates related motions which have to do with proximal functions.

Beyond the stimulation achieved during performance of related patterns, the techniques of proprioceptive neuromuscular facilitation may be specifically applied to the motions of the parts responsible or necessary to the vital functions. As with all movement, these functions may and should be stimulated in a variety of positions. For example, breathing motions may be resisted in prone and sidelying (lateral) positions as well as in supine. Swallowing is easier in the prone position than in supine. Tongue motions may be encouraged more effectively when the patient is prone with chest elevated by support on elbows and forearms. Where deficiency is marked, the most favorable position should be sought.

Analysis of individual muscles is not included, but study of these muscles will reveal that they are, in general, aligned in a spiral and diagonal fashion.

The illustrations (Figs. 3-1 through 3-17) present manual contacts for all functions except eye motions.

RESPIRATION

Techniques of proprioceptive neuromuscular facilitation may be applied as a means of stimulating response and strengthening muscles related to respiration. Strengthening of neck, trunk, and extremity patterns has a by-product of increased ability in respiration. The patterns most closely related to inspiration are neck extension, upper and lower trunk extension, and flexion patterns of the upper extremities. The patterns most closely related to expiration are neck flexion, upper and lower trunk flexion, and extension patterns of the upper extremities. Combinations of these patterns, such as upper trunk motions combined with bilateral asymmetrical upper extremity patterns (chopping and lifting), and bilateral symmetrical upper extremity patterns, stimulate stress situations. An increased demand is placed upon the accessory muscles of respiration that are normally used in deep respiration as well as on the respiratory mechanism itself (Fig. 3-1).

Stimulation of the intrinsic muscles of respiration and increased range of motion of the chest and diaphragm are achieved by direct application of techniques of facilitation. Resistance may be applied to the motions of the lateral chest walls, upper chest, sternum, and diaphragm. Correction of imbalances is approached by maximal resistance to a stronger area and

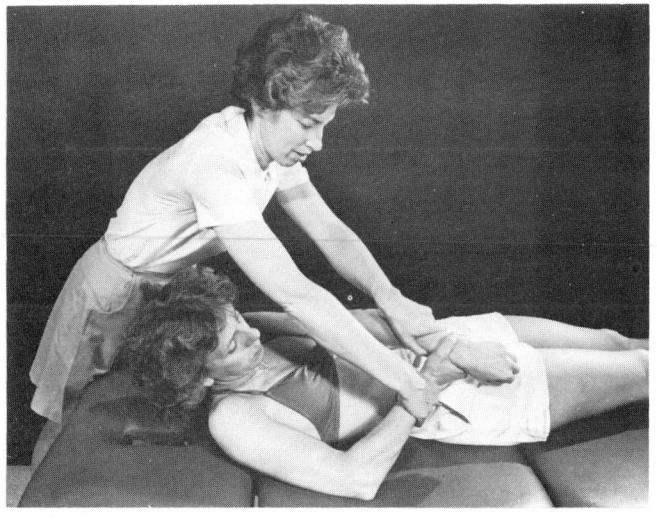

A

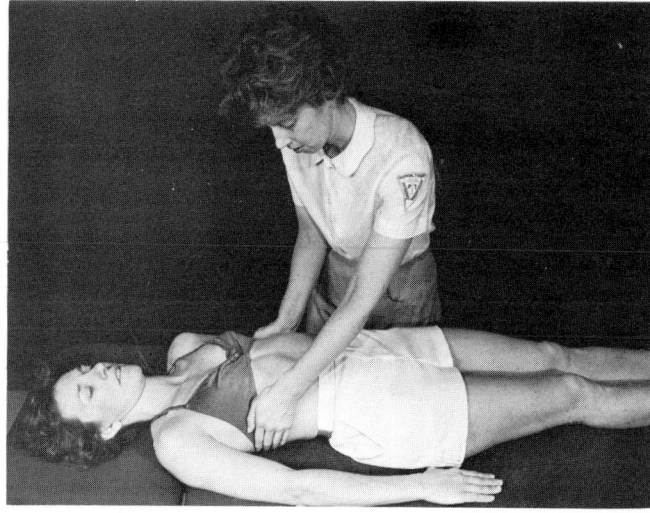

A

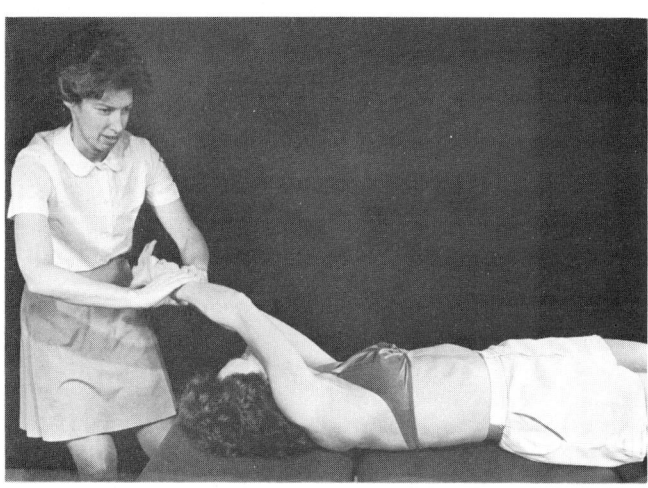

B

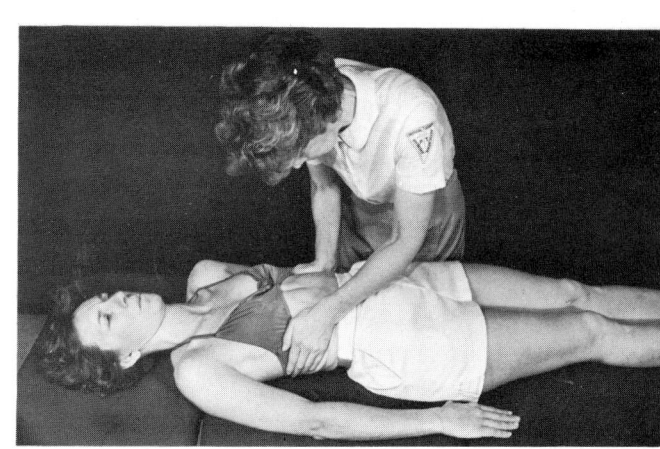

B

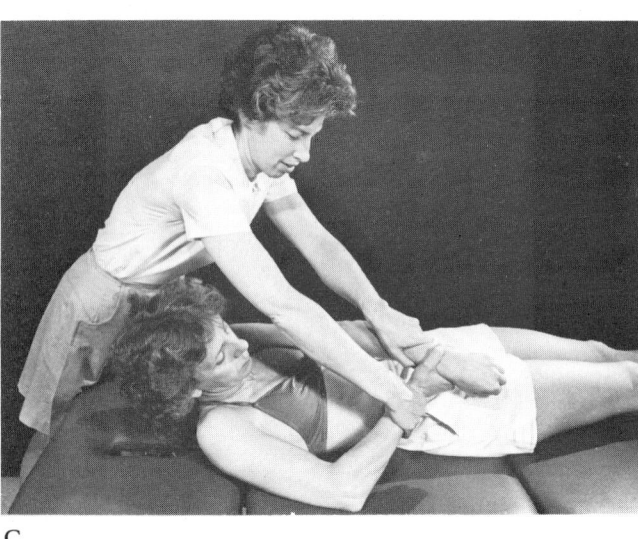

C

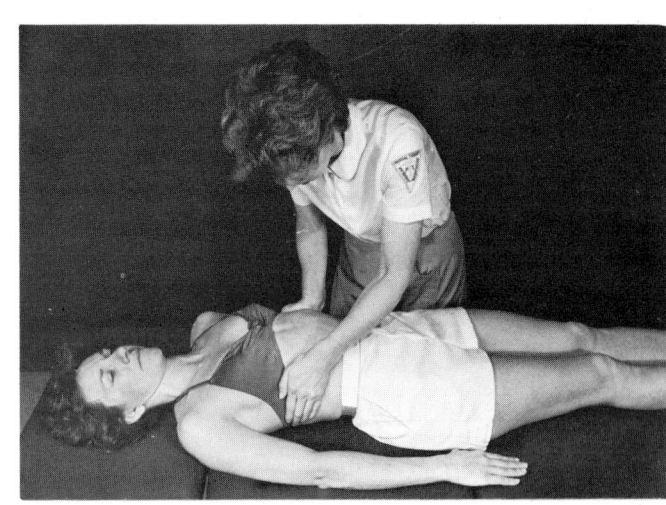

C

FIG. 3-2. Lateral expansion with RC, L.

A. "Ready?" (Hands in place)
B. "Blow it all out." (Compression, down and in)
C. "Breathe in. Hold it. Breathe in some more. And
   again. Relax." (L hand holds; R hand applies Str and
   MR)

FIG. 3-1. Rhythmic chopping and lifting.

A. "Lift up and breathe in." (Str for lift)
B. "Now pull down and blow out." (Str for chop)
C. "And ready! Lift, breathe in again." (Str for lift)

repeated contractions emphasizing the weaker area.

For example, if a patient has stronger response of the left lateral chest wall than of the right lateral chest wall, resistance is applied as follows: The physical therapist places her hands on the lateral chest walls with the bases of the palms near the apices of the lower ribs and with the fingers lying in close approximation in an upward and lateralward direction. The physical therapist instructs the patient to exhale ("Breathe out!") and applies pressure downward and medialward so as to achieve stretch on the intercostal muscles. The patient is then instructed, "Breathe in, as much as you can; hold it!" As the patient inhales, the physical therapist lessens the pressure and grades resistance so as to encourage range of motion. When the patient "holds" his breath, the physical therapist proceeds to repeated contractions. While the therapist maintains steady resistance to the stronger chest area, she repeatedly alternates increasing and decreasing pressure over the weaker area. The patient is instructed, "Breathe in again, and again, and again," and attempts to sustain his effort throughout the procedure. When the patient has repeated as many times as he is able, he exhales in a sustained manner (Fig. 3-2).

The above procedure may be applied to emphasize the upper region of the chest by using one hand in contact with the sternum and the other hand and arm over the lower lateral chest walls. The hand that is used for sternal contact is placed with the base of the palm on the manubrium sterni; the fingers are placed in close approximation to each other, extending downward toward the xiphoid process. Pressure is applied in a diagonal direction: downward and toward the abdomen. Pressure should not cause pain; if the patient experiences pain, the pressure has been too great in a directly downward direction. The other hand and arm are used to compress the lower chest, thereby channeling air to the upper region of the chest. Repeated contractions may be performed with the hand that is in sternal contact (Fig. 3-3).

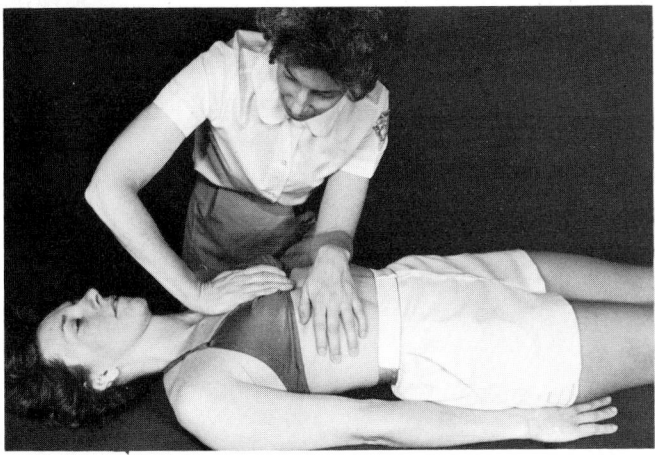

FIG. 3-3. Upper region reinforced by lateral compression. "Blow out." (Compress lateral walls.) "Breathe in. Hold it! And breathe in some more. And again. Now blow it all out. And relax." (MC on sternum, RC)

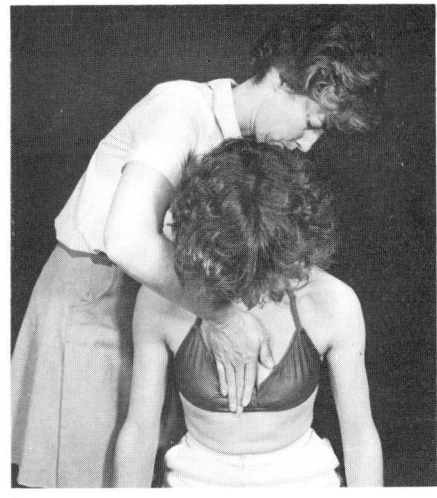

A

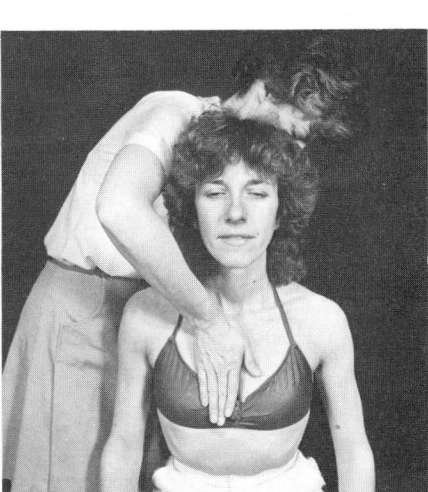

B

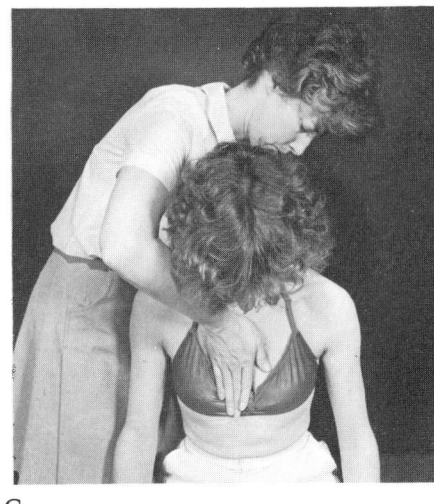

C

FIG. 3-4. Anteroposterior emphasis: sitting.

A. "Blow out!" (Hands apply Str: R downward, L upward)

B. "Breathe in. And hold! Breathe in again. And again."

C. "Now blow it out." (Hands repeat Str) "Breathe in again."

Emphasis of either side of the upper region of the chest may be performed by placing both hands with the bases of the palms near the sternum and the fingers pointing upward and outward toward the acromion processes. Various combinations of one area of the upper region of the chest and an area of the region of the lower chest may be used. The stronger area is used to reinforce the weaker area. This is done by preventing motion in the stronger area by pressure and resisting the weaker area, grading resistance through the range.

In the sitting posture respiration in the upper region may also be reinforced by flexion and extension of head and neck and upper trunk. The hand used for sternal contact is as shown in Figure 3-3. The hand for dorsal contact lies between the scapulae with fingers pointing upward (Fig. 3-4,A.). Following exhalation, stretch and pressure are applied in a diagonal direction downward toward the umbilicus by the hand in sternal contact, and upward on the trunk with the hand in dorsal contact (Fig. 3-4,B.). Techniques of SRH and RC are performed (Fig. 3-4,C.). This method of reinforcement can be applied in prone on elbows (Fig. 3-5) and in other developmental postures.

Stimulation of the diaphragm is accomplished by placing the thumbs and palms of the hands along the costal cartilages of the lower ribs. Pressure and stretch is applied with the thumbs pushed up and under the rib cage as far as possible without producing pain. The tips of the thumbs are pointed toward the xiphoid process. Repeated contractions may be performed to both sides simultaneously, or one side may be emphasized with sustained pressure to the other side. Resistance may be applied to forced expiration in this area by resisting the downward motion of the rib cage so as to prevent the patient from decreasing the diameter of his lower chest as he exhales.

Rhythmic stabilization may be performed as stimulation for the diaphragm by using the thumbs in contact as described above. The fingers are placed in contact with the lower chest walls. The patient is instructed, "Breathe in, hold it!" The patient sustains his breath while the physical therapist applies pressure and stretch alternately to the chest walls and the diaphragm. After two or three alternations, the patient is instructed, "Breathe in again! again! and again!" while the physical therapist repeats with increasing and decreasing pressure to the diaphragmatic area.

This procedure, performed in a symmetrical pattern (Fig. 3-6), may also be done in a reciprocal pattern. Pressure alternates from L hand on diaphragm and R hand on chest wall to R hand on diaphragm and L hand on chest all (Fig. 3-7).

Success of application of techniques to patterns of respiration will depend upon the physical therapist feeling the patient's response, synchronizing her demands with the patient's efforts, and carefully grading resistance to encourage response and range of motion.

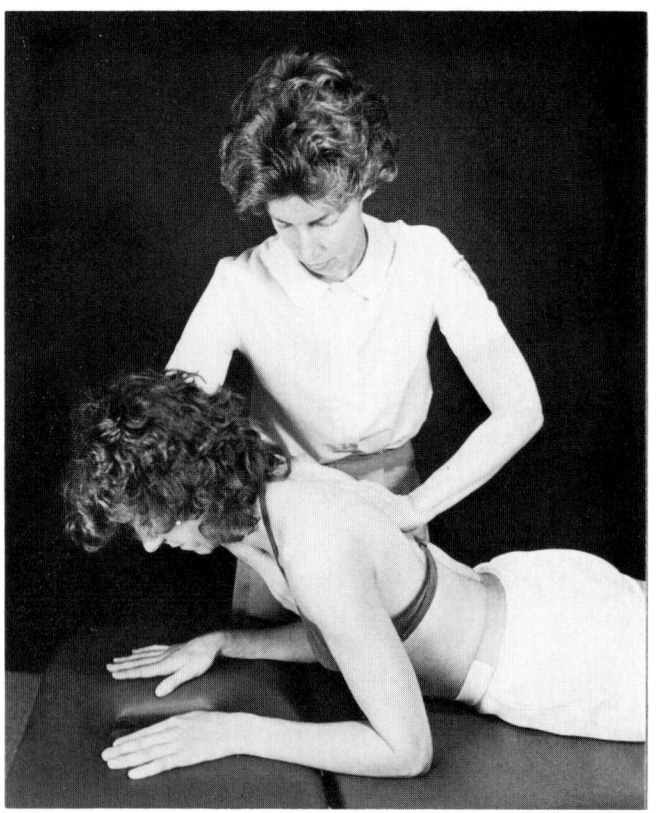

FIG. 3-5. Anteroposterior emphasis: prone. "Look down and blow out." (Str: R downward and L upward) "Look up and breathe in. And hold! Now relax."

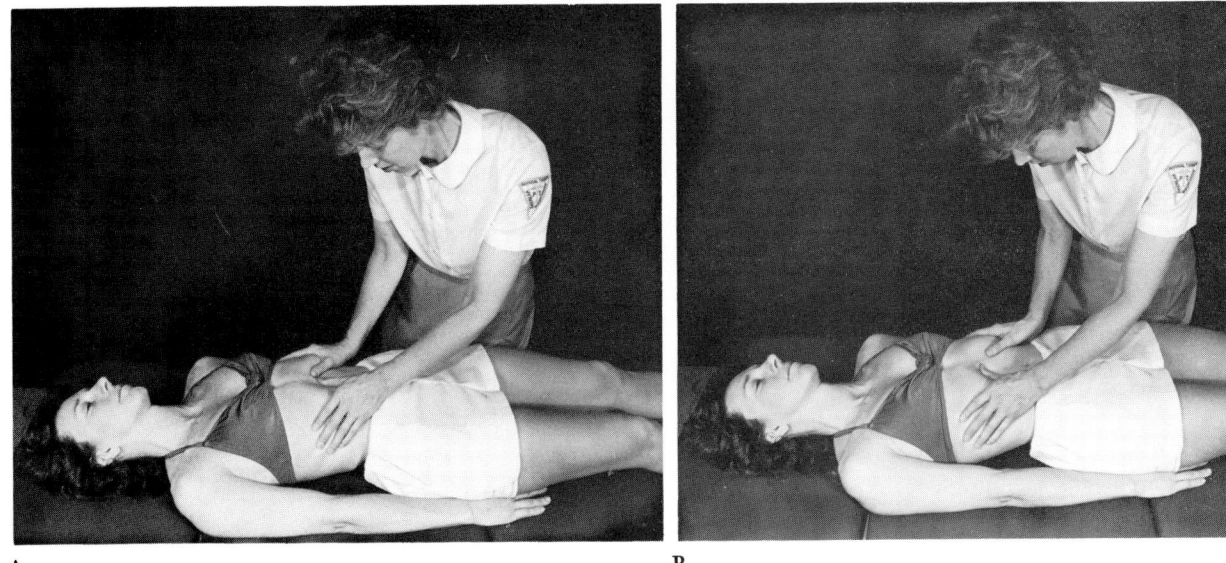

A   B

FIG. 3-6. Stimulation of diaphragm: BS, MC; RC.

A. "Breathe in. Hold it!" (Thumbs apply Str and pressure)
B. "Now breathe some more." (L holds; R repeats Str and MR) "And some more. And breathe out."

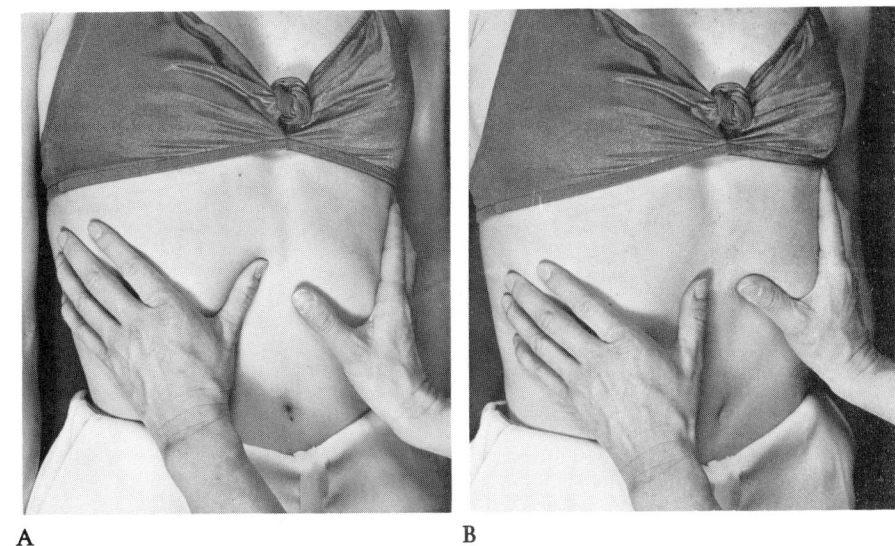

A   B

FIG. 3-7. Alternate pressure: L then, R, RS.

A. "Breathe in. Hold it!" (L hand resists diaphragm and R hand resists chest wall)
B. "And hold." (R hand resists diaphragm, L hand resists chest wall)

Repeat as in **A**, and as in **B**, then relax.

FACIAL MOTIONS

The normal facial motions are bilaterally symmetrical in character: both sides of the face move in identical motions. The normal subject is capable of innumerable combinations of facial motions, which include unilateral and bilaterally asymmetrical motions. Although the normal subject may isolate certain motions to a degree, in situations of emotional stress facial motions are usually bilaterally symmetrical in character. During vigorous physical activity, facial motions may take on a bilaterally asymmetrical character when facial motions are brought into play as reinforcement. Inability to perform bilaterally symmetrical motions voluntarily is an indication of weakness resulting in asymmetry of facial expression.

Facial motions may be grouped as antagonistic motions involving three pivots of action: the mouth, the nose, and the eyes. Extreme ranges of motion of any one pivot bring into play related movements of other pivots. Antagonistic motions may be considered as follows:

Elevation of eyebrows, upward and lateralward	Depression of eyebrows, downward and medialward (Fig. 3-8)
Opening of eyelids, lateralward	Closing of eyelids, medialward (Fig. 3-9)
Elevation and opening of nostrils, lateralward	Depression and closing of nostrils, medialward
Retraction of angles of mouth, upward	Protrusion of lips, downward (Fig. 3-10)
Retraction of angles of mouth, downward	Protrusion of lips, upward (Fig. 3-11)
Closing of lips with protrusion	Opening of lips with inversion (Fig. 3-12)

NOTE: Lip closure with protrusion combines with compression of the cheeks in the act of sucking and feeding. Patients who have weakness of facial muscles related to feeding may benefit from use of Str and MR as portrayed in Figure 3-12.

The facial muscles are spiral and diagonal in character and are arranged for symmetrical motions. Strong contraction of the circular muscles about the mouth and the eyes demands lengthening or shortening reactions of the other facial groups including those of the scalp. Strong contraction of the nasal groups in turn demands cooperation of the muscles responsible for motion about the eyes and the mouth.

The various techniques of proprioceptive neuro-

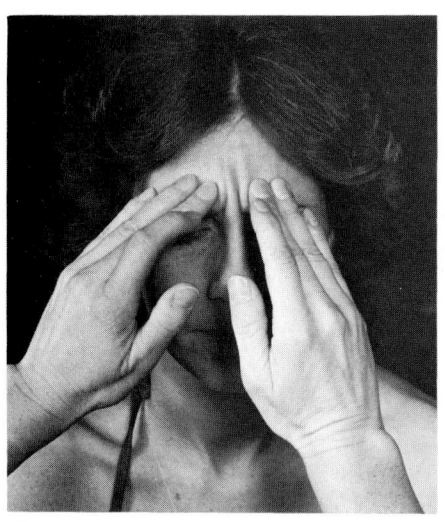 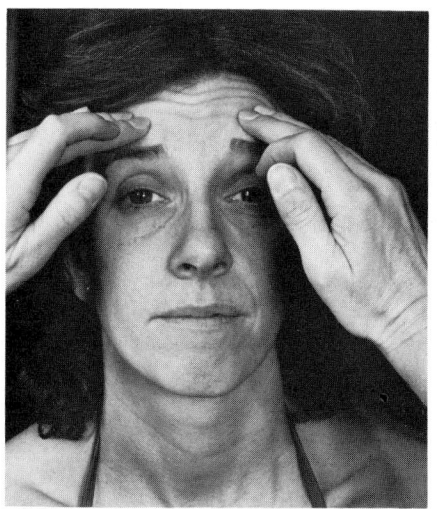 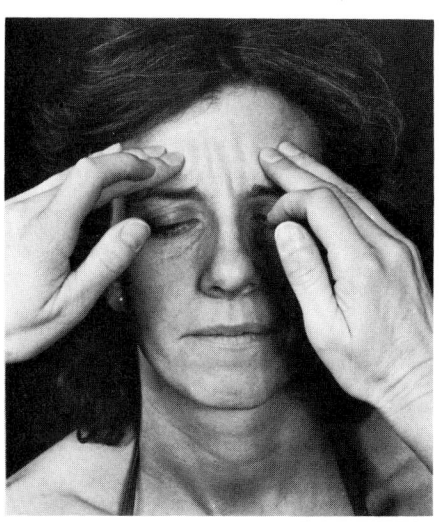

A   B   C

FIG. 3-8. Elevation and depression of eyebrows, diagonal direction.

A. "Ready!" (Str downward and medialward)
B. "Look up! Raise your eyebrows!"
C. "Hold it! Now look up some more! And higher! And higher! Now look down and in." (MR, RC, L)

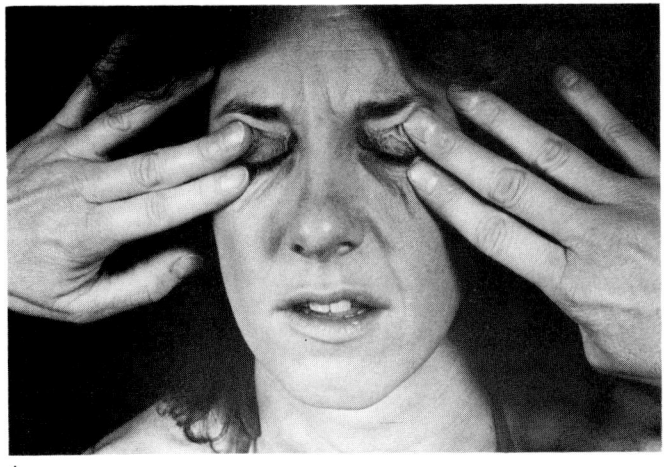
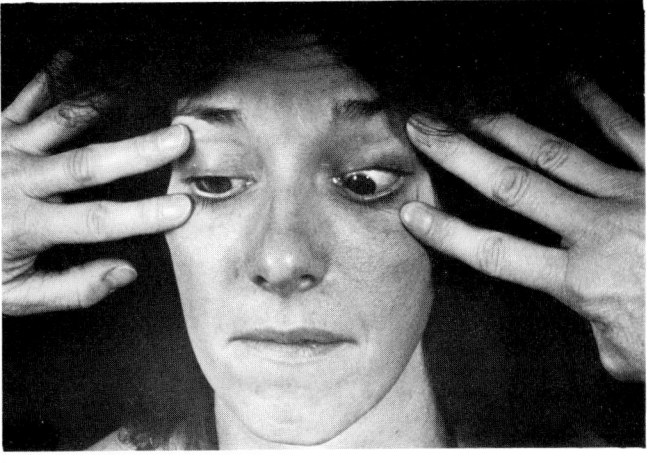

A **B**

FIG. 3-9. Opening and closing of the eyelids, diagonal direction.

A. "Open your eyes wide!" (Str) "Hold them open."
B. "Now, close your eyes! Don't let me open them!" (MR) "And relax."

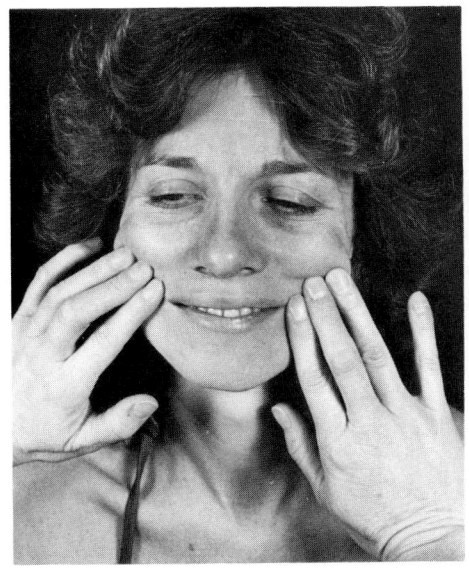
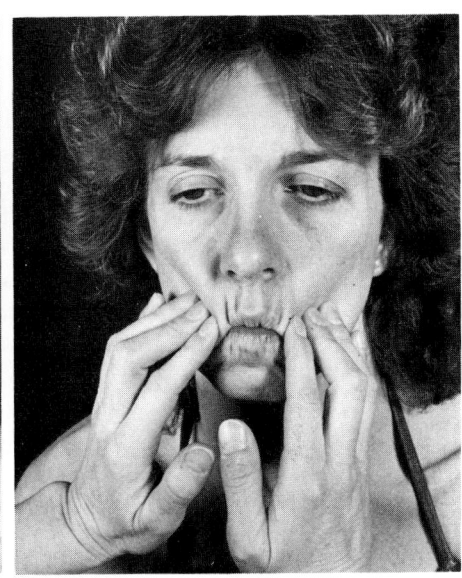

FIG. 3-10. Retraction of angles of mouth upward; protrusion of lips downward.

A. "Smile wide! Hold it there!" (Str)
B. "Pull your lips together forward and down! Hold it!" (MR, SR-H) "And smile again! And hold!"

A **B**

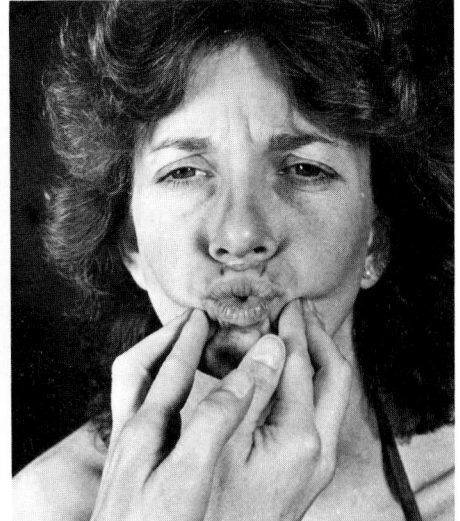

FIG. 3-11. Retraction of angles of mouth downward; protrusion of lips upward.

A. "Frown! Hold it!" (Str, MR)
B. "Pucker up and hold it! Now pucker up some more! And some more!" (MR, RC)

A **B**

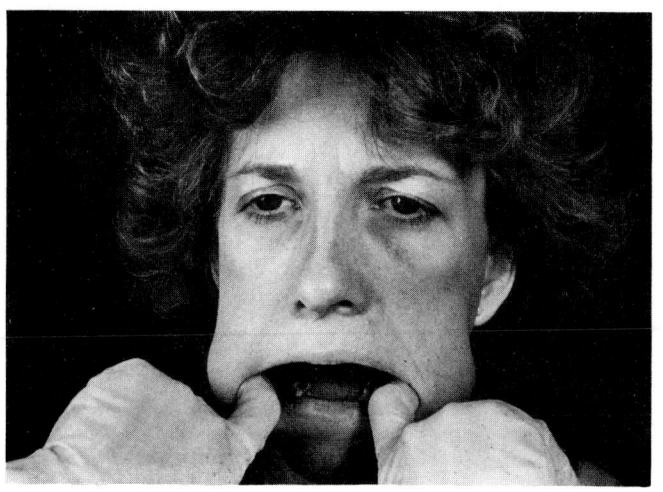

A

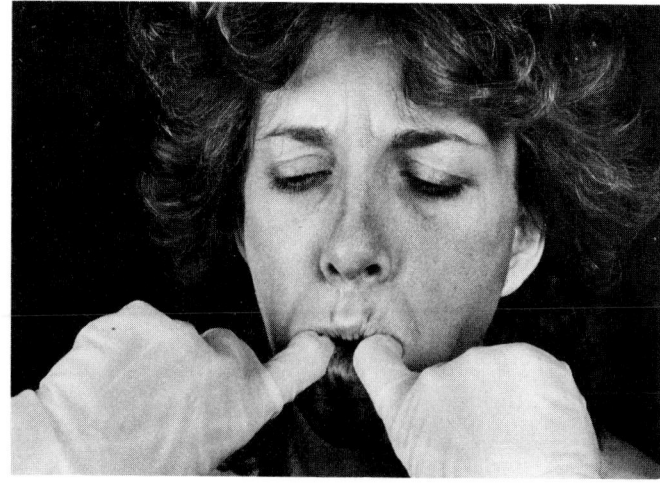

B

FIG. 3-12. Lips open with inversion, lips close with protrusion as cheeks compress.

    A. "Close your lips!" (Str, MR)

    B. "Hold it! Now close tightly! And again! And relax." (RC)

muscular facilitation that may be applied to facial motions include pressure, stretch, resistance, reinforcement, repeated contractions, and reversal of antagonists. Relaxation techniques may be used as indicated. The physical therapist uses the tips of the fingers as manual contacts. Stronger motions are resisted in order to stimulate and reinforce weaker motions.

For example, a patient may present weakness of elevation of the left eyebrow. The physical therapist places her fingertips on both sides of the patient's brow and applies pressure and stretch in a downward and medialward direction. Having achieved stretch, she instructs the patient, "Look up at me! Raise your eyebrows!" At this point the physical therapist resists strongly the motion on the right and allows range of motion to occur on the left. The patient is instructed to hold his eyebrows raised, and the physical therapist then applies the technique of repeated contractions. Reversing motions and relaxation techniques may be used to increase mobility of the elevation and depression of the brows.

Motions of the eyebrows may be used to reinforce opening and closing of the eyes; motions of the lips may be used to reinforce motions about the nose or the eyes. Study of the normal subject will reveal the relationship of facial motions. Neck patterns may be used as reinforcement. Any facial motion that requires elevation or upward motion is reinforced by neck extension. Facial motions that require depression or downward motions are reinforced by neck flexion. Neck rotation reinforces the motion of the side of the face to which the head is turned. If it is desired to reinforce a motion on the left, the head is turned to the left.

EYE MOTIONS

Performance of related neck and upper extremity patterns where the eye follows the hand provides stimulation for movement of the eyes. Neck extension with rotation patterns reinforce upward and lateralward eye movements. Neck flexion with rotation patterns reinforce downward and lateralward eye movements. Neck rotation reinforces lateral movements. The lateral movement of a given pattern determines the lateral direction of the eye movement, to the left or to the right.

Eye movements may be stimulated and certain movements or ranges of movement may be emphasized by application of techniques of facilitation. The physical therapist may use her index finger or a pencil and instruct the patient to follow the movement of the object. Motions may be upward, downward, or lateralward and in various combinations, such as upward and lateralward to the left or right, or downward and lateralward to the left or right. Reversing movements may be applied or repeated contractions may be performed. In order to perform repeated contractions, the physical therapist allows the patient to perform in one direction as far as possible. At this point, the physical therapist moves the pencil in the opposite direction very slightly, and just as the patient is about to follow with his eyes, the physical therapist quickly moves the pencil in the original direction. Related neck patterns may be performed actively or against resistance as reinforcement.

For the patient with nystagmus, SRH in decrements of range may be performed. The therapist moves a visual stimulus (finger or pencil) in one direction while the patient tracks the movement with his

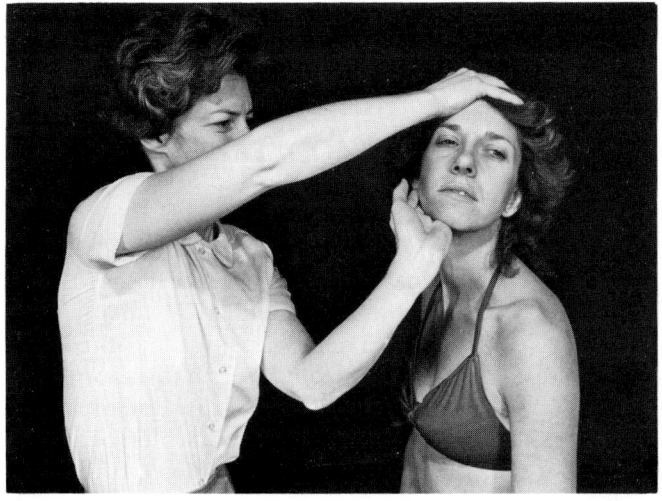

A

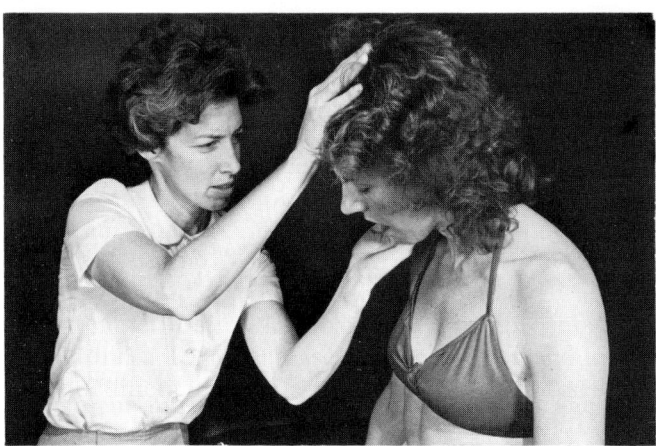

B

FIG. 3-13. Mouth opening to R, reinforced by head and neck D fl.

A. "Open your mouth and look down at your right hip." (Str, MR)
B. "Hold it! Now open some more. And again." (RC)

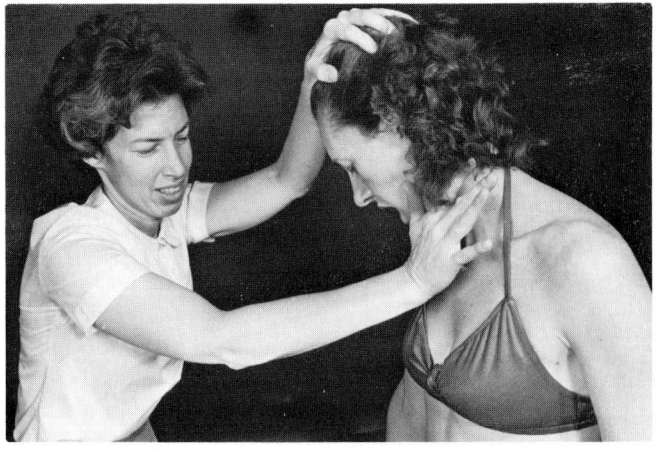

A

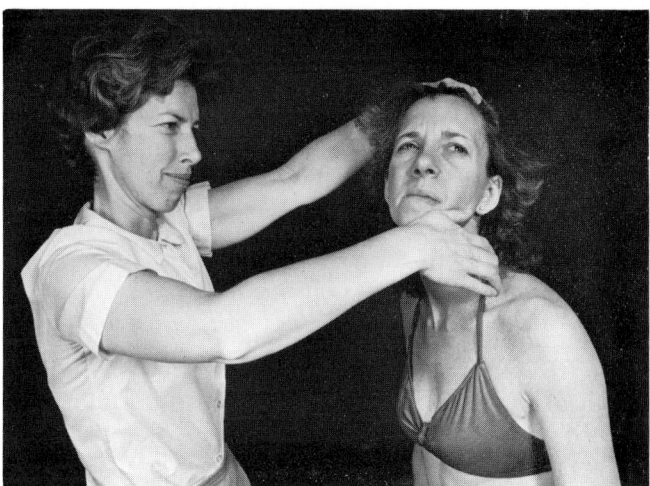

B

FIG. 3-14. Mouth closing to L, reinforced by head and neck D ex.

A. "Close your mouth and look up to your left." (Str, MR)
B. "Head up! Now hold!" (MR)

eyes. The therapist then halts the stimulus as the command, "Hold!" is given and the patient tries to fix his gaze. This sequence is repeated in the opposite direction, and then with decrements of range until motion ceases.

OPENING AND CLOSING OF THE MOUTH

Opening of the mouth requires depression with retraction of the mandible; closing of the mouth requires elevation with protrusion of the mandible. The mouth may be opened or closed in midline, or it may be opened and closed to one side or the other side, combining lateral movements with opening and closing (Figs. 3-13 and 3-14).

In patterns of facilitation, opening is related to neck flexion patterns and closing is related to neck extension. Lateral motion of the mandible is related to neck rotation. When opening of the mouth is reinforced by neck flexion with rotation to the right, depression with retraction and lateral motion of the mandible toward the right occurs. When closing of the mouth is reinforced by neck extension to the left, elevation with protrusion and lateral motion of the mandible toward the left occurs. When lateral motion of the mandible is reinforced by neck rotation, a certain amount of mandibular depression occurs. If reinforcement of mandibular motions by neck motions is attempted, the head should be free of hard surface contact, and the manual contacts described for the neck patterns may be used.

Techniques which may be used include pressure through manual contacts, stretch, resistance, rein-

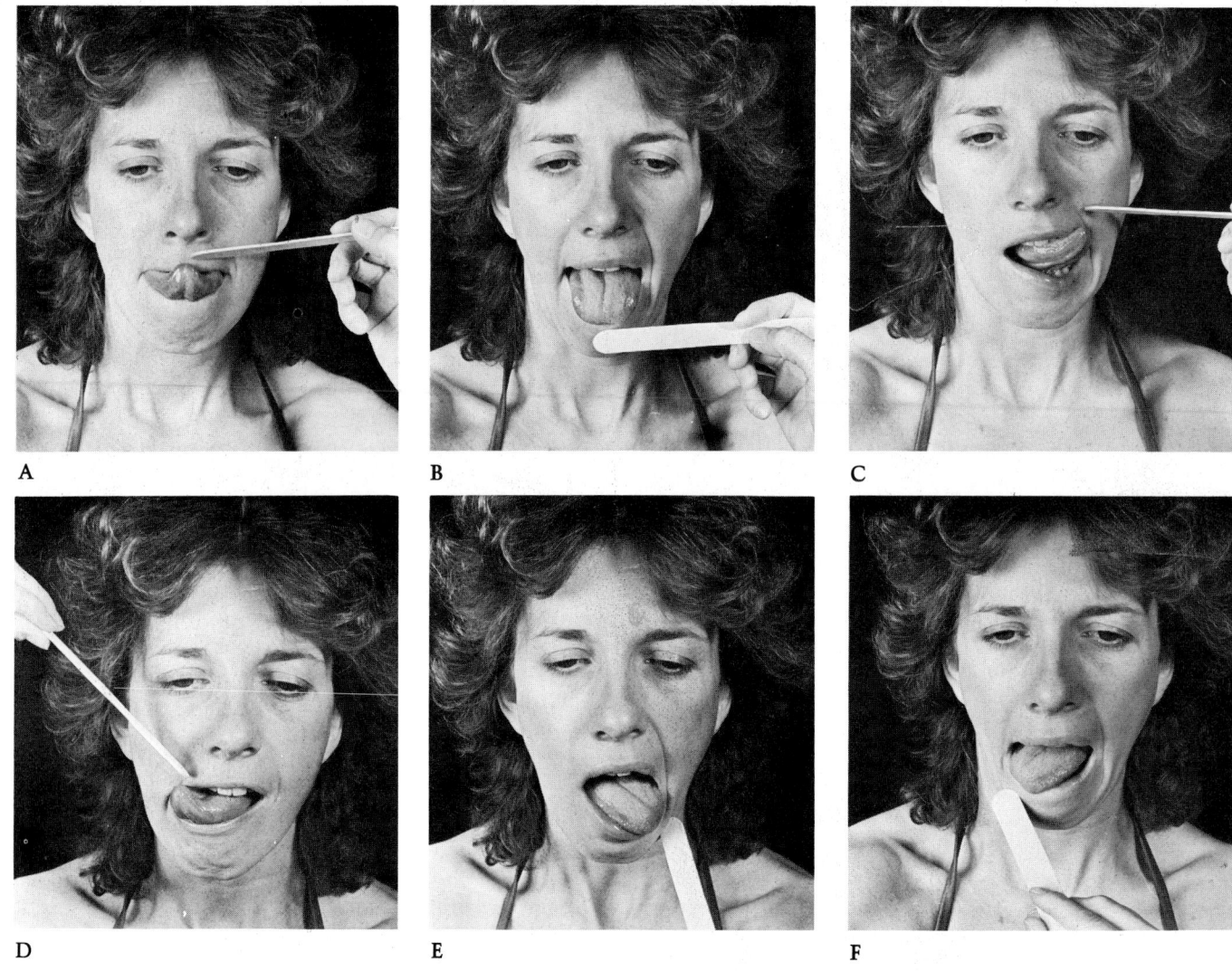

FIG. 3-15. Evaluation of tongue protrusion; midline and diagonal direction.

A. Protrusion in midline with elevation
B. Protrusion in midline with depression
C. Protrusion and elevation to L
D. Protrusion and elevation to R
E. Protrusion and depression L
F. Protrusion and depression R

forcement, repeated contractions, and reversal of antagonists. If range of motion is limited by adaptive shortening or contracture, relaxation techniques may be applied.

MOTIONS OF THE TONGUE

The tongue is an extremely versatile part of the body when its repertoire of motions and its dexterity are considered. Elevation, depression, protrusion, retraction, lateral motions, and rotatory motions are combined in various tongue motions. Combining several motions during evaluation will often disclose asymmetry of function or imbalance between the two sides. Protrusion straight forward may be combined with elevation and depression. Retraction straight backward may be combined with elevation and depression. Protrusion and elevation laterally to one side may be compared with protrusion and elevation laterally to the opposite side. Protrusion and depression laterally to one side may be compared with the same motion to the opposite side. In the same manner, retraction may be combined with depression, elevation, and lateral motions (Fig. 3-15).

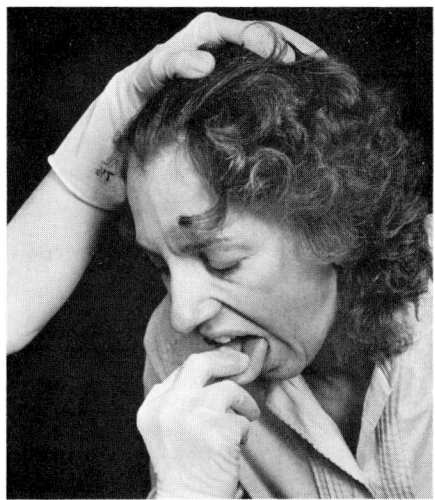

A

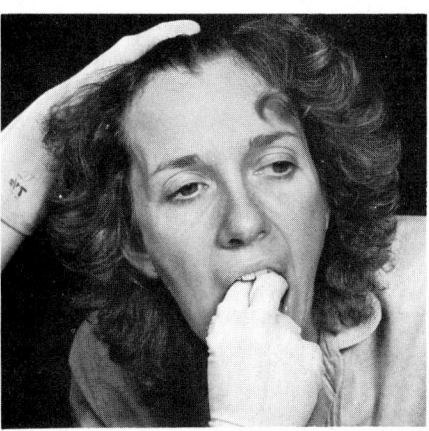

B

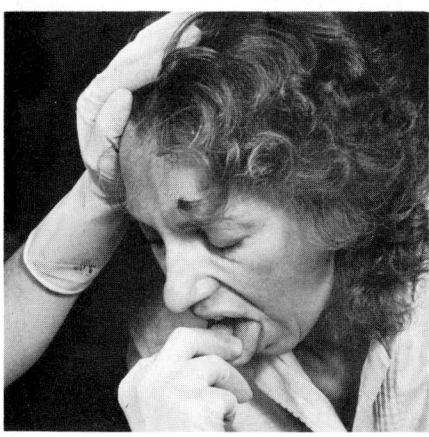

C

FIG. 3-16. Resisted protrusion of tongue L, reinforced by head and neck D fl.

A. "Stick out your tongue, so I can hold it with my fingers." (MC)
B. "Pull your tongue back and down to your right. Hold it!" (Str, MR)
C. "Push your tongue out toward me. Hold it there. Now, push some more. And some more. And relax." (MR, RC)

Resisted neck motions encourage reinforcement of those motions by motion of the tongue. Neck extension, in turn, reinforces elevation of the tongue, neck flexion reinforces depression, and neck rotation reinforces lateral motion. Opening of the mouth is related to depression of the tongue and closing is related to elevation.

Techniques of facilitation may be applied to tongue movements for the purpose of strengthening the movements of the tongue and correcting imbalances. The patient's tongue may be grasped by the physical therapist's gloved fingers or a piece of gauze. A tongue depressor blade may be used in resisting certain motions.

Quick repetitive stretch may facilitate tracking by the tongue. For example, if protrusion to the right is weak, the therapist asks the patient to stick his tongue out. The therapist, using a tongue blade, provides quick, repetitive stretch on the right lateral surface of the tongue. The tongue responds by tracking the stimulus and moving toward the right. Tongue elevation and depression may be stimulated similarly with tongue blade in light contact and with quick, brief motions on the upper and lower surfaces of the protruding tongue.

For example, if protrusion and elevation laterally to the left is weaker than that combination of motions to the right, the physical therapist places her fingers so as to push the patient's tongue backward, downward, and to the right. The patient is instructed to pull his tongue backward as the physical therapist places her fingers. After the tongue has been pushed backward, the physical therapist instructs the patient, "Push your tongue out and up to the left, and hold it there!" The physical therapist resists the motion and may perform repeated contractions as the patient sustains his efforts, or reversing motions may be performed. The physical therapist may resist related neck motions or opening and closing of the mouth as reinforcement, but caution must be used to prevent the patient from biting his tongue or the fingers of the physical therapist (Fig. 3-16).

SWALLOWING

Swallowing, or deglutition, is a complex act requiring interaction of the suprahyoid and infrahyoid muscle groups. These same muscle groups augment the neck flexion patterns and recieve stimulation when these patterns are performed. However, when neck patterns are performed against resistance, it is almost impossible for the normal subject to perform swallowing movements simultaneously. When the head is positioned in the lengthened range of either neck flexion or neck extension, swallowing becomes difficult. Thus, treatment of the patient with poor head control may begin with procedures to strengthen antagonistic

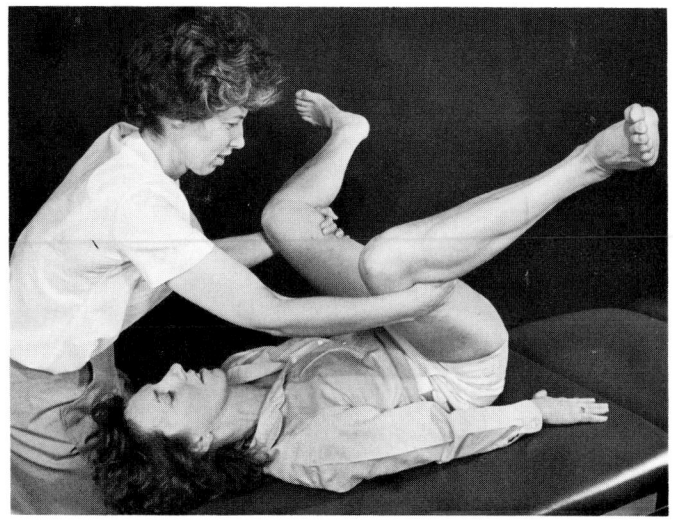 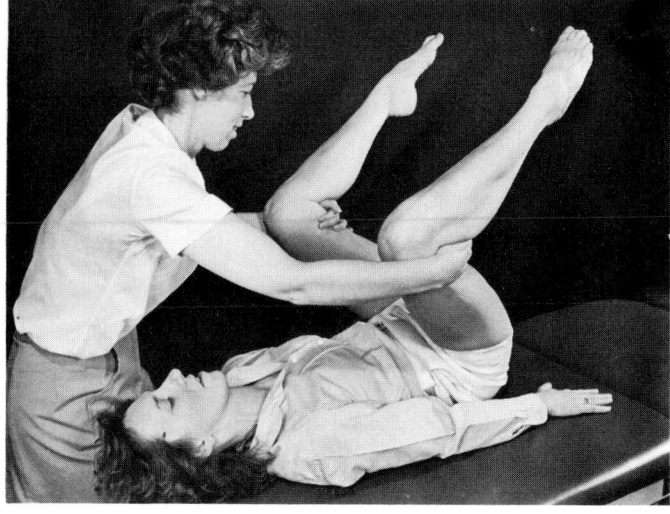

A   B

FIG. 3-17.   Stimulation of perineal muscles.

A. "Turn your feet down and in."
B. "Let go!" (Patient pulls down in D2 ex. Therapist resists external rotation
as it occurs before extension and adduction. These components of motion
are prevented by command, "Let go!").

muscle groups and to correct imbalances. With the head and neck in a neutral position, Ap and RS may be used.

Resistance may be applied to swallowing motions through the use of a simple device. A piece of sponge rubber, approximately $\frac{1}{2}'' \times \frac{1}{2}'' \times \frac{1}{2}''$, may be tied securely to a piece of stout cord or string. The rubber is placed upon the patient's tongue and he is instructed to "swallow" while the physical therapist provides resistance by tugging at the cord attached to the rubber.

Stimulation of elevation of the soft palate may be accomplished in the following manner. The patient opens his mouth widely and says, "Ah." The physical therapist touches the uvula or soft palate folds on either side with a cotton-tipped applicator stick, which stimulates a reflex contraction. The patient repeats "ah" as many times as possible. As a lag of response appears in an area, the physical therapist again stimulates the area by touching it lightly and as often as necessary.

Stimulation of the gag reflex is helpful because it demands response of the pharyngeal muscles with elevation of the soft palate and is followed automatically by a swallowing response.

MICTURITION AND DEFECATION

The voluntary performance and control of micturition and defecation may be enhanced by performance of related patterns of facilitation against maximal resist-ance. The act of emptying the bladder or bowel is most closely related to the flexion patterns of the lower trunk and lower extremities. Inhibition of these acts is most closely related to extension patterns of the lower trunk and lower extremities. In patients for whom incontinence is a problem, emphasis is placed on procedures to restore or develop control of bowel and bladder function.

The muscles of the perineal region may be stimulated during the performance of bilaterally symmetrical extension–adduction–external rotation patterns of the lower extremities. Specific stimulation of these muscles may be obtained through application of stretch and resistance. The patient should lie supine with the lower extremities flexed in abduction. If the patient is able, he may maintain his own extremities in the described position and may himself resist the extension–adduction–external rotation of his lower extremities. If he is not able to use his hands for the purpose of supporting and resisting his extremities, his feet may be supported on the table. The physical therapist may then apply stretch to the perineal region. Stretch is given in an upward and outward direction from the anus. The physical therapist instructs the patient to pull his extremities down and together. To stimulate muscles of the perineum, the extremely lengthened range of extension–adduction–external rotation patterns must be used. Preventing all movement except external rotation will achieve the desired effect. The physical therapist resists the contraction of the muscles, and repeated contractions may be performed while the patient sustains his effort (Fig. 3-17).

COUPLING PNF AND JOINT MOBILIZATION

Thomas S. Holland

After establishing the long-term goals in treatment of the orthopaedic patient, the therapist must determine a sequence of intermediate goals. The therapist must be aware of whether or not these intermediate goals relate to treatment of contractile or noncontractile tissue, or to a combination of both types. However, it would be a gross oversimplification to believe that PNF techniques relate specifically to innervated contractile tissues and joint mobilization techniques to noncontractile tissues.[52] The effectiveness of each treatment technique must be carefully assessed in relation to the specific intermediate treatment goal. Efficiency in orthopaedic patient care can often be achieved and carried to a more complete conclusion by proper selection of a sequence of techniques using both PNF and joint mobilization.

Obviously, the development of a patient care program begins with an appropriate, thorough examination and an assessment of those findings. Maitland offers much to the physical therapist in his discussion of assessment.[54] The examination of the orthopaedic patient must include testing of the physiological movements (osteokinematics) and the more intimate accessory movements of the joints (arthrokinematics); specific tests to identify potential involvement of structures; neurological testing; and testing of the patient's abilities to perform in total patterns of functional movement and posture. An analysis must be made of the total pattern; for example, in walking forward, the component patterns of the head and neck,

trunk, upper extremities, and lower extremities must be analyzed, and then specific joints involved, including the active, resisted, and passive biomechanical aspect of each.[53] The examination must also include a functional analysis of the articular mechanoreceptors of involved joints.[50,51] Most likely, the long-term treatment goal will be identified as the patient's ability to prevent loss of, to maintain, or to improve in his functional performance of a total pattern of movement or posture. The intermediate goals will relate to performance of specific component patterns and particular joint functions. It is not sufficient only to restore caudal glide of the glenohumeral joint to achieve improved elevation of the humerus if the functional goal is to increase the patient's ability in working overhead. The patient's ability to perform patterns of movement singly or in combination also serves as an effective tool for assessment. (See the section on free active motion in Chap. 1 for possible combinations of patterns of movement.)

The techniques selected must be directed toward an identified goal. The progression of techniques within the sequence is based on an assessment of their effectiveness. Maitland skillfully illustrates the selection and progression process as it relates to the clinical signs and symptoms in using techniques of passive movement.[54] A definition as well as indications and contraindications of PNF techniques are provided in Table 2-2.

SUMMARY OF TECHNIQUES

To achieve success in coupling PNF and joint mobilization, the therapist's knowledge and abilities must include the following:

Skills necessary for appropriate and adequate initial examination of the patient

Ability to identify intermediate goals and component aspects thereof

Skill in effective application and performance of a specific technique

Knowledge necessary to assess the effectiveness of the technique

Ability to apply sequence of techniques with progression for optimal effectiveness (See Weakness, under Signs/Symptoms in Table 4-1, for an example of progression.)

Table 4-1 outlines treatment techniques, and offers samples and examples of selection of a sequence, and progression in application. Of particular note is the use of rhythmic stabilization (RS), as we define it: a simultaneous, isometric co-contraction of antagonistic muscle groups, which produces relaxation. This allows mobilization techniques to be more effectively carried out at the limit of movement. Rhythmic stabilization is also effectively used to establish proprioceptive awareness of position and movement within the newly gained range following use of techniques of joint mobilization.

Coupling of PNF and joint mobilization results in successful treatment when goals relating to total patterns of posture and movement have been achieved. Through meticulous processes of selecting techniques, applying them in an appropriate progression, and then assessing their effectiveness, intermediate treatment goals should be effectively accomplished. Through these processes long-term goals may be met.

Table 4-1. Guidelines for Coupling PNF and Joint Mobilization (JM)

Sign/Symptoms	Joint Mobilization[55]	PNF		Sequence of Coupling
Pain	Degree of antigravity movement $<60\%$ | $>60\%$ A_N | Ph $I \to III^+$ | $II^- \to III^+$ (Short of P_1 at first)	Occurrence of pain At rest | During movement Position of comfort | $RS_{(P_1)} \to RS_{(Li)}$ RS Short of aggravation May follow with SR short of P_1)		Choose either a technique of JM or PNF at first and assess over 2–3 treatment sessions. The techniques must not aggravate the patient's condition during the first treatment session.
Stiffness	$Ph_{IV}/A_{IV@Li}$ Ph_{II} may be used to reduce treatment soreness.	RS (@ $R_1 \to R_2$) SR SRH HR CR		$RS \to Ph_{IV}/A_{IV} \to Ph_{II}$ Contractile Noncontractile Decrease lengthening lengthening treatment soreness $RS_{(Li)} \to SRH$ Contractile Muscular control activities through range in new range
Pain and stiffness	Treat first as pain alone, then progress as for stiffness.	Pain techniques, progressing to stiffness techniques		$RS \to A_N \to RS \to A_N$ Position of comfort $\to (P_1 \; P_2)$
Stiffness and pain	Short and gentle $\to$ vigorous; 3–4, 1–2 min. sessions; use movements associated with function loss.	Pain techniques, progressing to stiffness techniques		$RS \to Ph_{IV}/A_{IV} \to Ph_{II}$ (? CR, HR &/or SR)

Weakness: less than full passive ROM	Sequence: RS $\to$ A_N $\to$ Ph_{IV} $\to$ facilitation $\to RS \to SRH \to RC$
	     Shortened con- If appropriate If soft tissue *e.g.,* chopping
	     trolled range injury			

Spasm (limiting)	Sequence: $Ph_{IV} \to HR \to Ph_{IV} \to HR$			
Increased resting tone	Sequence: Rotational and transverse techniques, II, coupled with passive rotation and RS			

Acronyms

A	A passive accessory movement
CR	Contract relax
HR	Hold relax
Li	Limit of the available range
N	Neutral position
P_1	Point in range in which pain is first experienced
P_2	Pain at the limit of the available range
Ph	A passive physiological movement
R_1	Point in range in which resistance is first experienced
R_2	Resistance at the limit of the available range
RS	Rhythmic stabilization
SR	Slow reversal
SRH	Slow reversal–hold
I–IV	Grades of passive movement as described by Maitland

Table 4-1. Guidelines for Coupling PNF and Joint Mobilization (JM)

Sign/Symptoms	Joint Mobilization[55]	PNF		Sequence of Coupling
Pain	Degree of antigravity movement <60% | >60% A_N | Ph $I \rightarrow III^+$ | $II^- \rightarrow III^+$ (Short of P_1 at first)	Occurrence of pain At rest Position of comfort RS Short of aggravation May follow with SR short of P_1)	During movement $RS_{(P_1)} \rightarrow RS_{(Li)}$	Choose either a technique of JM or PNF at first and assess over 2–3 treatment sessions. The techniques must not aggravate the patient's condition during the first treatment session.
Stiffness	$Ph_{IV} / A_{IV@Li}$ Ph_{II} may be used to reduce treatment soreness.	RS (@ $R_1 \rightarrow R_2$) SR SRH HR CR		$RS \rightarrow Ph_{IV}/A_{IV} \rightarrow Ph_{II}$ Contractile Noncontractile Decrease lengthening lengthening treatment soreness $RS_{(Li)} \rightarrow SRH$ Contractile Muscular control activities through range in new range
Pain and stiffness	Treat first as pain alone, then progress as for stiffness.	Pain techniques, progressing to stiffness techniques		$RS \rightarrow A_N \rightarrow RS \rightarrow A_N$ Position of comfort $\rightarrow$ (P_1 P_2)
Stiffness and pain	Short and gentle $\rightarrow$ vigorous; 3–4, 1–2 min. sessions; use movements associated with function loss.	Pain techniques, progressing to stiffness techniques		$RS \rightarrow Ph_{IV}/A_{IV} \rightarrow Ph_{II}$ (? CR, HR &/or SR)
Weakness: less than full passive ROM	Sequence: RS $\rightarrow$ A_N $\rightarrow$ Ph_{IV} $\rightarrow$ facilitation $\rightarrow$ RS $\rightarrow$ SRH $\rightarrow$ RC Shortened con- If appropriate If soft tissue *e.g.,* chopping trolled range injury			
Spasm (limiting)	Sequence: $Ph_{IV} \rightarrow HR \rightarrow Ph_{IV} \rightarrow HR$			
Increased resting tone	Sequence: Rotational and transverse techniques, II, coupled with passive rotation and RS			

Acronyms

A   A passive accessory movement
CR   Contract relax
HR   Hold relax
Li   Limit of the available range
N   Neutral position
P_1 Point in range in which pain is first experienced
P_2 Pain at the limit of the available range
Ph   A passive physiological movement
R_1 Point in range in which resistance is first experienced
R_2 Resistance at the limit of the available range
RS   Rhythmic stabilization
SR   Slow reversal
SRH   Slow reversal–hold
I–IV   Grades of passive movement as described by Maitland

EVALUATION AND TREATMENT PROGRAM

Evaluation of Patient Performance

The evaluation of patient performance must be based upon knowledge of performance of normal subjects. Although normal subjects vary in their available range of motion, coordination, power, endurance, and rate of movement, the variations are within normal limits. These variations do not affect the subject's competence at ordinary motor activities, but may affect the subject's ability to perform highly skilled activities, his postural attitudes, his power, and his endurance.

The mature, normal subject is able, after verbal instruction, to

Initiate all patterns of facilitation from the lengthened range and proceed to the shortened range (isotonic contraction) in accordance with normal timing (see Chap. 1, Free Active Motion).

Perform all patterns against maximal resistance in accordance with normal timing.

"Hold" at any desired point in the range of motion (isometric contraction). In the shortened range he is able to hold so strongly that the hold cannot be broken unless derotation is used.

Perform all combinations of related patterns.

Perform reversals of patterns and the various techniques of facilitation against maximal resistance with a resultant buildup in power or gain in range of motion.

The physical therapist may defeat the performance of the subject by preventing rotation from occurring in the lengthened range of the patterns; by preventing normal timing through application of excessive resistance; or by derotating the part when a "hold" contraction is being performed.

It must be remembered that physical therapists as a group of normal individuals present variations of performance as clearly as any other group of normal subjects. While serving as a subject, the physical therapist must accept a goal of performance rather than a goal of self-analysis. If the subject directs his attention to such things as which muscles are contracting, he hinders his own performance and frustrates his physical therapist. Analysis and critical evaluation are helpful after performance.

GENERAL OBJECTIVES

The goal of evaluation or analysis of the patient is to ascertain his abilities, deficiencies, and potentialities accurately. Necessary general knowledge can be gleaned using the following questions:

Considering the patient's chronological age, are his motor abilities adequate?

If inadequate, are the deficiencies the result of

faulty development, trauma, or disease?

Are deficiencies evidenced by less or more than normal range of passive and active motion? incoordination? less than normal strength? lack of endurance? less or more than normal rate of movement? instability of posture?

Is deficiency generalized and profound, or is deficiency most evident in relation to the proximal parts (neck and trunk) or the distal parts (extremities)?

PATTERNS OF FACILITATION

Free active performance of patterns singly and in combinations should be assessed with the subject or patient in appropriate postures: standing, sitting, on hands and knees, and during activities such as walking in all directions. When necessary, detailed evaluation may be done most easily with the patient lying on a treatment table. However, those patterns which are not limited in range when performed on a flat surface may be evaluated as the patient lies on a gymnasium mat or as he performs total patterns of the developmental sequence.

Specific information can be gained using the following questions for evaluation:

Which patterns of facilitation are within normal limits? Which patterns are inadequate?

Is the available range of motion of specific patterns within normal limits?

Is passive range limited by adaptive shortening or contracture? spasticity? muscle spasm? pain?

Is passive range of motion excessive?

Are the muscles lengthened beyond their normal limits so that they do not serve as a range-limiting factor to the antagonistic pattern?

Have the ligaments, joint structures, and soft tissue contact become the only range-limiting factors?

Is active performance in keeping with the development level of the subject, considering his chronological age?

Is performance smooth, or is motion of the distal parts delayed?

Is performance in the "groove" of the pattern, or do bizarre movements occur?

Is performance of isotonic contraction possible through the available range of motion?

Is the active range less than the available range of passive motion?

Is active range limited by adaptive shortening or contracture, spasticity, muscle spasm, pain?

Are the major muscle components of less than normal strength?

Is deficiency present throughout the pattern, or is it most evident with relation to proximal, intermediate, or distal pivots?

Is a specific component of action more deficient than the other components, e.g., flexion, adduction, or external rotation of the hip in the flexion – adduction – external rotation pattern?

Is the performance of isometric contractions deficient?

Is a pattern more or less deficient than its directly antagonistic pattern, e.g., flexion – adduction – external rotation pattern of the lower extremity as compared with extension – abduction – internal rotation pattern of the same extremity?

Is imbalance most evident at proximal, intermediate, or distal pivots of action?

Is a pattern more or less deficient than its related pattern of the opposite diagonal, e.g., flexion – adduction – external rotation pattern as compared with flexion – abduction – internal rotation pattern of the same extremity? proximal, intermediate, or distal pivots?

Is a pattern more or less deficient than the antagonistic pattern of the opposite diagonal, e.g., flexion – adduction – external rotation pattern as compared with extension – adduction – external rotation pattern? proximal, intermediate, or distal pivots?

Plan of Approach

In order that abilities, deficiencies, and potentialities may be accurately disclosed, a systematic plan of approach is used. The following plan is general in nature and must be adapted for the individual patient. Contraindications for attempted full range of passive motion, active motion, or motion against resistance will necessarily alter the approach to evaluation.

The sequence of evaluation is from proximal to distal. The proximal parts and the function of these parts deserve first consideration since they are related to vital functions of the body. Whenever there is a possibility for deficiency of proximal function related to respiration, tongue motions, soft palate reactions, swallowing, and facial motions, these are evaluated first. Since the neck patterns are the key to the upper trunk, they receive the next consideration. The sequence of evaluation then proceeds as follows: upper trunk, upper extremities (proximal, intermediate, and distal pivots), lower trunk, lower extremities (proximal, intermediate, and distal pivots). See PNF Evaluation Forms: Sections 1 to 3.

Accurate evaluation requires considerable time and effort on the part of both the patient and the physical therapist. It may be necessary to devote several sessions to evaluation because of the time factor or the fatigue factor (physical therapists frequently tire before a patient will admit fatigue). The first session may be limited to evaluation of proximal parts and upper extremities. The second session may then be devoted to a brief review of the proximal parts and evaluation of the lower extremities.

Passive Movement

A specific pattern should first be checked for available range of passive motion. Limitation of range or excessive range should be noted for each pivot of motion and the part of the range where the variation becomes evident. The extremity patterns which demand complete lengthening of two-joint muscles should be compared with the pattern which does not require lengthening of these muscles. This comparison is necessary in order to determine the pivot of motion which is most limited. For example, evaluation of passive range of the flexion–adduction–external rotation pattern with reference to the hip pivot demands that the part be moved with the knee straight and the knee flexed. Unless this is done, normal length of the biceps femoris may mask a limitation in range of motion at the hip.

Passive movement of the part is performed in distal-to-proximal sequence. The distal pivots are moved into their shortened range, then intermediate pivots, then proximal pivots. Increased tension occurring at distal and intermediate pivots as the shortened range of the proximal pivot is approached should be noted. Such increase in tension may indicate intermediate and distal limitation. Movement may be repeated without demanding full range of the distal pivots in order to determine the degree to which distal tension limits proximal range of motion. This overlapping of tension is due to the topographical interrelationship of the major muscle components. Marked limitation of passive range of one pivot may influence passive range of the other pivots of motion. Excessive range of passive motion or hypermobility of a specific pivot of motion must also be noted and given due consideration in the treatment program.

Active Movement

The range of active motion of a specific pattern may be considered immediately following the evaluation of passive range. The patient should be instructed and asked to perform with all combinations of intermediate joint motion. Performance should be observed for variations in timing and range of active motion of each pivot of action. Comparison of active range and passive range should be made. Repetitions of performance may verify deficiencies or may reveal a lack of understanding by the patient of the physical therapist's instructions. Performance of a pattern against gravity may be considered as a basis for evaluation of active motion, and the patient may be positioned accordingly. Positioning must allow for the full range of motion to occur at the various pivots.

Resisted Movement

Unless contraindicated, maximal resistance may next be superimposed as a means of determining specific deficiencies. The patient should be required to perform with isotonic contraction through full range or as much range as possible, in accordance with normal timing, and should be required to perform an isometric contraction in the shortened range of the pattern. Resistance must be graded so as to permit normal timing to occur. Variations in timing, the range of motion of the specific pivots, and the strength of isotonic contraction and isometric contraction should be observed.

Facilitated Response

If the patient is unable to perform the full range of the pattern, or if a specific pivot fails to perform adequately, timing for emphasis and stretch stimulus may be used to determine potentials for increased response of the weaker pivots of action. The response of a weaker pivot during timing for emphasis should be compared with the response felt at this pivot when normal timing was performed against resistance. Increased response of a weaker pivot during timing for emphasis indicates potential for improvement, since overflow or reinforcement is apparently evident. This pivot may then be considered as a pivot for emphasis during the treatment program. If there is no increase in response of the weaker pivot during timing for emphasis, deficiency is great and emphasis of this pivot must be delayed until proximal parts, or the more proximal pivots, have been strengthened sufficiently to provide reinforcement for the weaker pivot.

DEVELOPMENTAL ACTIVITIES

Inasmuch as developmental activities are total patterns of movement with interaction of body segments, evaluation of the patient's abilities, disabilities, and potentials for performance is necessarily done on a gymnasium mat or in an open area. These activities demand space so that repetition of total patterns may be observed. In evaluation of the specific patterns of facilitation, interest is centered primarily upon one segment at a time. In evaluation of activities in the developmental sequence it is necessary to observe the total structure in a total pattern of movement. Furthermore, it is necessary to observe the coordination of component patterns. Having assessed the performance of patterns of facilitation, the therapist has gained a certain understanding of the patient's abilities and disabilities. This knowledge is useful in observation and assessment of a total pattern of movement.

In general, the objectives and the questions posed in evaluation of patterns of facilitation apply in evaluation of developmental activities. When the component patterns of a total pattern are individually assessed as patterns of facilitation, the information to be gained is the same. Yet the total pattern must be analyzed as a total pattern. The following questions should be raised during assessment of the three areas of use (mat activities, gait activities, and self-care activities):

Is the performance of a total pattern or activity in keeping with the developmental level of the subject, considering his chronological age?

Is the patient able to move in all directions? (See Table 1-6, Counterparts of Direction.)

If performance is inadequate, what are the major problems and areas of deficiency? Is performance limited by

Inability to respond to verbal commands or appropriate auditory stimuli, visual cues, or proprioceptive stimuli?

Generalized weakness, incoordination, spasticity, spasm, rigidity, pain, or multiple contractures?

Inadequacy of component patterns of head and neck, upper trunk and upper extremities, or lower trunk and lower extremities?

Inadequacy of ipsilateral component patterns, or of bilateral component patterns of upper or lower extremities?

Inadequacy of distal parts as compared with proximal parts?

Are those activities having flexor dominance more adequately performed than those activities having extensor dominance?

Is the maintenance of a balanced posture adequate or inadequate as compared with the ability to assume the position of balanced posture? Is the ability to move greater than the ability to sustain posture?

Considering the patient's ability to perform certain specific patterns of facilitation on the treatment table, is his ability to perform the same patterns during mat and gait activities more or less adequate?

Considering the patient's inability to perform certain specific patterns of facilitation on the treatment table, is he able or unable to perform the same patterns during mat and gait activities? Does alteration of position permit him to perform a certain pattern, that is, if he is unable to perform a certain pattern in the supine position, is he able or unable to perform in prone, lateral or sidelying, sitting, or standing positions?

Considering the patient's ability to perform a certain specific pattern of facilitation on a treatment table or during a mat activity, is he able to perform in a position of functional use? Is he able to combine and perform related component patterns necessary to a self-care activity?

Does the patient adequately reinforce his attempts to perform a total pattern of movement? Would external support for weak or inadequate segments permit him to better reinforce his attempts to move or to sustain posture?

Plan of Approach

The progression of activities as outlined in the developmental sequence, Table 1-8, serves as a guide for evaluation. Those activities which can best be performed on a mat should be evaluated as mat activities. Those related to gait may be performed on a mat, if possible, but severely disabled persons most often require the use of other equipment, such as wheelchairs, parallel bars, crutches, canes, braces, or assistive devices. Self-care activities should be assessed with the patient in a location appropriate to the activity: in bed; in his wheelchair, if he uses one; and in the bathroom. Special areas designated for practice of gait and self-care activities may be used for assessment, but the patient's specific problems may become more evident in the area where he actually lives, whether in hospital or at home.

Just as there is an overlapping between activities within the developmental sequence, so is there an overlapping of information gained by evaluation of various activities. The evaluator will learn which component patterns can be performed by the patient and those he cannot perform. She will interpret the patient's performance in relation to mat, gait, and self-care activities; sort and classify information about the patient; identify the patient's abilities and disabilities; seek realistic goals according to the patient's abilities and his potentials for increasing his abilities; and develop a plan of treatment for the patient or communicate as accurately as possible with those persons responsible for the planning and execution of the treatment program.

Detailed information gleaned by evaluation must be recorded for reference during program planning, for use as a guide in organizing a program, and for sharing with others responsible for the care of the patient.

The PNF Evaluation Forms (Figs. 5-1, 5-2, and 5-3) are intended to allow for interweaving of information about the patient's exercise program. Usually Section 1, Unilateral Patterns and Reinforcements (Fig. 5-1), should be completed first. Information recorded on Section 1 may be transferred or used in formulating Mat Activities, Section 2 (Fig. 5-2), and Pulley Program, Section 3 (Fig. 5-3). The Gradation of Responses key (opposite) will be most useful with Section 1 where grades (N,W,F,A) may be entered in the space following the numbered patterns. The acronyms listed below should be useful throughout.

(Text continues page 340)

GRADATION OF RESPONSES

N Pattern is performed in coordinate manner, actively, and then with good strength, against resistance. (Avoid use of stretch.)

W Overt voluntary response is present but weak, or range of movement is limited. (Do not enter W on chart; use ✓ and ⊘ as follows.)

F No overt voluntary response, but response can be facilitated.

A Voluntary response is absent and cannot be facilitated.

✓ In need of strengthening or increasing response, or increasing range.

⊘ In need of emphasis because of imbalance (stronger antagonist).

ACRONYMS

Reinforcements

BA	Bilateral asymmetrical
BS	Bilateral symmetrical
BR	Bilateral reciprocal
S,O	Same, opposite side
S,CD	Same, crossed diagonals
EH	Eyes follow hand(s)
HE	Hand(s) follow eyes

Range (R) for Initiation (I), Emphasis (E)

Le-RI, Le-RE	Lengthened
Mid-RI, Mid-RE	Middle
Sh-RI, Sh-RE	Shortened

Points in Range (R)

Le-R	Lengthened
Mid-R	Middle
Sh-R	Shortened

Total Patterns of Posture

Su	Supine
Pr	Prone
Sl	Sidelying
Si	Sitting
HK	Hands–knees
Kn	Kneeling
Sta	Standing

Directions

L	Left
R	Right
F	Forward
B	Backward
C	Circle
S	Sideward
DF	Diagonally forward
DB	Diagonally backward

Techniques

Ap	Approximation
CR	Contract–relax
HR	Hold–relax
HRA	Hold–relax–active motion
MC	Manual contact
MR	Maximal resistance
QR	Quick reversal
RC	Repeated contractions
RI	Rhythmic initiation
RRo	Rhythmic rotation
RS	Rhythmic stabilization
SR	Slow reversal
SRH	Slow reversal–hold
SRHR	Slow reversal–hold–relax
Str	Stretch
Str-R	Repetitive stretch
TE	Timing for emphasis
Tr	Traction

Diagonal Patterns

Upper Extremity

D1	fl	Flexion–adduction–external rotation
D1	ex	Extension–abduction–internal rotation
D2	fl	Flexion–abduction–external rotation
D2	ex	Extension–adduction–internal rotation

Lower Extremity

D1	fl	Flexion–adduction–external rotation
D1	ex	Extension–abduction–internal rotation
D2	fl	Flexion–abduction–internal rotation
D2	ex	Extension–adduction–external rotation

FIG. 5-1

PNF EVALUATION FORM, SECTION 1

Patient _____ Diagnosis _____ _____ M.D. Therapist _____ Date: _____

Unilateral Patterns and Reinforcements   Total Patterns of Movement and Posture

HEAD and NECK:	L	R	NOTE:
1. Fl, diag			Total patterns: (Indicate pattern numbers and total patterns or position to be used.)
2. Ex, "			Mat and pulley programs: (Indicate pattern numbers and reinforcements, BA, BS, etc.)
3. Rotation			

UPPER TRUNK:		L	R	Total patterns:
1. Fl, diag, arms BA ex				
2. Ex, " arms BA fl				
3. Rotation, arm(s) D1				
4. Resp:di( ) lch( ) st( )				Mats: Pulleys:

			NECK		ARM								ARMS		Total patterns:
	L	R	S	O	D1 fl		D1 ex		D2 fl		D2 ex		BA		
					S	O	S	O	S	O	S	O	S	O	
LOWER TRUNK:															
1. Fl, knees str															
2. Ex, knees str															
3. Fl, knees fl															
4. Ex, knees ex															
5. Fl, knees ex															
6. Ex, knees fl															
7. Rotation															Mats: Pulleys:

UPPER EXTREMITIES

Scapula, L __ R __ D1 _____ D2 _____

(Indicate nos. of shoulder patterns, reinforcements and position.)

SHOULDER:	L	R	BS	BA	BR		NECK		Total patterns:
					S	CD	S	O	
1. D1, fl; elb str									
2. D1, ex; " "									
3. D2, fl; elb str									
4. D2, ex; " "									
5. D1, fl; elb fl									
6. D1, ex; " ex									
7. D2, fl; elb fl									
8. D2, ex; " ex									
9. D1, fl; elb ex									
10. D1, ex; " fl									
11. D2, fl; elb ex									
12. D2, ex; " fl									Mats: Pulleys:

Total patterns:
Thrusting: D1, L __ R __ ; D2, L __ R __
Forearm: D1, sup, L __ R __ ; D1, pro, L __ R __
             D2, " L __ R __ ; D2, " L __ R __

ELBOW:	L	R	BS	BA	S	CD	S	O
1. Fl; D1, fl								
2. Ex; D1, ex								
3. Fl; D2, fl								
4. Ex; D2, ex								
5. Fl; D1, ex								
6. Ex; D1, fl								
7. Fl; D2, ex								
8. Ex; D2, fl								

Mats: Pulleys:

Thrusting: D1, L ___ R ___; D2, L ___ R ___

Total patterns:

WRIST:	L	R	BS	BA	BR S	BR CD	NECK S	NECK O
1. Fl; D1, fl								
2. Ex; D1, ex								
3. Fl; D2, ex								
4. ex; D2, fl								
HAND:								
1. Close, D1								
2. Open, D1								
3. Open, D2								
4. Close, D2								

Hand, individual digits:

Mats: Pulleys:

LOWER EXTREMITIES					BR	NECK		
HIP:	L	R	BS	BA	S	CD	S	O
1. D1, fl; knee str								
2. D1, ex; " "								
3. D2, fl; knee str								
4. D2, ex; " "								
5. D1, fl; knee fl								
6. D1, ex; " ex								
7. D2, fl; knee fl								
8. D2, ex; " ex								
9. D1, fl; knee ex								
10. D1, ex; " fl								
11. D2, fl; knee ex								
12. D2, ex; " fl								

Total patterns:

Mats: Pulleys:

KNEE:	L	R	BS	BA	BR S	BR CD	NECK S	NECK O
1. Fl; D1, fl								
2. Ex; D1, ex								
3. Fl; D2, fl								
4. Ex; D2, ex								
5. Fl; D1, ex								
6. Ex; D1, fl								
7. Fl; D2, ex								
8. Ex; D2, fl								

Total patterns:

Mats: Pulleys:

ANKLE and TOES:	L	R	BS	BA	BR S	BR CD	NECK S	NECK O
1. Dorsifl; D1, fl								
2. Pl flex; D1, ex								
3. Dorsifl; D2, fl								
4. Pl flex; D2, ex								

Total patterns:

Foot, individual digits:

Mats: Pulleys:

(Based on form used at Kabat-Kaiser Institutes, 1951.)

FIG. 5-2

PNF EVALUATION FORM, SECTION 2

Date: _____

Patient_____ Diagnosis _____ M.D. Therapist _____

Mat Activities: Facilitation of Total Patterns*

Total Patterns	Directions	Head and Neck	Techniques	Manual Contacts	Range; balance; assistance; equipment; individual patterns, Section 1
1. Rolling toward a. prone b. supine					
2. Lower trunk a. rotation b. elevation					
3. Prone Progression a. crawl b. circle-pivot c. on elbows d. creep e. plantigrade					
4. Rise and sit a. side-sit b. long-sit c. chair-sit					
5. Rise and kneel a. heel-sit b. hands-knees					
6. Rise and stand a. plantigrade b. kneeling c. chair-sit					
7. Walking a. level b. ramp c. stairs					
8. Run, skip, jump					
9. Other					

* To indicate those activities a patient should practice independently but with supervision, place an S in upper left corner of right-hand column. Incorporate suggestions noted in Section 1.

See Acronyms. Use ✓ and ⊘ where appropriate.

FIG. 5-3

PNF EVALUATION FORM, SECTION 3

Date: _____

Patient _____ Diagnosis _____ M.D. Therapist _____

Gym Activities: Supervised: Pulley Program

Patterns,* Combinations	Body Position Level & Weight**	Patterns,* Combinations	Body Position Level & Weight**
Upper Trunk 1. L, R, Arms BA 2. L, R, Arms BA 3. L, R, Arms, BA		Lower Extremities Hip(s) BA BS BR 1. L, R __ __ __ 2. L, R __ __ __ 3. L, R __ __ __ 4. L, R __ __ __ 5. L, R __ __ __ 6. L, R __ __ __ 7. L, R __ __ __ 8. L, R __ __ __ 9. L, R __ __ __ 10. L, R __ __ __ 11. L, R __ __ __ 12. L, R __ __ __	
Lower Trunk 1. L, R, Head, S, O 2. L, R, Head, S, O 3. L, R, Head, S, O			
Upper Extremities Shoulder(s) BA BS BR 1. L, R __ __ __ 2. L, R __ __ __ 3. L, R __ __ __ 4. L, R __ __ __ 5. L, R __ __ __ 6. L, R __ __ __ 7. L, R __ __ __ 8. L, R __ __ __ 9. L, R __ __ __ 10. L, R __ __ __ 11. L, R __ __ __ 12. L, R __ __ __		Knee(s) 1. L, R __ __ __ 2. L, R __ __ __ 3. L, R __ __ __ 4. L, R __ __ __ 5. L, R __ __ __ 6. L, R __ __ __ 7 .L, R __ __ __ 8. L, R __ __ __	
Elbow(s) 1. L, R __ __ __ 2. L, R __ __ __ 3. L, R __ __ __ 4. L, R __ __ __ 5. L, R __ __ __ 6. L, R __ __ __ 7. L, R __ __ __ 8. L, R __ __ __		Ankle(s) 1. L, R __ __ __ 2. L, R __ __ __ 3. L, R __ __ __ 4. L, R __ __ __	

Precautions: _____

* Section 1 for identification of unilateral patterns.

** Level of Pulleys: O Overhead; S Shoulder; F Floor

See Acronyms. Use ✓ and ⊘ where appropriate.

PNF EVALUATION FORMS: SECTIONS 1 TO 3   339

The diagnosis, indications for treatment, and goals of treatment are established by the member of the medical profession who is responsible for the patient. Exercise programs are planned with regard for the diagnosis, indications, and contraindications for exercise. Goals or objectives of treatment as established by the physician are usually general in nature. The overall objective of an exercise program is to hasten recovery of normal function, to attempt to establish or reestablish optimum function as quickly as possible. Given these facts, specific areas and pivots for emphasis must be established, and techniques must be selected as a means of helping to achieve or surpass the goals as outlined by the physician. The patient may be treated on a mat rather than on a table since resistance, repeated contractions, and reversal techniques may then be superimposed upon total patterns of movement of the developmental sequence. In this way initial power may be developed, and stimulation of mass patterns of flexion and extension may be achieved. A therapeutic pool provides an excellent opportunity for treatment of selected adult patients, since combinations of trunk motions may be performed with the body weight free of hard surface contact. Treatment in water enables the physical therapist to handle the adult patient as if he were a small child. Thus, the patient may be treated in whatever environment is appropriate for his condition and his needs.

AREAS FOR EMPHASIS

Selection of areas of emphasis and specific pivots of emphasis is based upon the evaluation of the patient, which provided an impression of the patient's abilities, deficiencies, and potentialities. Emphasis in treatment means that more time and effort is directed toward certain areas of the body or pivots of action than toward other areas or pivots of action. Shifting of emphasis from one pattern to another pattern and from one area of the body to another area serves the first area as recuperative motion and the second area as stimulation of neuromuscular response. In line with the process of development, selection of areas and pivots for emphasis is from proximal to distal. Any deficiency of proximal parts receives the first emphasis. As these parts improve, they provide reinforcement for the extremities. The proximal pivots of the extremities receive next emphasis, and then the more distal pivots. Available power in the distal parts may be used to reinforce weaker proximal pivots, but the emphasis is still proximal. If generalized weakness exists, the sequence from proximal to distal is mandatory.

If the neck, trunk, and extremities all present marked deficiency, the treatment program will include all combinations of neck, upper trunk, and lower trunk patterns. Consideration should be given to correction of imbalances, but the stronger patterns must be used as reinforcement of the weaker patterns. If a patient presents trunk deficiencies but has some available power in the extremities, the extremity patterns that are most closely related to the trunk patterns may be used as reinforcement.

If a patient presents greater strength in the lower trunk and limbs than he does in the upper trunk, neck, and upper extremities, the lower extremities and lower trunk are used to reinforce the upper trunk and neck. The upper trunk and neck are the areas for emphasis until such time that they will reinforce the upper extremities in their related patterns. The stronger lower extremities may be used to reinforce the upper extremities if such reinforcement enhances the response of the upper extremity pivots. It is frequently possible to achieve greater response of the neck and upper trunk by reinforcement of the lower extremities, if the patient is treated in a standing position. The patient automatically reinforces resisted motions of the neck and upper trunk by employing postural and righting reflexes. Rhythmic stabilization, reversal techniques, and repeated contractions for emphasis may be used with resistance applied to the head and neck.

A patient whose deficiencies are confined to one upper extremity has many potentials for reinforcement. Emphasis on the scapular motions or the proximal pivot is mandatory since scapular stability is essential to total function of the shoulder. The neck and opposite upper extremities provide the ideal reinforcements. The patient may be treated in any position that allows for performance of the desired patterns.

The above examples are given as a means of emphasizing the importance of proximal stimulation and the use of stronger areas as reinforcement for weaker areas. Areas for emphasis do not preclude overall stimulation. When large combinations of patterns are performed, mass stimulation occurs through irradiation and overflow. An extremity that presents response, however minimal, deserves stimulation, but that extremity cannot be considered as an area for emphasis if the trunk is also grossly deficient.

PIVOTS FOR EMPHASIS

The selection of specific pivots for emphasis proximal to distal. In the extremities, the should dle and hip receive first emphasis, then the inte diate and distal pivots. A balance of power betwe antagonistic patterns is of paramount importance, and imbalances are also corrected from proximal to distal. If the scapular motion is weak in the extension–abduction – internal rotation pattern and all other scapular motions are strong, the weak scapular motion is the first pivot for emphasis to be considered in the entire extremity. It is futile to emphasize weak opposition of the thumb unless any deficiency of internal rotation of the shoulder has been corrected. Opposition of the thumb is primarily a motion of rotation, and reinforcement for this distal rotation is dependent upon intrinsic internal rotation of the shoulder.

SELECTION OF TECHNIQUES

Selection of techniques cannot be made on an arbitrary basis except in relation to contraindications for a specific technique. Application of stretch stimulus is obviously contraindicated in the early treatment of fractures and postoperative conditions. Decision about a choice of techniques must be based upon the patient's response to that technique. The technique that facilitates a desired response to the greatest degree is the technique of choice. In general, if a patient needs to develop his ability to move, techniques that use isotonic contraction of muscle are employed; if he needs to develop postural control, techniques for isometric contraction are used. Coordinated performance of reversal of antagonists, through the full range of the patterns with normal power, is a response of the normal subject. Use of this technique should be a goal if it cannot be used initially. Decision on reinforcements, either of one pivot of action by another pivot of action, or one pattern by another pattern, must be based upon the relationship of the pattern, the available power, and the response of the reinforced pivot or pattern. Reinforcement may be limited to the use of stronger pivots of action within the weaker pattern of a single extremity, if imbalances within the pattern are so great that control of the motion requires both hands of the physical therapist. As soon as control of the part is possible, a larger combination of motion may be used.

In order that patient progress may proceed at an optimum rate the physical therapist should consider the following:

Proximal deficiencies should be corrected first, since proximal power provides more effective reinforcement.

Development of a balance of power in relation to all patterns and all pivots of action is of paramount importance. A balance of power implies adequate performance of isotonic and isometric contractions of antagonistic patterns.

Reinforcements should be selected in accordance with the increase in response they provide.

Correction and prevention of imbalances should be considered, but stronger motions must be used to stimulate weaker motions.

Wise selection of pivots for emphasis and rein-

forcement will prevent increase of imbalances. Selection of reinforcements may be influenced by the physical therapist's ability to control the combination of motions.

The choice of a technique should be determined by the patient's response. Arbitrary selection is undesirable except as indicated by contraindications.

Frequent reevaluation of the patient is essential, so that new areas of emphasis may be included and unnecessary ones eliminated.

Figure 5-4 is a sample form for planning a treatment program.

INTEGRATION OF ACTIVITIES

For optimum development or restoration of a patient's neuromuscular abilities, coordination of various phases of treatment is necessary. All activities must be integrated and directed toward the goals set for the individual patient. Goals may be expressed in terms of gait or self-care abilities, but the means to their accomplishment may be treatment on a table or on a mat, or in performance of mat class and pulley class activities.

Carefully selected activities are performed in the location that permits the patient to put forth maximum effort in order to learn at an optimum rate. Economy of the therapist's effort and time are factors. Performance of developmental activities on a mat may contribute more in less time than will performance of limited activities on a treatment table. Intensive emphasis on a specific pattern of facilitation during treatment on a table may produce a better gait pattern than will practice of a less adequate pattern during walking. Resisted plantigrade walking on a mat may more readily promote lengthening of posterior structures than will repeated and laborious attempts to relax hamstring muscles when the patient is lying supine on a table. Thus, integration of activities requires that goals be established, and that the proper time and the proper place be determined for emphasis of those activities that will hasten the patient's motor learning and integrate his neuromuscular abilities.

Integration of activities must extend beyond the physical therapy program.[47] In-bed activities on the ward, occupational therapy projects, recreational activities, and any other activity must be directed toward the goals established for the individual patient. Clearly defined long-term goals give direction. Specifically described short-term goals have the same direction but are phases of advancement. Long-term goals may have to be altered, raised, or lowered as the patient's potentialities become clearer. Short-term goals require constant alteration in keeping with the patient's status and his progress. A goal is a challenge to the patient and to the staff.

FIG. 5-4

PLANNING A TREATMENT PROGRAM

Patient: _____ Age _____ Onset _____ Today's Date _____

Diagnosis and primary problem: _____

A. Deficiency of vital functions: _____

B. Level of performance of total patterns: _____

   (Highest level: independence, coordination) _____

C. Mode of performance of total patterns of self-care, gait, and transfer activities: (Indicate type and degree of assistance

   including devices.) _____

_____

D. Mat work, total patterns to be emphasized to improve:

   Vital functions _____

   Self-care   _____

   Gait pattern   _____

   Transfer   _____

E. Table work, combining movements to be used to improve:

   Vital functions _____

   Self-care   _____

   Gait pattern   _____

   Transfer   _____

F. Unilateral patterns to be reinforced and emphasized to improve:

   Head and neck: flexion, L/R ____; extension, L/R ____; rotation, L/R ____

   Upper Trunk: flexion, L/R ____; extension, L/R ____; rotation, L/R ____

   Lower Trunk: flexion, L/R ____; extension, L/R ____; rotation, L/R ____

   Upper Extremity, L/R: Scapula ____, shoulder ____, elbow ____, forearm ____

                Wrist   ____, hand   ____, fingers ____, thumb ____

                D1: flexion ____, extension ____

                D2: flexion ____, extension ____

   Lower extremity, L/R: Hip ____, knee ____, ankle ____, foot ____

                D1: flexion ____, extension ____

                D2: flexion ____, extension ____

G. Suggestions for gait program: _____

_____

H. Suggestions for self-care program: _____

_____

I. Suggestions for pulley and self-conducted mat or home program:

_____

J. Major emphasis: mobility ____, stability ____, strength ____, endurance ____, timing ____

K. Techniques of choice: _____

_____

L. Additional comments: _____

_____

_____

SUGGESTIONS FOR TEACHING

6

PRACTICE AND MOTOR LEARNING

The motor learning process includes practice or repetition of the task to be learned. This is true of the infant learning to creep, of the youth learning to play tennis, of the patient learning or relearning the total patterns of self-care, gait, and work activities, and of the student learning to teach the patient.

Psychologists have studied and compared types of practice and rates of learning.[3] They have considered whole-task practice and part-task practice, which has been divided into forms such as pure part, progressive part, and repetitive part task. The use of the whole-task method has many advocates, especially among psychologists whose research problems have involved manipulative motor tasks. Trainers of athletes and teachers of sport skills, on the other hand, have relied largely upon part-task methods. Sport skills are essentially total patterns; the total structure is in action. Manipulative acts require repetitive use of fine movements; sport skills require repetitive use of gross movements. The patient who is to learn or relearn the motor tasks necessary to daily life needs to learn manipulative tasks such as feeding and dressing, and gross activities such as rising from bed and walking.

In training the patient to walk, the physical therapist has most surely used the whole-task method, and has used a part-task method when, for example, teaching the patient to shift his weight from one foot to the other. Beyond the teaching method of telling the patient and showing him what to do and how to do it, in the PNF method precise use of manual contacts and resistance are applied to hasten the patient's learning of a motor task. The whole-task type of practice is used with emphasis given to various phases and steps or parts within the task.[15]

The term *stepwise procedures* is descriptive of the emphasis of a part of the task during performance of the whole. An example of the use of stepwise procedures follows.

Whole task: Rising to standing from a wheelchair
Phases of the task: Total flexion followed by total extension, shifting from flexor dominance to extensor dominance
Steps or parts of the task, preparatory for rising: Placement of hands, or one hand, on arms (arm) of chair; locking brakes and lifting footrests; placement of feet to receive body weight; rocking and shifting weight forward in seat of chair
Steps or parts of the task, rising to standing: Flexion of head, neck, trunk, hips, and knees; extension of head, neck, trunk, hips, and knees

Preparatory steps may be trained by the part-task method, that is, several repetitions may be used to accomplish each step. Resistance is graded and serves to guide the patient's performance.

Rising to standing is the total pattern, the whole

task. As a stepwise procedure, the flexor phase may be repeated against resistance so as to increase the range and the degree of stretch of the extensor muscle groups. Without interruption or delay, the resistance, and the patient's effort, are shifted to the extensor phase. Repetitions and reversal of direction may be demanded at various points in the range.

The therapist's manual contact with the patient must be appropriate for his needs. The higher the level of contact (head and shoulder girdle as compared with pelvic girdle), the greater is the challenge to the patient and the lesser is the therapist's ability to control and protect the patient.

Facilitation techniques are selected according to the patient's needs. Those which may be appropriate and coupled with the use of stretch and resistance are slow reversal–hold, rhythmic stabilization, repeated contractions, and approximation.

As the patient's performance becomes smooth and coordinated, and of appropriate rate, repetitions for emphasis and the use of stepwise procedures become superfluous. The patient may have need to perform against resistance so as to promote the development of strength and endurance.

The PNF approach to teaching and training the patient also applies in the teaching and training of students who must become teachers of patients.

VARYING PRACTICE

Although repetition is a necessary ingredient of motor learning, its principal effect is to develop or establish habit patterns that do not require voluntary effort but rather occur automatically in performance of a motor task. In stepwise procedures, emphasis of a part of the whole task, repetition is used to teach, to improve strength and endurance, to develop skills, and to enhance the quality of performance. Repetition is practice. In a sense, the use of stepwise procedures is a form of varying practice.[49] The part of the task that was emphasized (practiced) is immediately used to proceed to the next step in the whole task. Repetition to the point of boredom or fatigue does not occur.

Varying practice is useful in, for example, gait training in the parallel bars. Several whole tasks are necessary: rising to standing; walking forward, backward, and stepping sideward by use of braiding*; turning or backing to wheelchair; and lowering to sitting.

The first task of rising to standing, facilitated by stepwise procedures coupled with stretch and resistance, should be given a "repeat performance." Following the sequence of activities in the parallel bars, the

---

* Example of braiding: The stronger side leads. Face and grasp one rail of the bars with both hands. Stepping or braiding to the right requires this sequence: L foot, D1 fl; R foot, D2 fl; L foot, D2 ex; R foot, D1 ex.

act of rising to standing may show marked improvement. Facilitation and varying practice (stepwise procedures, stretch and resistance, and change in activity) should have contributed to learning.

In the PNF method varying practice also includes combining patterns for reinforcement. The use of the opposite extremity, or the ipsilateral, or contralateral extremities provides reinforcement and reversal of fatigue. See Recuperative Motion.

The 2 × 2 Rule

In teaching students, working in pairs, varying practice follows the 2 × 2 rule. In teaching skills such as resisted rolling from supine toward prone using manual contacts at shoulder girdle and pelvis with techniques applied in sequence, the 2 × 2 rule is effective. The following sequence is an example:

Stretch, resist, hold at sidelying, stabilize (RS); emphasize (RC) shoulder (upper trunk), then pelvis (lower trunk), and reverse from sidelying to supine. Repeat the entire sequence once. Then, do the same sequence toward the opposite side, and repeat.

Next, the "therapist" becomes the "patient" for 2 × 2. This rule stresses the mind more than the body. Concentration is necessary, as in learning sport skills. The 2 × 2 change in activity reverses or avoids boredom and fatigue. Students become stimulated and eager to practice on their own.

Drilling is incompatible with the 2 × 2 rule. Instead of practicing a single technique many times, an appropriate sequence of three or four techniques should be taught as they might be used with a patient. A combination for a patient having pain would be RS, SRH, SR, and, as pain decreases, RC for strength and endurance throughout the range of motion. For patients having paresis Str, MR, and RC should be practiced. Changing the direction of a total pattern, changing to another activity, or shifting from one technique to another are ways of varying practice. Yet another is changing partners.

To apply the 2 × 2 rule with success requires that students be monitored closely, which, in turn, requires that there is a teaching assistant for each three pairs of students. Assistant instructors could include recent graduates who may welcome a review and an opportunity to teach.

The principal instructor should demonstrate each activity before the entire group, or should direct the demonstration using an assistant. Major points should be emphasized: position of therapist, placement of hands, and tracking or moving as the "patient" moves.

The principal instructor then monitors the group

and, as necessary, calls for attention to demonstrate correction of errors in performance. This is done in a positive way. That is, two of the best performers are asked to demonstrate. Thus, embarrassment is avoided along with the need to correct more errors. Time is saved.

If an assistant instructor finds it necessary to demonstrate to six students, it is likely that the entire class may benefit. Again, the principal instructor may direct or perform, or the assistant may do so. After a demonstration, the 2×2 rule applies. Practical application and correct practice are essential.

In teaching, "looking and seeing" is a skill. In order for the instructors to quickly identify the error — faulty manual contacts, incorrect posture and movement of the "therapist" — students must be positioned in an organized way. For example, pairs of students working on mats should have heads in the same position. Then, instructors can observe and correct errors far more readily. Little is to be gained if the student repeats an error four times, then is corrected, and performs correctly only three times. Rarely is the novice able to correct her own performance.

In summary, varying practice contributes to motor learning and provides a way to teach, a way to learn, and a way to treat.

REFERENCES AND SUGGESTED READING

REFERENCES FOR THE INTRODUCTION

1. Bouman HD (ed): Proceedings: An Exploratory and Analytical Survey of Therapeutic Exercise, Northwestern University. Am J Phys Med 46:3–1191, 1967
2. Dorland WAN: The Illustrated Medical Dictionary, 24th ed. Philadelphia, WB Saunders, 1965
3. Kabat H, Knott M: Proprioceptive facilitation technics for treatment of paralysis. Phys Ther Rev 33:53, 1953
4. Knott M: Neuromuscular facilitation in the child with central nervous system deficit. Phys Ther 46:721, 1966
5. Knott M: In the groove. Phys Ther 53:365, 1973
6. Knott M: Obituary. APTA Progress Report, February 1979
7. Knott M, Voss DE: Proprioceptive Neuromuscular Facilitation: Patterns and Techniques, 2nd ed. New York, Harper & Row, 1968
8. Legg AT, Merrill JB: Physical therapy in infantile paralysis. In Principles and Practice of Physical Therapy. Hagerstown, WF Prior Company, 1932
9. Simonds HC: The Inside Story: Kabat-Kaiser Institute. Vallejo, CA, Kabat-Kaiser Institute Publishers, 1951
10. Voss DE: Everything is there before you discover it. Phys Ther 62:1617, 1982

REFERENCES

1. Åstrand P, Rodahl K: Textbook of Work Physiology, 2nd ed, p 98. New York, McGraw-Hill, 1977
2. Buchwald JS: Exteroceptive reflexes and movement. Am J Phys Med 46:121, 1967
3. Cross KD: Role of practice in perceptual-motor learning. Am J Phys Med 46:487, 1967
4. Day MJ: Hypersensitive response to ice massage: Report of a case. Phys Ther 54:592, 1974
5. Diamond J: Your Body Doesn't Lie, p 161. New York, Warner Books, 1980
6. Dorland WAN: The Illustrated Medical Dictionary, 24th ed. Philadelphia, WB Saunders, 1965
7. Freeman JT: Posture in the aging and aged body. JAMA 165:843, 1957
8. Geldard FA: Some neglected possibilities of communication. Science 131:1583, 1960
9. Gellhorn E: Patterns of muscular activity in man. Arch Phys Med Rehabil 28:568, 1947
10. Gesell A: The Embryology of Early Motor Behavior. New York, Harper & Brothers, 1952
11. Gesell A, Amatruda CS: Developmental Diagnosis, 2nd ed. New York, Hoeber, 1947
12. Gray H: In Goss CM (ed): Anatomy of the Human Body, 27th ed., pp 32–46. Philadelphia, Lea & Febiger, 1959
13. Hagbarth KE: Excitatory and inhibitory skin areas for flexor and extensor motoneurones. ACTA Physiol Scand 26 (Suppl 94):1, 1952
14. Hagbarth KE, Eklund G: The effects of muscle vibration in spasticity, rigidity, and cerebellar disorders. J Neurol Neurosurg Psychiatry 31:207, 1968
15. Harlow HF, Harlow MR: Principles of primate learning. In The Spastics Society: Lessons from Animal Behavior, Little Club Clinics in Developmental Medicine, No. 7. London, Heinemann, 1962
16. Harrison VF: A review of the neuromuscular bases for motor learning. Research Quarterly 33:59, 1962
17. Hellebrandt FA: Physiology. In Delorme TL, Watkins AL: Progressive Resistance Exercise. New York, Appleton-Century-Crofts, 1951
18. Hellebrandt FA: Application of the overload principle to muscle training in man. Am J Phys Med 37:278, 1958

19. Hellebrandt FA, Houtz SJ, Eubank RNL: Influence of alternate and reciprocal exercise on work capacity. Arch Phys Med Rehabil 32:766, 1951

20. Hellebrandt FA, Houtz SJ, Hockman DE et al: Physiological effect of simultaneous static and dynamic exercise. Am J Phys Med 35:106, 1956

21. Hellebrandt FA, Schade M, Carns ML: Methods of evoking tonic neck reflexes in normal human subjects. Am J Phys Med 41:90, 1962

22. Hellebrandt FA, Waterland JC: Indirect learning: The influence of unimanual exercise on related muscle groups of the same and opposite side. Am J Phys Med 41:45, 1962

23. Hooker D: The Prenatal Origin of Behavior. Porter Lectures, Series 18. Lawrence, University of Kansas Press, 1952

24. Humphrey T: The trigeminal nerve in relation to early human fetal activity. Res Publ Assoc Res Nerv Ment Dis 33:127, 1954

25. Jacobs M: The development of normal motor behavior. Am J Phys Med 46:41, 1967

26. Kabat H: Analysis and therapy of cerebellar ataxia and asynergia. Arch Neurol Psychiatry 74:375, 1955

27. Kabat H: Proprioceptive facilitation in therapeutic exercise. In Licht S (ed): Therapeutic Exercise, 2nd ed. New Haven, E Licht, 1961

28. Kabat H, Knott M: Proprioceptive facilitation technics for treatment of paralysis. Phys Ther Rev 33:53, 1953

29. Kabat H, McLeod M, Holt C: Practical application of proprioceptive neuromuscular facilitation. Physiotherapy 45:87, 1959

30. Kimura D: Asymmetry of the human brain. Sci Am 228:70, 1973

31. Kravitz H, Goldenberg D, Neyhus A: Tactual exploration by normal infants. Dev Med Child Neurol 20:720, 1978

32. Levine MG, Knott M, Kabat H: Relaxation of spasticity by electrical stimulation of antagonistic muscles. Arch Phys Med Rehabil 33:668, 1952

33. Levine MG, Kabat H, Knott M, Voss DE: Relaxation of spasticity by physiological technics. Arch Phys Med Rehabil 35:214, 1954

34. Loomis JE, Boersma FJ: Training right brain-damaged patients in a wheelchair task: Case studies using verbal mediation. Can J Physiotherapy 34:204, 1982

35. McGraw MB: The Neuromuscular Maturation of the Human Infant. New York, Columbia University Press, 1943 (Reprinted edition: New York, Hafner Publishing Company, 1962)

36. Mead S: Personal communication, 1963

37. Morris W (ed): The American Heritage Dictionary. Boston/New York, Houghton Mifflin, 1969

38. Nicholas JA, Melvin M, Saraniti AJ: Neurophysiologic inhibition of strength following tactile stimulation of the skin. Am J Sports Med 8:181, 1980

39. O'Connell AL, Gardner EB: Ingredients of coordinate movement. Am J Phys Med 46:334, 1967

40. Peele TL: The Neuroanatomical Basis for Clinical Neurology. New York, McGraw-Hill, 1954

41. Robinson ME, Doudlah AM, Waterland JC: The influence of vision on the performance of a motor act. Am J Occup Ther 19:202, 1965

42. Rood MS: Neurophysiological mechanisms utilized in the treatment of neuromuscular dysfunction. Am J Occup Ther 10:220, 1956

43. Safranek MG, Koshland GF, Raymond G: Effect of auditory rhythm on muscle activity. Phys Ther 62:161, 1982

44. Sherrington C: The Integrative Action of the Nervous System, p. 340. New Haven, Yale University Press, 1961

45. Smith KU, Henry JF: Cybernetic foundations for rehabilitation. Am J Phys Med 46:379, 1967

46. Toussaint D, Knott M: The use of wall pulleys with mat activities. Phys Ther Rev 35:477, 1955

47. Voss DE: Proprioceptive neuromuscular facilitation: Application of patterns and techniques in occupational therapy. Am J Occup Ther 13:191, 1959

48. Waterland JC, Munson N: Involuntary patterning evoked by exercise stress. J Am Phys Ther Assoc 44:91, 1964

49. Williams ID: Evidence for recognition and recall schemata. J Motor Behavior 10:45, 1978 (Personal communication, Sept 30, 1980, regarding "To learn skills: Vary practice." Physiotherapy Canada 32:238, 1980)

References for Part 4: Coupling PNF and Joint Mobilization

50. Freeman MAR, Wyke BD: Articular contributions to limb muscle reflexes: The effects of partial neurectomy of the knee-joint on postural reflexes. Br J Surg 53:61–68, 1966

51. Freeman MAR, Wyke BD: Articular reflexes at the ankle joint: an electromyographic study of normal and abnormal influences of ankle–joint mechanoreceptors upon reflex activity in the leg muscles. Br J Surg 54:990–1001, 1967

52. Grieve GP: Common Vertebral Joint Problems, pp 384–387. London, Churchill Livingstone, 1981

53. Knott M, Voss DE: Proprioceptive Neuromuscular Facilitation: Patterns and Techniques, 2nd ed, pp 193–196. New York, Harper & Row, 1968

54. Maitland GD: Peripheral Manipulation, 2nd ed, pp 32–44; 45–60. London, Butterworth & Co, 1978

55. Wyke BD: Articular neurology: A review. Physiotherapy 58:94–99, 1972

SUGGESTED READING

Basic Information

Neurophysiology

Ashworth B, Grimby L, Kugelberg E: Comparison of voluntary and reflex activation of motor units: functional organization of motor neurones. J Neurol Neurosurg Psychiatry 30:91, 1967

Bouman HD: Some considerations of muscle activity. J Am Phys Ther Assoc 45:431–436, 1965

Bouman HD: Some considerations of the physiology of sensation. J Am Phys Ther Assoc 45:573–577, 1965

Brooks VB: Motor control: How posture and movement are governed. Phys Ther 63:664, 1983

Cohen LA: Role of eye and neck proprioceptive mechanisms in body orientation and motor coordination. J Neurophysiol 24:1, 1961

DENNY-BROWN D: Motor mechanisms — Introduction: The general principles of motor integration. In Field J, Magoun HW, Hall VE (eds): Handbook of Physiology, Section 1: Neurophysiology, Vol II, Chap 32. Washington, D.C., American Physiological Society, 1960

ELDRED E: The dual sensory role of muscle spindles. J Am Phys Ther Assoc 45:290–313, 1965

ELDRED E: Postural integration at spinal levels. J Am Phys Ther Assoc 45:332–344, 1965

ELDRED E: Posture and locomotion. In Field J, Magoun HW, Hall VE (eds): Handbook of Physiology, Section 1: Neurophysiology, Vol. II, Chap 41. Washington, D.C., American Physiological Society, 1960

FISCHER E: Neurophysiology a physical therapist should know. Phys Ther Rev 38:741–748, 1958

FISCHER E: Physiological basis of methods to elicit, reinforce, and coordinate muscle movement. Phys Ther Rev 38:468–473, 1958

FISCHER E: Physiological basis of volitional movement. Phys Ther Rev 38:405–412, 1958

GRANIT R: Receptors and Sensory Perception. New Haven, Yale University Press, 1962

GRIFFIN JW: Use of proprioceptive stimuli in therapeutic exercise. Phys Ther 54:1072, 1974

HARRISON VF: Review of skeletal muscle. Review of sensory receptors in skeletal muscles with special emphasis on the muscle spindle. Review of motor unit. Phys Ther Rev 41:17–40, 1961

LIPPOLD O: Physiological tremor. Sci Am 224:65, 1971

PAILLARD J: The patterning of skilled movement. In Field J, Magoun HW, Hall VE (eds): Handbook of Physiology, Section 1: Neurophysiology, Vol III, Chap 67. Washington, DC, American Physiological Society, 1960

RALSTON HJ: Recent advances in neuromuscular physiology. Am J Phys Med 36:94–120, 1957

RALSTON HJ: Some considerations of the physiological basis of therapeutic exercise. Phys Ther Rev 38:465–468, 1958

SCHADE JP: Neuromuscular integration. Prog Phys Ther 1:3, 1970

SCHOLZ JP, CAMPBELL SK: Muscle spindles and the regulation of movement. Phys Ther 60:1416, 1980

TWITCHELL TE: Attitudinal reflexes. J Am Phys Ther Assoc 45:411–418, 1965

Motor Development

AMES LB: Individuality of motor development. J Am Phys Ther Assoc 46:121–127, 1966

BOWER TGR: A Primer of Development. San Francisco, WH Freeman, 1977

GESELL A: Behavior patterns of fetal-infant and child. In Genetics and the inheritance of integrated neurological and psychiatric patterns. Proc Assoc Research Nerv Ment Dis 33:114–123, 1954

GESELL A, AMATRUDA CS: The Embryology of Behavior. New York, Harper, 1945

HELLEBRANDT, FA, RARICK L, GLASGOW R, CARNS ML: Physiological analysis of basic motor skills. I. Growth and development of jumping. Am J Phys Med 40:14–25, 1961

MONIE IW: Development of motor behavior. J Am Phys Ther Assoc 43:333–338, 1963

TWITCHELL TE: Normal motor development. J Am Phys Ther Assoc 45:419–423, 1965

TWITCHELL, TE: Variations and abnormalities of motor development. J Am Phys Ther Assoc 45:424–430, 1965

WEISZ S: Studies in equilibrium reaction. J Nerv Ment Dis 88:150–162, 1938

Motor Learning

BUCHWALD JS: Basic mechanisms of motor learning. J Am Phys Ther Assoc 45:314–331, 1965

FORWARD E: Implications of research in motor learning for physical therapy. J Am Phys Ther Assoc 43:339–344, 1963

GARDNER EB: The neurophysiological bases of motor learning: A review. Phys Ther 47:1115, 1967

HELLEBRANDT FA: Physiology of motor learning as applied to the treatment of the cerebral palsied. Q Rev Pediatr 7:5–14, 1952

HELLEBRANDT FA: Kinesthetic awareness of motor learning. Cerebral Palsy Rev 14:5–6, 1953

HELLEBRANDT FA: The physiology of motor learning. Cerebral Palsy Rev 19:9–14, 1958

HELLEBRANDT FA, PARRISH AM, HOUTZ SJ: Cross education: The influence of unilateral exercise on the contralateral limb. Arch Phys Med 28:76–85, 1947

MICHELS E: Associated movements and motor learning. Phys Ther 50:24, 1970

SMITH KU, ARNDT R: Self-generated control mechanisms in posture. Am J Phys Med 49:241, 1970

WALTERS CE: The effect of overload on bilateral transfer of a motor skill. Phys Ther Rev 35:567–569, 1955

WATERLAND JC, SHAMBES GM: Head and shoulder girdle linkage: Stepping in place. Am J Phys Med 49:279, 1970

Further Studies on Normal Subjects

BOHANNON RW: Cinematographic analysis of the passive straight-leg-raising test for hamstring muscle length. Phys Ther 62:1269, 1982

Hellebrandt FA: Cross education: Ipsilateral and contralateral effects of unimanual training. J Appl Physiol 4:136–144, 1951

HELLEBRANDT FA, HOUTZ SJ: Mechanisms of muscle training: The influence of pacing. Phys Ther Rev 38:319–322, 1958

HELLEBRANDT FA, HOCKMAN DE, PARTRIDGE MJ: Physiological effects of simultaneous static and dynamic exercise. Am J Phys Med 35:106–117, 1956

HELLEBRANDT FA, HOUTZ SJ, KRIKORIAN AM: Influence of bimanual exercise on unilateral work capacity. J Appl Physiol 2:446–452, 1950

HELLEBRANDT FA, HOUTZ SJ, PARTRIDGE MJ, WALTERS CE: Tonic neck reflexes in exercises of stress in man. Am J Phys Med 35:144–159, 1956

HELLEBRANDT FA, WATERLAND JC: Expansion of motor patterning under exercise stress. Am J Phys Med 41:56–66, 1962

HOLT LE, KAPLAN HM, OKITA TY, HOSHIKO M: Influence of antagonistic contractions and head position on the response of agonist muscles. Arch Phys Med Rehabil 50:279, 1968

LATIMER R: Utilization of tonic and labyrinthine reflexes for the facilitation of work output. Phys Ther Rev 33:237–241, 1953

MURRAY MP, DROUGHT AB, KORY RC: Walking patterns of normal men. J Bone Joint Surg (Am) 46:335–360, 1964

RICHARDS CL: Dynamic strength characteristics during iso-kinetic knee movements in healthy women. Can J Physiother 33:141, 1981

SURBURG PR: Interactive effects of resistance and facilitation patterning upon reaction and response times. Phys Ther 59:1513, 1979

TANIGAWA M: Comparison of the hold–relax procedure and passive mobilization on increasing muscle length. Phys Ther 52:725, 1972

WATERLAND JC, HELLEBRANDT FA: Involuntary patterning associated with willed movement performed against progressively increasing resistance. Am J Phys Med 43:13–30, 1964

WATERLAND JC, MUNSON N: Involuntary patterning evoked by exercise stress. J Am Phys Ther Assoc 44:91–97, 1964

WATERLAND JC, MUNSON N: Reflex association of head and shoulder girdle in nonstressful movements in man. Am J Phys Med 43:98–108, 1964

WELLOCK LM: Development of bilateral muscular strength through ipsilateral exercise. Phys Ther Rev 38:671–675, 1958

EMG Studies

HERMAN R: Electromyographic evidence of some control factors involved in the acquisition of skilled performance. Am J Phys Med 49:177, 1970

KELLY JL, BAKER MP, WOLF SL: Procedures for EMG biofeedback training in involved upper extremities of hemiplegic patients. Phys Ther 59:1500, 1979

KRAMER JF, REID DC: Backward walking: A cinematographic and electromyographic pilot study. Can J Physiother 33:77, 1981

MARKOS PD: Ipsilateral and contralateral effects of proprioceptive neuromuscular facilitation techniques on hip motion and electromyographic activity. Phys Ther 59:1366, 1979

O'CONNELL AL: Electromyographic study of certain leg muscles during movements of the free foot and during standing. Am J Phys Med 37:289–301, 1958

PARTRIDGE MJ: Elctromyographic demonstration of facilitation. Phys Ther Rev 34:227–233, 1954

PINK M: Contralateral effects of upper extremity proprioceptive neuromuscular facilitation patterns. Phys Ther 6:1158, 1981

SCHUNK MC: Electromyographic study of the peroneus longus muscle during bridging activities. Phys Ther 62:970, 1982

SINGH M, KARPOVICH PV: Effect of eccentric training of agonists on antagonistic muscles. J Appl Physiol 23:742, 1967

SULLIVAN PE, PORTNEY LG: Electromyographic activity of shoulder muscles during unilateral upper extremity proprioceptive neuromuscular facilitation patterns. Phys Ther 60:283, 1980

Selected Animal Studies

BIZZI E: The coordination of eye–head movements. Sci Am 231:100, 1975

LEVINE S: Stimulation in infancy. Sci Am 202:80, 1960

McCONNEL JK: Evolutionary factors in rehabilitation. Physiotherapy (London) 56:8, 1970

MENSCH G: Prosthetic gait observation: Comparison of bipedal and quadrupedal locomotion. Can J Physiother 31:269, 1979

OXNARD CE: Evolution of the human shoulder: Some possible pathways. Am J Phys Anthropol 30:319, 1969

TRAVIS AM, WOOLSEY CN: Motor performance of monkeys after bilateral partial and total cerebral decortication. Am J Phys Med 35:273, 1956

Related Information

General

CHRYSTAL M, ROSNER H: Mass movement patterns in neuromuscular reeducation. Phys Ther Rev 34:344–345, 1954

KABAT H: Central mechanisms for recovery of neuromuscular function. Science 112:2897:23–24, 1950

KABAT H: The role of central facilitation in restoration of motor function in paralysis. Arch Phys Med 33:521–533, 1952

KABAT H: Studies on neuromuscular dysfunction. In Payton OD, Hirt S, Newton RA (eds): Neurophysiologic Approaches to Therapeutic Exercise. Philadelphia, FA Davis, 1977

SULLIVAN PE, MARKOS PD, MINOR MAD: An Integrated Approach to Therapeutic Exercise. Reston, VA Reston Publishing, 1982

TODD JM: Facilitation of movement as taught at Vallejo. Physiotherapy (London) 58:416, 1972

WALTERS CE, GARRISON L, DUNCAN HJ, HOPKINS, FV, SYNDER JW: The effects of therapeutic agents on muscular strength and endurance. Phys Ther Rev 40:266–270, 1960

Clinical Applications

ARTHRITIS

AULT MM: Facilitation technics used to relieve contractures in a rheumatoid arthritis patient. Phys Ther Rev 40:657–658, 1960

IONTA MK: Facilitation technics in the treatment of early rheumatoid arthritis. Phys Ther Rev 40:119–120, 1960

NEUROLOGICAL CONDITIONS

BERMAN SR, LOGUE FE: Guillain-Barre syndrome. J Am Phys Ther Assoc 42:180, 1962

BOGARDH E, RICHARDS CL: Gait analysis and relearning of gait control in hemiplegic patients. Can J Physiother 33:223, 1981

BOHANNON RW: Results of resistance exercise on a patient with amyotrophic lateral sclerosis. Phys Ther 63:965, 1983

GRIFFIN J, REDDIN G: Shoulder pain in patients with hemiplegia. Phys Ther 61:1041, 1981

IRWIN-CARRUTHERS SH: An approach to physiotherapy for the patient with Parkinson's disease. Physiotherapy (South Africa), March 1971

KABAT H: Low Back and Leg Pain from Herniated Disk. St Louis, Warren H Green, 1980

KABAT H: Restoration of function through neuromuscular reeducation in traumatic paraplegia. AMA Arch Neurol Psychiatry 67:737–744, 1952

KABAT H: Analysis and therapy of cerebellar ataxia and asynergia. AMA Arch Neurol Psychiatry 74:375–382, 1955

KABAT H, McLEOD M, HOLT C: Neuromuscular dysfunction and treatment of corticospinal lesions. Physiotherapy 45:251–257, 1959

KNOTT M: Report of a case of Parkinsonism treated with proprioceptive facilitation technics. Phys Ther Rev 37:229, 1957

KNOTT M: Bulbar involvement with good recovery. J Am Phys Ther Assoc 42:38–39, 1962

TORP MJ: Adaptations of neuromuscular facilitation technics. Phys Ther Rev 36:577–586, 1956

TORP MJ: An exercise program for the brain-injured. Phys Ther Rev 36:644–675, 1956

TOUSSAINT D: Facilitation technics achieve self-care in poliomyelitis patient. Phys Ther Rev 37:590, 1957

VOSS DE: Proprioceptive neuromuscular facilitation. In Pearson PH, Williams CE (eds): Physical Therapy Services in the Developmental Disabilities. Springfield, IL, Charles C Thomas, 1972

CEREBRAL PALSY

KABAT H, McLEOD M: Athetosis: Neuromuscular dysfunction and treatment. Arch Phys Med 40:285–292, 1959

KABAT H, McLEOD M: Neuromuscular dysfunction and treatment of athetosis. Physiotherapy 46:125–129, 1960

KNOTT M: Specialized neuromuscular technics in the treatment of cerebral palsy. Phys Ther Rev 32:73–75, 1952

KNOTT M: Neuromuscular facilitation in the child with central nervous system deficit. J Am Phys Ther Assoc 46:721–724, 1966

VOSS DE: Proprioceptive neuromuscular facilitation: Demonstrations with cerebral palsied child, hemiplegic adult, arthritic adult, Parkinsonian adult. In Exploratory and Analytical Survey of Therapeutic Exercise (NU-STEP), Northwestern University Medical School, July 25–August 19, 1966. Am J Phys Med 46:838–898, 1967

VOSS DE: Proprioceptive neuromuscular facilitation. In Pearson PH, Williams CE (eds): Physical Therapy Services in the Developmental Disabilities. Springfield, IL, Charles C Thomas, 1972

ORTHOPAEDIC CONDITIONS

BROWN I: Intensive exercise for the low back. Phys Ther 50:487, 1970

KNOTT M: Avulsion of a finger with protracted disability. Phys Ther Rev 38:552, 1958

KNOTT J, BARUFALDI D: Treatment of whiplash injuries. Phys Ther Rev 41:573–577, 1961

KNOTT M, MEAD S: Facilitation technics in lower extremity amputations. Phys Ther Rev 40:587–589, 1960

NUNLEY RL, BEDINI SJ: Paralysis of the shoulder subsequent to a comminuted fracture of the scapula. Phys Ther Rev 40:442–447, 1960

VOSS DE, KNOTT M, KABAT H: Application of neuromuscular facilitation of shoulder disabilities. Phys Ther Rev 33:536–541, 1953

OTHER CONDITIONS

BOONE DC: Physical therapy aspects related to orthopedic and neurologic residuals of bleeding. J Am Phys Ther Assoc 46:1272, 1966

HUMPHREY TL, HUDDLESTON OL: Applying facilitation technics to self-care training. Phys Ther Rev 38:605, 1958

Equipment

JOHNSON MM, BONNER CD: Sling suspension techniques, demonstrating the use of a new portable frame. Phys Ther 51:524, 1971

SMITH WD: Combining wall pulleys and mat activities to total pattern movements. Phys Ther 54:746, 1974

TOUSSAINT D, KNOTT M: Use of wall pulleys with mat activities. Phys Ther Rev 35:477, 1956

VOSS DE, SLATINSKY JP: Textured cane handle. Phys Ther 53:1295, 1973

Adjuncts to Facilitation Techniques

COLD

BASSETT SW, LAKE BM: Use of cold applications in the management of spasticity. Phys Ther Rev 38:333–334, 1958

BOES MC: Reduction of spasticity by cold. J Am Phys Ther Assoc 42:29–32, 1962

BOYNTON BL, GARRAMONE PM, BUCA JT: Observations on the effects of cool baths for patients with multiple sclerosis. Phys Ther Rev 39:297–299, 1959

CONWAY B: Ice Packs in diabetic neuropathy. Phys Ther Rev 41:586–588, 1961

DAVIES EJ, PERRY JH, WAKEFIELD P: Afferent stimuli to facilitate or inhibit motor activity. (Techniques developed by M. Rood) In Decker R (ed): Motor Integration, Chap 5, pp 73–83. Springfield, IL, Charles C Thomas, 1962

JOHNSON DJ, MOORE S, MOORE J, OLIVER RA: Effect of cold submersion on intramuscular temperature of the gastrocnemius muscle. Phys Ther 59:1238, 1979

KELLY M: Effectiveness of a cryotherapy technique on spasticity. Phys Ther 49:349, 1969

LIGHTFOOT E, VERRIER M, ASHBY P: Neurophysiological effects of prolonged cooling of the calf in patients with complete spinal transection. Phys Ther 55:251, 1975

LORENZE DJ, CARANTONIS G, DE ROSA AJ: Effect on coronary circulation of cold packs to hemiplegic shoulders. Arch Phys Med 41:394–399, 1960

McGOWN HL: Effects of cold application on maximal isometric contraction. Phys Ther 47:185, 1968

MIGLIETTA OE: Evaluation of cold in spasticity. Am J Phys Med 41:148–151, 1962

OLSON JE, STRAVINO VD: A review of cryotherapy. Phys Ther 52:840, 1972

PETAJAN JH, WATTS N: Effects of cooling on the triceps surae muscle. Am J Phys Med 41:240–251, 1962

ROCKEFELLER LE: The use of cold packs for increasing joint range of motion. Phys Ther Rev 38:564–566, 1958

URBSCHEIT N, BISHOP B: Effects of cooling on the ankle jerk and H-response. Phys Ther 50:1041, 1970

WATSON, CW: Effect of lowering body temperature on the symptoms and signs of multiple sclerosis. N Engl J Med 261:1253–1259, 1959

WOLF BA: Effects of temperature reduction of multiple sclerosis. Phys Ther 50:808, 1970

ELECTRICAL STIMULATION

CURRIER DP, MANN R: Muscular strength development by electrical stimulation in healthy individuals. Phys Ther 63:915, 1983

LAINEY CG, WALMSLEY RP, ANDREW GM: Effectiveness of exercise alone versus exercise plus electrical stimulation in strengthening the quadriceps muscle. Can J Physiother 35:5, 1983

LIBERSON WT: Experiment concerning reciprocal inhibition of anatgonists elicited by electrical stimulation of agonists in a normal individual. Am J Phys Med 44:306–308, 1965

MELZACK R, JEANS ME, STRATFORD JG, MONKS RC: Ice massage and transcutaneous electrical stimulation: comparison of treatment for low-back pain. Pain 9:209, 1980

MECHANICAL VIBRATION

ARCANGEL CS, JOHNSTON R, BISHOP B: Achilles tendon reflex and the H-response during and after tendon vibration. Comments by discussant: Voss DE. J Am Phys Ther Assoc 51:889, 1971

deGAIL P, LANCE JW, NEILSON PO: Differential effects on tonic and phasic reflex mechanisms produced by vibration of muscles in man. J Neurol Neurosurg Psychiatry 29:1, 1966

EKLUND G, STEEN M: Muscle vibration therapy in children with cerebral palsy. Scand J Phys Med 1:35, 1969

GOODWIN GM, McCLOSKEY DI, MATTHEWS PBC: Proprioceptive illusions induced by muscle vibration: Contribution by muscle spindle to perception? Science 175:1382, 1972

HOCHREITER NW, JEWELL MJ, BARBER L, BROWNE P: Effect of vibration on tactile sensitivity. Phys Ther 63:934, 1983

JOHNSTON RM, BISHOP B, COFFEY GH: Mechanical vibration of skeletal muscle. Phys Ther 50:499, 1970

SPICER SD, MATYAS TA: Facilitation of the tonic vibration reflex (TVR) by cutaneous stimulation (abstr). Am J Phys Med 59:223, 1980

WALL PD, CRONLY-DILLON JR: Pain itch and vibration. AMA Arch Neurol 2:14, 1960

Related Fields

OCCUPATIONAL THERAPY

AYRES AJ: Proprioceptive neuromuscular facilitation elicited through the upper extremities. Part I. Background. Part II. Application. Part III. Specific application. Am J Occup Ther 9:1955

CARROLL J: Utilization of reinforcement in the program for the hemiplegic. Am J Occup Ther 4:211, 1950

COOKE DM: Effects of resistance on multiple sclerosis patients with intention tremor. Am J Occup Ther 12:89, 1958

KREWER S: The Arthritis Exercise Book. New York, Simon & Schuster, 1981

MYERS BJ: The proprioceptive neuromuscular facilitation (PNF) approach. In Trombly CA (ed): Occupational Therapy for Physical Dysfunction. Baltimore, Williams & Wilkins, 1983

MYERS BJ: Therapy Activities (videotape). Chicago, Rehabilitation Institute of Chicago, 1981

VOSS DE: Applications of patterns and techniques in occupational therapy. Am J Occup Ther 8:191, 1959

SPORTS PHYSICAL THERAPY

KRAMER PG: Restoration of dorsi flexion after injuries to the distal leg and ankle. J Ortho Sports Phys Ther 1:159, 1980

PENNY NJ, WELSH RP: Shoulder impingement syndromes in athletes and their surgical management. Am J Sports Med 9:11, 1981

RICHARDSON AB, JOBE FW, COLLINS HR: The shoulder in competitive swimming. Am J Sports Med 8:159, 1980

SADY SP, WORTMAN M, BLANKE D: Flexibility training: Ballistic, static or proprioceptive neuromuscular facilitation? Arch Phys Med Rehabil 63:261, 1982

SMITH MJ, STEWART MJ: Sports medicine and rehabilitation. In Nickel VL (ed): Orthopedic Rehabilitation. New York, Churchill Livingstone, 1982

SURBURG PR: Neuromuscular facilitation techniques in sports medicine. Physician and Sportsmedicine 9:115, 1981

Supportive Comments

DENKER H: Horowitz and Mrs. Washington. New York, GP Putnam Sons, 1979

GILLETTE HE: Changing concepts in the management of neuromuscular dysfunction. South Med J 52:1227–1229, 1959.

HIRT S: Progress is a relay race. Phys Ther 61:1609, 1981

KNOTT M: In the groove. Phys Ther 53:365, 1973

KREWER S: The Arthritis Exercise Book. New York, Simon & Schuster, 1981

MEAD S: A six-year evaluation of proprioceptive neuromuscular facilitation technics. In Proceedings of the Third International Congress of Physical Medicine, 1960. Chicago, American Congress of Physical Medicine and Rehabilitation and American Academy of Physical medicine and Rehabilitation, 1962

VOSS DE: Everything is there before you discover it. Phys Ther 62:1617, 1982

WATKINS AL: Medical progress: Physical medicine and rehabilitation. N Engl J Med 255:1233–1239, 1956

REFERENCE TABLES

PATTERN COMBINATIONS FOR REINFORCEMENT

Reference Table 1. Head and Neck Patterns Reinforced by Pattern Combinations of Upper Extremities

Pattern to be Reinforced	Upper Extremity Patterns (Eye Follows Hand)
Head and neck flexion with rotation (left/right)	Extension–adduction–internal rotation (contralateral) Bilateral asymmetrical (chopping; ipsilateral)
Head and neck extension with rotation (left/right)	Flexion–abduction–external rotation (ipsilateral) Bilateral asymetrical (lifting; ipsilateral)
Head and neck rotation (left/right)	Extension–abduction–internal rotation (ipsilateral) Flexion–adduction–external rotation (contralateral)

Reference Table 2. Upper Trunk Patterns Reinforced by Pattern Combinations of Head and Neck, Lower Trunk, and Upper Extremities

Pattern to be Reinforced	Neck Patterns (Ipsilateral)	Lower Trunk Patterns	Upper Extremity Patterns
Upper trunk flexion with rotation (left/right)	Head and neck flexion with rotation (ipsilateral)	1. Lower trunk flexion with rotation (ipsilateral)	1. Bilateral asymmetrical patterns (chopping, hands approximated), ipsilateral
		Flexion–abduction–internal rotation (ipsilateral lower extremity)	Extension–adduction–internal rotation (contralateral upper extremity)
		Flexion–adduction–external rotation (contralateral lower extremity)	Extension–abduction–internal rotation (ipsilateral upper extremity)
		2. Lower trunk flexion with rotation (contralateral)	2. Unilateral upper extremity patterns
		Flexion–abduction–internal rotation (contralateral lower extremity)	Extension–adduction–internal rotation (contralateral upper extremity)

(Continued)

Pattern to be Reinforced	Neck Patterns (Ipsilateral)	Lower Trunk Patterns	Upper Extremity Patterns
Upper trunk extension with rotation (left/right)	Head and neck extension with rotation (ipsilateral)	Flexion–adduction–external rotation (ipsilateral lower extremity) 1. Lower trunk extension with rotation (ipsilateral) Extension–abduction–internal rotation (ipsilateral lower extremity) Extension–adduction–external rotation (contralateral lower extremity) 2. Lower trunk extension with rotation (contralateral) Extension–abduction–internal rotation (contralateral lower extremity) Extension–adduction–external rotation (ipsilateral lower extremity) Note: All lower trunk patterns may be performed with bilateral knee flexion or knee extension, or the knees may remain straight. Extremities are held in close approximation.	1. Bilateral asymmetrical patterns (lifting, hands approximated), ipsilateral Flexion–abduction–external rotation (ipsilateral upper extremity) Flexion–adduction–external rotation (contralateral upper extremity) 2. Unilateral upper extremity pattern Flexion–abduction–external rotation (ipsilateral upper extremity) Note: Since neck patterns are the key to the upper trunk patterns, when upper extremity patterns are used to reinforce the upper trunk, the eyes follow the hands.
Upper trunk rotation (left/right)	Head and neck rotation (ipsilateral)	1. Lower trunk extension with rotation (ipsilateral) 2. Lower trunk flexion with rotation (contralateral)	1. Bilateral reciprocal patterns Extension–abduction–internal rotation (ipsilateral) Flexion–adduction–external rotation (contralateral) 2. Unilateral upper extremity patterns Extension–abduction–internal rotation (ipsilateral) Flexion–adduction–external rotation (contralateral)

Reference Table 3. Pattern Combinations for Reinforcement of Lower Trunk Patterns

Pattern to be Reinforced	Head and Neck and Upper Trunk Patterns	Bilateral Asymmetrical Upper Extremity Patterns	Unilateral Upper Extremity Patterns
Lower trunk flexion with rotation (left/right)	Flexion with rotation (ipsilateral)	1. Chopping (ipsilateral)	1. Flexion–adduction–external rotation (contralateral)
	Flexion with rotation (contralateral)	2. Chopping (contralateral)	2. Extension–adduction–internal rotation (ipsilateral)
Lower trunk extension with rotation (left/right)	Extension with rotation (ipsilateral)	1. Lifting (ipsilateral)	1. Extension–abduction–internal rotation (ipsilateral)
	Extension with rotation (contralateral)	2. Lifting (contralateral)	2. Flexion–abduction–external rotation (contralateral)

Reference Table 4. Upper Extremity Patterns Reinforced by Pattern Combinations of Head and Neck and Lower Extremities

Pattern to be Reinforced	Head and Neck Patterns (Eye Follows Hand)	Ipsilateral or Contralateral Lower Extremity Patterns
Flexion–adduction–external rotation	Extension with rotation (contralateral) Rotation (contralateral)	Flexion–adduction–external rotation Flexion–abduction–internal rotation
Extension–abduction–internal rotation	Flexion with rotation (ipsilateral)	Extension–abduction–internal rotation
	Rotation (ipsilateral)	Extension–adduction–external rotation
Flexion–abduction–external rotation	Extension with rotation (ipsilateral)	Extension–adduction–external rotation Extension–abduction–internal rotation
Extension–adduction–internal rotation	Flexion with rotation (contralateral) Rotation (contralateral)	Flexion–adduction–external rotation Flexion–abduction–internal rotation

Reference Table 5. Lower Extremity Patterns Reinforced by Pattern Combinations of Head and Neck and Upper Extremities

Pattern to be Reinforced	Head and Neck Patterns	Ipsilateral or Contralateral Upper Extremity
1. Flexion–adduction–external rotation	Flexion with rotation (ipsilateral) Rotation (ipsilateral)	Flexion–adduction–external rotation Extension–adduction–internal rotation
2. Extension–abduction–internal rotation	Extension with rotation (ipsilateral) Rotation (ipsilateral)	Extension–abduction–internal rotation Flexion–abduction–external rotation
3. Flexion–abduction–internal rotation	Flexion with rotation (ipsilateral) Rotation (ipsilateral)	Flexion–adduction–external rotation Extension–adduction–internal rotation
4. Extension–adduction–external rotation	Extension with rotation (contralateral) Rotation (contralateral)	Extension–abduction–internal rotation Flexion–abduction–internal rotation

Reference Table 6. Upper Extremity Pattern Combinations for Reinforcement of Opposite Upper Extremity

Pattern to be Reinforced	Bilateral Symmetrical	Bilateral Asymmetrical	Bilateral Reciprocal (Same Diagonal)	Bilateral Reciprocal (Opposite Diagonal)
Flexion–adduction–external rotation	Flexion–adduction–external rotation	Flexion–abduction–external rotation	Extension–abduction–internal rotation	Extension–adduction–internal rotation
Extension–abduction–internal rotation	Extension–abduction–internal rotation	Extension–adduction–internal rotation	Flexion–adduction–external rotation	Flexion–abduction–external rotation
Flexion–abduction–external rotation	Flexion–abduction–external rotation	Flexion–adduction–external rotation	Extension–adduction–internal rotation	Extension–abduction–internal rotation
Extension–adduction–internal rotation	Extension–adduction–internal rotation	Extension–abduction–internal rotation	Flexion–abduction–external rotation	Flexion–adduction–external rotation

Reference Table 7. Lower Extremity Pattern Combinations for Reinforcement of Opposite Lower Extremity

Pattern to be Reinforced	Bilateral Symmetrical	Bilateral Asymmetrical	Bilateral Reciprocal (Same Diagonal)	Bilateral Reciprocal (Opposite Diagonal)
1. Flexion–adduction–external rotation	Flexion–adduction–external rotation	Flexion–abduction–internal rotation	Extension–abduction–internal rotation	Extension–adduction–external rotation
2. Extension–abduction–internal rotation	Extension–abduction–internal rotation	Extension–adduction–external rotation	Flexion–adduction–external rotation	Flexion–abduction–internal rotation
3. Flexion–abduction–internal rotation	Flexion–abduction–internal rotation	Flexion–adduction–external rotation	Extension–adduction–external rotation	Extension–abduction–internal rotation
4. Extension–adduction–external rotation	Extension–adduction–external rotation	Extension–abduction–internal rotation	Flexion–abduction–internal rotation	Flexion–adduction–external rotation

OPTIMAL PATTERNS FOR INDIVIDUAL MUSCLES

Reference Table 8. Optimal Patterns for Muscles of the Head and Neck

Muscles (Left Muscles Considered)	Patterns	Muscles (Left Muscles Considered)	Patterns
Platysma	Flexion with rotation, left	Scalenus anterior	Flexion with rotation, left
		Scalenus medius	Rotation, left
Trapezius	Extension with rotation, left	Scalenus posterior	
Levator scapulae	Rotation, left	Rectus capitis posterior minor	Extension with rotation, left
Sternocleidomastoideus	Flexion with rotation, left, lengthened to middle range	Rectus capitis posterior major	
	Flexion with rotation, right, middle to shortened range	Obliquus capitis inferior	
	Rotation, left, lengthened to middle range	Obliquus capitis superior	
	Rotation, right, middle to shortened range	Splenius capitis	Extension with rotation, left
		Longissimus capitis	
		Splenius cervicis	
		Longissimus cervicis	
		Iliocostalis cervicis	
Suprahyoidei	Flexion with rotation, left	Interspinales	
Infrahyoidei		Intertransversarii	
Rectus capitis lateralis	Flexion with rotation, right	Semispinalis capitis	
Rectus capitis anterior	Flexion with rotation, left	Semispinalis cervicis	Extension with rotation, right
		Multifidus	
Longus colli	Flexion with rotation, left		
Longus capitis			

Muscles (Left Muscles Considered)	Patterns	Muscles (Left Muscles Considered)	Patterns
Spinalis thoracis Longissimus thoracis Iliocostalis thoracis Iliocostalis lumborum Sacrospinalis Interspinales Intertransversarii	Trunk extension with rotation, left	Rectus abdominis, left portion	Upper trunk flexion with rotation, left Lower trunk flexion with rotation, left
Semispinalis thoracis Multifidus Rotatores	Trunk extension with rotation, right	Transversus abdominis	Trunk extension with rotation, left Upper trunk rotation, left
Quadratus lumborum	Trunk extension with rotation, left Trunk flexion with rotation, left Trunk rotation, left	Intercostales externi Serratus posterior superior Diaphragma, descent of dome	Upper trunk extension with rotation, left
		Levators costarum Serratus posterior inferior	Upper trunk extension with rotation, right
Obliquus externus	Upper trunk flexion with rotation, right Lower trunk flexion with rotation, left	Intercostales interni Subcostales Diaphragma, ascent of dome	Upper trunk flexion with rotation, left
		Transversus thoracis	Upper trunk flexion with rotation, right
Obliquus internus	Upper trunk flexion with rotation, left Lower trunk flexion with rotation, right		

Reference Table 10.   Optimal Patterns for Muscles of Upper Extremity with Consideration for Action on Two or More Joints

Muscles	Patterns	Muscles	Patterns
Shoulder girdle Serratus anterior	Flexion–adduction–external rotation	Deltoideus, posterior portion Teres major Latissimus dorsi	Extension–abduction–internal rotation
Levator scapulae Rhomboideus major Rhomboideus minor Latissimus dorsi, inferior angle attachment	Extension–abduction–internal rotation	Latissimus dorsi, shortened range	Extension–adduction–internal rotation posteriorly
Trapezius	Flexion–abduction–external rotation	Supraspinatus Infraspinatus Teres minor Deltoideus, middle portion	Flexion–abduction–external rotation
Subclavius Pectoralis minor	Extension–adduction–internal rotation		
Pectoralis major, clavicular portion Deltoideus, anterior portion Coracobrachialis	Flexion–adduction–external rotation	Pectoralis major, sternal portion Subscapularis	Extension–adduction–internal rotation

(Continued)

Muscles	Patterns	Muscles	Patterns
Elbow Biceps brachii Brachialis	Flexion – adduction – external rotation with elbow flexion	Flexor digitorum profundus	Flexion – adduction – external rotation Extension – adduction – internal rotation
Triceps brachii Anconeus Subanconeus	Extension – abduction – internal rotation with elbow extension	Interossei palmares	Flexion – adduction – external rotation Extension – adduction – internal rotation
Forearm Supinator	Flexion – adduction – external rotation	Flexor digiti minimi brevis	Flexion – adduction – external rotation
Pronator quadratus	Extension – abduction – internal rotation	Opponens digiti minimi	Flexion – adduction – external rotation
Brachioradialis	Flexion – abduction – external rotation with elbow flexion	Extensor digitorum communis	Flexion – abduction – external rotation with elbow extension Extension – abduction – internal rotation with elbow extension
Pronator teres	Extension – adduction – internal rotation with elbow flexion		
Wrist Flexor carpi radialis	Flexion – adduction – external rotation with elbow flexion	Interossei dorsales	Flexion – abduction – external rotation Extension – abduction – internal rotation
Extensor carpi ulnaris	Extension – abduction – internal rotation with elbow extension	Extensor indicis proprius	Flexion – abduction – external rotation
		Extensor digiti minimi	Extension – abduction – internal rotation
Palmaris longus	Flexion – adduction – external rotation with elbow flexion Extension – adduction – internal rotation with elbow flexion	Abductor digiti minimi	Extension – abduction – internal rotation
		Lumbricales	All patterns of upper extremity
Flexor carpi ulnaris	Extension – adduction – internal rotation with elbow flexion	**Thumb** Flexor pollicis longus Flexor pollicis brevis Adductor pollicis	Flexion – adduction – external rotation
Extensor carpi radialis longus Extensor carpi radialis brevis	Flexion – abduction – external rotation with elbow extension	Abductor pollicis brevis	Extension – abduction – internal rotation
Hand and Fingers Flexor digitorum superficialis	Flexion – adduction – external rotation with elbow flexion Extension – adduction – internal rotation with elbow flexion	Abductor pollicis longus Extensor pollicis longus Extensor pollicis brevis First interosseus dorsalis	Flexion – abduction – external rotation
		Opponens pollicis Palmaris brevis	Extension – adduction – internal rotation

Reference Table 11. Optimal Patterns for Muscles of Lower Extremity with Consideration for Action on Two or More Joints

Muscles	Patterns	Muscles	Patterns
Hip Psoas major Psoas minor Iliacus Obturatorius externus Pectineus Adductor longus Adductor brevis Gracilis Sartorius	} Flexion–adduction–external rotation } With knee flexion	Semitendinosus Semimembranosus	} Extension–adduction–external rotation with knee flexion Flexion–adduction–external rotation with knee flexion
		Articularis genus	All patterns with knee extension
Gluteus medius Gluteus minimus	} Extension–abduction–internal rotation	**Ankle and Foot** Tibialis anterior	Flexion–adduction–external rotation
Tensor fasciae latae	Flexion–abduction–internal rotation	Peroneus longus Gastrocnemius, lateral portion Soleus, lateral portion	} Extension–abduction–internal rotation
Gluteus maximus Piriformis Obturatorius internus Gemellus superior Gemellus inferior Quadratus femoris Adductor magnus	} Extension–adduction–external rotation	Peroneus brevis Peroneus tertius	} Flexion–abduction–internal rotation
		Tibialis posterior Gastrocnemius, medial portion Soleus, medial portion Plantaris	} Extension–adduction–external rotation
Knee Rectus femoris, medial portion	Flexion–adduction–external rotation with knee extension	**Foot and Toes** Extensor hallucis longus Extensor digitorum longus Extensor digitorum brevis Interossei dorsales	} Flexion–abduction–internal rotation Flexion–adduction–external rotation
Vastus medialis	} Extension–adduction–external rotation with knee extension Flexion–adduction–external rotation with knee extension	Flexor hallucis longus Flexor digitorum longus Flexor digitorum brevis Flexor hallucis brevis Interossei plantares	} Extension–adduction–external rotation Extension–abduction–internal rotation
Biceps femoris Popliteus	} Extension–abduction–internal rotation with knee flexion Flexion–abduction–internal rotation with knee flexion	Flexor digiti minimi brevis Adductor hallucis Quadratus plantae, lateral portion	} Extension–abduction–internal rotation
Rectus femoris, lateral portion	Flexion–abduction–internal rotation with knee extension	Quadratus plantae, medial portion	Extension–adduction–external rotation
Vastus intermedius Vastus lateralis	} Extension–abduction–internal rotation with knee extension Flexion–abduction–internal rotation with knee extension	Lumbricales	All patterns of lower extremity

OPTIMAL PATTERNS ACCORDING TO PERIPHERAL INNERVATION

Reference Table 12. Optimal Patterns for Muscles of Upper Extremity According to Peripheral Innervation

Nerve	Flexion–Adduction–External Rotation	Extension–Abduction–Internal Rotation	Flexion–Abduction–External Rotation	Extension–Adduction–Internal Rotation
Spinal accessory and C3–4				
Trapezius	– – –	– – –	xxx	– – –
Dorsal scapular C3–4				
Levator scapulae	– – –	xxx	– – –	– – –
Dorsal scapular C5				
Rhomboideii major and minor	– – –	xxx	– – –	
Suprascapular nerve C5–6				
Supraspinatus	– – –	– – –	xxx	– – –
Infraspinatus	– – –	– – –	xxx	– – –
Subclavius C5–6				
Subclavius	– – –	– – –	– – –	xxx
Subscapular nerves C5–6				
Subscapularis	– – –	– – –	– – –	xxx
Teres major	– – –	xxx	– – –	– – –
Long thoracic nerve C5–6–7				
Serratus anterior	xxx	– – –	– – –	– – –
Axillary nerve, C5–6				
Deltoid	xxx	xxx	xxx	– – –
Teres minor	– – –	– – –	xxx	– – –
Musculocutaneous nerve, C5–6–7	xxx			
Coracobrachialis	xxx	– – –	– – –	– – –
Biceps	xxx Elbow flexion	– – –	– – –	– – –
Brachialis	xxx Elbow flexion	– – –	– – –	– – –
Anterior thoraciclateral C5–6–7				
Pectoralis major, clavicular	xxx	– – –	– – –	– – –
Anterior thoracicmedial C8–T1				
Pectoralis minor	– – –	– – –	– – –	xxx
Pectoralis major, sternal	– – –	– – –	– – –	xxx
Thoracodorsal nerve C6–7–8				
Latissimus dorsi	– – –	xxx	– – –	Posteriorly with elbow flexion
Radial nerve C6–7–8				
Triceps bchii	– – –	xxx Elbow extension	– – –	– – –
Brachioradialis	– – –	– – –	xxx Elbow flexion	– – –
Extensor carpi radialis longus	– – –	– – –	xxx	– – –
Anconeus	– – –	xxx Elbow extension	– – –	– – –
Extensor carpi radialis brevis	– – –	– – –	xxx	– – –
Extensor digitorum communis	– – –	xxx	xxx	– – –
Extensor digiti quinti proprius	– – –	xxx	– – –	– – –
Extensor carpi ulnaris	– – –	xxx	– – –	– – –
Supinator	xxx	– – –	– – –	– – –
Abductor pollicis longus	– – –	– – –	xxx	– – –
Extensor pollicis brevis	– – –	– – –	xxx	– – –
Extensor pollicis longus	– – –	– – –	xxx	– – –
Extensor indicis proprius	– – –	– – –	xxx	– – –
Median nerve C6–7–8, T1				

Nerve	Flexion–Adduction–External Rotation	Extension–Abduction–Internal Rotation	Flexion–Abduction–External Rotation	Extension–Adduction–Internal Rotation
Flexor digitorum profundus, 1 and 2	xxx	– – –	– – –	xxx
Pronator teres	– – –	– – –	– – –	xxx
Palmaris longus	xxx	– – –	– – –	xxx
Flexor carpi radialis	xxx	– – –	– – –	– – –
Flexor digitorum superficialis	xxx	– – –	– – –	xxx
Flexor pollicis longus	xxx	– – –	– – –	– – –
Pronator quadratus	– – –	xxx	– – –	– – –
Abductor pollicis brevis	– – –	xxx	– – –	– – –
Opponens pollicis	– – –	– – –	– – –	xxx
Flexor pollicis brevis	xxx	– – –	– – –	– – –
Lumbricales 1 and 2	Mass closing of hand	Mass opening of hand	Mass opening of hand	Mass closing of hand
Ulnar nerve C8, T1				
Flexor carpi ulnaris	– – –	– – –	– – –	xxx
Flexor digitorum profundus 3 and 4	xxx	– – –	– – –	xxx
Flexor pollicis brevis	xxx	– – –	– – –	xxx
Palmaris brevis	– – –	– – –	– – –	xxx
Abductor digiti quinti	– – –	xxx	– – –	– – –
Opponens digiti quinti	xxx	– – –	– – –	– – –
Flexor digiti quinti	xxx	– – –	– – –	– – –
Dorsal interossei	– – –	xxx	xxx	– – –
Palmar interossei	xxx	– – –	– – –	xxx
Adductores pollicis	xxx	– – –	– – –	– – –
Lumbricales 3 and 4	Mass closing of hand	Mass opening of hand	Mass opening of hand	Mass closing of hand

Note: Scapular motions are more easily controlled if the elbow remains straight. Elbow flexion may be allowed in the flexion patterns; elbow extension may be allowed in the extension patterns.

Note: Involvement of triceps is indication for performing patterns with elbow straight when distal components are emphasized.

Note: Distal components are more easily controlled if the elbow remains straight although two-joint action of muscles may be considered. Maximal reeducation requires all combinations of elbow joint motion.

(After Gray H: Anatomy of the Human Body, 23rd ed. Philadelphia, Lea & Febiger, 1936)

Reference Table 13. Optimal Patterns for Lower Extremity Muscles According to Peripheral Innervation

Nerve	Flexion–Adduction–External Rotation	Extension–Abduction–Internal Rotation	Flexion–Abduction–Internal Rotation	Extension–Adduction–External Rotation
L1–2–3				
Psoas minor	xxx	– – –	– – –	– – –
Psoas major	xxx	– – –	– – –	– – –
Femoral, L2–3–4				
Iliacus	xxx	– – –	– – –	– – –
Pectineus	xxx	– – –	– – –	– – –
Sartorius	xxx Knee flexion	– – –	– – –	– – –
Rectus femoris	xxx Knee extension	– – –	xxx Knee extension	– – –
Vastus medialis	xxx Knee extension	– – –	– – –	xxx Knee extension
Vastus lateralis	– – –	xxx Knee extension	xxx Knee extension	– – –
Vastus intermedius	– – –	xxx Knee extension	xxx Knee extension	– – –
Articularis genus	xxx Knee extension	xxx Knee extension	xxx Knee extension	xxx Knee extension
Obturator nerve, L3–4				
Obturator externus	xxx	– – –	– – –	– – –
Adductor magnus	– – –	– – –	– – –	xxx
Adductor longus	xxx	– – –	– – –	– – –
Adductor brevis	xxx	– – –	– – –	– – –
Gracilis	xxx Knee flexion	– – –	– – –	– – –
Superior gluteal L4–5, S1				
Gluteus medius	– – –	xxx	– – –	– – –
Gluteus minimus	– – –	xxx	– – –	– – –
Tensor fasciae latae	– – –	– – –	xxx	– – –
L5, S1				
Quadratus femoris	– – –	– – –	– – –	xxx
Gemellus inferior	– – –	– – –	– – –	xxx
S1,2,3				
Obturator internus	– – –	– – –	– – –	xxx
Gemellus superior	– – –	– – –	– – –	xxx
S1,2				
Piriformis	– – –	– – –	– – –	xxx
Inferior gluteal L5, S1–2				
Gluteus maximus	– – –	– – –	– – –	xxx
Sciatic nerve, L4,5; S1,2,3				
Semitendinosus	xxx Knee flexion	– – –	– – –	xxx Knee flexion
Semimembranosus	xxx Knee flexion	– – –	– – –	xxx Knee flexion
Biceps femoris, long & short heads	– – –	xxx Knee flexion	xxx Knee flexion	– – –
Common peroneal nerve L4–5; S1–2				
Tibialis anterior	xxx	– – –	– – –	– – –
Extensor digitorum longus	xxx	– – –	xxx	– – –
Extensor hallucis longus	xxx	– – –	xxx	– – –
Peroneus longus	– – –	xxx	– – –	– – –
Peroneus brevis	– – –	– – –	xxx	– – –
Extensor digitorum brevis	xxx	– – –	xxx	– – –
Peroneus tertius	– – –	– – –	xxx	– – –
Tibial nerve, L4–5, S1–2				
Gastrocnemius	– – –	xxx Knee flexion	– – –	xxx Knee flexion
Popliteus	– – –	xxx Knee flexion	xxx Knee flexion	– – –
Plantaris	– – –	– – –	– – –	xxx Knee flexion
Soleus	– – –	xxx	– – –	xxx

Reference Table 13. Optimal Patterns for Lower Extremity Muscles According to Peripheral Innervation *(Continued)*

Nerve	Flexion–Adduction–External Rotation	Extension–Abduction–Internal Rotation	Flexion–Abduction–Internal Rotation	Extension–Adduction–External Rotation
Tibialis posterior	– – –	– – –	– – –	xxx
Flexor digitorum longus	– – –	xxx	– – –	xxx
Flexor hallucis longus	– – –	xxx	– – –	xxx
Medial plantar nerve L5 – S1				
Flexor digitorum brevis	– – –	xxx	– – –	xxx
Abductor hallucis	xxx	– – –	– – –	– – –
First lumbrical	xxx	xxx	xxx	xxx
Flexor hallucis brevis	– – –	xxx	– – –	xxx
Lateral plantar nerve L5 – S1 – 2				
Quadratus plantae	– – –	xxx	– – –	xxx
Abductor digiti quinti	– – –	– – –	xxx	– – –
Flexor digiti quinti brevis	– – –	xxx	– – –	– – –
Opponens digiti quinti	– – –	xxx	– – –	– – –
Adductors hallucis	– – –	xxx	– – –	– – –
Plantar interossei	– – –	xxx	– – –	xxx
Dorsal interossei	xxx	– – –	xxx	– – –
Three lateral lumbricales	xxx	xxx	xxx	xxx

Note: Distal parts may be more easily controlled if the knee remains straight. Unless flexion or extension of the knee is specified, any combination of the knee motion may be used.
(After Gray H: Anatomy of the Human Body, 23rd ed. Philadelphia, Lea & Febiger, 1936)

INDEX

Neck. *See also* Head and neck
  motion patterns of, 2, 2t–3t
  washing of, 275t
Newborns
  range of movement in, 211
  stepping movements as reflexive
    response of, 210

Occupational therapy
  goals and, 340–341
  physical therapist and, 291
Orthopaedic patients
  examination of, 327
  joint mobilization techniques for,
    327–328, 329t
Overlapping
  overlapping to integrative motor
    development, 211
  provided by muscles, 4

Pain
  pressure for, 291
  in stretch reflex, 294
Parallel bars, 261f–262f
Passive motion
  antagonistic pattern imbalances in, 299
  for determination of range, 7
Patients
  ataxia in, 302
  evaluation of. *See* Evaluation, of
    patient's performance
  fracture of head of radius in, 305
  goals for, 340–341
  lack of endurance in, 299
  with lengthened range weakness, 299
  limitation of active motion in, 305
  muscle imbalances in, 299–300
  orthopaedic, 327
  posture of. *See* Posture
  quadriparetic, with flexor reflexes
    dominant, 306
  rhythmic initiation with, 300
  stretch reflex, and voluntary movement
    of, 298
  sustained effort by, 295
  teaching to "hold," 302
  training of. *See* Training
  voluntary efforts of. *See* Voluntary
    movements
Patterns of facilitation
  adjuncts to techniques of, 312–314
  patient performance and, 332–333
  patient postures for evaluation, 332
  pressure for agonistic and antagonistic
    patterns, 291
Patterns of motion
  bilateral asymmetrical lower extremity,
    2, 2t
  components of action and, 1, 4
  consistency of components in, 2–3
  diagonal, 1–5, 2t–3t
  of extremities, 2–4, 2t–3t
  groove of, 5
  head and neck. *See* Head and neck
  key to lower trunk, 2
  mass movement. *See* Mass movement
  motion components, 1–4, 2t–3t
  range of, 4–5

spiral and diagonal, 1–5, 2t–3t
straight motion, 1
total. *See* Total pattern, of movement
Pelvic elevation, supine, 233f
Performance, 9
  evaluation of. *See* Evaluation, of
    patient's performance
  positioning for, 7
Perineal muscle stimulation, 326, 326f
Physical therapist
  patient interaction with, 291. *See also*
    Commands
  positioning of, 218, 291
Physician, treatment goals of, 340
Pivots of action, 1–4, 2t–3t
  emphasis on, 300, 333, 340–341
  muscle contractions and, 5–6
Point of completion, of movement, 216
Point of initiation, of movement, 216
Positioning
  for facilitation, 7–8
  for performance, 7
  of physical therapist, 218, 291
Posture
  erect. *See* Standing; Standing balance
  for evaluation, 332
  prone, 98, 212, 234f–246f
  reflexes, postural, 210, 219t, 294
Practice
  motor learning and, 9, 343–344
  part-task, 343
  stepwise procedures, 341
  2 × 2 rule in, 344–345
  varying, 9, 344–345
  whole-task, 343
Preparatory activities, 259
Preparatory commands, 292
Pressure. *See also* Manual contact
  as facilitation mechanism, 291
  as sensory cue, 291
Primitive responses, to stress, 214. *See
  also* Reflexes
Pronation, 1
Prone progression, 212, 234f–246f
  crawling, 212, 234f–235f
  creeping, 212, 240f–244f
  on elbows and knees, 236f–237f
  on hands and feet, 245f–246f
  on hands and knees, 238f–244f
Psoas major muscles, 5
Pulleys. *See* Wall pulley exercises

Quadriparetic patients, 306
Quick reversal, 303

Radial extensor thrust, 98, 100f–101f
Range of initiation, 4–5
Range of motion, 4–5. *See also*
  Movement, range of
Recreational activities, 341
  sports, 1
Recuperative motion, 136–137
  techniques of PNF and, 136
Reflexes
  antagonistic, 300
  flexor, 298, 306
  hyperactive, 300
  imbalance between flexor and extensor,
    298
  in infants, 212–213
  and mature movements, 214

in newborns, 210
postural, 210, 219t, 294
  approximation and, 294
  and righting, 259
primitive responses, 214
stretch. *See* Stretch reflex
support and, 219t
tonic labyrinthine, 7
tonic vibration, 314
Reinforcement. *See also* Practice
  developmental level of subject and, 135
  motions of, 134
  pattern combinations for, 353t–356t
  vision as, 292
Relaxation
  electric stimulation for, 313
  of spasticity, 313
  voluntary effort, 303–306
Repeated contractions, 216, 218t, 298–299
  standing balance training and, 259
Repetition
  avoidance of, 295
  mass extension, 306
  in motor learning, 279, 343
Resistance, 1, 333. *See also* Muscles
  for deficiency of innervation, 295
  maximal, 295
Respiration, stimulation of, 315–318,
  316f–319f
Reversal
  of antagonists, 259, 300–303
  quick, 303
  slow, 301–302, 305–306
  techniques, 300–306
Rhythm
  auditory, 292–293
  weakening, 292
Rhythmic initiation, 300
Rhythmic rotation, 306
Rhythmic stabilization, 302–303
  for diaphragm stimulation, 318, 319f
  and standing balance, 259
Rhythmic timing, 292–293
Righting response
  in fetus, 210
  rolling as component of, 211
Rising to stand, 7
Rock beat, 292–293
Rocking, of lower trunk, 250f
Rolling
  in fetus, 211
  and gait pattern training, 259
  prone toward supine, 228f–231f
  supine toward prone, 221f–227f
Rotation
  components in standing balance, 259
  consistency of, 3
  rhythmic, 306
  rotational movement, 4–5
  of upper extremities, 2t–3t, 90–96

Scratching, of skin, and agonist inhibition,
  291
Segments, interaction of, 212t
Self-care activities, 275–276, 277f–278f
  analysis of component patterns of, 275
  evaluation of, 334
  superiority of left hand in, 275
Self-direction, 293
  through verbal mediation, 293
Self-touching, 279, 293
  chopping and lifting, 293